I10627306

2007
YEAR BOOK OF
PEDIATRICS®

The 2007 Year Book Series

Year Book of Allergy, Asthma, and Clinical Immunology™: Drs Rosenwasser, Boguniewicz, Milgrom, Routes, and Weber

Year Book of Anesthesiology and Pain Management™: Drs Chestnut, Abram, Black, Gravlee, Lee, Mathru, and Roizen

Year Book of Cardiology®: Drs Gersh, Cheitlin, Elliott, Graham, Sundt, and Waldo

Year Book of Critical Care Medicine®: Drs Dellinger, Parrillo, Balk, Bekes, Dorman, and Dries

Year Book of Dentistry®: Drs McIntyre, Belvedere, Buhite, Davis, Henderson, Johnson, Jureyda, Ohrbach, Olin, Scott, Spencer, and Zakariasen

Year Book of Dermatology and Dermatologic Surgery™: Drs Thiers and Lang

Year Book of Diagnostic Radiology®: Drs Osborn, Birdwell, Dalinka, Gardiner, Levy, Elster, Oestreich, and Rosado de Christenson

Year Book of Emergency Medicine®: Drs Hamilton, Handly, Quintana, Werner, and Bruno

Year Book of Endocrinology®: Drs Mazzaferri, Bessesen, Clarke, Howard, Kennedy, Leahy, Meikle, Molitch, Rogol, and Schteingart

Year Book of Family Practice®: Drs Bowman, Apgar, Dexter, Neill, Scherger, and Zink

Year Book of Gastroenterology™: Drs Lichtenstein, Burke, Campbell, Dempsey, Drebin, Jaffe, Katzka, Kochman, Morris, Rombeau, Shah, and Stein

Year Book of Hand and Upper Limb Surgery®: Drs Chang and Steinmann

Year Book of Medicine®: Drs Barkin, Berney, Frishman, Garrick, Loehrer, Mazzaferri, Phillips, and Snydman

Year Book of Neonatal and Perinatal Medicine®: Drs Fanaroff, Ehrenkranz, and Stevenson

Year Book of Neurology and Neurosurgery®: Drs Kim and Verma

Year Book of Nuclear Medicine®: Drs Coleman, Blaufox, Royal, Strauss, and Zubal

Year Book of Obstetrics, Gynecology, and Women's Health®: Dr Shulman

Year Book of Oncology®: Drs Loehrer, Arceci, Glatstein, Gordon, Hanna, Morrow, and Thigpen

Year Book of Ophthalmology®: Drs Rapuano, Cohen, Eagle, Flanders, Hammersmith, Myers, Nelson, Penne, Sergott, Shields, Tipperman, and Vander

Year Book of Orthopedics®: Drs Morrey, Beauchamp, Peterson, Swiontkowski, Trigg, and Yaszemski

Year Book of Otolaryngology-Head and Neck Surgery®: Drs Paparella, Gapany, and Keefe

Year Book of Pathology and Laboratory Medicine®: Drs Raab, Parwani, Bejarano, and Bissell

Year Book of Pediatrics®: Dr Stockman

Year Book of Plastic and Aesthetic Surgery™: Drs Miller, Bartlett, Garner, McKinney, Ruberg, Salisbury, and Smith

Year Book of Psychiatry and Applied Mental Health®: Drs Talbott, Ballenger, Buckley, Frances, Jensen, and Markowitz,

Year Book of Pulmonary Disease®: Drs Phillips, Barker, Lewis, Maurer, Tanoue, and Willsie

Year Book of Rheumatology, Arthritis, and Musculoskeletal Disease™: Drs Panush, Furst, Hadler, Hochberg, Lahita, and Paget

Year Book of Sports Medicine®: Drs Shephard, Pierrynowski, Cantu, Feldman, McCrory, Nieman, Rowland, Jankowski, and Shrier

Year Book of Surgery®: Drs Copeland, Bland, Cerfolio, Daly, Eberlein, Fahey, Mozingo, Pruett, and Seeger

Year Book of Urology®: Drs Andriole and Coplen

Year Book of Vascular Surgery®: Dr Moneta

2007

The Year Book of
PEDIATRICS®

Editor

James A. Stockman III, MD

President, The American Board of Pediatrics; Clinical Professor of Pediatrics, University of North Carolina Medical School at Chapel Hill, and Duke University Medical Center, Durham, North Carolina

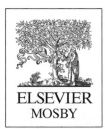

ELSEVIER
MOSBY

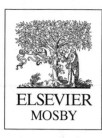

ELSEVIER
MOSBY

Vice President, Continuity: John A. Schrefer
Developmental Editor: Timothy Maxwell
Senior Issue Manager: Donna M. Adamson
Illustrations and Permissions Coordinator: Linda Jones

2007 EDITION

Printed in the United States of America
Composition by Thomas Technology Solutions, Inc
Printing/binding by Sheridan Books, Inc.

Editorial Office:
Elsevier
Suite 1800
1600 John F. Kennedy Blvd.
Philadelphia, PA 19103-2899

International Standard Serial Number: 0084-3954
International Standard Book Number: 0-323-04652-5
                                    978-0-323-04652-7

Table of Contents

Journals Represented

Journals represented in this YEAR BOOK are listed below.

Acta Paediatrica
American Journal of Ophthalmology
Annals of Internal Medicine
Archives of Disease in Childhood
Archives of Otolaryngology-Head and Neck Surgery
Archives of Pediatrics and Adolescent Medicine
Blood
British Medical Journal
Clinical Infectious Diseases
Clinical Pediatrics
Journal of Adolescent Health
Journal of Clinical Endocrinology and Metabolism
Journal of Developmental and Behavioral Pediatrics
Journal of Pediatric Gastroenterology and Nutrition
Journal of Pediatric Hematology/Oncology
Journal of Pediatric Orthopaedics
Journal of Pediatric Orthopaedics Part B
Journal of Pediatrics
Journal of Urology
Journal of the American Medical Association
Lancet
New England Journal of Medicine
Pediatric Cardiology
Pediatric Emergency Care
Pediatric Infectious Disease Journal
Pediatrics

STANDARD ABBREVIATIONS

The following terms are abbreviated in this edition: acquired immunodeficiency syndrome (AIDS), cardiopulmonary resuscitation (CPR), central nervous system (CNS), cerebrospinal fluid (CSF), computed tomography (CT), deoxyribonucleic acid (DNA), electrocardiography (ECG), health maintenance organization (HMO), human immunodeficiency virus (HIV), intensive care unit (ICU), intramuscular (IM), intravenous (IV), magnetic resonance (MR) imaging (MRI), ribonucleic acid (RNA), ultrasound (US), and ultraviolet (UV).

NOTE

To facilitate the use of the YEAR BOOK OF PEDIATRICS® as a reference tool, all illustrations and tables included in this publication are now identified as they appear in the original article. This change is meant to help the reader recognize that any illustration or table appearing in the YEAR BOOK OF PEDIATRICS® may be only one of many in the original article. For this reason, figure and table numbers will often appear to be out of sequence within the YEAR BOOK OF PEDIATRICS.®

Introduction

"Why abandon a belief merely because it ceases to be true? Cling to it long enough and...it will turn true again, for so it goes. Most of the change we think we see in life is due to truths being in and out of favor."—Robert Frost (1874-1963)

One could paraphrase the words of poet Frost by saying "what goes around comes around." One wonders, however, whether Frost's reflections on reality will ever apply to quality of care improvements in medicine in general, and in pediatrics in particular. One cannot abandon a truth only to see it reborn again if that truth has not yet come into its first reality. The truth referred to here is a genuine commitment to create the resources necessary to improve the care we provide to our patients. Most of us believe we are doing a decent job in this regard. We certainly want to. Nonetheless, most of us actually do not know how well we are doing, either as individuals or as groups of individuals. We have little means to compare ourselves with others. What is missing, in part, is a health care delivery system that collects data on quality in a seamless fashion, one that transcends the handwritten chart, a process that we can all buy into, one that is intended not to penalize those who practice behind the quality curve, rather one that helps shift the entire curve for the better for all. The key, in part, is an electronic health record, one that is integrated into a common secure database linked to efficiently organized quality improvement initiatives at the local, state, and national levels.

In this year's YEAR BOOK OF PEDIATRICS, you will find articles and commentaries on topics such as paper versus computerized medical records, prescription errors in the pediatric setting, how Britain established as a national priority that all primary care physicians utilize a common integrated electronic medical record (and actually implemented this in fewer than half a dozen years), and how we here in the United States have struggled to do so with astoundingly little success or financial commitment. You will learn that the investment of as little as 2% of our current annual health care budget over the next 5 years could replicate the British achievement.

Consider the following 2 scenarios. A 6 year old comes to your office having just moved into your community. She is about to enter a new school system and needs an immunization update. The only "Permanent" record of her immunizations is a handwritten record that the child's mother has brought with her. Unfortunately, coffee has spilled on it and it is illegible. Prior immunizations were given in a disparate series of public health clinics, except for one set of immunizations given by a pediatrician who has since passed away and whose spouse cannot find the old chart. What is a practitioner to do in this all-too-common circumstance?

Contrast the above with the following true situation. This editor is out and about looking for a used car. He finds one, a 7-year-old model said to be a 1-owner vehicle with just 20,000 miles on the odometer, looking like new. The dealer has no service records, having bought the car at an auction. So what to do? I write down the vehicle identification number (VIN) and excuse myself, retreating to my old car. There I pull out my laptop, beam up to a satellite Internet provider, type in www.carfax.com, give a credit card number to cover the $19.95 fee, and in literally less than 5 nanoseconds verify the entire history on the desired car including the following information: where it was originally delivered, the facts that it indeed was a 1 owner vehicle, that it had never been salvaged, junked, rebuilt, nor had it sustained fire/flood or hail damage and had never been declared a lemon. Indeed, the mileage indicated appeared to be accurate and all prior service records were available instantaneously. I had all the information needed to make an informed decision.

Two scenarios: one where absence of a national database could result in an incorrect decision affecting the life of a child, the other one in which the presence of a national database allows an informed decision regarding the purchase of a piece of metal. What is wrong with this picture? We have to do better than this for our progeny—starting by reading the YEAR BOOK cover to cover.

James A. Stockman III, MD

1 Adolescent Medicine

The Impact of School Daily Schedule on Adolescent Sleep
Hansen M, Janssen I, Schiff A, et al (Evanston Township High School, Ill; Northwestern Univ, Chicago; Northwestern Univ, Evanston, Ill)
Pediatrics 115:1555-1561, 2005   1–1

Objectives.—This study was initiated to examine the impact of starting school on adolescent sleep, to compare weekday and weekend sleep times, and to attempt to normalize the timing of the circadian sleep/wake cycle by administering bright light in the morning. This was a collaborative project involving high school students and their parents, as well as high school and university faculty members, for the purpose of contributing information to the scientific community while educating students about research processes and their own sleep/wake cycles and patterns.

Methods.—Sixty incoming high school seniors kept sleep/wake diaries beginning in August and continuing through 2 weeks after the start of school in September. Sleep diaries were also kept for 1 month in November and 1 month in February. Early-morning light treatments were given to 19 students in the last 2 weeks of November and the last 2 weeks of February. Neuropsychologic performance was measured with computer-administered tests. Paper-and-pencil tests were used for assessment of mood and vigor. A testing period consisted of 2 consecutive days at the beginning and end of November and at the beginning and end of February. Tests were given 3 times per day, ie, in the morning before school (6:30-8:00 AM), during midday lunch periods (11:30 AM to 1:00 PM), and in the afternoon (3:00-4:30 PM), on each of the test days.

Results.—Adolescents lost as much as 120 minutes of sleep per night during the week after the start of school, and weekend sleep time was also significantly longer (approximately 30 minutes) than that seen before the start of school (August). No significant differences were found between weekday sleep in the summer and weekend sleep during the school year. Early-morning light treatments did not modify total minutes of sleep per night, mood, or computer-administered vigilance test results. All students performed better in the afternoon than in the morning. Students in early morning classes reported being wearier, being less alert, and having to expend greater effort.

Conclusions.—The results of this study demonstrated that current high school start times contribute to sleep deprivation among adolescents. Consistent with a delay in circadian sleep phase, students performed better later in the day than in the early morning. However, exposure to bright light in the morning did not change the sleep/wake cycle or improve daytime performance during weekdays. Both short-term and long-term strategies that address the epidemic of sleep deprivation among adolescents will be necessary to improve health and maximize school performance.

▶ The data from this article speak for themselves. In the morning, at school, most teens are zombies. One might assume that during the summer, when there may not be obligations to get up on time, a normal sleep pattern is established by teens. When they go back to school, however, in late summer/early fall, they wind up sleeping, on average, 2 hours less per night on weekdays while school is in session. There is a little bit of catch-up on the weekend but not much. The consequence of this is that, over time, teens become increasingly sleep deprived. The psychological studies performed here show how significant the problem is. In the morning at school, many teens are truly "flaked out." It is not until early afternoon that they begin to wake up and are at their sharpest. This problem is not eliminated by exposure on a regular basis to bright lights, which is a common therapy for certain sleep disorders. In other words, the pattern exhibited by these kids is not a sleep disorder but rather a simple problem of just too little time to sleep.

An interesting study would be to see how our offspring perform in high school on all the standardized tests if they were given first thing in the morning, late in the morning, or in the afternoon. One could bet confidently from the evidence of this study that those who would perform best are those who took their examinations later in the day.

It is unlikely that our youngsters will significantly change their sleep habits. Maybe we should begin classes at 10:00 AM and end at 6:00 PM and see how our progeny perform. Then again, maybe our teachers would not be at their best at such times. In any event, it would be an interesting experiment. Also, please do not look to melatonin as a panacea for the sleep problem that teenagers face when they start back to school. One might think that part of the problem is not too dissimilar to jet lag or to a change in hours for those who have to engage in shift work. Unfortunately, a large meta-analysis of the world's literature looking at the effectiveness of melatonin shows that there is no evidence that melatonin is useful in treating secondary sleep disorders or sleep disorders accompanying sleep restriction, such as jet lag and shift work sleep disorders.[1]

Some people swear by melatonin, and if there is any good news in the meta-analysis regarding melatonin, it is that the drug appears to be safe. If you are a believer in melatonin, recognize that the most popular misconception underlying the widespread use of this drug is that it induces sleep pharmacologically. It does not. Melatonin acts as a regulating switch, pushing the body's circadian phase forward or backward, depending on when the drug is taken. If exogenous melatonin is taken at or after the onset of darkness, it substitutes for the endogenous melatonin secretion, which normally starts then and the phase shifts forward toward the sleep phase. The effect is greater because the dosage used is vastly greater than the amount naturally secreted. If exogenous melatonin is taken on waking, phase change is delayed—in physiologic terms, the nocturnal period of lowered alertness and performance tends to be prolonged. So, taken in the morning on arrival, for example, after a long flight eastward, melatonin delays circadian adaptation. Thus, if you are going to use melatonin in an experimental trial in high school students to see how to improve school performance in the first weeks after re-entry following a summer vacation, use the drug properly in an experimental design. That would be an interesting study.

One final comment about sleepiness and teenagers. If all else fails, dial up Lindsay Wagner and order a Sleep Number® bed for your offspring; it's a little more expensive than melatonin, but perhaps more effective.

J. A. Stockman III, MD

Reference

1. Buscemi N, Vandermeer B, Hooton N, et al: Efficacy and safety of exogenous melatonin for secondary sleep disorders and sleep disorders accompanying sleep restriction: Meta-analysis. *BMJ* 332:385-388, 2006.

Childhood Sexual Abuse and Early Menarche: The Direction of Their Relationship and Its Implications

Zabin LS, Emerson MR, Rowland DL (The Johns Hopkins Univ Bloomberg School of Public Health, Baltimore, Md; Valparaiso Univ, Ind)
J Adolesc Health 36:393-400, 2005   1–2

Purpose.—A relationship between childhood sexual abuse (CSA) and early menarche previously has been proposed and psychobiological mechanisms for the association have been suggested. Because it has serious implications for many disciplines, we attempted to confirm that association and explore its direction, first with hypothesis 1: the negative relationship between pubertal age and CSA is based on victims' increased target gratifiability at ages of high target vulnerability, and then with hypothesis 2: CSA and circumstances surrounding it are related causally to early menarche.

Methods.—African-American and multi-ethnic Caucasian women (N = 323) were interviewed at several women's clinics at Johns Hopkins Bayview Medical Center; 64 women reported premenarcheal abuse. We assessed (1) ages of CSA and menarche to determine their relationships, (2) household characteristics and their relationships with CSA, (3) variables associated with CSA, to determine the independent effect of CSA and explore potential dose response (i.e., effects of increased stress).

Results.—CSA and menarcheal age are related negatively ($p < .05$). Hypothesis 1 need not be rejected totally, but with most CSA events occurring long before puberty, hypothesis 2 is supported. Theoretically, stressful CSA characteristics increase victim/nonvictim differences in menarcheal age. Stress may derive from household characteristics often related to CSA but, even controlling for them, CSA has independent effects on menarcheal age.

Conclusions.—Hypothesis 1 may apply when CSA occurs within 2 years premenarche but, because hypothesis 2 is supported, continuing psychobiological effects and stress engendered by CSA are underscored. Mechanisms through which they impact the developing child require further exploration, and medical and psychological attention.

► In 2006, approval was obtained from the American Board of Medical Specialties to develop a board certification process in the area of child abuse. The development of this subspecialty to the point of board certification comes none too soon given the expanding understanding we have of the spectrum of child abuse. Approximately 150,000 cases of CSA are reported each year in the United States, with as many as 20% of adult women and 5% to 10% of adult men having experienced sexual abuse during childhood. One risk factor for this, as the abstract reports, is a child who has early sexual development themselves. This appears to be especially true in girls. Many years ago, there was reported a relationship between age of puberty and age at first intercourse among inner-city African-American females and males. These data were reported by the same investigators who have now studied the relationship of age of CSA and age of onset of sexual maturation.

So, what do we know about CSA? This is generally defined as a form of sexual activity involving a child under conditions ranging from physical coercion to deceit, including but not necessarily restricted to penetration. There is no strict definition of what a "child" means with respect to age. The literature on this has ranged from an upper age limit of 11 to 18 years. The peak of reported childhood assaults are between the ages of 7 and 13 years. There seems to be a very strong correlation between age of sexual development and the age of onset of CSA. Menarche, a relatively late stage of puberty, occurs at an average age of 12.8 years here in the United States, with maturation considered being late if menarche has not occurred by 14 and early if before 11.5 years (in a mixed US population). In most cases, the onset of pubertal development is 2 years before this. As noted elsewhere in the YEAR BOOK OF PEDIATRICS, the age of onset of puberty may be declining, at least until recently.

The authors of this report are probably correct in their assessment that early age of sexual development in a girl does put that child at greater risk for CSA, all other factors taken into consideration. The authors also hypothesize why this might be true, but in the final analysis, your guess is as good as anyone else's. It should also be noted that there are data to indicate that earlier age at first date is associated with sexual violence among female adolescents.[1]

One final comment having to do with child abuse in general: there is a lot to be learned from animal species other than us about the problem. Take Rhesus monkeys, for example. It is bad enough that some Rhesus monkey mothers regularly kick, hit, bite, and otherwise brutalize their babies, but to make matters worse, females exposed to such abusive behavior as infants more frequently than not grow up to become abusive parents themselves, perpetuating a primate cycle of family violence. A study of Rhesus monkeys shows that being abused as an infant outweighs any primarily genetic trait in fostering abusive parenting by female monkeys.[2]

It appears that Rhesus monkeys are an excellent animal model of human child abuse. Rhesus moms frequently mistreat their babies after having themselves been raised by abusive parents, either biological or adoptive. Contrarily, females born to abusive mothers uniformly become caring parents after having been raised by non-abusive adoptive mothers. In a study of Rhesus monkeys, the population investigated included some mothers who had been observed to abuse their offspring. The researchers transferred some newborns between mothers to create 4 groups of female infants: 6 infants born to physically abusive mothers and given as newborns to unrelated, non-abusive mothers; 8 infants born to non-abusive mothers and adopted as newborns by abusive mothers; 8 infants born to abusive mothers and raised by them; and 9 infants born to non-abusive mothers and raised by them. Each infant then was tracked into adulthood and observed for 3 or 4 months after she gave birth to her first child. Nine of the 16 females raised by abusive mothers—including 4 born to non-abusive females—abused their own offspring. None of the 15 females reared by non-abusive mothers became an abusive parent.

These findings make a strong case for non-human models of child abuse. It may just be possible to understand why some female monkeys repeat the cycle of child abuse and with that information perhaps we can apply it to the human situation. You can decide whether monkeys have free will; however, we humans do, meaning that there is no excuse for parents to abuse a child, even if they were abused themselves.

J. A. Stockman III, MD

References

1. Rickert VI, Vaughan RD, Wiemann CW: Adolescent dating violence and date rape. *Curr Opin Obstet Gynecol* 14:495-500, 2002.
2. Bower B. Mother knows worst: Abusive parenting spans generations in monkeys. *Science News* 168:5-6, 2005.

Adolescents Tell Us Why Teens Have Oral Sex

Cornell JL, Halpern-Felsher BL (Univ of California, San Francisco)
J Adolesc Health 38:299-301, 2006   1–3

Background.—Several studies have found that substantial number of adolescents, including younger adolescents, engage in oral sex and that oral sex in many cases precedes the first vaginal sex experience. It has been suggested that adolescents engage in oral sex for pleasure and intimacy while avoiding pregnancy and sexually transmitted diseases, and there is evidence that oral sex is thought by teenagers to be more acceptable, less risky, and more prevalent among their peers than vaginal sex. However, no study has specifically asked adolescents about their reasons for engaging in oral sex. Adolescents' perceptions of reasons for having oral sex and any differences in these perceptions by gender, race/ethnicity, and sexual experience were investigated.

TABLE 1.—Adolescents' Perceptions of Reasons for
Having Oral Sex

Reason	Participants Who Listed Reason (N = 452)	
	%	n
Pleasure	35.1	149
Improve relationship	29.9	127
Popularity, reputation	24.9	106
Curiosity, for experience	16.0	68
Less risk than vaginal sex	15.8	67
Wants to, can't wait	12.9	55
Peer pressure, friends are doing it	10.6	45
Fun, bored	8.5	36
Pressure, force, fear	7.8	33
Low self esteem, stupid	3.1	13
Under alcohol or drug influence	2.6	11
Family problems	1.9	8
Don't know	1.9	8
To rebel	1.6	7
Media	1.4	6

Methods.—The study participants included 425 ninth-grade adolescents (mean age = 14.53 years, 64% female) participating in the second wave of a longitudinal school-based study on the relationship between risk perceptions and sexual activity. Only participants who answered the open-ended survey question concerning reasons for oral sex were included in this report. All study participants were asked one open-ended question regarding their perception of the reasons why teens of their age have oral sex. The responses were then collapsed into thematic categories reached by consensus between the authors.

Results.—The most frequently cited perceived reasons for adolescents' engaging in oral sex were pleasure and to improve a relationship (Table 1). Females suggested significantly more often than males that a reason to have oral sex is to improve an intimate, romantic relationship. Males were not more likely than females to list any of the reasons. With the exception of popularity/reputation, there were no differences in listed reasons for having oral sex between participants with and without sexual experiences. There were no significant differences in response listing by race/ethnicity.

Conclusions.—This report can provide a general understanding of adolescents' perceptions of why teenagers engage in oral sex. It is suggested that a combination of social benefits and risk avoidance factors may have a role in the decision to engage in oral sex. Health care educators and providers should discuss oral sex in clinical risk assessments and sexual health education and should ensure that adolescents are prepared to make sexual decisions that include both oral and vaginal sex.

▶ This report shows us how one table is worth a thousand words in explaining what is in an adolescent's mind when they engage in a certain form of activity.

It has been suggested that adolescents engage in oral sex to achieve sexual pleasure and intimacy while avoiding pregnancy and sexually transmitted infections. This study of 425 ninth graders seems to verify this assumption. As importantly, we learn that engaging in oral sex is designed also to increase one's popularity and one's social reputation.

Any parent will tell you it is hard to get inside the head of a teenager. Absent that ability, perhaps every parent should read this report. It may help them understand their offspring a little bit better.

J. A. Stockman III, MD

Factors Associated With Time of Day of Sexual Activity Among Adolescent Women

Fortenberry JD, Katz BP, Blythe MJ, et al (Mid-America Adolescent STD Cooperative Research Ctr, Indianapolis, Ind; Indiana Univ, Indianapolis; Regenstrief Inst, Indianapolis, Ind)
J Adolesc Health 38:275-281, 2006   1–4

Background.—Our objective was to describe familial, intrapersonal, and partner-related factors associated with time of day of sexual activity among adolescent women.

Methods.—Annual questionnaires and daily diaries were collected from 106 adolescents. Participants contributed up to 3 questionnaires and 5 12-week diary periods over 27 months. Predictor variables included type of day (weekend, school day, vacation day); partner variables (argument with partner, partner emotional support, time spent with partner); parent/family variables such as supervision, monitoring, and attitudes about adolescent sexual behavior; and mood and behavior variables such as negative mood, positive mood, and sexual interest. The outcome variable for each diary day was no coitus, coitus between noon and 6 PM, or coitus after 6 PM.

Results.—Coitus occurred on 12.0% of the diary days. Coital events were more than twice as likely to occur after 6 PM (8.5% of days) than in the afternoon (3.5% of days). Afternoon sex was least likely to occur on school days whereas evening sex occurred most often on weekends. An argument with a partner, partner emotional support, time spent with partner, sexual interest, and coital frequency were associated with increased likelihood of afternoon sex, whereas parental supervision and negative mood were associated with decreased likelihood of afternoon sex. For school days, skipping school was associated with increased likelihood of afternoon sex. Evening/night sexual activity was not associated with any parent/family variables.

Conclusion.—Afternoon sex on school days is relatively uncommon. Direct parental supervision may decrease afternoon sexual activity but relationship and intrapersonal factors also are important factors in the timing of sexual activity on any given day.

▶ The preceding article (Abstract 1–3) told us why teenagers rationalize their oral sexual activity. This report tells us the time of day that teens engage in sexual activity. There are no surprises here. When there is no supervision, there will be sexual activity, although unsupervised afternoons do not seem to be the hotbed of such activity. The findings from this report show that sexual intercourse among adolescent girls occurs at a rate of 1 per 12 days, and such activity occurring in unsupervised afternoon times accounts for less than one third of all coital events and is least common on afternoons of school days. Most of the sexual activity seen in the sample studied occurred after 6 PM or before noon. Parent supervision was associated with a decreased likelihood of afternoon sex, but did not affect the likelihood of evening/night sex.

Anyone attempting to study adolescent sexuality will find themselves in a very complex situation. There are no rules of thumb except that when the sun goes down, the trouble begins or, as my mother used to say, "Nothing good happens after midnight."

J. A. Stockman III, MD

Systematic Review: Noninvasive Testing for *Chlamydia trachomatis* and *Neisseria gonorrhoeae*

Cook RL, Hutchison SL, Østergaard L, et al (Univ of Pittsburgh, Pa; Aarhus Univ, Denmark)
Ann Intern Med 142:914-925, 2005   1–5

Background.—Testing of urine samples is noninvasive and could overcome several barriers to screening for chlamydial and gonococcal infections, but most test samples are obtained directly from the cervix or urethra.

Purpose.—To systematically review studies that assessed the sensitivity and specificity of nucleic acid amplification tests for *Chlamydia trachomatis* and *Neisseria gonorrhoeae* in urine specimens and to compare test characteristics according to type of assay, site of sample collection, presence of symptoms, disease prevalence, and characteristics of the reference standard.

Data Sources.—Relevant studies in all languages were identified by searching the MEDLINE database (January 1991 to December 2004) and by hand-searching the references of identified articles and relevant journals.

Study Selection.—Studies were selected that evaluated 1 of 3 commercially available nucleic acid amplification tests, included data from tests of both a urine sample and a traditional sample (obtained from the cervix or urethra), and used an appropriate reference standard.

Data Extraction.—From 29 eligible studies, 2 investigators independently abstracted data on sample characteristics, reference standard, sensitivity, and specificity.

Data Synthesis.—Articles were assessed qualitatively and quantitatively. Summary estimates for men and women were calculated separately for chlamydial and gonococcal infections and were stratified by assay and presence of symptoms. The pooled study specificities of each of the 3 assays exceeded 97% when urine samples were tested, for both chlamydial infection and gonorrhea and in both men and women. The pooled study sensitivities for the polymerase chain reaction, transcription-mediated amplification, and strand displacement amplification assays, respectively, were 83.3%, 92.5%, and 79.9% for chlamydial infections in women; 84.0%, 87.7%, and 93.1% for chlamydial infections in men; and 55.6%, 91.3%, and 84.9% for gonococcal infections in women. The pooled specificity of polymerase chain reaction to gonococcal infections in men was 90.4%. In subgroup analyses, the sensitivity did not vary according to the prevalence of infection or the presence of symptoms but did vary according to the reference standard used.

Limitations.—Few published studies present data on the transcription-mediated amplification or strand displacement amplification assays, and few studies report data from asymptomatic patients or low-prevalence groups.

Conclusions.—Results of nucleic acid amplification tests for *C. trachomatis* on urine samples are nearly identical to those obtained on samples collected directly from the cervix or urethra. Although all 3 assays can also be used to test for *N. gonorrhoeae*, the sensitivity of the polymerase chain reaction assay in women is too low to recommend its routine use to test for gonorrhea in urine specimens.

▶ Here in the United States, experts estimate an annual incidence of 2.8 million new chlamydial infections. Most of these infections are asymptomatic. It is generally accepted that genital infection with *C trachomatis* is the most widespread bacterial sexually transmitted disease here and elsewhere in the world. It is associated with annual costs that exceed $2 billion. Nearly every major US public health organization now recommends routine screening of sexually active young women for chlamydia infection. This screening has been shown to be cost-effective in the prevention of pelvic inflammatory disease, the major cause of infertility and chronic pelvic pain. Fewer than 60% of teens and women at risk undergo such testing.

Several important developments have recently enlarged the potential scope of screening programs and have modified thinking about whom and how to screen. Many studies of young women have drawn attention to the high rate of recurrent infection (15% to 25%) within 6 months of treatment. Most of these recurrences probably represent reinfection from untreated partners, but a proportion may also represent persistent infection or ineffective treatment. Given the high prevalence of recurrent infection, the Centers for Disease Control and Prevention has recommended retesting 3 to 4 months after initial infection. This recommendation has remarkably expanded the numbers of women who need to be screened and has identified the highest at risk in our patient population. In addition to this, nucleic acid amplification tests for chlamydia are significantly more sensitive than previously available diagnostic tests and can be used on first-void urine specimens and on self-collected vaginal swabs—techniques that no longer require painful urethral swabs in men and pelvic examinations in women. Such assays have made highly sensitive chlamydia testing more widely available and have facilitated the implementation of community-based testing outside of traditional clinics. Nucleic acid amplification tests have also created a huge number of large population-based investigations of chlamydia prevalence and adequacy of treatment. These tests can also be adapted to home testing kits and the testing of adolescents in sites, such as schools or community centers.

If you wish to read more about how cost-effective newer methods are for screening for *Chlamydia trachomatis*, see the excellent report of Hu et al.[1] Annual screening of all women here in the United States between 15 and 29 years old, followed by selective semi-annual screening for women with a history of infection, turns out to be the most cost-effective strategy. In the Hu et al study, risk estimates after chlamydia infections were developed for pelvic inflammatory disease, ectopic pregnancy, tubal infertility, and chronic pelvic pain. The figures for these complications were 15% to 80%, 5% to 25%, 10% to 20%, and 18% to 30%, respectively. These estimates confirm previous studies showing how bad chlamydia can be in the long term for those who become infected.

So what is the current recommendation for chlamydia screening? It is that all sexually active individuals be tested annually using a nucleic acid amplification technique. In those who initially test positive and who receive treatment, rescreening 3 to 4 months later is recommended, followed by continued 6-month screening in groups with a high prevalence or a history of previous infection. However, despite data and recommendations that strongly support the benefits and cost-effectiveness of screening in this high priority group that includes teenagers, actual practice falls far short of this recommended practice. Public-based screening programs in many communities are underfunded, and too many of them offer screening to less than half of the target population. Our medical community is no better than the public health system itself: few physicians offer screening to their sexually-active patients 15 to 24 years old.[2] This problem needs to be solved. While screening should continue in traditional clinic-based sites, such as sexually transmitted disease clinics, gynecology clinics, contraceptive clinics, and juvenile detention clinics, the real opportunity for improved detection is within each of our communities: our primary care practices, schools, community centers, and teen clinics.

Last, we should not forget about the adolescent male when referring to chlamydia. Boys are also an important reservoir of infection within our communities. Unfortunately, few data are available to directly support the screening of adolescent males. It seems only logical to conclude that widespread screening and treatment of adolescent males would probably substantially reduce recurrences in women and reduce the overall prevalence in the community. The problem with nucleic acid amplification tests, as good as they are, is that they are somewhat costly and do not give an immediate result at the point of initial contact. An accurate, rapid, and inexpensive point-of-care test will be the next technical breakthrough.

To read more about this important topic, see the excellent editorial of Stamm.[3]

J. A. Stockman III, MD

References

1. Hu D, Hook EW, Goldie SJ: Screening for *Chlamydia trachomatis* in women 15 to 29 years of age: A cost-effectiveness analysis. *Ann Intern Med* 141:501-513, 2004.

2. Mangione-Smith R, McGlynn EA, Hiatt L: Screening for chlamydia in adolescents and young women. *Arch Pediatr Adol Med* 154:1108-1113, 2000.
3. Stamm WE: Chlamydia screening: Expanding the score. *Ann Intern Med* 141:568-572, 2005.

Coercive Sexual Experiences and Subsequent Human Papillomavirus Infection and Squamous Intraepithelial Lesions in Adolescent and Young Adult Women

Kahn JA, Huang B, Rosenthal SL, et al (Cincinnati Children's Hosp Med Ctr, Ohio; Univ of Texas, Galveston; Albert Einstein College of Medicine, Bronx, NY)
J Adolesc Health 36:363-371, 2005   1–6

Purpose.—The purpose of this study was to examine the associations between coercive sexual experiences and subsequent human papillomavirus (HPV) infection and/or squamous intraepithelial lesion (SIL) in adolescent and young adult women, and to determine whether risk behaviors mediate and sociodemographic factors moderate any observed associations.

Methods.—Data were obtained from a longitudinal cohort study of female university students (N = 608). χ^2 and Wilcoxon rank-sum tests were used to determine associations between history of a coercive sexual experience and subsequent risk behaviors, and between risk behaviors and HPV or SIL. Logistic regression models were used to determine whether a coercive sexual experience was associated with HPV or SIL and whether the association was mediated by risk behaviors and/or moderated by sociodemographic factors.

Results.—Twenty-two percent of participants reported a prior coercive sexual experience. Report of a prior coercive sexual experience was associated with a higher lifetime number of sexual partners ($p < .0001$), which in turn was associated with subsequent HPV infection ($p < .0001$) and SIL ($p < .0001$). In logistic regression models, coercive sexual experience was associated significantly with HPV (odds ratio [OR], 1.84; 95% confidence interval [CI], 1.19–2.84) and at a marginal significance level with SIL (OR, 1.90; 95% CI, .97–3.70). When the number of sexual partners was included in the first model, the association between coercive sexual experience and HPV infection became nonsignificant and the β coefficient decreased by 49%. Race and age did not appear to moderate the association between coercive sexual experience and HPV.

Conclusions.—The number of sexual partners is an important mechanism through which adolescent and young adult women who report a coercive sexual experience acquire HPV.

▶ Back in 2003, a report showed that almost 9% of adolescents indicated they had been hit, slapped, or physically abused by a boyfriend or girlfriend in the past 12 months. Black and Hispanic adolescents reported higher rates of abuse than whites, with no significant difference between boys and girls. In addition, some 9% of adolescents report they have been forced to have sex when they did not want to. More girls (11.9%) than boys (6.1%) report that they had been forced to have sex, with black and Hispanic youth reporting higher rates of abuse than whites.[1] This problem is not unique to the United States. From a global perspective, the World Health Organization has documented high rates of sexual assault in such diverse countries and regions as Cameroon, the Caribbean islands, Peru, New Zealand, South Africa, and Tanzania.

The article by Kahn et al is the first prospective study to document subsequent acquisition of HPV infection in young women who reported a history of coercive sexual experience earlier in life, usually during adolescence. A positive relationship was seen between coercive sexual experiences and the development of SILs. A history of coercive sexual experience is associated with behavioral factors that increase the risk for exposure to HPV, largely through an increase in the number of sexual partners over time. In fact, studies have shown that women who report a history of forced sexual intercourse early in life are more likely to have multiple sex partners, unprotected sex, and heavy cigarette use.[2]

Many professional organizations, including the American Academy of Pediatrics, the American College of Obstetrics and Gynecology, and the World Health Organization, have issued policy statements reflecting the need for universal screening for partner violence for women. It is up to us to detect violent experiences in order to implement strategies to help adolescents deal with the consequences, many of which can be lifelong. Dr Charles Irwin,[3] editor-in-chief of the *Journal of Adolescent Health*, recently stated the case very clearly: "Given the prevalence data from the United States and globally, the issue is not whether health providers should be screening adolescents for coercive relationships, but how and when this information should be gathered." Screening during visits for routine care should be part of our visit checklist. We should also not be asking questions that have answers we are not prepared to deal with. We have to be aware of services for both boys and girls that can assist them in working through the difficult circumstances they may find themselves in.

J. A. Stockman III, MD

References

1. Centers for Disease Control and Prevention: Youth risk behavior surveillance: United States, 2003, http://www.cdc.gov/healthyyouth/YRBS\, accessed January 16, 2006.
2. Howard DE, Wang MQ: Psychosocial correlates of US adolescents who report a history of forced sexual intercourse. *J Adolesc Health* 36:372-379, 2005.
3. Irwin CE: Coercive sexual experiences during adolescence and young adulthood: A public health problem. *J Adolesc Health* 36:359-361, 2005.

Lifetime Effects, Costs, and Cost Effectiveness of Testing for Human Papillomavirus to Manage Low Grade Cytological Abnormalities: Modelling Study

Legood R, Gray A, Wolstenholme J, et al (Univ of Oxford, England; Inst of Cancer Research, Sutton, England)
BMJ 332:79-83, 2006   1–7

Objectives.—To predict the incremental lifetime effects, costs, and cost effectiveness of using human papillomavirus testing to triage women with borderline or mildly dyskaryotic cervical smear results for immediate colposcopy.

Design.—Modelling study.

Setting.—Three centres participating in NHS pilot studies, United Kingdom. Population Women aged 25-64 with borderline or mildly dyskaryotic cervical smear results.

Interventions.—Screening using conventional cytology, liquid based cytology, and four strategies with different age cut-off points and follow up times that used combined liquid based cytology and human papillomavirus testing (adjunctive human papillomavirus testing).

Results.—The model predicts that compared with using conventional cytology without testing for human papillomavirus, testing for the virus in conjunction with liquid based cytology for women with borderline or mildly dyskaryotic cervical smear results (aged 35 or more) would cost £3735 (€5528; $6474) per life year saved. Extending adjunctive human papillomavirus testing in combination with liquid based cytology to include women aged between 25 and 34 costs an additional £4233 per life year saved. Human papillomavirus testing is likely to reduce lifetime repeat smears by 52%-86% but increase lifetime colposcopies by 64%-138%.

Conclusions.—Testing for human papillomavirus to manage all women with borderline or mildly dyskaryotic cervical smear results is likely to be cost effective. The predicted increase in lifetime colposcopies, however, deserves careful consideration.

Effect of Testing for Human Papillomavirus as a Triage During Screening for Cervical Cancer: Observational Before and After Study

Moss S, for the Liquid Based Cytology/Human Papillomavirus Cervical Pilot Studies Group (Inst of Cancer Research, Sutton, England; et al)
BMJ 332:83-85, 2006   1–8

Objective.—To assess the effect of introducing testing for human papillomavirus combined with liquid based cytology in women with low grade cytological abnormalities.

Design.—Observational before and after study.

Setting.—Three cervical screening laboratories, England.

Participants.—5654 women aged 20-64 with low grade cytological abnormalities found at routine cervical screening in a pilot; 5254 similar women in the period before the pilot.

Interventions.—Human papillomavirus testing combined with liquid based cytology in the management of women with borderline or mildly dyskaryotic cervical smear results compared with conventional smear tests, with immediate referral to colposcopy of women positive for human papillomavirus.

Results.—57.9% (3187/5506) of women tested in the pilot were positive for human papillomavirus. The rate of repeat smears fell by 74%, but the rate of referral to colposcopy for low grade cytological abnormalities more than doubled. The estimated negative predictive value of human papillomavirus testing varied between 93.8% and 99.7%.

Conclusion.—The addition of testing for human papillomavirus in women with low grade cytological abnormalities resulted in a reduction in the rate of repeat smears, but an increase in rates of referral to colposcopy.

▶ These 2 reports (Abstracts 1–7 and 1–8) document that DNA testing for human papillomavirus (HPV) is a cost-effective way to clarify the meaning of equivocal results of cervical cytology. HPV infections are quite common in teens and clearly represent sexual transmission. In most cases, HPV infections of the cervix clear within 1 to 2 years in terms of cervical pathology. Persistent infections leading to a risk of cancer do occur, however, with invasive cancer typically presenting approximately 2 decades after first exposure to HPV.

When the results of screening cytology are equivocal, HPV testing is cost-effective in deciding whether colposcopy is needed, as confirmed by the reports by Legood et al (Abstract 1–7) and Moss et al (Abstract 1–8). HPV testing is useful to clarify results for the cytologic categories that harbor true uncertainty. Technical efficacy of triage is no longer questioned, but the cost-effectiveness of triage by HPV testing compared with cytologic or colposcopic methods will vary between populations and regions.

One thing is clear: after excisional or ablative treatments of the cervix for precancerous lesions, the absolute risk of recurrence of cervical pathology is about 5% to 10%. Testing for HPV 4 to 6 months after treatment is highly sensitive and specific for this risk of recurrence and is better than cytology alone for monitoring cure.

To read more about HPV testing as a component of cervical screening, see the superb commentary by Schiffman and Castle.[1]

J. A. Stockman III, MD

Reference

1. Schiffman MS, Castle PE: When to test women for human papillomavirus: Cervical screening using HPV testing shows great promise but warrants caution. *BMJ* 332:61-62, 2006.

Sustained Efficacy Up to 4.5 Years of a Bivalent L1 Virus-like Particle Vaccine Against Human Papillomavirus Types 16 and 18: Follow-up From a Randomised Control Trial
Harper DM, for the HPV Vaccine Study Group (Dartmouth Med School, Lebanon, NH; et al)
Lancet 367:1247-1255, 2006   1–9

Background.—Effective vaccination against HPV 16 and HPV 18 to prevent cervical cancer will require a high level of sustained protection against infection and precancerous lesions. Our aim was to assess the long-term efficacy, immunogenicity, and safety of a bivalent HPV-16/18 L1 virus-like particle AS04 vaccine against incident and persistent infection with HPV 16 and HPV 18 and their associated cytological and histological outcomes.

Methods.—We did a follow-up study of our multicentre, double-blind, randomised, placebo-controlled trial reported in 2004. We included women who originally received all three doses of bivalent HPV-16/18 virus-like particle AS04 vaccine (0.5 mL; n=393) or placebo (n=383). We assessed HPV DNA, using cervical samples, and did yearly cervical cytology assessments. We also studied the long-term immunogenicity and safety of the vaccine.

Findings.—More than 98% seropositivity was maintained for HPV-16/18 antibodies during the extended follow-up phase. We noted significant vaccine efficacy against HPV-16 and HPV-18 endpoints: incident infection, 96.9% (95% CI 81.3-99.9); persistent infection: 6 month definition, 94.3 (63.2-99.9); 12 month definition, 100% (33.6-100). In a combined analysis of the initial efficacy and extended follow-up studies, vaccine efficacy of 100% (42.4-100) against cervical intraepithelial neoplasia (CIN) lesions associated with vaccine types. We noted broad protection against cyto-histological outcomes beyond that anticipated for HPV 16/18 and protection against incident infection with HPV 45 and HPV 31. The vaccine has a good long-term safety profile.

Interpretation.—Up to 4.5 years, the HPV-16/18 L1 virus-like particle AS04 vaccine is highly immunogenic and safe, and induces a high degree of protection against HPV-16/18 infection and associated cervical lesions. There is also evidence of cross protection.

Pediatricians' Intention to Administer Human Papillomavirus Vaccine: The Role of Practice Characteristics, Knowledge, and Attitudes
Kahn JA, Zimet GD, Bernstein DI, et al (Cincinnati Children's Hosp Med Ctr, Ohio; Indiana Univ, Indianapolis; Univ of Cincinnati, Ohio; et al)
J Adolesc Health 37:502-510, 2005   1–10

Purpose.—The objective of this study was to examine pediatrician characteristics and attitudes associated with intention to recommend two hypothetical human papillomavirus (HPV) vaccines.

Methods.—A survey instrument mailed to a random sample of 1000 pediatricians assessed provider characteristics, HPV knowledge, and attitudes about HPV vaccination. Intention to administer each of two HPV vaccines types (a cervical cancer/genital wart vaccine and a cervical cancer vaccine) to girls and boys of three different ages (11, 14, and 17 years) was assessed. Linear mixed modeling for repeated measures and multivariable linear regression models were performed to identify variables associated with intention to recommend vaccination.

Results.—The mean age of participants (n = 513) was 42 years and 57% were female. Participants were more likely to recommend vaccination to girls vs. boys and older vs. younger children, and were more likely to recommend a cervical cancer/genital wart vaccine than a cervical cancer vaccine ($p < .0001$). Variables independently associated with intention to recommend a cervical cancer/genital wart vaccine were: higher estimate of the percentage of sexually active adolescents in one's practice (β .084, $p = .002$), number of young adolescents seen weekly (β 1.300, $p = .015$), higher HPV knowledge (β 1.079, $p = .015$), likelihood of following the recommendations of important individuals and organizations regarding immunization (β .834, $p = .001$), and fewer perceived barriers to immunization (β −.203, $p = .001$).

Conclusions.—Vaccination initiatives directed toward pediatricians that focus on modifiable predictors of intention to vaccinate, such as HPV knowledge and attitudes about vaccination, may facilitate adherence to emerging national immunization guidelines.

▶ The subject of this report is vaccination as a prevention strategy for HPV-related diseases. Here in the United States, HPV is among the most common sexually transmitted infections, and sexually active adolescents are at particularly high risk for HPV acquisition. Genetic and epidemiologic studies have clearly demonstrated that HPV infection is a necessary cause of both cervical cancer and genital warts. More than 99% of cervical cancers contain at least one high-risk HPV type, and approximately 70% contain HPV types 16 or 18. Moreover, low-risk HPV types 6 or 11 are responsible for approximately 90% of congenital warts and almost all cases of recurrent respiratory papillomatosis. Thus, a vaccine that could prevent HPV acquisition would have the potential to significantly reduce the incidence of both childhood and adult diseases.

All of us have heard the recent developments in the introduction of HPV vaccines. Pediatricians will play a critical role in HPV vaccine delivery because early adolescents are more likely to visit a pediatrician than any other care provider and because a pediatrician's recommendation is likely to influence strongly a parent's or adolescent's decision to receive the vaccine. For these reasons, the report abstracted is important because it gives us some insights regarding our attitudes about HPV immunizations and factors associated with the intention to recommend immunization. From the report of Kahn et al we begin to learn a little bit about the roadblocks that we present ourselves with in potentially moving forward with vaccination of teens. It is obvious that some are hesitant to discuss issues related to sexuality with preadolescents. There is also some concern that adolescents who receive vaccines to prevent sexually transmitted infections may perceive sexual intercourse to be safer and perhaps practice riskier behaviors. Hopefully, this issue can be adequately addressed with anticipatory guidance. Care providers also have expressed concern about negative parent reactions to discussing sexually transmitted infections with their child or adolescent. Since about one third of adolescents initiate sexual intercourse by the first year of high school, it is clear that discussions of this type will have to take place fairly early. They need to take place with both boys and girls since both should be immunized.

Once the HPV vaccine is recommended by the Centers for Disease Control and Prevention for administration to all preadolescents, the complexity of the office visit for this patient population will increase tremendously given the need to discuss in some detail the indications for vaccination and the rationale associated with the need for vaccination. You can be guaranteed that there will be much more to this than simply giving a shot.

J. A. Stockman III, MD

Early Puberty and Adolescent Pregnancy: The Influence of Alcohol Use
Deardorff J, Gonzales NA, Christopher FS, et al (Univ of California, San Francisco; Arizona State Univ, Tempe)
Pediatrics 116;1451-1456, 2005   1–11

Objective.—Early pubertal timing predicts deleterious outcomes for young girls, including substance use, risky sexual behavior, and pregnancy. In turn, adolescent pregnancy predicts long-term negative consequences such as reduced educational attainment and income-earning potential. Despite evidence of the direct links between early puberty and negative outcomes, this study is the first to examine the role that alcohol plays in the timing of sexual intercourse and pregnancy among early-maturing females.

Design.—Participants were 666 females, aged 18 to 22 years, from 4 major ethnic groups in Arizona (non-Hispanic white, black, Latino, and Native American). All women included in the sample had experienced a pregnancy in their teens or early 20s. Participants completed a self-administered questionnaire that inquired about their timing of menarche, sexual initiation, first alcohol use, and age at first pregnancy. A mediating model predicting age at pregnancy was tested by using path modeling.

Results.—Early puberty was found to be associated with earlier age of alcohol use and sexual initiation, which in turn predicted early pregnancy. Age at first sexual intercourse and age at first substance use significantly mediated the relation between age at menarche and age at first pregnancy. The results did not vary by ethnic group.

Conclusions.—Girls who mature early are more likely to engage in early substance use and sexual intercourse, which in turn puts them at greater risk for adolescent pregnancy. It is important that health care providers are sensitive to the risks associated with early maturation among young girls and provide preventive screening, education, and counseling related to alcohol use and sexual initiation for this group.

▶ The results of this study out of California and Arizona speak for themselves. Without question, there are many factors that lead to unintended pregnancy during teenage years. Such pregnancies are the major reason for the relatively high abortion rates here in the United States in the teen population.

The Centers for Disease Control and Prevention have recently provided us with interesting information regarding abortion rates here in the United States. See if you can answer the following three questions:

1. As a percentage of all legal abortions in the United States, have abortions in the pediatric population increased or decreased over the period 1973 to 2001?
2. 2001 is the last full year for which the CDC has reported complete information on legal abortion rates in the United States. Ten states have reported abortion rates (expressed as numbers of abortions per 1000 live births) in excess of 300; which states are these?
3. In 2001, 12 states reported legal abortion rates of less than 150 per 1000 live births. Which states were these?

The answer to the above questions are as follows: As a percentage of all legal abortions performed in the US, those occurring in the age group ≤19 years have declined steadily and significantly so, from 32.7% to 18.1% in the period 1973 to 2001. The absolute numbers of abortions in this age group has also declined from 201,377 to 154,481.[1] As far as the average number of abortions performed in the United States overall per 1000 live births in 2001, this number was 246.

The highest rates of abortion were seen in the following states:[a]

State	Legal Abortion Rates[b] (≥300/1000 Live Births) Rate
New York	500 (New York City 767; remainder of state 263)
Delaware	453
Rhode Island	429
Florida	416
Massachusetts	324
Nevada	322
Washington	322
Kansas	316
Oregon	315
Connecticut	311

[a]Excludes data from Alaska, California, and New Hampshire, which did not provide reporting information.
[b]Rate expressed as numbers of legal abortions per 1000 live births.

Of the 12 states reporting legal abortion rates under 150 per 1000 live births, the following table lists those states (among the 47 that provided data):

State	Rate
Legal Abortion Rates[a] (≤150/1000 Live Births)	
Oklahoma	140
Indiana	137
South Carolina	126
Kentucky	115
West Virginia	114
Maryland	103
South Dakota	85
Mississippi	84
Utah	75
Colorado	69
Idaho	36

J. A. Stockman III, MD

Reference

1. Strauss LT, Herndon J, Chang J, et al: Abortion surveillance—United States, 2001. *MMWR Surveill Summ* 54:1-32, 2005.

2 Allergy and Dermatology

Evidence of a Role of Tumor Necrosis Factor α in Refractory Asthma
Berry MA, Hargadon B, Shelley M, et al (Univ Hosp of Leicester Natl Health
Service Trust, England)
N Engl J Med 354:697-708, 2006   2–1

Background.—The development of tumor necrosis factor α (TNF-α) antagonists has made it feasible to investigate the role of this cytokine in refractory asthma.

Methods.—We measured markers of TNF-α activity on peripheral-blood monocytes in 10 patients with refractory asthma, 10 patients with mild-to-moderate asthma, and 10 control subjects. We also investigated the effects of treatment with the soluble TNF-α receptor etanercept (25 mg twice weekly) in the patients with refractory asthma in a placebo-controlled, double-blind, crossover pilot study.

Results.—As compared with patients with mild-to-moderate asthma and controls, patients with refractory asthma had increased expression of membrane-bound TNF-α, TNF-α receptor 1, and TNF-α–converting enzyme by peripheral-blood monocytes. In the clinical trial, as compared with placebo, 10 weeks of treatment with etanercept was associated with a significant increase in the concentration of methacholine required to provoke a 20 percent decrease in the forced expiratory volume in one second (FEV_1) (mean difference in doubling concentration changes between etanercept and placebo, 3.5; 95 percent confidence interval, 0.07 to 7.0; P=0.05), an improvement in the asthma-related quality-of-life score (by 0.85 point; 95 percent confidence interval, 0.16 to 1.54 on a 7-point scale; P=0.02), and a 0.32-liter increase in post-bronchodilator FEV_1 (95 percent confidence interval, 0.08 to 0.55; P=0.01).

Conclusions.—Patients with refractory asthma have evidence of upregulation of the TNF-α axis.

▶ This report reminds us that there is asthma and there is asthma. Mild to moderate asthma has a major component of bronchospasm and some airway inflammation. Cases of refractory asthma tend to have much more in the way of airway inflammation. There is a greater involvement of neutrophils. TNF-α plays a role in this. TNF-α is an inflammatory cytokine that is produced in large amounts by mast cells and is present in very large quantities in the bronchoalveolar fluid in the airways of patients with asthma.

If you are not all that familiar with TNF, including the origins of its name, it is one of the major inflammatory mediators. It was originally discovered and named on the basis of its tumor regression activity. A number of therapies have been developed that specifically target cytokines to diminish inflammation. Currently available inhibitors include the monoclonal antibodies against TNF-α, infliximab and adalimumab, and the soluble TNF receptor fused to human IgG, etanercept. TNF-α inhibitors have been used with some success in patients with rheumatoid arthritis, ankylosing spondylitis, psoriasis, and Crohn's disease. Now we see from the study of Berry et al that the soluble TNF inhibitor etanercept can be of benefit in patients with chronic refractory asthma.

Clearly etanercept is not for everyone. Inhaled and oral steroids remain the mainstay of anti-inflammatory treatment of patients with asthma. Unfortunately, there is a small subset of both children and adults in whom inflammation is so refractory that steroids alone or in combination with other anti-inflammatory agents do not seem to do the job. That is where TNF inhibitors come in. TNF-α is stored by mast cells and is rapidly released during IgE-mediated reactions that typify the asthmatic response to allergens. TNF-α causes a rapid migration of eosinophils and neutrophils into the airways. TNF-α also releases cytotoxic mediators resulting in airway injury. The end result of this is a chronic, unresolved inflammation that causes structural damage to the lung. This expression of TNF-α is directly related to the severity of asthma, and this has been documented in several studies. Thus, activation of TNF-α is fundamental to the process causing asthma, particularly to the development of persistent airflow limitation and bronchial hyperreactivity in patients with refractory asthma, despite the use of high-dose steroids.

No one is saying that we should jump quickly on the bandwagon of using TNF-α inhibitors for children with refractory asthma. In spite of the excitement generated by the news of this novel therapy, it would be premature to conclude that we should be using it willy-nilly. TNF-α inhibitors can cause serious adverse side effects including injection-site reactions, demyelinating disorders, lymphoproliferative diseases, and reactivation of tuberculosis with dissemination to the miliary form.

Although the incidence of adverse effects with etanercept was low in this study by Berry et al in adults, longer-term studies of patients with asthma are needed to determine whether TNF-α inhibitors can be safely used in adults or in children. It could be that the risk of recurrent respiratory tract infections or immunogenic adverse effects will preclude its routine use in all but the most seriously affected of patients, if then.

In a commentary by Erzurum[1] that accompanied this report, it was noted that the total annual cost of asthma care in the United States for adults and children is approximately $10 billion, with the majority of the economic impact related to hospitalization and emergency department costs. TNF-α inhibitors are expensive, but if it is determined that there is a niche role for them to play, the benefit/cost-effectiveness ratio may favor their selective use in highly selected cases. Time and further research will tell us whether this is true.

This commentary closes with a couple of facts having to do with risk factors for the development of reactive airway disease or worsening of existing reactive airway disease. If there is a single thing you might look for in a home that is an identifier of an unhealthy indoor environment, it is windowpane condensation. A number of studies have shown that window condensation is associated with an increased risk of asthma in preschool children.[2,3] In homes, windowpane condensation, all other things being equal, is an indication of an unhealthy indoor environment, with increased relative air humidity and an air exchange rate below the current ventilation standard of the Environmental Protection Agency. This standard is a minimum of 0.5 air exchanges per hour. In addition, window condensation is associated with an increased risk for mite allergen and mold exposure. As with martinis, the dryer the better.

Finally, recognize that if you live along a highway where there is a lot of truck and automobile traffic, you will also experience a higher risk for reactive airway disease. This has been demonstrated in infants less than one year of age.[4] It seems that infants who reside less than 100 m from a major highway or intersection are likely to receive high doses of particulate matter in the air they breathe. Diesel exhaust particles in particular seem to be the agents that exacerbate both asthma and allergic rhinitis. This is because of their unique ability to enhance those T-helper cells that direct allergic immune responses and the production of IgE. Studies have shown that these particles are inhalable and have a relatively large surface area per unit mass, which is an excellent medium for absorbing and transporting proteins into the peripheral airways of children, especially infants. These particles tend to bind grass pollen allergen and effectively deliver the pollen into the airway. If you live within 100 m of a highway, your increased risk of wheezing runs 2.5-fold.

J. A. Stockman III, MD

References

1. Erzurum SC: Inhibition of tumor necrosis α for refractory asthma. *N Engl J Med* 354:754-758, 2006.
2. Asher MI, Keil U, Anderson HR, et al: International study of asthma and allergies in children (ISAAC): Rationale and methods. *Eur Respir J* 8:483-491, 1995.
3. Lindfors A, Wickman M, Hedlin G, et al: Indoor environmental risk factors in young asthmatics: a case-controlled study. *Arch Dis Child* 73:408-412, 1995.
4. Ryan PH, LeMasters G, Biagini J, et al: Is it traffic type, volume or distance? Wheezing in infants living near truck and bus traffic. *J Allergy Clin Immunol* 116:279-284, 2005.

Use of Exhaled Nitric Oxide Measurements to Guide Treatment in Chronic Asthma

Smith AD, Cowan JO, Brassett KP, et al (Univ of Otago, Dunedin, New Zealand)
N Engl J Med 352:2163-2173, 2005   2–2

Background.—International guidelines for the treatment of asthma recommend adjusting the dose of inhaled corticosteroids on the basis of symptoms, bronchodilator requirements, and the results of pulmonary-function tests. Measurements of the fraction of exhaled nitric oxide (FE_{NO}) constitute a noninvasive marker that may be a useful alternative for the adjustment of inhaled-corticosteroid treatment.

Methods.—In a single-blind, placebo-controlled trial, we randomly assigned 97 patients with asthma who had been regularly receiving treatment with inhaled corticosteroids to have their corticosteroid dose adjusted, in a stepwise fashion, on the basis of either FE_{NO} measurements or an algorithm based on conventional guidelines. After the optimal dose was determined (phase 1), patients were followed up for 12 months (phase 2). The primary outcome was the frequency of exacerbations of asthma; the secondary outcome was the mean daily dose of inhaled corticosteroid.

Results.—Forty-six patients in the FE_{NO} group and 48 in the group whose asthma was treated according to conventional guidelines (the control group) completed the study. The final mean daily doses of fluticasone, the inhaled corticosteroid that was used, were 370 µg per day for the FE_{NO} group (95 percent confidence interval, 263 to 477) and 641 µg per day for the control group (95 percent confidence interval, 526 to 756; P=0.003), a difference of 270 µg per day (95 percent confidence interval, 112 to 430). The rates of exacerbation were 0.49 episode per patient per year in the FE_{NO} group (95 percent confidence interval, 0.20 to 0.78) and 0.90 in the control group (95 percent confidence interval, 0.31 to 1.49), representing a nonsignificant reduction of 45.6 percent (95 percent confidence interval for mean difference, −78.6 percent to 54.5 percent) in the FE_{NO} group. There were no significant differences in other markers of asthma control, use of oral prednisone, pulmonary function, or levels of airway inflammation (sputum eosinophils).

Conclusions.—With the use of FE_{NO} measurements, maintenance doses of inhaled corticosteroids may be significantly reduced without compromising asthma control.

▶ Patients as young as 12 years of age were included in this article, which clearly indicates the value of the conclusions, at least to a substantial part of the pediatric population. All of us need help in caring for patients with asthma. National and international guidelines recommend that patients with persistent symptoms use inhaled steroids as first-line therapy. Based on findings such as daytime or nighttime symptoms and impaired pulmonary functioning, guidelines also provide algorithms for increasing the doses of these medications and adding other forms of treatment. The rub is a lack of a solid biological marker to tell us how well patients are actually doing. Thus, it becomes more art than science when attempting to titrate the appropriate level of therapy to an individual patient's needs.

The most recent addition to the list of biological markers that might be able to tell us how well patients are doing is the amount of NO in exhaled air. In the article abstracted, we learn the value of exhaled NO as a yardstick in the treatment of chronic asthma. Other studies have come to similar conclusions, that is, an inverse relationship exists between how well a patient is managing with asthma and the amount of exhaled NO. The lower the levels of NO, the better the clinical condition.

Read the editorial by Deykin[1] before jumping on the exhaled NO bandwagon to judge how well your patients with asthma are doing. Deykin points out that much more research in this area is needed and that the data from the study abstracted require cautious interpretation and application. The NO study involved only patients with mild to moderate asthma, and we have no idea whether the findings can be applied to patients with either milder or more severe disease. Nonetheless, it is important to identify what the appropriate level of treatment is for each asthmatic patient and to use as little in the way of steroids as is reasonable. We need a good litmus test for this purpose, and it may well be that the measurement of NO in exhaled air will turn out to be a less invasive and technically simpler way to make an assessment of airway responsiveness than are other tools in our treatment bag. Please see the Newborn chapter for how NO is increasingly being used as a therapeutic agent in the management of preterm babies.

Last, if you are interested in purchasing a nitric oxide analyzer, it is available from Aerocrine AB Stockholm, Sweden. Make sure you have deep pockets. Elevated breath nitric oxide levels are seen in many different conditions in addition to those associated with reactive airway disease. For example, school children who report having a cold also have significantly higher nitric oxide airway levels than children not having a cold.[2] Homes that have high formaldehyde levels may have healthy appearing children, who nonetheless, also have high exhaled nitric oxide levels. Also, cat-sensitized children tend to have higher nitric oxide levels than non-cat-sensitized children when studied with a nitric oxide breath analyzer. If indeed there is any relationship between exhaled nitric oxide level and reactive airways disease, it is the fact that the relationship between the two is the 1741st reason not to have a cat in the house. When it comes to cats, homes, and children, just say NO.

J. A. Stockman III, MD

References

1. Deykin A: Targeting biological markers in asthma: Is exhaled nitric oxide the bull's eye? *N Engl J Med* 352:2233-2235, 2005.
2. de Gouw HW, Grunberg K, Schot R, et al: Relationship between exhaled nitric oxide and airway hyperresponsiveness following experimental rhinovirus infection in asthmatic subjects. *Eur Respir J* 11:126-132, 1998.

Sun Exposure and Risk of Melanoma
Oliveria SA, Saraiya M, Geller AC, et al (Mem Sloan-Kettering Cancer Ctr, New York; Ctrs for Disease Control and Prevention, Atlanta, Ga; Boston Univ)
Arch Dis Child 91:131-138, 2006   2–3

Background.—As skin cancer education programmes directed to children and adolescents continue to expand, an epidemiological basis for these programmes is necessary to target efforts and plan for further evaluation.

Aims.—To summarise the epidemiological evidence on sun exposure during childhood and adolescence and melanoma risk.

Methods.—A literature review was conducted using Medline (1966 to December 2004) to identify articles relating to sun exposure and melanoma. The review was restricted to studies that included sun exposure information on subjects 18 years of age or younger.

Results.—Migrant studies generally indicate an increased melanoma risk in individuals who spent childhood in sunny geographical locations, and decreasing melanoma risk with older age at arrival. Individuals who resided in geographical locations close to the equator or close to the coast during childhood and/or adolescence have an increased melanoma risk compared to those who lived at higher latitudes or never lived near the coast. The intermittent exposure hypothesis remains controversial; some studies indicate that children and adolescents who received intermittent sun exposure during vacation, recreation, or occupation are at increased melanoma risk as adults, but more recent studies suggest intermittent exposure to have a protective effect. The majority of sunburn studies suggest a positive association between early age sunburn and subsequent risk of melanoma.

Conclusion.—Future research efforts should focus on: (1) clarifying the relation between sun exposure and melanoma; (2) conducting prospective studies; (3) assessing sun exposure during different time periods of life using a reliable and quantitative method; (4) obtaining information on protective measures; and (5) examining the interrelations between ability to tan, propensity to burn, skin type, history of sunburns, timing and pattern of sun exposure, number of nevi, and other host factors in the child and adolescent populations.

▶ It is estimated that there will be over 60,000 new cases of invasive melanoma and almost 8000 deaths from this malignancy in the United States each year. The lifetime risk for melanoma in any one individual seems to run about 1.5%. This risk has been rising. The incidence of melanoma has escalated at a rate of about 3% per year in the United States. At one time, melanoma was thought to be rare in those younger than 20 years, but current evidence indicates a rapidly rising incidence of melanoma in both children and teenagers. We see from this report from Memorial Sloan-Kettering Cancer Center in New York City more precise information than we have had previously about the risk of sun exposure during childhood and the subsequent risk of malignancy. Children spend an estimated 2.5 to 3 hours outdoors each day and thus receive several times more annual UV-B rays than adults because of a greater opportunity to be outdoors midday. If there has been any benefit to society with the increasing popularity over the last decade or so of electronic games and computers that children and adolescents utilize, it has been a decrease in this amount of sun exposure. We do see from this report a correlation in children and adolescents between sun exposure and the risk of melanoma, inasmuch as individuals residing in geographic locations closer to the equator and close to the coast manifest an increased melanoma risk compared with those who live at higher latitudes and who never lived near the coast during the same age period.

As time passes, we are learning much, much more about who gets melanoma and who seems to be more protected from it. All melanomas are not the same. The report that follows (Abstract 2–4) gives us insights into why melanomas develop where they develop on the body and documents the fact that not all melanomas are triggered by exposure to sunlight.

J. A. Stockman III, MD

Clinicopathological Features of and Risk Factors for Multiple Primary Melanomas

Ferrone CR, Porat LB, Panageas KS, et al (Mem Sloan-Kettering Cancer Ctr, New York)

JAMA 294:1647-1654, 2005   2–4

Context.—The incidence of multiple primary melanomas ranges from 1.3% to 8.0% in large retrospective reviews; however, the impact of certain risk factors is not understood.

Objectives.—To determine the incidence of multiple primary melanomas (MPM) from a prospective, single-institution, multidisciplinary database, and to describe the clinical and pathological characteristics and risk factors specific to these patients.

Design and Setting.—Review of a prospectively maintained database at Memorial Sloan-Kettering Cancer Center in New York, NY.

Patients.—A total of 4484 patients diagnosed with a first primary melanoma between January 1, 1996, and December 31, 2002.

Main Outcome Measures.—Incidence of and risk factors for MPM.

Results.—Three hundred eighty-five patients (8.6%) had 2 or more primary melanomas, with an average of 2.3 melanomas per MPM patient. Seventy-eight percent had 2 primary melanomas. For 74% of patients, the initial melanoma was the thickest tumor. Fifty-nine percent presented with their second primary tumor within 1 year. Twenty-one percent of MPM patients had a positive family history of melanoma compared with only 12% of patients with a single primary melanoma (SPM) (*P*<.001). Thirty-eight percent of MPM patients had dysplastic nevi compared with 18% of SPM patients (*P*<.001). The estimated cumulative 5-year risk of a second primary tumor for the entire cohort was 11.4%, with almost half of that risk occurring within the first year. For patients with a positive family history or dysplastic nevi, the estimated 5-year risk of MPM was significantly higher at 19.1% and 23.7%, respectively. The most striking increase in incidence for the MPM population was seen for development of a third primary melanoma from the time of second primary melanoma, which was 15.6% at 1 year and 30.9% at 5 years.

Conclusions.—The incidence of MPM is increased in patients with a positive family history and/or dysplastic nevi. These patients should undergo intensive dermatologic screening and should consider genetic testing.

▶ We as pediatricians should be aware that children and adults who have melanoma can develop more melanomas. Among patients with a history of primary melanoma, retrospective reviews report the incidence of a second primary tumor to range from 0.2% to 8.6%. It has been known for over 50 years that the phenomenon of MPM occurs. Most individuals with more than 1 melanoma have just 2 primary tumors, but a patient has been described who has had as many as 48 separate primary melanomas.[1]

We learn from the report of Ferrone et al that the estimated cumulative 5-year risk of a second primary melanoma in their series of over 4000 patients was 11.4%, somewhat higher than reported in the literature. Of the 11.4%, roughly half of the risk was accrued during the first year after diagnosis of the first skin malignancy. After the first year, the other half of second malignancies accrued over years 2 through 5 at a rate somewhat higher than the yearly risk calculated in previous series. One thing is clear: 1 melanoma puts a patient at risk of a second primary melanoma, and a second primary melanoma puts a patient at even higher risk of a third primary melanoma. After a second primary melanoma, the incidence of a third malignancy is almost tripled. The 1- and 5-year incidences of a third primary melanoma from the date of the second primary melanoma are 15.6% and 30.9%, respectively.

Please recognize that the development of more than 1 melanoma is directly related to one's family history. The risk of subsequent primary melanoma is high for patients with a positive family history of melanoma, dysplastic nevi, or both, at 19.0%, 23.6%, and 29.9% at 5 years from initial diagnosis of melanoma, respectively. Interestingly, the risk for patients with no family history of melanoma or dysplastic nevi is still roughly 1.2% per year after the first year.

The substantially higher rate of positive family history of melanoma and dysplastic nevi in patients who develop more than 1 melanoma offers a unique opportunity to further characterize melanoma risk at a genetic level. Mutations in the tumor suppressor gene CDKN2A and the proto-oncogene CDK4 have been identified in patients with a positive family history and multiple melanomas. The relevance of these mutations, however, remains unclear.

If there is a bottom line to this report, it is that children, adolescents, and adults who develop a melanoma must be counseled to undergo not only life-long annual dermatologic follow-up for the detection of additional primary melanomas, but also to perform self-examinations and behavior modifications. In the higher-risk cohorts with multiple melanomas, positive family history, or dysplastic nevi, it may be prudent for patients to be seen more frequently than annually. For patients with multiple atypical nevi, photographically assisted follow-up may be indicated.

Without saying, the information provided from this report means full employment for dermatologists into the indefinite future.

J. A. Stockman III, MD

Reference

1. Slingluff CL, Vollmer RT, Seigler HF: Multiple primary melanoma: Incidence and risk factors in 283 patients. *Surgery* 113:330-339, 1993.

Clinical Recognition of Meningococcal Disease in Children and Adolescents

Thompson MJ, Ninis N, Perera R, et al (Univ of Oxford, England; Imperial College, London)
Lancet 367:397-403, 2006   2–5

Background.—Meningococcal disease is a rapidly progressive childhood infection of global importance. To our knowledge, no systematic quantitative research exists into the occurrence of symptoms before admission to hospital.

Methods.—Data were obtained from questionnaires answered by parents and from primary-care records for the course of illness before admission to hospital in 448 children (103 fatal, 345 non-fatal), aged 16 years or younger, with meningococcal disease. In 373 cases, diagnosis was confirmed with microbiological techniques. The rest of the children were included because they

TABLE 3.—Overall Frequency and Time of Onset of Clinical Features of Meningococcal Disease in Children Before Hospital Admission

	Percentage of Children (95% CI)	Median Hour of Onset
Clinical features present in >50% of children		
Fever	93·9% (89-98)	1
Drowsiness	81·1% (74-88)	7
Nausea or vomiting	76·4% (67-84)	4
Irritability	66·6% (57-75)	4
Haemorrhagic rash	61·0% (51-70)	13
Poor appetite or feeding	59·9% (50-70)	5
Clinical features present in 20-50%		
General aches	48·5% (39-58)	7
Confusion or delirium*	45·1% (36-55)	16
Cold hands and feet	43·2% (33-53)	12
Headache*	40·5% (31-50)	0
Leg pain	36·7% (28-47)	7
Neck pain or stiffness	35·0% (26-44)	13
Photophobia	27·5% (19-36)	15
Sore throat or coryza	23·6% (15-32)	5
Clinical features present in <20%		
Abnormal skin colour	18·6% (11-27)	10
Floppy muscle tone†	18·3% (12-26)	13
Bulging fontanelle‡	11·5% (5-18)	15
Breathing difficulty	10·8% (5-18)	11
Seizure	9·8% (4-16)	17
Unconsciousness	9·5% (4-15)	22
Increased thirst	8·1% (3-14)	8
Diarrhoea	6·6% (2-12)	9

Percentages and median hours of onset are standardized to UK case-fatality rate.
*Data only available for children aged >1 year.
†Data only available for children aged <5 years.
‡Data only available for children aged <1 year.
(Courtesy of Thompson MJ, Ninis N, Perera R, et al: Clinical recognition of meningococcal disease in children and adolescents. *Lancet* 367:397-403, 2006. Reprinted with permission from Elsevier.)

had a purpuric rash, and either meningitis or evidence of septicaemic shock. Results were standardised to UK case-fatality rates.

Findings.—The time-window for clinical diagnosis was narrow. Most children had only non-specific symptoms in the first 4–6 h, but were close to death by 24 h. Only 165 (51%) children were sent to hospital after the first consultation. The classic features of haemorrhagic rash, meningism, and impaired consciousness developed late (median onset 13–22 h). By contrast, 72% of children had early symptoms of sepsis (leg pains, cold hands and feet, abnormal skin colour) that first developed at a median time of 8 h, much earlier than the median time to hospital admission of 19 h (Table 3).

Interpretation.—Classic clinical features of meningococcal disease appear late in the illness. Recognising early symptoms of sepsis could increase the proportion of children identified by primary-care clinicians and shorten the time to hospital admission. The framework within which meningococcal disease is diagnosed should be changed to emphasise identification of these early symptoms by parents and clinicians.

▶ This report reminds us how quickly children become critically ill and potentially die of meningococcal disease. A petechial rash is often an early sign of the condition, thus the reason for including this topic in this chapter. Anyone who watched *ER* on March 16, 2006, saw how precipitously a couple of teens with meningococcemia crashed within a brief period of presentation. Unfortunately, the features of meningococcal disease that appear earliest are common to many self-limiting viral illnesses. Fever is the first symptom noticed in children younger than 5 years; headache is the first symptom seen in those older than 5. Ninety-four percent of children develop fever at some point, and most young children are irritable. Loss of appetite, nausea, and vomiting are early features for all age groups, with many children also having upper respiratory tract symptoms, usually a sore throat or runny nose. These features, hardly specific to meningococcal disease, last for about 4 hours in younger children, but as long as 8 hours in adults, before more typical and prominent features of the disease become apparent. The first specific clinical features are usually signs of sepsis—leg pain, abnormal skin color, cold hands and feet, and in older children, thirst. Parents of younger children also report drowsiness and difficulty in breathing. Less commonly, younger children can have diarrhea at this stage. Most sepsis symptoms appear before the first contact with a primary care provider. The first classic sign of meningococcal disease to emerge is rash, although at onset, this is sometimes nonspecific and only developed, in this report, into a petechial and then a large hemorrhagic rash over several hours. Specific signs of meningitis, including neck stiffness, photophobia, and bulging fontanel, occur somewhat later at around 12 to 15 hours from the onset of the first nonspecific signs and symptoms. The last signs, such as unconsciousness, delirium, or seizures, are seen at a median of 15 hours in infants (<1 year of age) and at about 24 hours in older children. Hemorrhagic rash, the most commonly recognized classic feature of the disease, is seen in fewer than two thirds of patients.

This report is worth reading in some detail since it is the first comprehensive description of the time course of the clinical features of meningococcal disease in children and adolescents before admission to the hospital. The report also gives us 3 clinical features that should put a chill up our spines in identifying many of these children as having meningococcal disease: leg pain, cold hands and feet, and abnormal skin color. These occur, in most children, before the onset of rash, meningism, and impaired consciousness. Obviously, cold hands and feet and abnormal skin color are signs of early sepsis and should be recognized as such. Meningococcal disease should never be excluded by clinical examination in the first 4 to 6 hours of illness at presentation.

J. A. Stockman III, MD

A Vaccine to Prevent Herpes Zoster and Postherpetic Neuralgia in Older Adults

Oxman MN, for the Shingles Prevention Study Group (VA San Diego Healthcare System, Calif; et al)
N Engl J Med 352:2271-2284, 2005   2–6

Background.—The incidence and severity of herpes zoster and postherpetic neuralgia increase with age in association with a progressive decline in cell-mediated immunity to varicella–zoster virus (VZV). We tested the hypothesis that vaccination against VZV would decrease the incidence, severity, or both of herpes zoster and postherpetic neuralgia among older adults.

Methods.—We enrolled 38,546 adults 60 years of age or older in a randomized, double-blind, placebo-controlled trial of an investigational live attenuated Oka/Merck VZV vaccine ("zoster vaccine"). Herpes zoster was diagnosed according to clinical and laboratory criteria. The pain and discomfort associated with herpes zoster were measured repeatedly for six months. The primary end point was the burden of illness due to herpes zoster, a measure affected by the incidence, severity, and duration of the associated pain and discomfort. The secondary end point was the incidence of postherpetic neuralgia.

Results.—More than 95 percent of the subjects continued in the study to its completion, with a median of 3.12 years of surveillance for herpes zoster. A total of 957 confirmed cases of herpes zoster (315 among vaccine recipients and 642 among placebo recipients) and 107 cases of postherpetic neuralgia (27 among vaccine recipients and 80 among placebo recipients) were included in the efficacy analysis. The use of the zoster vaccine reduced the burden of illness due to herpes zoster by 61.1 percent (P<0.001), reduced the incidence of postherpetic neuralgia by 66.5 percent (P<0.001), and reduced the incidence of herpes zoster by 51.3 percent (P<0.001). Reactions at the injection site were more frequent among vaccine recipients but were generally mild.

Conclusions.—The zoster vaccine markedly reduced morbidity from herpes zoster and postherpetic neuralgia among older adults.

▶ It is not uncommon that the YEAR BOOK OF PEDIATRICS includes articles dealing solely with adults. There is much to be learned from such articles. The study abstracted tells us the benefits of administering the same varicella vaccine that is given in early childhood to adults so that herpes zoster and postherpetic neuralgia can be prevented. Zoster affects literally hundreds of thousands of people annually here in our country. Most are individuals older than 50 years. Because VZV becomes latent in cranial nerve ganglia, dorsal root ganglia, and autonomic ganglia along the entire neuraxis, zoster can crop up anywhere on the body. The pain associated with herpes zoster can be long lasting. Half of patients older than 70 years who experience zoster say their pain lasts for more than 1 year. It is a pain that is not easily controlled.

After an episode of varicella in childhood (and presumably after immunization), as we grow older, antibody titers to varicella tend to persist, but cellular-based immunity gradually wanes. What we see in the article by Oxman et al is an impressive reduction in morbidity from herpes zoster and postherpetic neuralgia in adults who are given the VZV vaccine. In this study, almost 40,000 adults 60 years or older were followed up over a period of slightly more than 3 years. These adults were divided into a placebo group and a group that received the varicella zoster vaccine. A total of 957 confirmed cases of herpes zoster were observed in the follow-up period. The use of the zoster vaccine reduced the burden of illness due to zoster by more than 60%. The actual incidence of herpes zoster was cut in half. Side effects were minimal.

As much as we now know about the pros and cons of VZV vaccine when administered to children, we still have to understand the implications of the widespread use of this vaccine for middle-aged and older adults who are otherwise healthy but seropositive for this virus. There are 2 main factors that affect the issue of whether the vaccine should be recommended for otherwise healthy adults. By 2047, most, if not close to all, middle-aged Americans will have received the VZV vaccine during childhood. Like the wild-type varicella virus, the vaccine virus will become latent in ganglia. If the viral burden is less in the ganglia of adults who were vaccinated in infancy, then the incidence of zoster may be reduced in those adults who received the vaccine in childhood. Alternatively, the cell-mediated immunity to VZV in the vaccine recipients may be reduced by their exposure to fewer cases of varicella, which would normally boost immune responsiveness, thus supporting the need to vaccinate middle-aged adults. Also, before any recommendation can be made about vaccination of adults, the cost-effectiveness of such vaccination will need to be carefully studied. The current cost of vaccination runs between $50 and $100 if one includes the cost of the vaccine plus a facility fee for its administration. Rough estimates suggest that vaccine administration to adults would be highly cost-effective (in the range of $2000 per quality-adjusted life-year gained). It seems a no-brainer that the vaccine would fall well within the traditional cutoff point of $50,000 per quality-adjusted life-year used to evaluate new therapies, and it would appear to be at least as cost-effective as virtually any other currently used vaccine.

Sure as shooting, most of us are in an age group that will clearly benefit, or possibly benefit, from being given the VZV vaccine. The US Census Bureau projects that, by the year 2040, as many as 13 million Americans will be 85 years or older. One can hope that the use of a zoster vaccine will reduce or eradicate zoster and its related complications, just as the measles vaccine has wiped out not only measles but also measles-associated postinfectious encephalomyelitis and subsequent sclerosing panencephalitis in regions in which the vaccine has been used. Is it worth dipping into one's pocket, if need be, to reduce one's risk of the development of zoster by 50%? I, for one, have my checkbook ready and waiting. It just may be that grown-ups will ultimately need the varicella vaccine more than children do.

To read about therapies for chronic postherpetic neuralgia, see the excellent commentary on this topic by Hampton.[1]

J. A. Stockman III, MD

Reference

1. Hampton T: When shingles wanes but pain does not. *JAMA* 293:2459-2460, 2005.

Rocky Mountain Spotted Fever From an Unexpected Tick Vector in Arizona
Demma LJ, Traefer MS, Nicholson WL, et al (Ctrs for Disease Control, Atlanta, Ga; Indian Health Service, Whiteriver, Ariz; Indian Health Service, Albuquerque, NM)
N Engl J Med 353:587-594, 2005   2–7

Background.—Rocky Mountain spotted fever is a life-threatening, tick-borne disease caused by *Rickettsia rickettsii*. This disease is rarely reported in Arizona, and the principal vectors, *Dermacentor* species ticks, are uncommon in the state. From 2002 through 2004, a focus of Rocky Mountain spotted fever was investigated in rural eastern Arizona.

Methods.—We obtained blood and tissue specimens from patients with suspected Rocky Mountain spotted fever and ticks from patients' homesites. Serologic, molecular, immunohistochemical, and culture assays were performed to identify the causative agent. On the basis of specific laboratory criteria, patients were classified as having confirmed or probable Rocky Mountain spotted fever infection.

Results.—A total of 16 patients with Rocky Mountain spotted fever infection (11 with confirmed and 5 with probable infection) were identified. Of these patients, 13 (81 percent) were children 12 years of age or younger, 15 (94 percent) were hospitalized, and 2 (12 percent) died. Dense populations of *Rhipicephalus sanguineus* ticks were found on dogs and in the yards of patients' homesites. All patients with confirmed Rocky Mountain spotted fever had contact with tick-infested dogs, and four had a reported history of tick bite preceding the illness. *R. rickettsii* DNA was detected in nonengorged *R. sanguineus* ticks collected at one home, and *R. rickettsii* isolates were cultured from these ticks.

Conclusions.—This investigation documents the presence of Rocky Mountain spotted fever in eastern Arizona, with common brown dog ticks (*R. sanguineus*) implicated as a vector of *R. rickettsii*. The broad distribution of this common tick raises concern about its potential to transmit *R. rickettsii* in other settings.

▶ When you live in North Carolina, as I do, you come to fully appreciate Rocky Mountain spotted fever, which seems to be as common here in the North Carolinas as it ever has been in the Rocky Mountains. There are few illnesses, infection wise, that remain as virulent. While it may not kill as many people who contract it as, say rabies, the mortality rate with Rocky Mountain spotted fever still runs as high as 20%. It is now more than 100 years since Howard T. Ricketts first described the pathogen transmitted by Montana ticks that killed up to 75% of patients it infected. A century later, we still continue to learn much about Rocky Mountain spotted fever and the organism(s) that cause it, as evidenced by the information provided in the article from the Centers for Disease Control and Prevention.

Rocky Mountain spotted fever occurs when *R rickettsii* in the salivary glands of a vector tick is transmitted into the dermis, spreading and replicating in the cytoplasm of endothelial cells and eliciting widespread vasculitis, hypoperfusion, and organ damage induced by vascular permeability, which is most dangerous in the lungs and brains. For those who do not see a lot of Rocky Mountain spotted fever, the diagnosis is sometimes difficult because of the nonspecific presentation of the disease, which includes a fever, headaches, myalgia, and, usually after a 3- to 5-day period, a rash that evolves from macular to maculopapular to petechial. Patients frequently have nausea, vomiting, abdominal pain, and coughing, which further serve to distract one from diagnosing the total symptom complex as Rocky Mountain spotted fever. Early suspicion is critical because severe illness and death are associated with a delayed diagnosis. This is especially a problem when a small but real percentage of patients present with an absence of a rash or present during a season with a low level of tick activity.

Here in the United States, the American dog tick (*D variabilis*) and the Rocky Mountain wood tick (*D andersoni*) are the ticks harboring *R rickettsii*. A tick that becomes infected with the organism can pass the organism on to its progeny once a tick ovary is infected. There have been distinct peaks in the incidence of Rocky Mountain spotted fever occurring in 1920, 1939-1949, and again from 1974-1984. The reason for this cyclical waxing and waning is unknown. The last 10 years has also seen another peak during the period 1998 through 2004 when 1514 cases were reported, which is an increase of a factor of 4 during any other 6-year period reported in US history. Similar increases are being reported in Canada, Mexico, Costa Rica, Panama, Colombia, Brazil, and Argentina, where the infection is re-emerging after years of dormancy.

If you suspect Rocky Mountain spotted fever, promptly start therapy with doxycycline. The laboratory confirmation is a weak link. The most widely applied diagnostic tool, serologic analysis, is not useful during active infection. Polymerase chain reaction analysis is insensitive, and immunohistochemical analysis of a skin biopsy for *R rickettsii* antigen is not widely or promptly available. When in doubt, treat. If you are afraid to use doxycycline because of the patient's age, check with the "Red Book."

J. A. Stockman III, MD

Near Strangulation as a Result of Hair Tourniquet Syndrome
Chegwidden HJ, Poirier MP (Eastern Virginia Med School, Norfolk)
Clin Pediatr (Phila) 44:359-361, 2005   2–8

Background.—Hair tourniquet syndrome has been a recognized clinical entity for many years. In this situation, hair becomes tightly wrapped around an appendage. The syndrome is usually seen in infants. Body parts involved typically include the finger, toe, penis, clitoris, and uvula. There have also been many reports of necrosis as an end result of hair tourniquet syndrome. A case of hair tourniquet syndrome in an infant, which caused signs and symptoms of acute strangulation, was described.

Case Report.—Girl, 11 months, was brought to the emergency department (ED) after she was found struggling to breathe while in bed with her 5-year-old sister. The infant had become entangled in the knee-length hair of her sister, and several strands of hair were reportedly wrapped around the infant's neck. The father reported that the infant had purple lips and bluish skin and difficulty breathing. The father cut hair from the older child's head to unwrap the hair from the infant and free her.

The emergency medical system was activated, and rescue personnel responded within minutes. The patient had no respiratory distress en route to the hospital. On arriving at the ED, the patient was generally playful and in no distress. Her vital signs were stable, and pulse oximetry was 100%. The infant had ligature marks around her neck and several long hairs on her body and clothing consistent with the history. Petechiae was evident on her face and neck, and there was some edema of the facial tissues.

There were no signs of airway compromise or difficulty in swallowing. Results of the rest of the examination were normal. The patient was monitored in the ED for several hours and then discharged when no complications surfaced. Follow-up with her pediatrician showed no long-term complications.

Conclusion.—Hair tourniquet syndrome is often considered in the medical evaluation of the irritable or crying infant. The exact mechanism of entanglement of the hair is unknown, and most cases are thought to be accidental. Once a hair tourniquet is identified, the recommended treatment is immediate removal. Prolonged conservative management of the distal tissue is often sufficient, but surgical exploration is sometimes indicated. Increased physician and parent awareness of accidental strangulation from the hair tourniquet syndrome is important for the prevention of potentially tragic outcomes.

► This is the first time this editor has heard of the hair tourniquet syndrome in someone as old as the girl reported here. Most cases of the problem are reported in much younger babies who present with irritability or crying. For example, one early report was that of a baby who had a hair tourniquet syndrome of the penis. This was in a 4-week-old boy who had the hair wrapped around his penis by a vengeful family nurse.[1] This classic, almost 2-century-old case has been followed by numerous subsequent reports in the literature, mostly involving a single human hair wrapped around some appendage. Appendages are not the only organs that have been affected by hair tourniquet syndrome. Case reports have shown hair wrapped around the uvula. Entwined hairs can cause autoamputation of the uvula.[2,3]

Actually, this baby is not the oldest baby to have been reported with strangulation of the neck as a result of hair tourniquet syndrome. A 27-month-old boy was accidentally strangled by his mother's unbraided waist-length hair while he co-slept with her.[4] In the latter report, the mother was awakened from sleep and her husband found the child suspended by hair wound around his neck, back to back with his wife. The baby was deeply blue and the father pulled the hair out from the mother by its roots. Fortunately, the child survived. There is even a gruesome report of a homicidal strangulation of an adult woman using her hair as the ligature.[5]

The report abstracted of this 11-month-old baby is the first and only report of strangulation of a child as the result of a sibling's hair becoming accidentally entwined around the neck. The child described in the report had signs of facial petechiae, swelling, and ligature marks around the neck, all consistent with the history that the father recounted. It was not clear from this report exactly how the sister's hair got wrapped around the baby's neck.

If there is any one risk factor for hair tourniquet syndrome, it is the sleeping arrangement of infants and children. Co-sleeping seems to be the problem in many instances. If a parent wishes to allow co-sleeping of their children, with themselves or their siblings, it is strongly suggested that proper precautions be taken to limit the potential risk of hair tourniquet strangulation, despite the rarity of this event.

J. A. Stockman III, MD

References

1. Dr. G: Ligature of the penis. *Lancet* 2:136, 1832.
2. McNeal RM, Cruickshank JC: Strangulation of the uvula by hair wrapping. *Clin Pediatr* 26:599-600, 1987.
3. Trocinski DR: The crying infant. *Emerg Med Clin North Am* 16:895-910, 1998.
4. Kindley AD, Rodd RM: Accidental strangulation by mother's hair. *Lancet* 11:565, 1978.
5. Ruzkiewicz AR, Lee KA, Landgren AG: Homicidal strangulation by victim's own hair presenting as natural death. *Am J Forensic Med Pathol* 15:340-343, 1994.

Single Blind, Randomised, Comparative Study of the Bug Buster Kit and Over the Counter Pediculicide Treatments Against Head Lice in the United Kingdom
Hill N, Moor G, Cameron MM, et al (London School of Hygiene and Tropical Medicine; Rothamsted Research, Hertfordshire, England)
BMJ 331:384-386, 2005   2–9

Objective.—To compare the effectiveness of the Bug Buster kit regimen with a single treatment of over the counter pediculicides for eliminating head lice.

Design.—Single blind, multicentre, randomised, comparative clinical study.

Setting.—Four counties in England and one county in Scotland.

Participants.—133 young people aged 2-15 years with head louse infestation: 56 were allocated to the Bug Buster kit and 70 to pediculicide treatment.

Interventions.—Home use of proprietary pediculicides (organophosphate or pyrethroid) or the Bug Buster kit.

Main Outcome Measure.—Presence of head lice 2-4 days after end of treatment: day 5 for the pediculicides and day 15 for the Bug Buster kit.

Results.—The cure rate using the Bug Buster kit was significantly greater than that for the pediculicides (57% v 13%; relative risk 4.4, 95% confidence interval 2.3 to 8.5). Number needed to treat for the Bug Buster kit compared with the pediculicides was 2.26.

Conclusion.—The Bug Buster kit was the most effective over the counter treatment for head louse infestation in the community when compared with pediculicides.

▶ Here is another report on the Bug Buster Kit. Head lice have been around for ages. Described in ancient Egyptian and Greek medical texts, this little critter is one that attracts a lot of attention. If you go on Google, you will find almost a million links to the topic of head lice. It is interesting to see that though several millennia have passed since the first descriptions of infestation of one's scalp by lice, we continue to learn much about its treatment.

Hill et al report the most complete assessment of the nonpharmacologic approach utilizing the Bug Buster, testing it against traditional pediculicides. The findings seem to show that Bug Buster, a kit comprised of 4 fine-tooth combs with instructions to use them 4 times over 2 weeks, is more effective in eradicating head lice than a single treatment of a pediculicide that is available over-the-counter (this in Great Britain): cure rates were almost 60% vs 13%. The latter cure rate is remarkably low in comparison with what we would expect to see, which makes some of the findings of this article a bit suspect.

Even if this study from Great Britain underestimates the effectiveness of pediculicide, it still shows that manual removal of head lice can be, in and of itself, quite effective in the right hands. For more on this lousy topic, see the editorial by Dawes.[1]

This is the last entry in the Allergy and Dermatology chapter, so we will close with a "who-dunnit" question for you. A 16-year-old girl comes to your office with a complaint of an itchy lower lip for the past 5 months. Her symptoms also have included oozing, soreness, and scab formation on her lower lip. Physical examination shows superficial crusted plaques with erosion of the lower lip. The only significant historical fact is that 5 months ago, she began playing the clarinet when she joined the school band. Your diagnosis?

If you make a diagnosis of "clarinet lip," you would be correct. Clarinet lip is a condition brought about by sensitivity to Aurndo donax. Aurndo donax is the grass (related to bamboo) used to make traditional clarinet reeds. If you do not believe there is such a thing as "clarinet lip," read the case history of a young woman who presented with the symptoms described above. She was advised to use synthetic polystyrene reeds. Her lip lesions healed within 2 weeks.[2] Such a remedy would probably also apply to those who have problems with the saxophone. Polystyrene reeds, in such a circumstance, would allow one to engage in safe sax.

J. A. Stockman III, MD

References

1. Dawes M: Combing and combating head lice: Choosing between four successive combings or two applications of pediculicide. *BMJ* 331:362-363, 2005.
2. Duke A: Clarinet lip. *BMJ* 332:558, 2006.

3 Blood

The Cost-Effectiveness of Screening the US Blood Supply for West Nile Virus

Custer B, Busch MP, Marfin AA, et al (Univ of California, San Francisco; Ctrs for Disease Control and Prevention, San Francisco; Natl Ctr for Infectious Diseases, Fort Collins, Colo)
Ann Intern Med 143:486-492, 2005   3–1

Background.—The spread of West Nile virus across North America and evidence of transmission by transfusion prompted the U.S. Food and Drug Administration to encourage the development of methods to screen the blood supply.

Objective.—To assess the cost-effectiveness of nucleic acid amplification testing for West Nile virus in the U.S. blood supply.

Design.—Markov cohort simulation.

Data Sources.—Outcome probabilities estimated from nucleic acid testing done for West Nile virus in 2003, data from the Centers for Disease Control and Prevention, and published literature. Costs were taken from an economic study of West Nile virus infection and from estimated test costs.

Target Populations.—Transfusion recipients, 60 years of age or older, with and without underlying immunocompromise.

Time Horizon.—Lifetime.

Perspective.—Societal.

Interventions.—The authors compared 6 strategies, taking into consideration minipool (pools of 6 to 16 donations) versus individual donation testing, and the geographic and seasonal nature of West Nile virus activity.

Outcome Measures.—Costs and effects of each strategy based on the prevention of transfusion-transmitted West Nile virus.

Results of Base-Case Analysis.—The cost-effectiveness of annual, national minipool testing was $483 000 per quality-adjusted life-year (QALY), whereas the cost-effectiveness of annual, national individual donation testing was $897 000/QALY. The cost-effectiveness of targeted individual donation testing in an area experiencing an outbreak coupled with minipool testing elsewhere was 520 000/QALY.

Results of Sensitivity Analysis.—In 1-way analyses, the most important influences were the prevalence of West Nile virus and the cost of minipool testing and individual donation testing. The 95% range of results from

West Nile Virus Among Blood Donors in the United States, 2003 and 2004
Stramer SL, Fang CT, Foster GA, et al (American Red Cross, Gaithersburg, Md; American Red Cross, Rockville, Md; Quality Analytics, Riverwoods, Ill)
N Engl J Med 353:451-459, 2005   3–3

Background.—West Nile virus first appeared in the United States in 1999 and has since spread throughout the contiguous states, resulting in thousands of cases of disease. By 2002, it was clear that the virus could be transmitted by blood transfusion, and by the middle of 2003, essentially all blood donations were being tested for West Nile virus RNA with the use of investigational nucleic acid amplification tests; testing was performed on individual samples or on "minipools" of up to 16 donations.

Methods.—We analyzed data from the West Nile virus testing program of the American Red Cross for 2003 and 2004 to identify geographic and temporal trends. In areas with a high incidence of infection, individual donations were tested to increase the sensitivity of testing. Donors with reactive results participated in follow-up studies to confirm the original reactivity and to assess the natural history of infection.

Results.—Routine testing in 2003 and 2004 identified 540 donations that were positive for West Nile virus RNA, of which 362 (67 percent) were IgM-antibody–negative and most likely infectious. Of the 540 positive donations, 148 (27 percent) were detectable only by testing of individual donations, but only 15 of the 148 (10 percent) were negative for IgM antibody. The overall frequencies of RNA-positive donations during the epidemic periods were 1.49 per 10,000 donations in 2003 and 0.44 per 10,000 in 2004. In 2004, 52 percent of the positive donations were from donors in four counties in southern California.

Conclusions.—Rapid implementation of a nucleic acid amplification test led to the prospective identification of 519 donors who were positive for West Nile virus RNA and the removal of more than 1000 potentially infectious related components from the blood supply of the Red Cross. No cases of transfusion-transmitted infection were confirmed among recipients of the tested blood.

► It has been almost 8 years since the West Nile virus first appeared on our shores and 6 years since it was apparent that the virus could be transmitted by blood transfusions. In 2003, screening for this virus in blood donations began. This article and the article by Busch et al (see Abstract 3–2) analyze the results of screening of some 7.1 million donations for West Nile virus and tell us just how effective screening is for this infectious agent.

When screening for West Nile virus was first begun back in 2003, the screening was done only on pooled blood samples from 16 donors. This is known as minipool screening. Such an approach to screening is quite cost-effective when the prevalence of "bad" units is low. Remarkably, viral contamination began to be documented in as many as 1 in 150 donors in some areas of the country during epidemics. From among approximately 27.2 million donations screened nationwide during the first 2 years of screening, slightly more than

1000 donor units were detected as being positive for West Nile virus (a yield of 1 in 26,200), but marked variations in yields were found, depending on the season of the year and the location within the United States. This yield compares with yields ranging from 1 in 100 to 1 in 1000 donations for HIV, hepatitis B virus, and hepatitis C virus when screening for those viruses began. Soon after the screening began, it became quite clear that antibody screening was not going to be effective by itself and that screening for viremia with the use of nucleic acid amplification was going to be necessary. Best estimates now are that minipool screening was about 93% sensitive in picking up infectious donations, which translates into a residual risk of less than 1 in 350,000, calculated according to the following formula: $[(1039 \div 0.93) - 1039] \div 27.2$ million. This risk can be compared with contemporary risks of transfusion-transmitted hepatitis B virus of 1 in 220,000 donations, transfusion-transmitted hepatitis C virus of 1 in 1,600,000 donations, and transfusion-transmitted HIV of 1 in 1,800,000 donations. The difference with West Nile virus infection and these other bloodborne infections is that units of blood are infectious only for relatively short periods of time, and a wide variation exists, based on seasonality.

So just how effective has West Nile virus screening been when performed on donor units of blood? Apparently, it has been extremely effective because not a single case of transfusion-transmitted infection has been confirmed in recipients of blood from donors who have been screened. Is it worth the cost? If you were the one getting West Nile virus from a unit of blood, you would say yes, and the cost-effective data analysis also seem to say yes. Not until this virus fades away will we likely stop screening for it in blood donors.

J. A. Stockman III, MD

A New Formula for Blood Transfusion Volume in the Critically Ill

Morris KP, Naqvi N, Davies P, et al (Birmingham Children's Hosp, England)
Arch Dis Child 90:724-728, 2005   3–4

Background.—Published formulae, frequently used to predict the volume of transfused red cells required to achieve a desired rise in haemoglobin (Hb) or haematocrit (Hct), do not appear to have been validated in clinical practice.

Aims.—To examine the relation between transfusion volume and the resulting rise in Hb and Hct in critically ill children.

Methods.—Phase 1: Sample of 50% of children admitted during 1997; 237 of these 495 patients received at least one packed red cell transfusion; 82 children were transfused without confounding factors that could influence the Hb/Hct response to transfusion and were analysed further. Actual rise in Hb concentration or haematocrit was compared to that expected from use of existing formulae. A new formula was developed. Phase 2: In 50 children receiving a packed red cell transfusion during 2001, actual rise in Hb concentration was compared to expected rise in Hb with use of the new formula.

Results.—Phase 1: Existing formulae performed poorly; median ratio of actual/predicted rise in Hb or Hct ranged from 0.61 to 0.85. Using the regression coefficients new formulae were developed for both Hb and Hct. These formulae were applicable across all age and diagnostic groups. Phase 2: Median ratio of actual/predicted rise in Hb improved to 0.95 with use of the new formula.

Conclusions.—Existing formulae underestimate the volume of packed red cells required to achieve a target Hb or Hct. Adoption of the new formulae could reduce the number of transfusion episodes in PICU, cutting costs and reducing risk.

▶ This article reinforces what many of us have come to believe: the current formula that most of us use to determine the volume of blood necessary for a transfusion tends to undershoot the final Hb level after the transfusion. The formula that most use is: volume of packed red blood cells to transfuse = total blood volume × (target Hb − current Hb) divided by Hb of donor unit.

We believe in this formula because it should theoretically work, but, in fact, the formula has not been validated in clinical practice. The article from England attempts to do this. The article shows us that, far more often than not, the formula fails to achieve the desired Hb level. The authors of this article propose a new formula: Hb (g/dL). You will have to read the article in some detail to see how this new formula was derived, but the math does appear to be accurate.

There are probably a number of reasons why the currently used formula underestimates the actual volume of transfused blood needed to produce a rise in Hb. Once removed from the body, red blood cells undergo a progressive loss of viability that leads to a decline in posttransfusion survival. The age of blood is important: the 24-hour posttransfusion survival index of preserved blood is 90% or greater if blood is transfused within 1 week of collection but may fall below 80% if transfused later in its shelf life. Current textbooks state that a newborn has a circulating blood volume of 80 mL/kg to 90 mL/kg and that a teen has a circulating blood volume of about 70 mL/kg, but remarkably little supporting literature based on studies of red cell mass exist to substantiate these blood volumes. The concentration of red cells in packed red cell transfusions also varies somewhat.

Whether the results of this article from Great Britain will lead to revolutionary, evolutionary, or no change in transfusion practice remains to be seen. One suspects that the article will have little impact. Most of us seem satisfied with a less than predicted rise in Hb. We are simply happy that the Hb has moved in the right direction.

One additional comment about transfusion, this regarding transfusion early in life. If you think a baby who is about to be born needs a boost in his or her hemoglobin, one of the easiest ways to do this is to plan for a placental transfusion of the baby's own blood. Theoretically, one can transfer a baby's blood that is in the baby's side of the placental circulation by one or more techniques, which include delayed cord clamping, holding an infant below the placenta, and administering an oxytocic agent to the mother. Recently, a study was undertaken to determine whether any of these techniques actually work.[1] It would appear that the only effective way of transferring blood from the placenta to a baby during delivery is to delay clamping the umbilical cord by 30 seconds. With this technique, the infant's mean blood volume will be increased from 62.7 mL/kg to 74.4 mL/kg. This procedure seems to work effectively for both vaginal and cesarean section deliveries. Holding an infant below the mother or administering an oxytocic agent to the mother seems to do little in the way of delivering placental blood to a newborn baby.

J. A. Stockman III, MD

Reference

1. Aladangady N, McHugh S, Aitchison TC, et al: Infant's blood volume in a controlled trial of placental transfusion at preterm delivery. *Pediatrics* 117:93-98, 2006.

The Influence of High-Altitude Living on Body Iron

Cook JD, Boy E, Flowers C, et al (Kansas Univ, Kansas City; The Micronutrient Initiative, Ottawa, Ontario, Canada; Pan American Health Organisation, La Paz, Bolivia)
Blood 106:1441-1446, 2005   3–5

Abstract.—The quantitative assessment of body iron based on measurements of the serum ferritin and transferrin receptor was used to examine iron status in 800 Bolivian mothers and one of their children younger than 5 years. The survey included populations living at altitudes between 156 to 3750 m. Body iron stores in the mothers averaged 3.88 ± 4.31 mg/kg (mean $\pm$ 1 SD) and 1.72 ± 4.53 mg/kg in children. No consistent effect of altitude on body iron was detected in children but body iron stores of 2.77 ± 0.70 mg/kg (mean $\pm$ 2 standard error [SE]) in women living above 3000 m was reduced by one-third compared with women living at lower altitudes ($P < .001$). One half of the children younger than 2 years were iron deficient, but iron stores then increased linearly to approach values in their mothers by 4 years of age. When body iron in mothers was compared with that of their children, a striking correlation was observed over the entire spectrum of maternal iron status ($r = 0.61$, $P < .001$). This finding could provide the strongest evidence to date of the importance of dietary iron as a determinant of iron status in vulnerable segments of a population.

▶ The authors of this article describe the effect of living at high altitude on body iron in 800 Bolivian mothers and their children. A lot can be learned from this study. We see that body iron in women is significantly lower in subjects living at altitudes above 3000 m. At the same time, there is a linear increase in body iron with increasing age in children 0 to 4 years of age, and body iron reaches the same level as mothers by about the age of 4 years. However, the most interesting finding in this study was the close correlation between mother and child in terms of total body iron throughout the entire range of body iron values. The authors of this article choose to interpret this correlation as an indication of the importance of dietary iron, which is a factor common to mem-

Discontinuing Prophylactic Transfusions Used to Prevent Stroke in Sickle Cell Disease

Adams RJ, for The Optimizing Primary Stroke Prevention in Sickle Cell Anemia (STOP 2) Trial Investigators (Medical College of Georgia, Augusta; Med Univ of South Carolina, Charleston; Univ of Miami, Fla; et al)
N Engl J Med 353:2769-2778, 2005   3–7

Background.—Prophylactic transfusion prevents strokes in children with sickle cell anemia who have abnormalities on transcranial Doppler ultrasonographic examination. However, it is not known how long transfusion should be continued in these children.

Methods.—We studied children with sickle cell disease who had a high risk of stroke on the basis of a transcranial Doppler screening examination and who had received transfusions for 30 months or longer, during which time the Doppler readings became normal. The children were randomly assigned to continued transfusion or no continued transfusion. Children with severe stenotic lesions on cerebral magnetic resonance angiography were excluded. The composite primary end point was stroke or reversion to a result on Doppler examination indicative of a high risk of stroke.

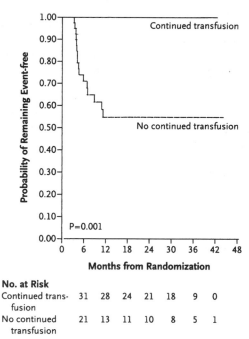

No. at Risk							
Continued transfusion	31	28	24	21	18	9	0
No continued transfusion	21	13	11	10	8	5	1

FIGURE 2.—Kaplan–Meier estimates of the probability of no end point event among patients assigned to continued transfusion or no continued transfusion. *P* values were determined by the log-rank test. (Reprinted by permission of *The New England Journal of Medicine* from Adams RJ, for The Optimizing Primary Stroke Prevention in Sickle Cell Anemia (STOP 2) Trial Investigators: Discontinuing prophylactic transfusions used to prevent stroke in sickle cell disease. *N Engl J Med* 353:2769-2778. Copyright 2005, Massachusetts Medical Society. All rights reserved.)

Results.—The study was stopped after 79 children of a planned enrollment of 100 underwent randomization. Among the 41 children in the transfusion-halted group, high-risk Doppler results developed in 14 and stroke in 2 others within a mean (±SD) of 4.5±2.6 months (range, 2.1 to 10.1) of the last transfusion. Neither of these events of the composite end point occurred in the 38 children who continued to receive transfusions. The average of the last two transcranial Doppler results before transfusion was started was the only predictor of the composite end point (P=0.05).

Conclusions.—Discontinuation of transfusion for the prevention of stroke in children with sickle cell disease results in a high rate of reversion to abnormal blood-flow velocities on Doppler studies and stroke (Fig 2).

▶ Clearly, we have come a long way in understanding why children with sickle cell disease develop strokes. When I was a resident at the Children's Hospital of Philadelphia, a 9-year-old was admitted to service with a stroke. He had sickle cell disease. The resident group, as naive as we were, asked ourselves the question, why would sickle cell disease cause someone to have a stroke? Previously, the teaching had been that sickle blood forms occlude small blood vessels, which then causes painful crises, splenic infarctions, and other conditions. We asked ourselves, if that were the pathophysiology in the brain of patients with sickle cell anemia, why would they be presenting with classic strokes in the form of hemiplegia, which sounded more like large blood vessel occlusive disease. This was back in 1970 when no one had actually performed a cerebral angiogram on a patient with sickle cell disease for fear that the high osmolar contrast material used in cerebral angiography might cause even greater sickling. With the support of the hematology division and the neuroradiology department at the University of Pennsylvania, we performed exchange transfusion on a number of patients with sickle cell anemia who had previously experienced strokes so that cerebral angiography could be safely performed and found that these patients had major blood vessel occlusive disease. This finding ultimately led others to the conclusion that patients with sickle cell anemia who had previously experienced strokes should begin maintenance transfusion programs, which essentially eliminated the recurrence of stroke. Not only did transfusion programs prevent a recurrence of strokes but they also seemed to improve the actual anatomy of the diseased cerebral blood vessels.

We now know why patients with sickle cell disease have strokes. The blood vessels of these patients show evidence of proliferative intimal hyperplasia, reminiscent of the inflammatory vascular lesions so commonly seen in other disorders. The genesis of these lesions most likely relates to the well-described tendency of sickle cells to adhere to, activate, and damage endothelial cells. Sticky oxidant-generating sickle cells attach to vascular endothelial cells in the turbulent environment of the carotid artery circulation. This results in activation and damage of the endothelial cell, which stimulates these endothelial cells and white cells to produce inflammatory cytokines, chemoattractants, adhesion molecules, procoagulants, and growth factors. White blood cells and platelets then adhere, amplifying the overall process. Over time and with sufficient stimulation, smooth muscle cells in the blood vessel migrate into the wall, proliferate, and, ultimately, narrow the arterial lumen. Transcranial Doppler US can detect these lesions if they are large enough. The coup de grace, a stroke (occurring when the tipping point is reached in the delicate relationship between oxygenation and perfusion, on the one hand, and inflammation and coagulation, on the other), happens when deoxygenated red cells containing sickle hemoglobin get caught up in the damaged vessel and obstruct blood flow.

Previous studies[1] have shown that if children with stenotic extracranial and intracranial lesions (as demonstrated by transcranial Doppler US) undergo a regular program of transfusion that is designed to suppress erythropoiesis so that no more than 30% of their circulating red cells are sickle cells, then about 90% of strokes in such children will be prevented. As we see in the current article, this high risk of a stroke returns if one discontinues a transfusion program. Not only does transfusion simply prevent a stroke but it also reverses the stenotic lesion. Blood vessels can, given sufficient time and protection, repair themselves. Unfortunately, this protection probably needs to be forever. Long-term transfusion programs are not without their risks, but the risk–benefit ratio in terms of prevention of a stroke clearly favors continuation.

J. A. Stockman III, MD

Reference

1. Adams RJ, McKie VC, Shu L, et al: Prevention of a first stroke by transfusions in children with sickle cell anemia and abnormal results on transcranial Doppler ultrasonography. *N Engl J Med* 339:5-11, 1998.

Dysregulated Arginine Metabolism, Hemolysis-Associated Pulmonary Hypertension, and Mortality in Sickle Cell Disease

Morris CR, Kato GJ, Poljakovic M, et al (Children's Hosp & Research Ctr at Oakland, Calif; Natl Institutes of Health, Bethesda, Md; Univ of Pittsburgh School of Medicine, Pa; et al)
JAMA 294:81-90, 2005   3–8

Context.—Sickle cell disease is characterized by a state of nitric oxide resistance and limited bioavailability of L-arginine, the substrate for nitric oxide synthesis. We hypothesized that increased arginase activity and dysregulated arginine metabolism contribute to endothelial dysfunction, pulmonary hypertension, and patient outcomes.

Objective.—To explore the role of arginase in sickle cell disease pathogenesis, pulmonary hypertension, and mortality.

Design.—Plasma amino acid levels, plasma and erythrocyte arginase activities, and pulmonary hypertension status as measured by Doppler echocardiogram were prospectively obtained in outpatients with sickle cell disease. Patients were followed up for survival up to 49 months.

Setting.—Urban tertiary care center and community clinics in the United States between February 2001 and March 2005.

Participants.—Two hundred twenty-eight patients with sickle cell disease, aged 18 to 74 years, and 36 control participants.

Main Outcome Measures.—Plasma amino acid levels, plasma and erythrocyte arginase activities, diagnosis of pulmonary hypertension, and mortality.

Results.—Plasma arginase activity was significantly elevated in patients with sickle cell disease, with highest activity found in patients with secondary pulmonary hypertension. Arginase activity correlated with the arginine-ornithine ratio, and lower ratios were associated with greater severity of pulmonary hypertension and with mortality in this population (risk ratio, 2.5; 95% confidence interval [CI], 1.2-5.2; $P = .006$). Global arginine bioavailability, characterized by the ratio of arginine to ornithine plus citrulline, was also strongly associated with mortality (risk ratio, 3.6; 95% CI, 1.5-8.3; $P<.001$). Increased plasma arginase activity was correlated with increased intravascular hemolytic rate and, to a lesser extent, with markers of inflammation and soluble adhesion molecule levels.

Conclusions.—These data support a novel mechanism of disease in which hemolysis contributes to reduced nitric oxide bioavailability and endothelial dysfunction via release of erythrocyte arginase, which limits arginine bioavailability, and release of erythrocyte hemoglobin, which scavenges nitric oxide. The ratios of arginine to ornithine and arginine to ornithine plus citrulline are independently associated with pulmonary hypertension and increased mortality in patients with sickle cell disease.

▶ The more we learn about the pathophysiology of sickle cell anemia, the more we learn how complicated that pathophysiology is. The story is much more complicated than deoxygenation causing sickling causing blood vessel obstruction. The previous article (see Abstract 3–7) showed us how sickle cells, through a complex mechanism, stick to vascular endothelial cells, which initiates a process of blood vessel wall damage, particularly in certain blood vessels, including cranial arteries. The current article expands our knowledge of sickle cell disease pathophysiology by looking at the mechanism of hemolysis-associated pulmonary hypertension, a common problem in youngsters and adults with sickle cell anemia. We learn that L-arginine, the substrate for nitric oxide (NO) synthesis, is deficient in sickle cell disease. Increased NO consumption by free plasma hemoglobin and reactive oxygen species leads to decreased NO bioavailability that is exacerbated by decreased availability of the NO synthase substrate L-arginine. This reduced NO bioavailability enhances oxidative stress, which is further complicated by the elevated arginase activity found in patients with sickle cell disease. Arginase is an enzyme that degrades NO.

The authors of this article theorize that because endothelial dysfunction may contribute to the pathogenesis of pulmonary hypertension through impaired production, bioavailability, and responsiveness of NO, elevated arginase activity and dysregulated arginine metabolism might contribute to the endothelial dysfunction syndrome that occurs in the lungs of patients with sickle cell disease. Indeed, they found that plasma arginase activity was significantly elevated in patients with sickle cell disease, and the highest activity was found in patients with secondary pulmonary hypertension.

So what does all this mean? It likely means that elevated plasma arginase activity in sickle cell disease is the prime mechanism of disease that links oxidative stress, chronic organ damage, and hemolysis to endothelial dysfunction and pulmonary hypertension. This enzyme is normally contained only within cells and appears in the plasma only after cell damage or death. Thus, inflammation, chronic end organ damage, and hemolysis are all potential sources of the elevated arginase activity seen in sickle cell disease. The abnormalities found in this study are clearly associated with pulmonary hypertension and the prospective risk of death in patients with sickle cell disease. One can measure arginine and the enzyme in question as well as other metabolites, and one can calculate a ratio of these substances. This just may provide clinicians with an objective index of disease severity and may help identify patients at exceptional risk of pulmonary complications of sickle cell disease. Patients at high risk could begin transfusion programs to intervene in the pathophysiology described, perhaps preventing the occurrence of a life-threatening complication of sickle cell disease.

J. A. Stockman III, MD

Identification of Unrelated Cord Blood Units for Hematopoietic Stem Cell Transplantation in Children With Sickle Cell Disease
Adamkiewicz TV, Boyer MW, Bray R, et al (Emory Univ, Atlanta, Ga; Columbus Children's Hosp, Ohio; Arizona Cancer Ctr, Tucson)
J Pediatr Hematol Oncol 28:29-32, 2006   3–9

Summary.—This study examined the theoretical availability of compatible unrelated umbilical cord blood (UCB) units for hematopoietic stem cell transplantation (HSCT) of children with sickle cell disease (SCD), matched for DRB1 at high resolution. UCB units registered via Bone Marrow Donors Worldwide were matched with patients who had been previously typed for possible HSCT. Suitable matching was determined after typing at antigen level at A and B loci and allele-level typing at DRB1. Forty patients met criteria for analysis. All matched at four of six loci with at least two UCB units, and 50% (n = 20) matched at five of six loci with at least one unit. In patients matched at four loci or more, significantly more units per patient (median 19 vs. 2 units; $P = 0.03$) at higher cell dose (median 205 vs. 113 best nucleated cell dose per unit; $P < 0.01$) were identified compared with patients matched at five loci or more. Hypothetically, at a dose of at least 5×10^7 nucleated cells/kg, 54% of patients weighing 40 kg would match with units at four or more of six loci and 5% at five or more of six loci. This study suggests that cord blood units matching at four or more of six HLA loci at acceptable cell doses can be identified for a majority of children with SCD weighing 40 kg or less. Availability of units matched at five or more of six HLA loci was more limited. Defining procedure-related risks and benefits remains a challenge.

▶ It is clear that some children with SCD should be considered for stem cell transplantation to cure their disease. Such transplantation is not without its risks (mortality rate, 10%-20%), but it is a treatment well worth thinking about. The treatment option, however, is available to less than 20% of children with SCD because of a lack of donors. This raises the question about the availability of publicly banked unrelated UCB units that are able to be matched to children with SCD. This report provides us with the needed information.

The report by Adamkiewicz et al gives us an important update by demonstrating that UCB units are likely to be available for the majority of patients with SCD. Somewhere between 54% and 100% of patients weighing 10 to 40 kg will match with 1 or more UCB units at 4 or more HLA loci. As many as 40% of patients will match with 1 or more UCB units at 5 or more HLA loci. Currently, the minimum acceptable criteria for the use of a cord blood transplant is considered to be a match in at least 4 HLA loci, assuming an adequate number of cells in the donor unit.

UCB is now an alternative to bone marrow as a source of hematopoietic stem cells, and UCB transplantation is a potentially important therapy for use in SCD. Ready availability, lack of donor attrition, and a lower incidence of severe graft-versus-host disease make UCB transplantation an attractive alternative to bone marrow transplantation. Indeed, there have been several reports of the successful use of UCB as the stem cell source for patients undergoing transplantation for hemoglobinopathies. Among 44 patients who received UCB as the source of transplanted stem cells from an HLA-identical sibling for either thalassemia or sickle cell anemia, the 2-year probability of event-free survival was 79% and 90%, respectively.[1]

Having an UCB transplantation is not a cakewalk. With a chance of dying in the first year or two running as high as 20%, one must consider carefully the benefits of such a transplantation. Recognize, however, that between 5% and 10% of untransplanted patients with SCD will not survive to 18 years of age, and half will die before 40 to 50 years of age. One must choose carefully the patients who will benefit the most from this risky procedure, but at the same time we should not shy away from using the therapeutic modality that can best serve the patient over the long haul.

J. A. Stockman III, MD

Reference

1. Locatelli F, Rocha V, Reed W, et al: Related UCB transplantation in patients with thalassemia and SCD. *Blood* 101:2137-2143, 2003.

Leukocyte Aggregation-related Pseudoleukopenia in Pediatrics: A Sporadic Event or a Systematic Error?

Urbach J, Rogowski O, Branski D, et al (Hadassah Univ, Jerusalem; Tel Aviv Univ, Israel)

Pediatr Infect Dis J 24:717-720, 2005   3–10

Objective.—To determine whether electronic counter-related pseudoleukopenia is a rare phenomenon or a systematic underestimation in children with acute infection/inflammation.

Methods.—We have used a simple slide test and image analysis to reveal the number of white blood cells and their degree of aggregation. The number of leukocytes counted by an electronic cell analyzer was divided by the number of cells counted on the slides creating an electronic cell-to-slide leukocyte count ratio.

Results.—A significant ($P < 0.0005$) negative ($r = -0.314$) correlation between the above mentioned ratios and the percent of aggregated leukocytes in the peripheral blood was found in a group of 239 children with various acute infections. Thus elevated leukocyte aggregation is associated with a relatively lower electronic analyzer cell count.

Conclusions.—The appearance of aggregated leukocytes in the peripheral blood during acute infections might be associated with pseudoleukopenia. This phenomenon has been extensively described in the adult population and seems to exist in children as well.

▶ It has been known for some time that adults frequently manifest pseudoleukopenia particularly in the situation in which inflammation or acute infection is present. Pseudoleukopenia is an artifact of electronic counting equipment technology. For whatever reason, in the presence of acute infection or inflammation, some individuals will experience a high degree of leukocyte aggregation. When several white cells stuck together go through electronic counting equipment, they are counted as 1 cell, artifactually decreasing what might have otherwise been a significantly increased white count. Although well documented in adults, the occurrence of pseudoleukopenia in children has been infrequently studied, except by the authors of this report. They, for example, have evaluated the subject of electronic counter underestimation of white blood cell counts in a group of patients after the IV administration of high-dose immunoglobulins. This resulted in an almost 25% artifactual decrease in the white blood cell count.[1] In another study, these investigators found that about one third of patients with nonviral acute febrile illnesses had a normal electronic counter-based white blood cell count, despite obvious evidence of inflammation as judged by fever, C-reactive protein, fibrinogen concentrations, and erythrocyte sedimentation rates, again suggesting the possibility that the "normal" white blood cell count may have been due to a pseudoleukopenia.[2]

This study by Urbach et al is the first to study the subject of pseudoleukopenia in pediatrics in an organized way. The investigators studied the ratio of electronic counter leukocyte counts divided by the directly visualized count showing that the ratio is hardly 1 in all patients with active infection. In addition, they were able to visualize leukocyte adhesion by a technique that they developed. Their leukocyte adhesiveness or aggregation test actually turns out to be a nonspecific marker of infection, correlating significantly with markers of the acute phase response, including fibrinogen, erythrocyte sedimentation rate, and the concentration of C-reactive protein. Most likely, leukocyte adhesion results from the presence of bridging molecules like fibrinogen.

If there is a bottom line to the implications of this report, it is that we should not always believe a normal white blood cell count in the presence of inflammation. Pseudoleukopenia is a real phenomenon in children. What we need, however, is to know whether a patient does, in fact, manifest evidence of white cell aggregation that might artifactually decrease the white blood cell count. Interestingly, this phenomenon has been studied with red blood cells. For example, if a patient has a *Mycoplasma pneumoniae* infection and an increased titer of cold agglutinins, macroagglutination of red blood cells may be seen. This causes a spuriously low red blood cell count as reported with electronic counting equipment. What it also does, however, is to spuriously increase the red blood cell mean corpuscular volume (MCV). One knows that there is a spurious decrease in the red cell count simply by looking at the MCV and seeing that it is much too high to be explained by anything other than an artifact. It would be extremely helpful if some investigator were to study a similar correlation between the white blood cell count and the white blood cell size. Electronic counting equipment is capable of measuring white blood cell size as it does with red blood cells and platelets. Someone, please, do a study of white blood cell size as an indicator of pseudoleukopenia.

See the Infectious Disease chapter for a report on the significance of extreme leukocytosis in the evaluation of febrile children. This report will convince you that it is important to know how accurate your white blood cell counts are.

J. A. Stockman III, MD

References

1. Zeltser D, Fusman R, Chapman Y, et al: Increased leukocyte aggregation induced by gamma globulin: A clue to the presence of pseudoleukopenia. *Am J Med Sci* 320:177-182, 2000.
2. Mahrashak N, Kassirer M, Zeltser D, et al: The inflammation meter: Novel technology to detect the presence of inflammation/infection in patients without leukocytosis but with increased leukocyte adhesiveness/aggregation. *Acta Haematol* 104:16-21, 2000.

Prospective Phase 1/2 Study of Rituximab in Childhood and Adolescent Chronic Immune Thrombocytopenic Purpura

Neufeld EJ, for the Pediatric Rituximab/ITP Study Group and the Glaser Pediatric Research Network (Harvard Med School, Boston; et al)

Blood 107:2639-2642, 2006   3–11

We assessed safety and efficacy of rituximab in a prospective study of 36 patients, age 2.6 to 18.3 years, with severe chronic immune thrombocytopenic purpura (ITP). The primary outcome of sustained platelets above 50×10^9/L (50 000/mm^3) during 4 consecutive weeks, starting in weeks 9 to 12, was achieved by 11 of 36 patients (31%, confidence interval [CI], 16% to 48%). Median response time was 1 week (range, 1 to 7 weeks). Attainment of the primary outcome was not associated with age, prior pharmacologic responses, prior splenectomy, ITP duration, screening platelet count, refractoriness, or IgM reduction. First-dose, infusion-related toxicity was common (47%) despite premedication. Significant drug-related toxicities included third-dose hypotension (n = 1) and serum sickness (n = 2). Peripheral B cells were depleted in all subjects. IgM decreased 3.4% per week, but IgG did not significantly decrease. Rituximab was well tolerated, with manageable infusion-related side effects, but 6% of subjects developed serum sickness. Rituximab is beneficial for some pediatric patients with severe, chronic ITP.

▶ Most patients with ITP require no therapy. When there is a decision to use therapy, the usual ones include steroids, IV immunoglobulin, anti-D immune globulin, or splenectomy. These therapies are generally reserved for children with chronic ITP. Splenectomy, while usually effective, carries with it the risk of infection. Therefore, it is infrequently used as part of the current therapeutic armamentarium. Unfortunately, some children with chronic ITP do not respond to any traditional therapy, and their platelet count is low enough to be of some danger to them. This is where monoclonal antibody therapy comes into play.

Rituximab is a monoclonal antibody directed against the CD20 antigen expressed on pre-B and mature B lymphocytes that is approved for use in the treatment of B-cell lymphoma. Rituximab rapidly eliminates most circulating B cells, with subsequent recovery of B-cell counts some 6 to 12 months after the initiation of therapy. Such a reduction of B cells may be effective in the treatment of a variety of autoimmune diseases including ITP. The study by Neufeld et al is the first report of rituximab therapy that is widely comprehensive in the information provided. A response rate of 31% (defined by producing a sustained platelet count above 50,000/mm^3) was observed. The median response time was just 1 week. This response rate is somewhat lower than previously reported in both adult and pediatric patients with severe chronic ITP. In a retrospective study of rituximab therapy in children with severe chronic ITP, 63% of 24 patients achieved a stable platelet count (more than 150,000/mm^3) without additional therapy.[1]

There seems to be no uniform way in which hematologists use rituximab. Some use it always before splenectomy, to exactly the opposite. Approaches are largely based on the high cost and variable reimbursement for this therapy, uncertain long-term effects, and the feeling on the part of patients about the pros and cons of splenectomy in terms of the risk of subsequent infection. There are insufficient data to conclude that rituximab is preferable to splenectomy in younger patients, but chances are this is the way it will be used.

Please do not think that treatment with monoclonal antibody is free of problems. As we see in this report, there is an extraordinarily high rate of first infusion–related complications in terms of serum sickness–type illness. We also do not know anything about the durability of the response to rituximab over the long haul. Last, neither the optimal dose, frequency of administration, nor duration of treatment has been thoroughly delineated for children.

Despite all the caveats about rituximab as part of the management of ITP in children, it is good to see that we do have, what some would otherwise consider, a last-ditch agent that does salvage a substantial proportion of children with a chronic life-threatening illness.

J. A. Stockman III, MD

Reference

1. Wang J, Wiley JM, Luddy R, et al: Chronic immune thrombocytopenic purpura in children: Assessment of rituximab treatment. *J Pediatr* 146:217-221, 2005.

Oral Contraceptives and DDAVP Nasal Spray: Patterns of Use in Managing vWD-associated Menorrhagia: A Single-Institution Study
Amesse LS, Pfaff-Amesse T, Leonardi R, et al (Wright State Univ, Dayton, Ohio)
J Pediatr Hematol Oncol 27:357-363, 2005   3–12

Summary.—The purpose of this study was to examine patterns of use for oral contraceptive and desmopressin acetate nasal spray, both used in managing menorrhagia in adolescents with von Willebrand disease (vWD). Hospital records of adolescents with documented vWD and menorrhagia were reviewed retrospectively. Subjects with vWD type 1 (n = 36) administered either oral contraceptives (OC) or intranasal desmopressin acetate (DDAVP) and followed from 6 months to 4 years were selected for inclusion. Treatment outcomes were examined with respect to effectiveness and safety. Assessing menstrual blood loss using PBAC scores from pretreatment and treatment periods determined effectiveness. Safety was evaluated by monitoring reported adverse events. No significant differences were identified in treatment effectiveness for controlling menorrhagia in vWD adolescents in the OC and intranasal DDAVP group comparisons: 86% versus 77% ($P > 0.05$), respectively. When combining both treatment groups, the majority of vWD adolescents, 81% ($P > 0.05$), experienced alleviation of menorrhagia symptoms. Treatment failures were attributed to either the inability of a regimen to control bleeding or to adverse events, including severe headaches and flushing with DDAVP. Safety outcomes were not significantly greater in vWD patients with menorrhagia when OC were compared with intranasal DDAVP. Both medical approaches, OC and DDAVP nasal spray, used in managing menorrhagia in adolescents with documented type I vWD were well tolerated and showed equivalent effectiveness, and no serious adverse events were reported.

► Anyone who has cared for a teenage girl with vWD knows how problematic the menstrual cycle can be for these young ladies. vWD-associated menorrhagia is a significant and sometimes serious problem. When one considers that somewhere between 1% and 3% of the American population has vWD, you can see the magnitude of the problem, actually first described by Dr von Willebrand himself back in 1926. In detail, he wrote about a young adolescent with his disease who presented with menorrhagia and who subsequently died after her fourth menses at age 13 years.[1]

We have learned much about its inheritance, presentation, and management in the three quarters of a century since Dr von Willebrand described his disease. vWD is usually an inherited genetic defect, although acquired mutations account for some cases. Types 1 and 2 are most often inherited in an autosomal dominant pattern with variable penetrance, whereas type 3 is characteristically transmitted as an autosomal recessive. Type 1 is the most common, representing 70% of all vWD cases and exhibits the mildest symptoms. Type 3 is the least common and the most severe. The bleeding manifestations in vWD are quite variable and inconsistent and display significant phenotypic heterogeneity such that no single distinguishing symptom defines the disease. The clinical symptoms can encompass various types of mucocutaneous hemorrhage, including nose bleeds, gum bleeds, gastrointestinal and genitourinary bleeding, easy bruisability, menorrhagia, and/or excessive bleeding at the time of dental procedures, child birth, or surgery. Indeed, many cases of vWD are not detected until a patient undergoes surgery or experiences an episode of trauma.

Exactly what causes the clotting defect in vWD remains a complex issue. Either qualitative or quantitative abnormalities of the multimeric glycoprotein vWD factor can be involved, depending on the type of vWD. This factor is synthesized predominantly by endothelial cells and megakaryocytes and functions as both a carrier protein and a stabilizing factor for the clotting factor VIII in the coagulation cascade. vWD factor also supports platelet adhesion and aggregation at the site of vascular injury during thrombus formation. In normal people during menstruation, endometrial glands and stroma are shed into the endometrial cavity while intravascular fibrin-platelet plugs form, facilitating hemostasis. In subjects with vWD, there is insufficient microvascular thrombosis, and coagulation and menorrhagia results.

Without question, most teens will have menorrhagia for reasons unrelated to vWD. However, statistics show that approximately 15% of young women diagnosed with menorrhagia are likely to have vWD. For some reason, this remains a little-known statistic since a survey reported 4 years ago indicated that only 16.5% of gynecologists—the specialists most commonly seen by women for menorrhagia—consider vWD in the differential diagnosis of menorrhagia in the young adolescent.[2] Thus, it is up to the primary care provider to, more often than not, think of vWD in teens observed with menorrhagia.

If you make a diagnosis of vWD as a cause of menorrhagia, be aware that there is no uniform consensus regarding the most efficacious form of therapy. Two different medical approaches are usually used in adolescents: OCs and the administration of intranasal DDAVP. Some patients with vWD are unresponsive to DDAVP. In others, OCs are ineffective. In these cases, less commonly used is antihemophilic factor/vWD complex and aminocaproic acid.

In this report by Amesse et al, we see just how effective DDAVP and OCs are in the management of all individuals with vWD type 1. Both forms of therapy seem to be comparable, with success rates running about 80%. Some treatment failures were related to adverse drug effects, such as severe headaches and flushing, with DDAVP.

It should be noted that DDAVP is not effective for vWD type 3. Also, in the rare subtype of vWD type 2b and the platelet-type, pseudo-vWD, administration of DDAVP may actually result in thrombocytopenia. For this reason, DDAVP should be used in subjects with vWD only when the molecular nature of their disorder has been adequately evaluated by a hematology team.

See the report which follows (Abstract 3–13) that warns us about DDAVP-induced hyponatremia in young children who are treated with this drug as part of the management of vWD.

J.A. Stockman III, MD

References

1. Nielsson IM: von Willebrand's disease: 50 years old. *Acta Med Scand* 201:497-508, 1977.
2. Dilley A, Drews C, Lally C, et al: A survey of gynecologists concerning menorrhagia: Perceptions of bleeding disorders as a possible cause. *J Women's Health Gend Based Med* 11:39-44, 2002.

DDAVP-Induced Hyponatremia in Young Children

Das P, Carcao M, Hitzler J (Univ of Toronto)
J Pediatr Hematol Oncol 27:330-332, 2005

3–13

Background.—Desmopressin (DDAVP) is used to improve hemostasis in patients with bleeding disorders. The side effects of DDAVP in adults and children are benign. However, there has been concern regarding the development of hyponatremia and seizures after DDAVP administration in young children. Three cases were presented in which hyponatremia (and in 2 cases, seizures) developed in children under 3 years of age after IV DDAVP administration.

Case 1.—Boy, 17 months, (weight, 10 kg) with mild hemophilia A underwent a DDAVP challenge test to assess responsiveness to DDAVP 1 month before an elective placement of myringotomy tubes. The FVIII:C levels 1 hour and 4 hours after administration of IV DDAVP (0.3 µg/kg) were 0.35 U/mL and 0.22 U/mL, respectively.

The patient was sent home. The parents noted that he was irritable and gave him frequent bottles of milk to settle him. The child began vomiting 8 hours after the administration of DDAVP, and at 16 hours post administration he experienced a brief generalized tonic-clonic seizure. He was rushed to the hospital where his serum sodium level was determined to be 123 mmol/L. The boy was treated with a combination of fluid restriction and IV saline solution. He had no additional seizures.

Case 2.—Boy, 2.7 years, (weight, 14 kg) with a diagnosis of a nonspecific platelet dysfunction was admitted for elective bilateral laparoscopic orchidopexy. The boy's serum sodium level was 144 mmol/L before surgery. He received 0.3 µg/kg DDAVP IV before the start of the procedure and achieved good hemostasis. A brief period of hypotension and tachycardia was treated with a 2/3-1/3 solution of dextrose with saline and an intraoperative bolus infusion of Ringer's lactate.

Postoperatively, the patient was placed on 5% dextrose with 0.45% saline at a rate equivalent to 150% maintenance fluid requirement. In the 24 hours after surgery, the patient was permitted unrestricted oral fluids. At 25 hours after administration of DDAVP, a generalized tonic-clonic seizure developed. It was treated with IV lorazepam and phenobarbital. The patient was treated with an infusion of hypertonic (3%) saline solution and fluid restriction. No further seizures occurred and the serum sodium level returned to normal over the subsequent 12 hours.

Case 3.—Girl, 13 months, (weight, 10.4 kg) with type I von Willebrand disease was admitted for excision of a dermoid cyst. A prior DDAVP challenge test had shown an excellent response to DDAVP. Preoperatively, the girl received 0.3 µg/kg of IV DDAVP when the serum sodium level was 140 mmol/L. Perioperatively, she received Ringer's lactate at 90% maintenance rate for 2.5 hours. After surgery she was placed on a 2/3-1/3 solution equivalent to 100% maintenance fluids requirement. Her serum sodium level at 8 hours after surgery was 133 mmol/L. She then drank a total of 520 mL of a combination of sugar water and a soy-based formula.

The child became irritable and agitated approximately 14 hours after the administration of DDAVP. Her serum sodium level at this time was measured at 126 mmol/L. She was treated with fluid restriction and IV infusion of hypertonic (3%) saline and was transferred to the ICU because of marked irritability and agitation. With additional infusion of normal saline and fluid restriction, her serum sodium level normalized at 23 hours after DDAVP administration, and she was no longer irritable.

Conclusion.—The reasons why young children are particularly predisposed to hyponatremia after administration of DDAVP have not been determined. It is likely that the increased risk of hyponatremia is related to the small size and large fluid intake in relation to total plasma volume, compared with adults. Fluid restriction, avoidance of hypo-osmolar fluid, and close monitoring of fluid and electrolytes for 12 to 24 hours after DDAVP administration is recommended for children younger than 3 years of age.

▶ It was some 30 years ago that Mannucci et al first prescribed the use of DDAVP to improve clotting in patients with bleeding disorders.[1] In the interim 30 years, DDAVP has been successfully used to manage subjects with mild hemophilia and patients with von Willebrand disease. It has also been successful in the management of bleeding in certain patients with congenital platelet function disorders. The drug releases preformed factor VIII/von Willebrand disease factor complex from endothelial tissues into plasma. It also is thought to increase platelet adhesion and aggregation while leading also to the release of tissue plasminogen activator.

The effect of DDAVP is somewhat temporary, with benefits lasting 12 to 24 hours, but this is usually a period of time that is all that is necessary to control most bleeding in most patients. Unlike the administration of clotting factors, there are very few complications associated with DDAVP, except for mild and transient facial flushing, headache, tachycardia, and (in a few patients) hypotension. The most significant complication of DDAVP, however, is the development of hyponatremia, which can lead to seizures and even death.

The report abstracted reminds us that we cannot use DDAVP cavalierly for any disorder for which we give it. Two youngsters are presented who were given DDAVP prior to minor surgical procedures. Both youngsters developed seizures in the hours after drug administration. A third child developed significant hyponatremia associated with irritability and agitation. She, fortunately, did not develop seizures.

For some reason, young children appear to be particularly susceptible to the hyponatremic effects of DDAVP. If DDAVP is administered to control or prevent bleeding, careful attention must be made to not allow excess fluids to be given. The authors who reported these 3 children make a series of recommendations that all of us should follow when administering DDAVP IV to children under the age of 3. These recommendations are as follows:

1. Normal saline is the IV fluid of choice. Hypotonic IV fluids (eg, 2/3-1/3, 5% dextrose/0.45 normal saline) should not be used during the first 24 hours after the administration of DDAVP.
2. Total fluid intake should be restricted to 75% of maintenance requirements in the 24 hours following the administration of DDAVP.
3. Large amounts of hypo-osmolar oral fluids should not be given during the first 24 hours following the administration of DDAVP.
4. The patient's fluid balance should be monitored closely for 24 hours following the administration of DDAVP.
5. Serum sodium and osmolality should be measured and monitored prior to

and every 6 hours for 24 hours following the administration of DDAVP, preferably in an inpatient setting.

See the Genitourinary chapter for a study reporting the frequency of DDAVP-associated symptomatic hyponatremia when used for such common problems as nocturnal enuresis.[2]

J. A. Stockman III, MD

References

1. Mannucci PM, Ruggeri ZM, Pareti FI, et al: DDAVP: A new pharmacological approach to the management of hemophilia and von Willebrand disease. *Lancet* 1:869-872, 1977.
2. Thumfart J, Roehr C-C, Kapelari K, et al: Desmopressin associated symptomatic hyponatremic hypovolemia in children. Are there predictive factors? *J Urol* 174:294-298, 2005.

Activation of Coagulation System During Air Travel: A Crossover Study
Schreijer AJM, Cannegieter SC, Meijers JCM, et al (Academic Med Ctr, Amsterdam; Leiden Univ Med Ctr, The Netherlands)
Lancet 367:832-838, 2006   3–14

Background.—There is an increased risk of venous thrombosis after air travel, but the underlying mechanism is unclear. Our aim was to ascertain whether flying leads to a hypercoagulable state.

Methods.—We did a crossover study in 71 healthy volunteers (15 men, 56 women), in whom we measured markers of activation of coagulation and fibrinolysis before, during, and after an 8-h flight. The same individuals participated in two control exposure situations (8-h movie marathon and daily life) to separate the effect of air travel on the coagulation system from those of immobilisation and circadian rhythm. To study the effect of risk factors for thrombosis, we included participants with the factor V Leiden mutation (n=11), those who took oral contraceptives (n=15), or both (n=15), as well as 30 individuals with no specific risk factors.

Findings.—After the flight, median concentrations of thrombin-antithrombin (TAT) complex increased by 30.1% (95% CI 11.2-63.2), but decreased by 2.1% (−11.2 to 14) after the cinema and by 7.9% (−16.2 to −1.2) after the daily life situation. We recorded a high response in TAT levels in 17% (11 of 66) of individuals after air travel (3% [2 of 68] for movie marathon; 1% [1 of 70] in daily life). These findings were most evident in the group with the factor V Leiden mutation who used oral contraceptives. We noted a high response in all variables (prothrombin fragment 1 and 2, TAT, and D-dimer) in four of 63 (6.3%) volunteers after the flight, but in no-one after either of the control situations (Table 3).

Interpretation.—Activation of coagulation occurs in some individuals after an 8-h flight, indicating an additional mechanism to immobilisation underlying air travel related thrombosis.

TABLE 3.—Proportion of High-Responders per Exposure, for Whole Group and by Number of Risk Factors (Oral Contraceptive Use, Factor V Leiden Mutation, or Both)

	High Responders (Total Number [%, 95% CI])	0 Risk Factors (Number, %)	1 Risk Factor (Number, %)	2 Risk Factors (Number, %)
TAT				
Flight	11/66 (17%, 8·6-27·9)	3/29 (10%)	2/23 (9%)	6/14 (43%)
Cinema	2/68 (3%, 0·4-10·2)	0/28	1/25 (4%)	1/15 (7%)
Daily life	1/70 (1%, 0·0-7·7)	0/29	0/26	1/15 (7%)
TAT and F1 + 2				
Flight	6/66 (9%, 3·4-18·7)	2/29 (7%)	2/23 (9%)	2/14 (14%)
Cinema	1/68 (2%, 0·0-7·9)	0/28	0/25	1/15 (7%)
Daily life	0/70 (0%, 0·0-5·1)	0/29	0/26	0/15
TAT, F1 + 2, and D-dimer				
Flight	4/63 (6%, 1·8-15·5)	2/29 (7%)	1/23 (4%)	1/14 (7%)
Cinema	0/68 (0%, 0·0-5·3)	0/28	0/25	0/15
Daily life	0/70 (0%, 0·0-5·1)	0/29	0/26	0/15

Proportions of high responders tested by χ^2 without continuity correction of Fisher's exact test when there were cells with 5 or less counts. Proportion of high responders after flight compared with daily life: TAT (p=0.002), TAT and F1 + 2 (p=0.01), TAT and F1 + 2 and D-dimer (p=0.048). Within response to flight, proportion of high responders with 2 *vs* 0 risk factors: TAT (p=0.04), TAT and F1 + 2 (p=0.58), TAT and F1 + 2 and D-dimer (p=1.0)

(Courtesy of Schreijer AJM, Cannegieter SC, Meijers JCM, et al: Activation of coagulation system during air travel: A cross-over study. *Lancet* 367:832-838, 2006. Reprinted with permission from Elsevier.)

▶ This report looks at activation of the coagulation system during air travel. While the study was done in adult men and women, the data should equally apply to the older end of the pediatric population as well, a population, particularly for those who are on oral contraceptives, that is of some relevance when it comes to excess clotting.

It has been known for some time that those who sit still have a higher risk of developing venous thrombosis. Venous thrombosis was first linked to air travel back in 1954. The report in the *Lancet* adds important new information to the mosaic of travel-induced thrombosis. The Dutch group compared the concentrations of markers of coagulation activation in blood samples of healthy volunteers drawn before, during, and immediately after an 8-hour flight, with those taken at the same time points during 8 hours of immobilization in a movie theater and during normal daily activities. By doing so, the conditions of immobilization and hypobaric hypoxia in flight could be disentangled from immobilization alone (spending a long day in a movie theater) and also be controlled for daily activities. By including almost 40% of participants with the factor V Leiden mutation and women on oral contraceptives, it was also possible for the Dutch investigators to assess the effect of these risk factors on the coagulation system.

The results of this study showed increased concentrations of clotting markers during flight compared with the other 2 situations, especially in volunteers with genetic disorders such as factor V Leiden or in those on oral contraceptives. It was clear that immobilization during air travel was somewhat different in its clotting effects than was immobilization resulting from sitting in a movie theater. Altitude, therefore, does make a difference.

In the study by Schreijer et al, most of the individuals showed downregulation, during immobilization, of prothrombin fragments 1 + 2, which parallels thrombin formation. However, in some susceptible individuals, possibly after an initial decrease of thrombin generation, the protein C system became overrun and thrombin formation was enhanced, leading to a rise in thrombin markers.

Previous commentaries in the YEAR BOOK OF PEDIATRICS have noted how to prevent, or at least decrease, the risk of air flight–associated thrombosis. Intermittent calf contraction might improve blood return and reduce venous stasis. Excessive sedation caused by alcohol or sedative drugs favors immobility and thus venous stasis and should be avoided. Compressive stockings further improve venous return and reduce the incidence of thrombosis. Although aspirin use for 3 days before flying has not been shown to be effective, single-dose, weight-adjusted, low-molecular-weight heparin does reduce flight-associated thrombosis in those at special risk. It is not recommended for routine use since deep venous thrombosis is estimated to occur in less than 4% of individuals after long-haul flights, and fatal pulmonary embolism is in fact rare, with an estimated death rate of just 1 per 2 million passengers on international flights terminating in Australia. Those at particular risk are individuals with a history of prior thrombosis, active cancer, recent surgery of any type, and minor surgery of the lower extremities. The study of Schreijer et al shows us that women on oral contraceptives and individuals with a mutation of factor V Leiden should be offered the possibility of extended prophylactic measures, including low-molecular-weight heparin or compressive stockings.

One concluding, unrelated comment having to do with clotting, if you are a coagulationist, you probably think everything is due to a clotting disorder, even the death of Jesus by crucifixion. Then again, was this a possible mechanism of Jesus' death? A letter to the editor in the *Journal of Thrombosis and Haemostasis* and further letters[1-3] does, in fact, suggest that Jesus' Jewish heritage may have endowed him with a hypercoagulable state making pulmonary embolus from deep vein thrombosis due in part to dehydration and immobilization the most likely cause of his relatively rapid death. Unlike most who were nailed to the cross to die, Jesus is said to have died in less than 6 hours, whereas most crucifixions took some days before death occurred. The genetic mutation in question is common throughout Israel, especially in people who live in the Galilee area.

J. A. Stockman III, MD

References

1. Brenner B: Did Jesus Christ die of pulmonary embolism? *J Thromb Haemost* 3:2131-2133, 2005.
2. ur Rehman H: Did Jesus Christ die of pulmonary embolism? A rebuttal. *J Thromb Haemost* 3:2130-2131, 2005.
3. Saliba WR: Did Jesus Christ die of pulmonary embolism? *J Thromb Haemost* 4:891-892, 2006.

Correction of Factor XI Deficiency by Liver Transplantation

Ghosh N, Marotta PJ, McAlister VC (London Health Sciences Centre, Ont, Canada)
N Engl J Med 352:2357-2358, 2005   3–15

Background.—Liver transplantation is now considered an appropriate option for the treatment of hemophilia complicated by cirrhosis. The correction of deficiencies of factor VIII and factor IX by liver transplantation is well known. Factor XI deficiency is a less common form of hemophilia that is associated with prolonged bleeding during surgery. The first case report of correction of factor XI deficiency by liver transplantation was reported.

> *Case Report.*—Man, 48, with hepatitis C virus cirrhosis and hepatocellular carcinoma and who had previously been found to have factor XI deficiency underwent liver transplantation. After removal of the patient's liver, a split-liver graft from a cadaveric donor was orthotopically transplanted. The procedure was complicated by intraoperative bleeding at the cut margin of the liver, which was controlled by local measures. Fresh-frozen plasma was used to correct his coagulopathy during surgery. The patient had a smooth postoperative course and has remained well. Factor XI levels returned to the normal range by day 7 after transplantation and have remained normal.

Conclusions.—The transfer of factor XI deficiency from donor to recipient of an orthotopic liver transplant has been documented previously, and that observation suggests that factor XI production is confined to the liver. This case, in which factor XI deficiency was corrected by liver transplantation, provides further support for the hypothesis that this coagulation factor is produced mainly in the liver.

▶ It is not often that we include in the YEAR BOOK OF PEDIATRICS a letter to the editor. We make an exception, however, for this tidy brief case report since it adds significant information regarding one of the inherited coagulation disorders and since it was sufficiently meritorious to be published in *The New England Journal of Medicine*. In this report, we learn of a man with hepatitis C virus who was also known to have factor XI deficiency. This fellow presumably got his hepatitis C infection from a blood transfusion he had received some 20 years previously as part of the management of unexpected bleeding after an inguinal hernia repair. His liver disease progressed to cirrhosis followed soon thereafter by the detection of hepatocellular carcinoma. For these disorders he had a liver transplant performed, and in the postsurgical period he was found to have a cure of his factor XI deficiency.

This case report is important for it teaches us 2 things. The first is that factor XI is most likely produced in the liver. The second is that deficiencies of this factor are treatable by liver transplantation, a rather dramatic therapy.

This is the last entry in the Blood chapter so we will close with a quiz question having to do with blood. You are seeing a teenager who comes to you with a history of having turned green over the past couple of months. Specifically, the teen's hands, face, and fingers are said to have developed a green sheen. The patient and her mother deny excessive consumption of green-colored foods or vegetables or items with green food coloring. There is no history of jaundice, discolored urine, melena, hematochezia, menorrhagia, pallor, or fever. The teen is a star athlete but has recently complained of some mild fatigue. Physical examination shows an otherwise healthy teenaged girl with normal vital signs. The teen demonstrates a remarkable and unmistakable green complexion of the forehead, nasal bridge, and the medial aspects of both cheeks and chin. The green color is evident on the dorsum of both hands and fingers. The color of the remainder of the body is normal. There is no conjunctival icterus and the oral and nasal mucosal membranes are unremarkable. The rest of the physical examination is entirely within normal limits. If you have one study or set of studies to perform to determine what is going on, what would that be and what is the likely diagnosis?

You would be correct if you chose to do a complete blood count including red cell indices to determine if this young lady were likely to have iron deficiency anemia. A young girl was recently report to have developed a green color to her skin in the presence of iron deficiency, a phenomenon which for many years has been called "chlorosis."[1] Medical chlorosis, the "green sickness," has been recognized as a sign of iron deficiency for many years although it is now quite rare. Chlorosis rapidly diminished in the early 20th century as nutrition improved and hemoglobin determinations easily performed in outpatient laboratories enabled care providers to judiciously prescribe iron therapy at an early, preclinical stage of iron deficiency. By 1930, the abrupt disappearance of chlorosis led to speculation that the characteristic green complexion associated with the condition had been largely imagined by overzealous or copycat physicians, poets, and novelists. In 1987, Dr Bill Crosby, a well-recognized hematologist, wrote a commentary titled: Whatever became of chlorosis?[2] Chlorosis, in fact, had been a highly popular diagnosis in the 18th, 19th, and early 20th century for young women with a number of psychological, gynecologic, and/or gastrointestinal complaints. Its linkage to iron deficiency came in the early 20th century.

If you do not believe there is such a thing as chlorosis, see the report of Perdahl-Wallace and Schwartz,[1] which includes a wonderful photograph of the disease. If you still do not believe there is such a thing as chlorosis, at least read the botanical literature which shows the linkage to iron deficiency. Specifically, chlorosis is the name of a common botanical disease of iron-deficient chlorophylls-containing plants. Why things change color in the face of iron deficiency remains an enigma.

J. A. Stockman III, MD

References

1. Perdahl-Wallace E, Schwartz RH: A girl with green complexion and iron deficiency: Chlorosis revisited. *Clin Pediatr* 45:187-189, 2006.
2. Crosby WH: Whatever became of chlorosis? *JAMA* 257:2799-2800, 1987.

4 Child Development

Aircraft and Road Traffic Noise and Children's Cognition and Health: A Cross-National Study
Stansfeld SA, for the RANCH study team (Univ of London; Karolinska Inst, Stockholm; Consejo Superior De Investigaciones Científicas, Madrid; et al)
Lancet 365:1942-1949, 2005   4–1

Background.—Exposure to environmental stressors can impair children's health and their cognitive development. The effects of air pollution, lead, and chemicals have been studied, but there has been less emphasis on the effects of noise. Our aim, therefore, was to assess the effect of exposure to aircraft and road traffic noise on cognitive performance and health in children.

Methods.—We did a cross-national, cross-sectional study in which we assessed 2844 of 3207 children aged 9-10 years who were attending 89 schools of 77 approached in The Netherlands, 27 in Spain, and 30 in the UK located in local authority areas around three major airports. We selected children by extent of exposure to external aircraft and road traffic noise at school as predicted from noise contour maps, modelling, and on-site measurements, and matched schools within countries for socioeconomic status. We measured cognitive and health outcomes with standardised tests and questionnaires administered in the classroom. We also used a questionnaire to obtain information from parents about socioeconomic status, their education, and ethnic origin.

Findings.—We identified linear exposure-effect associations between exposure to chronic aircraft noise and impairment of reading comprehension (p=0.0097) and recognition memory (p=0.0141), and a non-linear association with annoyance (p<0.0001) maintained after adjustment for mother's education, socioeconomic status, longstanding illness, and extent of classroom insulation against noise. Exposure to road traffic noise was linearly associated with increases in episodic memory (conceptual recall: p=0.0066; information recall: p=0.0489), but also with annoyance (p=0.0047). Neither aircraft noise nor traffic noise affected sustained attention, self-reported health, or overall mental health.

Interpretation.—Our findings indicate that a chronic environmental stressor—aircraft noise—could impair cognitive development in children, specifically reading comprehension. Schools exposed to high levels of aircraft noise are not healthy educational environments.

▶ No one will question that prolonged exposure to excessive noise levels in the workplace can be a cause of permanent high-frequency hearing loss, but less is known about the health effects of exposure to lower levels of noise in our environment. The latter is the type of environment many of us find ourselves in if we live near an airport. Think about what it is like to be living in Alexandria, Virginia, a stone's throw away from Reagan Airport, if you are 10 years old. The study of Stansfeld et al tells exactly what it is like by examining some 2800 children 9 to 10 years of age attending schools located near 3 major airports in Spain, The Netherlands, and the United Kingdom. They assessed noise levels around schools resulting from aircraft and traffic and compared these levels to the results of cognitive performance testing and health questionnaires. They found that chronic exposure to aircraft noise had deleterious effects on reading comprehension and reported annoyance, even after an adjustment was made for socioeconomic differences between high noise and low noise schools. This study adds to the developing literature about the negative effect of noise on learning.

This is not the first article of its type. For example, 326 German school children were matched for socioeconomic status and were followed up prospectively as the old Munich Airport was replaced by a new international facility. Children attending schools near the old airport improved their reading scores and cognitive memory performance when the airport was shut down, whereas children going to school near the new airport experienced a decrease in testing scores.[1]

The $64 question is how environmental noise, from aircraft, for example, is capable of interfering with a child's acquisition of learning skills. The supposition is that children react to noise stress by "tuning out" unwanted noise stimuli and, in the process, also pay less attention to other inputs, such as from their teacher. In fact, it has been shown that, for children to adequately hear a teacher, the background noise in a classroom should be at least 10 dB below the level of the teacher's voice.[2] Also, children with hearing loss require an even greater signal-to-noise ratio. Some have also suggested that the school environment can contribute to this problem if it was not well designed with respect to ventilation and air conditioning unit background noise.

While Stansfeld et al theorize that living in a noisy environment leads to "learned helplessness," in some areas, there is encouraging news that noise can be reduced and its ill effects prevented. Switzerland has placed a nighttime curfew on aircraft departures, except in special circumstances. Also, the American National Standards Institute has published a standard for classroom acoustics, stipulating that noise levels in an empty classroom should be less than 35 dB[A] and that reverberation or echoes should be controlled.

The only major noise-controlled airport in the United States after dark is Reagan Airport in Washington, DC. The limitation there of aircraft landing and departing after 10:00 PM was not put into place for security reasons but rather to let the President sleep better (or at least that's the urban myth). Is aircraft noise during the day one possible explanation for lapses in presidential cognition, from time to time, in the last half century?

J. A. Stockman III, MD

References

1. Hygge S, Evans GW, Bullinger M: A prospective study of some effects of aircraft noise on cognitive performance in school children. *Psychol Sci* 13:469-474, 2002.
2. Wetherill EA: Classroom design for good hearing. Montpelier Vermont Noise Pollution Clearinghouse, Quiet Zone Newsletter, Fall 2002, http://www.nonoise.org/library/qz3, accessed May 23, 2005.

Use of a Dummy (Pacifier) During Sleep and Risk of Sudden Infant Death Syndrome (SIDS): Population Based Case-Control Study
Li D-K, Willinger M, Petitti DB, et al (Kaiser Permanente Northern California, Oakland; Kaiser Permanente Southern California, Pasadena)
BMJ 332:18-21, 2006   4–2

Objectives.—To examine the association between use of a dummy (pacifier) during sleep and the risk of sudden infant death syndrome (SIDS) in relation to other risk factors.

Design.—Population based case-control study.

Setting.—Eleven counties in California.

Participants.—Mothers or carers of 185 infants whose deaths were attributed to SIDS and 312 randomly selected controls matched for race or ethnicity and age.

Main Outcome Measure.—Use of a dummy during sleep determined through interviews.

Results.—The adjusted odds ratio for SIDS associated with using a dummy during the last sleep was 0.08 (95% confidence interval 0.03 to 0.21). Use was associated with a reduction in risk in every category of sociodemographic characteristics and risk factors examined. The reduced risk associated with use seemed to be greater with adverse sleep conditions (such as sleeping prone or on side and sleeping with a mother who smoked), although the observed interactions were not significant. In addition, use of a dummy may reduce the impact of other risk factors for SIDS, especially those related to adverse sleep environment. For example, infants who did not use a dummy and slept prone or on their sides (*v* on their back) had an increased risk of SIDS (2.61, 1.56 to 4.38). In infants who used dummies, there was no increased risk associated with sleeping position (0.66, 0.12 to 3.59). While cosleeping with a mother who smoked was also associated with increased risk of SIDS among infants who did not use a dummy (4.5, 1.3 to 15.1), there was no such association among those who did (1.1, 0.1 to 13.4).

Conclusions.—Use of a dummy seems to reduce the risk of SIDS and possibly reduces the influence of known risk factors in the sleep environment.

▶ There is no question that sleep environment has been consistently reported to be an influencing effect on the risk of SIDS. Previous studies have suggested that the use of a pacifier during sleep will reduce the risk of SIDS. This study underscores this. It shows that the use of a pacifier during sleep does reduce the risk of SIDS consistently across a wide range of socioeconomic characteristics and risk factor profiles. Even in circumstances where the risk of SIDS is higher (such as infants put to sleep in the prone position, who sleep with the mother, who live in a household where there is smoking, or who sleep in a crib with soft bedding), the use of a pacifier still diminishes the overall risk of SIDS, at least in this one report.

Not everyone believes that pacifier use reduces the risk of SIDS. In fact, letters to the editor cautioning against too much credence in the conclusions of the report by Li et al came fast and furious. It is clear that SIDS researchers still need to determine what the protective mechanism of pacifiers might be, if indeed any protection exists, or whether pacifier use is simply a marker for something else.[1]

Your guess is as good as this editor's about whether the use of an infant pacifier does anything at all to reduce the incidence of SIDS. For now, manufacturers of dummies are content in thinking that their products do more than just pacify. Are we dummies in thinking that pacifiers have other medical indications?

This report and the one that follows (Abstract 4–3) tell us that there is still much to be learned about SIDS. In the developed world, SIDS has been responsible for more infant deaths beyond the neonatal period than any other cause. In retrospect, we should have concluded long ago that an epidemic of SIDS pandemic prevailed. The prone sleeping position was identified as a risk factor for SIDS as early as 1944 in New York.[2] Nonetheless, despite the harsh effects of SIDS on parents and professionals, it took a long time to change medical and parental practice. Hence, the back-to-sleep campaign—in 1991 in the United Kingdom and 1994 in the United States—was too late for 10,000 infants in the United Kingdom and 50,000 babies in the rest of Europe, the United States, and Australasia.[3] Hopefully the next major advancement in the health of children will not take 50 years to take root.

J. A. Stockman III, MD

References

1. Blair PS, Fleming PJ: Dummies and SIDS: Causality has not been established. *BMJ* 332:178, 2006.
2. Abramson H: Accidental mechanical suffocation in infants. *Pediatrics* 25:404-413, 1944.
3. Gilbert R, Salanti G, Hareden M, et al: Infant sleeping position and the sudden infant death syndrome: Systematic review of observational studies and historical review of recommendations from 1940 to 2002. *Int J Epidemiol* 34:874-887, 2005.

Bedsharing, Roomsharing, and Sudden Infant Death Syndrome in Scotland: A Case-Control Study
Tappin D, Ecob R, Brooke H (Univ of Glasgow, Yorkhill, Scotland, England; Ecob Consulting)
J Pediatr 147:32-37, 2005   4–3

Objective.—To examine the hypothesis that bedsharing with an infant is associated with an increased risk of sudden infant death syndrome (SIDS).

Study Design.—A 1:2, case:control study in Scotland UK, population 5.1 million, including 123 infants who died of SIDS between January 1, 1996 and May 31, 2000, and 263 controls. The main outcome measure was sharing a sleep surface during last sleep.

Results.—Sharing a sleep surface was associated with SIDS (multivariate OR 2.89, 95% CI 1.40, 5.97). The largest risk was associated with couch sharing (OR 66.9, 95% CI 2.8, 1597). Of 46 SIDS infants who bedshared during their last sleep, 40 (87%) were found in the parents' bed. Sharing a bed when <11 weeks (OR 10.20, 95% CI 2.99, 34.8) was associated with a greater risk, $P = .010$, compared with sharing when older (OR 1.07, 95% CI 0.32, 3.56). The association remained if mother did not smoke (OR 8.01, 95% CI 1.20, 53.3) or the infant was breastfed (OR 13.10, 95% CI 1.29, 133).

Conclusions.—Bedsharing is associated with an increased risk of SIDS for infants <11 weeks of age. Sharing a couch for sleep should be strongly discouraged at any age.

▶ There was a firestorm of protest in 2005 when the American Academy of Pediatrics produced a strong statement against bed sharing. This protest came from a number of sectors that found it difficult to believe that having babies share a bed with a parent was bad. That statement came shortly before this report appeared. The stakes are high in this vehement debate as studies suggest that up to 50% of sudden infant deaths occurs in infants sleeping in adult beds (about 2000 deaths per year here in the United States), and an even higher percentage of these deaths (67%) are occurring in the African-American population where bed sharing tends to be somewhat higher in prevalence. The debate, as one might suspect, pits those who feel that bed sharing is essential for optimal breast feeding and the enhancement of maternal bonding against those who believe that there are definitive risks associated with bed sharing.

The American Academy of Pediatrics' position on bed sharing can be traced back to a statement from its Task Force on Infant Positioning and SIDS that was published in 1997.[1] This early statement included the following: "While bed sharing may have certain benefits (breast feeding) there are no scientific studies demonstrating that bed sharing reduces SIDS risk. Conversely, there are studies suggesting that bed sharing under certain conditions may actually increase the risk of SIDS."

So what do we learn from this most recent study of Tappin et al? We learn that, statistically, there is a substantial SIDS risk associated with bed sharing in nonsmoking mothers. Previous studies had failed to clearly separate out smoking from nonsmoking mothers, an important distinction since maternal smoking itself is associated with an increased risk of SIDS.

Without question, the controversy over bed sharing will continue, perhaps ad infinitum. A word of wisdom, perhaps, to new parents would be to encourage mothers who are interested in bed sharing to breast feed their babies in bed, but before the mother is ready to fall asleep, to place the baby back in a crib. Almost all cases of SIDS have occurred while a mother was asleep. Whether this suggestion represents the Wisdom of Solomon or an editor's hunch is for you to decide. In any event, read the superb editorial on this topic by Thach.[2]

J. A. Stockman III, MD

References

1. Kattwinkel J, Brooks J, Keenan M, et al: American Academy of Pediatrics Task Force on Infant Positioning and SIDS: Does bed sharing affect the risk of SIDS? *Pediatrics* 100:272, 1997.
2. Thach BT: Where should baby be put back to sleep (editorial)? *J Pediatr* 147:6-7, 2005.

Burnout, Psychological Morbidity, Job Satisfaction, and Stress: A Survey of Canadian Hospital Based Child Protection Professionals
Bennett S, Plint A, Clifford TJ (Univ of Ottawa, Ontario, Canada)
Arch Dis Child 90:1112-1116, 2005   4–4

Aims.—(1) To measure the prevalence of burnout, psychological morbidity, job satisfaction, job stress, and consideration of alternate work among multidisciplinary hospital based child and youth protection (CYP) professionals; (2) to understand the relations between these variables; and (3) to understand the reasons for leaving among former programme members.

Methods.—Mailed survey of current and former members of all Canadian academic hospital based CYP programmes. Surveys for current members contained validated measures of burnout, psychological morbidity, job satisfaction/stress, and questions about consideration of alternate work. Surveys for former members examined motivation(s) for leaving.

Results.—One hundred and twenty six of 165 current members (76.4%) and 13/14 (92.9%) former members responded. Over one third (34.1%) of respondents exhibited burnout while psychological morbidity was present in 13.5%. Job satisfaction was high, with 68.8% finding their job "extremely" or "quite" satisfying, whereas 26.2% found their job "extremely" or "quite" stressful. Psychological morbidity, job satisfaction, and job stress were not associated with any of the demographic variables measured, but burnout was most prevalent among non-physician programme members. Almost two thirds of current members indicated that they had seriously considered a change in work situation. Former members indicated that burnout and high levels of job stress were most responsible for their decision to leave and that increasing the number of programme staff and, consequently, reducing the number of hours worked would have influenced their decision to stay.

Conclusions.—Current levels of burnout and the large proportion of individuals who have contemplated leaving the service suggest a potential crisis in Canadian hospital based CYP services.

▶ My hat has always been off to those who dedicate themselves to the protection of children. This is not an easy task, as the article from Canada indicates. In the last few years, a series of child abuse tragedies and fiercely contested murder trials have put pediatricians under the spotlight as never before with respect to their expertise in the area of child abuse and neglect. In the United States, in Canada, and in Great Britain, in particular, reluctance to get involved with child protection has been growing among health professionals. The article by Bennett et al tells us a lot about this, at least from one aspect. These investigators attempted to measure and analyze the stress and burnout among child protection professionals. They found a lot of both. This report is the first comprehensive examination of Canadian hospital-based multidisciplinary child protection professionals' experiences. It does support the concept that these practitioners are experiencing high levels of burnout and job stress and that, consequently, many have considered changing the focus of their work.

We have every reason to believe that what is described in Canada applies equally to circumstances in the United States. These findings are disturbing, particularly in such a demanding and highly specialized area of practice in which training programs are few and experts are in short supply. Recently, the American Board of Pediatrics decided to develop a certificate-defining competency in the area of child abuse and neglect, which, hopefully, will place greater emphasis on and perhaps create a greater interest in training in this area. Something has to be done to make workloads more manageable.

We should take inspiration from those who commit their lives to helping children. Recently we learned of a little known champion of children's causes, Gustave Rau, that we now share with you. Gustave Rau was born into a wealthy family in the 1920s. He never married and had no children of his own. As an only child, he was groomed to take over the family's auto parts manufacturing business near Stuttgart, Germany. He ran the company for a number of years. By age 40, however, he had had it and made an unusual career move. He left the business world, entered medical school, and became a pediatrician. Following completion of his residency training, he sold off all of his factories and used some of the proceeds to set up a medical foundation dedicated to reducing the burden of disease in the underdeveloped world. He moved to Africa and worked as a kind of pediatric Albert Schweitzer, building and working in a hospital in a remote village in Zaire near the Rwandan border. He developed one of the largest pediatric units in Africa. During more than 2 decades in Africa, Dr Rau lived simply in spite of his considerable wealth. However, he allowed himself one expensive diversion: he collected art. A few times a year, he flew out of the bush in a rickety plane and made his way to Europe or America to bid and buy at art auctions. He served as his own art advisor, favoring European art from the Renaissance to post-Impressionism. Over the years, his art collection gradually grew to 423 paintings, plus sculpture and other works. In 1986, he purchased the pastel drawing by Mary Cassatt, Louise Breastfeeding Her Child (1899), a well-known piece of artwork very relevant to pediatrics. There being no suitable space for displaying a large, expensive art collection in a remote African village, the Rau collection was kept in storage in Switzerland for many years. Finally, at age 70 and in failing health, Dr Rau retired and returned to his native Germany. In 2001, he authorized a worldwide public tour of highlights from his collection. By then it was valued at $0.6 billion, one of the largest and best private art collections in the world.

Dr Gustave Rau, pediatrician, died in 2002. His art collection, including the Cassatt painting, was left to the German chapter of UNICEF. Dr Rau directed that his collection be sold over a period of some years to fund the cause to which he devoted much of his life: providing assistance to underprivileged children.[1]

J. A. Stockman III, MD

Reference

1. Kooepsell TD: Mary Cassatt (1844-1926). *Arch Pediatr Adolesc Med* 159:314, 2005.

Bed-Wetting and Its Association With Developmental Milestones in Early Childhood
Touchette E, Petit D, Paquet J, et al (Hôpital du Sacré-Coeur de Montréal; Université de Montréal; Université Laval, Quebec City)
Arch Pediatr Adolesc Med 159:1129-1134, 2005   4–5

Objective.—To evaluate the relationship between bed-wetting and various developmental milestones in a large and representative sample of young children.

Design.—A randomized 3-level stratified survey design.

Setting.—Data were collected by questionnaires, and interviews were scheduled at home with the mother.

Participants.—A representative sample of children born from 1997 to 1998 in Quebec. A complete set of data on bed-wetting was obtained for 1666 children at the ages of 29, 41, and 53 months.

Main Outcome Measures.—Percentage of children who bed-wet and developmental factors associated with bed-wetting.

Results.—Approximately 10% of the children were bed-wetting at the age of 53 months. Bed-wetting cessation occurred for most children studied between the ages of 29 and 41 months. Motor skills were achieved by fewer boys who bed-wet compared with boys who did not (had sat up without support for 10 minutes at 5 months, $P = .05$; and had started crawling at 5 months, $P < .01$). More girls who bed-wet were prematurely born and had hyperactivity and inattention ($P < .01$ for all) compared with those who did not. Language milestones were achieved by fewer children who bed-wet compared with those who did not (boys: $P = .04$; girls: $P = .02$). No between-group difference was found for physical growth and sleep variables.

Conclusions.—These findings show an association between bed-wetting and developmental milestones in early childhood. This study supports that bed-wetting could be indicative of a possible delay in the development of the central nervous system and could act as a noticeable indicator for parents and pediatricians.

▶ The authors of this article pose a very interesting possibility: bed-wetting could be the result of a delay in the development of the CNS. They show that motor skills are achieved by fewer boys who bed-wet compared with boys who had not and that girls who bed-wet were born more immaturely and tended to exhibit more evidence of hyperactivity and inattention. These findings might empirically suggest that the management of bed-wetting would be best fostered with methods that were behavioral, as opposed to pharmacologic. All too often, we tend to resort to medicines as a quick fix—as a way to solve problems that really do need to be managed in a more comprehensive manner with the use of behavioral therapy. This may be one reason why desmopressin, while effective for the short haul, does little to alter the natural history of enuresis in comparison with the use of behavioral techniques such as the urine alarm. Too few of us use the latter when, in fact, it probably is the most efficacious method to help a family manage nighttime wetting for the long haul.

For more on the topic of enuresis and evidence-based approaches to its management, see the review by Christophersen.[1]

J. A. Stockman III, MD

Reference

1. Christophersen E: Is evidence-based treatment sufficient to manage nighttime wetting problems (enuresis)? *Arch Pediatr Adolesc Med* 159:1182-1183, 2005.

Children's Television Viewing and Cognitive Outcomes: A Longitudinal Analysis of National Data
Zimmerman FJ, Christakis DA (Univ of Washington, Seattle; Children's Hosp and Regional Med Ctr, Seattle)
Arch Pediatr Adolesc Med 159:619-625, 2005   4–6

Objective.—To test the independent effects of television viewing in children before age 3 years and at ages 3 to 5 years on several measures of cognitive outcomes at ages 6 and 7 years.

Design.—Using data from a nationally representative data set, we regressed 4 measures of cognitive development at ages 6 and 7 years on television viewing before age 3 years and at ages 3 to 5 years, controlling for parental cognitive stimulation throughout early childhood, maternal education, and IQ.

Results.—Before age 3 years, the children in this study watched an average of 2.2 hours per day; at ages 3 to 5 years, the daily average was 3.3 hours. Adjusted for the covariates mentioned earlier, each hour of average daily television viewing before age 3 years was associated with deleterious effects on the Peabody Individual Achievement Test Reading Recognition Scale of 0.31 points (95% confidence interval [CI], −0.61 to −0.01 points), on the Peabody Individual Achievement Test Reading Comprehension Scale of 0.58 points (95% CI, −0.94 to −0.21 points), and on the Memory for Digit Span assessment from the Wechsler Intelligence Scales for Children of −0.10 points (95% CI, −0.20 to 0 points). For the Reading Recognition Scale score only, a beneficial effect of television at ages 3 to 5 years was identified, with each hour associated with a 0.51-point improvement in the score (95% CI, 0.17 to 0.85 points).

Conclusions.—There are modest adverse effects of television viewing before age 3 years on the subsequent cognitive development of children. These results suggest that greater adherence to the American Academy of Pediatrics guidelines that children younger than 2 years not watch television is warranted.

Association of Television Viewing During Childhood With Poor Educational Achievement

Hancox RJ, Milne BJ, Poulton R (Univ of Otago, Dunedin, New Zealand)
Arch Pediatr Adolesc Med 159:614-618, 2005   4–7

Background.—Excessive television viewing in childhood has been associated with adverse effects on health and behavior. A common concern is that watching too much television may also have a negative impact on education. However, no long-term studies have measured childhood viewing and educational achievement.

Objective.—To explore these associations in a birth cohort followed up to adulthood.

Design.—Prospective birth cohort study.

Setting.—Dunedin, New Zealand.

Participants.—Approximately 1000 unselected individuals born between April 1, 1972, and March 31, 1973. Ninety-six percent of the living cohort participated at 26 years of age.

Main Outcome Measures.—Educational achievement by 26 years of age.

Results.—The mean time spent watching television during childhood and adolescence was significantly associated with leaving school without qualifications and negatively associated with attaining a university degree. Risk ratios for each hour of television viewing per weeknight, adjusted for IQ and sex, were 1.43 (95% confidence interval [CI], 1.24-1.65) and 0.75 (95% CI, 0.67-0.85), respectively (both, $P<.001$). The findings were similar in men and women and persisted after further adjustment for socioeconomic status and early childhood behavioral problems. Television viewing during childhood (ages 5-11 years) and adolescence (ages 13 and 15 years) had adverse associations with later educational achievement. However, adolescent viewing was a stronger predictor of leaving school without qualifications, whereas childhood viewing was a stronger predictor of nonattainment of a university degree.

Conclusions.—Television viewing in childhood and adolescence is associated with poor educational achievement by 26 years of age. Excessive television viewing in childhood may have long-lasting adverse consequences for educational achievement and subsequent socioeconomic status and well-being.

▶ This report and the one that precedes it are not the only ones on the topic that link television viewing during early childhood with poor educational achievement, but they are probably among the very best articles on the topic. The American Academy of Pediatrics has strongly come out against extended TV viewing by young children, which everyone should consider bubble gum for the eyes. Nonetheless, significant debate about the linkage between television viewing and poor educational achievement continues. Even a few distinguished pediatricians have suggested that quality TV time is in fact good for babies.

While the debate about television viewing rages on, so too is the debate about whether listening to Mozart really makes babies more intelligent. Thus far we do not know whether exposure to classical music, including Mozart, makes smart babies smarter. In the not too distant future, however, we will know whether exposure to classical music helps to minimize stress in newborn babies. Physicians at Weill Medical College of Cornell University have decided to run a trial to see whether the music of Mozart affects levels of stress, heart rate, and motor activity in preterm babies. This study is ongoing and is based on preliminary reports that have described the beneficial effects of Mozart's music. Newly arrived babies at a hospital in eastern Slovakia are enrolled in this study. They are listening to works of the Austrian composer to help them recover from the trauma of birth. In the Cornell University trial, Mozart's music will be played through a small speaker in the baby's incubator, and the volume of the music will be set at 10 dB above average ambient noise, which is usually around 55 dB or about the same as the noise produced by a running refrigerator. A monitoring device will record movement, while a video camera will capture the reaction of the infants to the music.

If you want to read more details on the Mozart trial, go to the Clinical Trials Government website (http://ClinicalTrials.gov and refer to NCT00224211). Please note that even reflecting on Mozart's accomplishments can, in fact, be stressful. This editor recognized this phenomenon when first watching the film "Amadeus." I realized that when Mozart was my age, he had already been dead 9 years.

J. A. Stockman III, MD

The Remote, the Mouse, and the No. 2 Pencil: The Household Media Environment and Academic Achievement Among Third Grade Students

Borzekowski DLG, Robinson TN (Johns Hopkins Bloomberg School of Public Health, Baltimore, Md; Stanford Univ, Calif)
Arch Pediatr Adolesc Med 159:607-613, 2005   4–8

Background.—Media can influence aspects of a child's physical, social, and cognitive development; however, the associations between a child's household media environment, media use, and academic achievement have yet to be determined.

Objective.—To examine relationships among a child's household media environment, media use, and academic achievement.

Methods.—During a single academic year, data were collected through classroom surveys and telephone interviews from an ethnically diverse sample of third grade students and their parents from 6 northern California public elementary schools. The majority of our analyses derive from spring 2000 data, including academic achievement assessed through the mathematics, reading, and language arts sections of the Stanford Achievement Test. We fit linear regression models to determine the associations between variations in household media and performance on the standardized tests, adjusting for demographic and media use variables.

Results.—The household media environment is significantly associated with students' performance on the standardized tests. It was found that having a bedroom television set was significantly and negatively associated with students' test scores, while home computer access and use were positively associated with the scores. Regression models significantly predicted up to 24% of the variation in the scores. Absence of a bedroom television combined with access to a home computer was consistently associated with the highest standardized test scores.

Conclusion.—This study adds to the growing literature reporting that having a bedroom television set may be detrimental to young elementary school children. It also suggests that having and using a home computer may be associated with better academic achievement.

▶ No one any longer argues that watching a lot of television is detrimental to a child's academic achievement. A recent nationally representative survey found that 8- to 18-year-olds watch an average of 3 hours of television a day compared with 1 hour a day spent on recreational computer use.[1] Without question, children spend more time watching TV than they do reading. Despite the fact that the American Academy of Pediatrics recommends that children younger than 2 years not watch any TV, the majority in this age group actually not only have access to a television, but do watch TV every day.

This year's YEAR BOOK OF PEDIATRICS contains 3 articles (Abstracts 4–6, 4–7, and 4–8), all appearing in the same issue of the *Archives of Pediatrics and Adolescent Medicine*, dealing with the effects of TV viewing. These studies, in the aggregate, inform us that it is not so much about how much time is spent before the television, as it is the content that affects a child's development. For example, educational TV generally turns out to be beneficial to the average child. Overall, however, TV viewing is negatively associated with academic achievement. The report of Zimmerman and Christakis (Abstract 4–6) suggests that the negative associations found between early TV viewing (younger than 3 years) and children's scores on 2 subscales of the Peabody Individual Achievement Test can be explained, at least in part, by the fact that the children in their sample had been exposed to inappropriate TV content.

So, what do we learn from the 3 reports that appear in this year's YEAR BOOK OF PEDIATRICS dealing with TV and academic achievement? Sitting in front of the boob tube means children have less time to participate in more valuable activities, such as reading and doing homework. No surprise there. We also get a sense from these reports that it is time to move beyond the simple debate about whether TV use is good or bad. There is good content to be found on TV that is entirely appropriate for children, should they choose (or their parents choose) to tune into it. There is every reason to think that good TV would be good for a child, since good time spent on the computer has been demonstrated to be of educational value. It is up to us and to parents to encourage TV viewing of well-produced, age-appropriate, educational TV. A commentary that also appeared in the *Archives of Pediatric and Adolescent Medicine* concluded that such programs can represent a valuable tool for stimulating children's cognitive development.[2]

Anything that stimulates quality thinking, including quality time on the computer, should be good for us at both ends of the age spectrum. There is even a link described between higher levels of education and a lower risk of Alzheimer's disease. Over the years, several studies have shown that formal education seems to protect against Alzheimer's disease. For example, a 1997 study of 642 elderly people, conducted in Chicago, found that each year of education reduces a person's risk of Alzheimer's disease by some 17%. It could very well be that education protects against Alzheimer's disease by increasing the number and strength of neuronal connections in the brain, thus improving an individual's so-called cognitive reserve. According to this theory, later in life when Alzheimer's pathology begins to eat away at one's brain neurons, folks with larger number of reserves would be better able to cope with the onslaught. The analogy is hair loss, where if you start with many more hair follicles, you can lose the same amount per day, but not show as much hair loss over time as someone with fewer follicles, but at some point the problem becomes more and more obvious quite rapidly. Since the mid 1990s, researchers have been following a group of older Catholic priests, nuns, and brothers who have agreed to donate their brains after death in order to study the relationship between education and Alzheimer's disease. These were compared with controls, and it has been shown that highly educated participants did not develop Alzheimer's disease until they had about 5 times as many plaques and tangles as less educated study subjects.

Thus it is that exercising one's mind (the only beneficial form of exercise) produces long lasting benefits that cannot be achieved in other ways.[3]

J. A. Stockman III, MD

References

1. Roberts DF, Foehr UG, Rideout V, et al: Media in the lives of 8- to 18-year-olds, http://www.kff.org/entmedia/7251.cfm, accessed January 18, 2006.
2. Chernin AR, Linebarger DL: The relationship between children's television viewing and academic performance. *Arch Pediatr Adolesc Med* 159:687-689, 2005.
3. Marx J: Preventing Alzheimer's: A lifelong commitment? *Science News* 309:864-866, 2005.

Iron and Zinc Supplementation Does Not Improve Parent or Teacher Ratings of Behavior in First Grade Mexican Children Exposed to Lead

Kordas K, Stoltzfus RJ, Lóopez P, et al (Cornell Univ, Ithaca, NY; UNAM, Mexcio City; School of Natural Sciences, UAQ, Querétaro, Mexico)
J Pediatr 147:632-639, 2005   4–9

Objective.—To determine the efficacy of iron and zinc supplementation on behavior ratings of lead-exposed children.

Study Design.—In this double-blind, randomized trial, 602 first-grade children received 30 mg ferrous fumarate, 30 mg zinc oxide, both, or placebo daily for 6 months. Lead, iron, and zinc status were determined at baseline and follow-up. Parents and teachers provided ratings of child behavior using the Conners Rating Scales.

Results.—The baseline mean (SD) blood lead concentration was 11.5 (6.1) µg/dL, with 51% of children $\geq$10 µg/dL. The prevalence of attention deficit hyperactivity disorder, estimated by combined parent and teacher ratings, was 6%. At follow-up, parent ratings of oppositional, hyperactive, cognitive problems, and attention deficit hyperactivity disorder decreased by 1.5, 1.2, 2.5, and 3.4 points, respectively ($P < .05$). Teacher ratings of hyperactivity increased by 1.1 points ($P = .008$), and the mean cognitive problem score declined by 0.7 points ($P = .038$). There were no treatment effects on mean change in scores, but children receiving any zinc had a higher likelihood of no longer receiving clinically-significant teacher ratings of oppositional behaviors.

Conclusions.—This regimen of supplementation did not result in consistent improvements in ratings of behavior in lead-exposed children over 6 months.

▶ This report is an interesting example of voodoo medicine. If you practice voodoo medicine, you are going to get voodoo results, such as in this report. These comments are not intended to be overly critical of the intentions of the design of this study, which indeed are admirable. For a long time, there has been a great deal written about the link between lead exposure and childhood behavior. Some have suggested that children exposed to significant burdens of lead not only have developmental quotient abnormalities but also have a problem with inattention mimicking attention-deficit/hyperactivity disorder (ADHD). It has also been shown that those who are lead overburdened tend to be iron deficient, and iron deficiency itself is known to decrease levels of CNS monoamine oxidase, also producing symptoms of ADHD. Lastly, zinc, either alone or as an adjunct to traditional therapies, has been used to treat children with ADHD with some modest success. Putting all these assorted pieces of relationships together, the investigators in Mexico decided to treat first-grade children who had been exposed to lead with both iron and zinc to see whether there would be improvement in their behavior. There was no consistent improvement found.

Despite the negative results of this study, there is much to be learned by reading this report in detail. It teaches us much about the subtleties of the long-term consequences of micronutrient deficiency in children and its impact on childhood behavior.

J. A. Stockman III, MD

Masturbation in Infancy and Early Childhood Presenting as a Movement Disorder: 12 Cases and a Review of the Literature
Yang ML, Fullwood E, Goldstein J, et al (Children's Hosp of Pittsburgh, Pa; Children's Hosp Boston; Children's Mem Hosp, Chicago; et al)
Pediatrics 116:1427-1432, 2005   4–10

Purpose.—Infantile masturbation (gratification behavior) is not commonly identified as a cause of recurrent paroxysmal movements. Extensive and fruitless investigations may be pursued before establishing this diagnosis. Sparse literature is available regarding masturbatory behavior as a whole, but literature available as case reports describes common features. The purpose of this case series is to describe consistent features in young children with posturing accompanying masturbation.

Methods.—Twelve patients presenting to a pediatric movement disorders clinic with a suspected movement disorder were determined to have postures and movements associated with masturbation. We reviewed the clinical history, examination, and home videotapes of these patients.

Results.—Our patients had several features in common: (1) onset after the age of 3 months and before 3 years; (2) stereotyped episodes of variable duration; (3) vocalizations with quiet grunting; (4) facial flushing with diaphoresis; (5) pressure on the perineum with characteristic posturing of the lower extremities; (6) no alteration of consciousness; (7) cessation with distraction; (8) normal examination; and (9) normal laboratory studies.

Conclusions.—The identification of these common features by primary care providers should assist in making this diagnosis and eliminate the need for extensive, unnecessary testing. Direct observation of the events is crucial, and the video camera is a useful tool that may help in the identification of masturbatory behavior.

▶ It is interesting to note how many reports have appeared over the years describing how masturbatory activity in infancy and young childhood can easily mimic movement disorders, including seizures. It was back in 1909 that the first medical literature begin to appear on the concept of childhood masturbation, and it has taken us a solid century to finally figure out that this is part of normal childhood development even though it can at times present in bizarre ways.[1] Although a normal behavior in childhood, it is often unrecognized by families and care givers, especially because genital manipulation is frequently totally absent. In young children, unusual posture and movements can occur during masturbation and may lead us to infer that seizures, abdominal pain, colic, or other neurological or medical problems are present. All too often in such circumstances, a medical evaluation is undertaken that is both wasteful in time and economic resources.

Since this editor has little else to say on the topic of masturbation in infancy and young childhood, we close with the observation that the Social Security Administration posts on its website (www.ssa.gov) a listing of the top 100 names that parents give their children at the time they register for Social Security (which is usually done not long after birth). If you want to be an expert in child development on the "must" list of knowledge are the contemporary names given to boys and girls. What follows are the top 10 names that recently were most commonly given by parents to their new offspring:

The top 10 names given by parents to their sons:

1. Jacob
2. Michael
3. Joshua
4. Matthew
5. Ethan
6. Andrew
7. Daniel
8. William
9. Joseph
10. Christopher

The top 10 names given by parents to their daughters:

1. Emily
2. Emma
3. Madison
4. Olivia
5. Hannah
6. Abigail
7. Isabella
8. Ashley
9. Samantha
10. Elizabeth

. . . who would have thought 10 years ago that Isabella would have made the short list?

J. A. Stockman III, MD

Reference

1. Still GF: Common disorders in diseases of childhood. London, United Kingdom: Oxford University Press, 1909:336-380.

5 Dentistry and Otolaryngology (ENT)

Association of Amoxicillin Use During Early Childhood With Developmental Tooth Enamel Defects

Hong L, Levy SM, Warren JJ, et al (Univ of Iowa, Iowa City)
Arch Pediatr Adolesc Med 159:943-948, 2005   5–1

Background.—It has been speculated that amoxicillin use could be associated with dental enamel defects.

Objective.—To assess the association between dental fluorosis, one of the most common developmental tooth enamel defects, and amoxicillin use during early childhood.

Design, Setting, and Participants.—As participants in the Iowa Fluoride Study, subjects were followed up from birth to 32 months using questionnaires every 3 to 4 months to gather information on fluoride intake and amoxicillin use.

Methods.—Early-erupting permanent teeth of 579 subjects were assessed for fluorosis using the Fluorosis Risk Index at approximately the age of 9 years. Relationships between fluorosis and amoxicillin use were assessed using relative risk (RR), Mantel-Haenszel stratified analyses, and multivariable logistic regression.

Results.—Amoxicillin use was reported by 75% of subjects by 12 months and 91% by 32 months. Overall, 24% had fluorosis on both maxillary central incisors. Amoxicillin use from 3 to 6 months significantly increased the risk of fluorosis on the maxillary central incisors (RR = 2.04; 95% confidence interval [CI], 1.49-2.78). After adjusting for fluoride intake and otitis media, the risk of fluorosis on the maxillary central incisors from amoxicillin use during 3 to 6 months (Mantel-Haenszel RR = 1.85; 95% CI, 1.20-2.78) was still statistically significant. Multivariable logistic regression analyses confirmed the increased risk of fluorosis from amoxicillin use during 3 to 6 months (odds ratio = 2.50; 95% CI, 1.21-5.15); fluoride intake was also statistically significant.

Conclusion.—The findings from this study suggest a link between amoxicillin use during infancy and developmental enamel defects of permanent teeth; however, further research is needed.

▶ Most of us are more than familiar with the fact that tetracyclines adversely affect the development of teeth. What is less well-known are the suggestions in the literature that amoxicillin use can also be associated with developmental tooth enamel defects.[1] The article by Hong et al is part of a long-running comprehensive study of oral health in children in Iowa. The article describes a provocative finding of the possible association between fluorosis of permanent teeth and amoxicillin use in early childhood. Some of the first rumblings about a relationship between amoxicillin and fluorosis came from an isolated community in Missouri that had largely anecdotal support.

So has a real link been proven between amoxicillin use and dental fluorosis? This remains to be seen. The implications of a proven amoxicillin–fluorosis link could be enormous, but it is unlikely that pediatric care patterns would quickly change given the effectiveness of amoxicillin as a treatment for the infections for which it is now used. If one looks back through the decades of repeated dental cautions about tetracycline use, it took years and alternative drug choices to reshape clinical practice to reduce what was a far more common problem. If the choice is hearing loss and its sequelae versus the possible risk of a minor cosmetic outcome, there is little doubt of what choice a practitioner will make. For now, any association between amoxicillin use and fluorosis requires, at best, extensive further study, but stay tuned for such studies. We do not want to be in the same boat practitioners were a generation or more ago, who were just waking up to the problems of tetracycline use in children.

One other comment: pigmented gums are a well-established sign of active smoking. Now we see that parents who smoke can indirectly be a cause of pigmented gums in their children. A case-control study using oral photographs from 59 nonsmoking children found excessive gingival pigmentation in up to 78%. Seventy-one percent of these children had at least one parent who smoked, whereas only 35% of those without pigmentation had a parent who smoked. Although these data need to be confirmed, this series of data suggest that there is a more than 2-fold increased risk of having pigmentation of the gums if you are a child living in a household where there is a smoker. The next time you are doing a physical examination, pay careful attention to the patient's gums. It might be a good segue into talking to a parent about a very tangible manifestation of a bad habit they may have.[2]

J. A. Stockman III, MD

References

1. Fuchs DJ: Enamel defects: Hypocalcification and hypoplasia: The "amoxicillin generation" display defects in enamel rod development. *ADA News* 31:9, 2000.
2. Hanioka T, Tanaka K, Ojima M, et al: Association of melanin pigmentation in the gingiva of children with parents who smoke. *Pediatrics* 116:e186-e190, 2005.

Neuropsychological and Renal Effects of Dental Amalgam in Children: A Randomized Clinical Trial

Bellinger DC, Trachtenberg F, Barregard L, et al (Harvard Med School, Boston; New England Research Insts, Watertown, Mass; Goteborg Univ, Sweden; et al)
JAMA 295:1775-1783, 2006   5–2

Context.—No randomized trials have been published that address the concern that inhalation of mercury vapor released by amalgam dental restorations causes adverse health effects.

Objective.—To compare the neuropsychological and renal function of children whose dental caries were restored using amalgam or mercury-free materials.

Design and Setting.—The New England Children's Amalgam Trial was a 2-group randomized safety trial involving 5 community health dental clinics in Boston, Mass, and 1 in Farmington, Me, between September 1997 and March 2005.

Participants and Intervention.—A total of 534 children aged 6 to 10 years at baseline with no prior amalgam restorations and 2 or more posterior teeth with caries were randomly assigned to receive dental restoration of baseline and incident caries during a 5-year follow-up period using either amalgam (n=267) or resin composite (n=267) materials.

Main Outcome Measures.—The primary neuropsychological outcome was 5-year change in full-scale IQ scores. Secondary outcomes included tests of memory and visuomotor ability. Renal glomerular function was measured by creatinine-adjusted albumin in urine.

Results.—Children had a mean of 15 tooth surfaces (median, 14) restored during the 5-year period (range, 0-55). Assignment to the amalgam group was associated with a significantly higher mean urinary mercury level (0.9 vs 0.6 µg/g of creatinine at year 5, $P<.001$). After adjusting for randomization stratum and other covariates, no statistically significant differences were found between children in the amalgam and composite groups in 5-year change in full-scale IQ score (3.1 vs 2.1, $P=.21$). The difference in treatment group change scores was 1.0 (95% confidence interval, −0.6 to 2.5) full-scale IQ score point. No statistically significant differences were found for 4-year change in the general memory index (8.1 vs 7.2, $P=.34$), 4-year change in visuomotor composite (3.8 vs 3.7, $P=.93$), or year 5 urinary albumin (median, 7.5 vs 7.4 mg/g of creatinine, $P=.61$).

Conclusions.—In this study, there were no statistically significant differences in adverse neuropsychological or renal effects observed over the 5-year period in children whose caries were restored using dental amalgam or composite materials. Although it is possible that very small IQ effects cannot be ruled out, these findings suggest that the health effects of amalgam restorations in children need not be the basis of treatment decisions when choosing restorative dental materials.

▶ Most medical students do not learn what most dental students learn early in their training, namely, that dental amalgam, which contains 50% mercury by weight, has been used now for at least 150 years. Because mercury is an acknowledged neurotoxin, concerns about health effects of exposure to this chemical have been widespread, and many individuals have voluntarily submitted to removal of amalgam dental fillings, an uncomfortable and expensive procedure that is not entirely free of hazard.

This study by Bellinger et al and the one that follows by DeRouen et al (Abstract 5–3) report the neuropsychological and renal effects of dental amalgam in children. In their study of 534 New England children aged 6 to 10 years, Bellinger found that at 5-year follow-up, children randomly assigned to an amalgam filling group had higher mean mercury levels than those in the resin-based (white fillings) composite group, but there were no statistically significant differences between the groups in terms of 5-year full-scale IQ score, 4-year change in general memory index, visuomotor composite score, or urinary albumin levels. In the report by DeRouen et al, 507 children aged 8 to 10 years from Lisbon, Portugal, were randomly assigned to receive dental restorations using amalgam or resin composite. At 7 years of follow-up, children in the amalgam group also had higher mercury levels, but there were no statistically significant differences between groups of children on neurobehavioral assessments of memory, attention/concentration, or motor/visuomotor performance.

Thus, the reports of Bellinger et al and DeRouen et al bring us good news, news about which we should be somewhat cautious, however, with respect to overinterpretation. The follow-up duration of these 2 reports was limited to only 5 to 7 years. The delayed effects of early toxic exposure may not show up for many more years. We just do not know. Mercury has been suggested as a risk factor for the development of multiple sclerosis and Alzheimer's disease.[1] Also, it is possible that neither of these studies had enough children in them to truly detect very subtle differences in neurologic outcomes. Last, we now know that sensitivity to mercury toxicity may have a genetic basis, with certain children and adults being more susceptible to its toxic effects at the same levels of exposure. Approximately 25% of the US population is polymorphic for coproporphyrinogen oxidase (*CPOX4*). This is the gene encoding urinary porphyrin excretion, including the handling of heavy metal byproducts such as mercury. It has been reported that those with *CPOX4* do not handle mercury as well as others.

As nicely done as these reports on dental amalgam are, given the numbers of children exposed to dental amalgam, it is critical that there be further, even more rigorous, studies that examine the outcomes of those exposed to mercury fillings. One last comment, completely unrelated to fillings, having to do with dental care. We are gradually seeing more and more preventive dentistry being performed by pediatricians. Medicaid currently pays for pediatricians to apply fluoride varnish during well-child visits in many states. A recent study of this trend by Quinonez et al has shown the cost effectiveness of pediatrician-applied fluoride varnish in children 3½ years of age and younger.[2] In North Carolina, all pediatric residents in training are now taught how to apply fluoride varnish to the teeth of children. The practice of pediatrics continues to evolve.

J. A. Stockman III, MD

Reference

1. Thompson CM, Markesbery WR, Ahmann WD, et al: Regional brain trace-element studies in Alzheimer's disease. *Neurotoxicology* 9:1-7, 1988.
2. Quinonez RB, Stearns SC, Talekar BS, et al: Simulating cost-effectiveness of fluoride varnish during well-child visits for Medicaid-enrolled children. *Arch Pediatr Adolesc Med* 160:164-170, 2006.

Neurobehavioral Effects of Dental Amalgam in Children: A Randomized Clinical Trial

DeRouen TA, Martin MD, Leroux BG, et al (Univ of Washington, Seattle; Universidade de Lisboa, Lisbon, Portugal; Universidade Catolica Portuguesa, Lisbon, Portugal)

JAMA 295:1784-1792, 2006   5–3

Context.—Dental (silver) amalgam is a widely used restorative material containing 50% elemental mercury that emits small amounts of mercury vapor. No randomized clinical trials have determined whether there are significant health risks associated with this low-level mercury exposure.

Objective.—To assess the safety of dental amalgam restorations in children.

Design.—A randomized clinical trial in which children requiring dental restorative treatment were randomized to either amalgam for posterior restorations or resin composite instead of amalgam. Enrollment commenced February 1997, with annual follow-up for 7 years concluding in July 2005.

Setting and Participants.—A total of 507 children in Lisbon, Portugal, aged 8 to 10 years with at least 1 carious lesion on a permanent tooth, no previous exposure to amalgam, urinary mercury level <10 µg/L, blood lead level <15 µg/dL, Comprehensive Test of Nonverbal Intelligence IQ ≥67, and with no interfering health conditions.

Intervention.—Routine, standard-of-care dental treatment, with one group receiving amalgam restorations for posterior lesions (n=253) and the other group receiving resin composite restorations instead of amalgam (n=254).

Main Outcome Measures.—Neurobehavioral assessments of memory, attention/concentration, and motor/visuomotor domains, as well as nerve conduction velocities.

Results.—During the 7-year trial period, children had a mean of 18.7 tooth surfaces (median, 16) restored in the amalgam group and 21.3 (median, 18) restored in the composite group. Baseline mean creatinine-adjusted urinary mercury levels were 1.8 µg/g in the amalgam group and 1.9 µg/g in the composite group, but during follow-up were 1.0 to 1.5 µg/g higher in the amalgam group than in the composite group ($P<.001$). There were no statistically significant differences in measures of memory, attention, visuomotor function, or nerve conduction velocities (average z scores were very similar, near zero) for the amalgam and composite groups over all 7 years of follow-up, with no statistically significant differences observed at any time point (P values from .29 to .91). Starting at 5 years after initial treatment, the need for additional restorative treatment was approximately 50% higher in the composite group.

Conclusions.—In this study, children who received dental restorative treatment with amalgam did not, on average, have statistically significant differences in neurobehavioral assessments or in nerve conduction velocity when compared with children who received resin composite materials without amalgam. These findings, combined with the trend of higher treatment need later among those receiving composite, suggest that amalgam should remain a viable dental restorative option for children.

The Treatment of Posterior Drooling by Botulinum Toxin in a Child With Cerebral Palsy

Jongerius PH, van Hulst K, van den Hoogen FJA, et al (Otorhinolaryngology Univ, Nijmegen, The Netherlands)
J Pediatr Gastroenterol Nutr 41:351-353, 2005   5–4

Background.—Anterior drooling is the unintentional loss of saliva from the mouth. It must be distinguished from posterior drooling, which is the spilling of saliva over the tongue through the faucial isthmus. Posterior drooling can occur whenever the trigger to swallow is impaired or missing. This form of drooling is associated with significant adverse consequences, including congested breathing, coughing, gagging, vomiting, and possibly aspiration into the trachea. Unrecognized and silent pneumonia can occur. The risk of posterior drooling may be increased in many disabled children because they are often cared for in a supine position for most of the day. Many children with cerebral palsy (CP) suffer from gastroesophageal reflux. In these children, pH-sensitive receptors in the mucosa of the distal esophagus are stimulated, which activates the esophageal–salivary reflex, leading to increased salivation. This may, in turn, exacerbate anterior and posterior drooling. Botulinum neurotoxin (BoNT) injections in the salivary glands have shown promise in the treatment of anterior drooling. Repeated bilateral single-dose BoNT injections into the submandibular glands were given to a patient with CP with severe drooling, aspiration, and recurrent pneumonia.

Case Report.—Male child, 9 years, with a diagnosis of CP, and quadriplegic spastic athetosis was referred to an outpatient clinic because he drooled constantly in such a way that clothes, furniture, and objects became wet. The drooling caused him to withdraw from peer activities. In the previous 2 years, he experienced an average of 7 bouts of pneumonia per year. Congested breathing during restless sleep caused him to choke on his own saliva. The first BoNT injection was administered with the patient under general anesthesia. Baseline submandibular flow was reduced by 47% in the first 2 weeks after injection and by 36% at 24 weeks after injection. The parents reported a significant improvement in drooling at 8 weeks after the injection. At 6 months after the injection, the parents reported that drooling appeared to be on the increase again. A second BoNT injection was administered 7 months after the initial injection. Symptoms of posterior drooling disappeared again after the second injection, and the pulmonary condition improved. Pneumonia was reported at 10 months after the first injection, and a third BoNT injection was administered. After the third injection, the patient's tongue movements were stronger, and he showed no refusal to swallow. Pooling in the valleculae still occurred but was followed by an efficient swallow act.

Conclusions.—BoNT injections in this patient with posterior drooling resulted in significant reductions in the submandibular salivary flow rate. The most important findings were a reduction of posterior drooling and the absence of recurrent pneumonia.

▶ It has been known for some time that botulinum toxin injected into submandibular glands is effective in reducing drooling. The type of drooling we are talking about here is what is known as anterior drooling. Anterior drooling is largely a cosmetic problem in those who have it, usually children with CP. However, anterior drooling has to be distinguished from posterior drooling, which refers to saliva that is spilled over the tongue through the faucial isthmus. This type of drooling is very common in youngsters with CP who also have gastroesophageal reflux, which is also a common problem in such youngsters. Exposure of the distal esophagus to acid results in an immediate increase in salivary secretion. Such saliva, if not handled properly, can lead to recurrent aspiration pneumonia, a problem seen in the 9-year-old patient reported here.

Many children with CP have difficulty handling excessive saliva. Those affected with posterior drooling have very congested and noisy breathing as well as aspiration-associated pneumonias. While 1 case with this set of problems successfully treated does not a series make, it does seem reasonable to consider the use of botulinum toxin for posterior drooling in such circumstances.

J. A. Stockman III, MD

Abnormal Oral Vascular Network Pattern Geometry: A New Clinical Sign of Down Syndrome

Latini G, Bianciardi G, Parrini S, et al (Perrino Hosp, Brindisi, Italy; Univ of Siena, Italy; Univ Hosp, Lund, Sweden)

J Pediatr 148:132-137, 2006   5–5

Background.—Down syndrome (trisomy 21, DS) has an incidence of approximately 1:700 live births and is a leading cause of mental retardation. Antenatal diagnosis of DS is important not only for making a decision regarding termination of the pregnancy but also in assisting parents who wish to complete a DS pregnancy in receiving adequate support. Preconception identification of couples potentially at risk for an infant with DS would be advisable, but, with the exception of advanced age at conception, the parental risk factors for meiotic nondisjunction leading to the DS chromosomal aberration are not well established. Extracellular matrix (ECM) changes have been previously reported in DS, and the key role of ECM in angiogenesis and blood vessel geometry have been well-established. However, many biologic systems have no characteristic length scale and thus have fractal or self-affine properties. The hypothesis that a change in the fractal geometry of the oral mucosal vascularization is present in both patients with DS and in their healthy parents was tested.

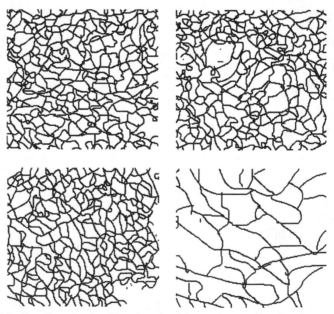

FIGURE 4.—Two-dimensional oral vascular network lattices from unaffected mother (*top left*) and father of patients with DS (*top right*), as compared with control adult subject (*bottom right*) are shown. Vascular network pattern of child with DS is also shown (*bottom left*). Binary forms were generated after conversion from original networks. (Original magnification × 30.) (Courtesy of Latini G, Bianciardi G, Parrini S, et al: Abnormal oral vascular network pattern geometry: a new clinical sign of Down syndrome. *J Pediatr* 148:132-137. Copyright 2006 by Elsevier.)

Methods.—The study was conducted in 14 genetically unrelated patients with DS, their unaffected parents, and 42 genetically unrelated sex- and age-matched control families. The lower gingival and vestibular oral mucosa was selected for study because of the high vasculature pattern visibility and easy accessibility. A 32- × 22-mm area of the lower gingival and vestibular oral mucosa was photographed for each subject. The images were then converted into binary skeletonized form for geometric pattern analysis.

Results.—The scaling plots for the D(1-15) and D(1-46) fractal dimensions exhibit a power-low scaling relationship. The vascular networks of patients with DS and their healthy parents showed significantly higher fractal dimensions than the control networks (Fig 4). Other statistically significant differences were found, including lower *Dmin* values in patients with DS than in DS fathers and mothers, higher D 1-46, D 1-15, and L-Z in patients with DS than DS mothers.

Conclusions.—There is a previously unrecognized change in the microvascular architecture of the oral mucosa in both patients with DS and their healthy parents. This newly recognized sign may prove to be a useful marker for identification of couples who may be at risk for children with Down syndrome.

▶ The findings of this report seem to make sense. Extracellular matrix changes have been previously reported in children with Down syndrome. One example of this is the joint hyperflexibility that has been so well documented in those affected with Down syndrome. It is also known that the extracellular matrix plays a key role in angiogenesis and the geometry of the layout of blood vessels within one's body. Thus one might think that those who have extracellular matrix problems might have peculiar distributions of their blood vessels. This is exactly what was seen in the oral mucosa of subjects with Down syndrome in this report (and to some degree in their parents as well). Why the parents of children with Down syndrome might show these findings is inexplicable.

For more on the topic of Down syndrome and neonatal screening, see the Miscellaneous chapter.

J. A. Stockman III, MD

Easy Removal of Nasal Magnets
Starke L (Wright State Univ, Kettering, Ohio)
Pediatr Emerg Care 21:598-599, 2005   5–6

Background.—Magnet-backed earrings have been increasing in popularity for several years, particularly in the pediatric population. Complications, including pain and necrosis, can occur from the use of these earrings when they are placed on or in body areas other than the ears. In this case report, magnets that had become lodged in the nasal cavity as a result of the use of magnet-backed earrings to decorate the alae were removed.

Case Report.—Boy, 13, was seen at the emergency department (ED) with 2 magnets in the nose, 1 on either side of the septum. The boy had placed flashing-light magnetic-backed earrings on both alae. The external portion of the earrings had fallen off, and the patient had pain in his nose as the magnets became attached through his septum and he was unable to remove them. Removal in the ED was first attempted with a Fogarty balloon catheter. However, the balloon slipped past the magnets without changing their position. This procedure increased the patient's pain; however, no topical anesthetic was available. Two physicians attempted simultaneous removal of the magnets with bayonet forceps, 1 in each nostril. The magnets strongly attracted the forceps, which limited the grip of the forceps on each magnet. This procedure added to the patient's discomfort. The patient was discharged and referred to an otolaryngologist, who also attempted unsuccessfully to remove the magnets with a 2-operator forceps removal. The patient was scheduled for removal under general anesthesia, but before surgery, the boy's father removed the magnets with a heavy-duty pocket magnet pickup, which can be purchased from an auto supply store.

Conclusions.—Delay in removal of magnets adhered across the nasal septum can be minimized and tissue trauma reduced if the magnets are removed in the ED, which avoids the delay for otolaryngology referral. Removal in the ED can be accomplished with a simple household magnet, which can be purchased for less than $10 from an auto supply store. Pretreatment of the nasal mucosa with 4% lidocaine with a 1:1000 concentration of epinephrine spray is recommended to minimize pain and bleeding in the patient.

▶ If you have not seen magnets lodged in the nose, you must have been on Mars for a period of time. Teens and preteens are now using magnet-based earrings to decorate their nostrils. Sometimes the magnets do not come out as easily as they go in. A review of the literature shows a number of different methods for the removal of nasal magnets that include bayonet forceps and Hartmann forceps. Bayonet forceps will usually easily remove a magnet because the magnet is attracted to the forceps. Better yet, as this article shows, is the use of a pocket magnet.

The most significant difficulty with lodged nasal magnets occurs when a youngster has put a magnet in each nostril for bi-alar decoration to keep 2 earrings on opposite nostrils in place. These magnets attract each other through the septum of the nose. A pocket magnet works particularly well in such circumstances. The tip of the pocket magnet is placed inside the naris by pressing laterally with the magnet as the naris is entered. This avoids contact with the sensitive septum. Once the first magnet is removed, the second can be dislodged by placing the magnet tip at the opening of the naris, whereupon, the second magnet usually easily comes out of the nose. The second magnet rarely falls out on its own because of edema.

Please know that delay in removal of nasal magnets that are attracted to one another across the nasal septum can cause necrosis of the nasal septum. A "heavy-duty pocket magnet pickup" can be purchased for about $10 in any auto supply store and turns out to be a very effective medical instrument. Although the method of removal described in this article is relatively atraumatic, pretreatment of the nasal mucosa with 4% lidocaine with a 1:1000 concentration of epinephrine spray is recommended to minimize patient discomfort and bleeding.

While on the topic of things having to do with the nose, see how you might address the following smelly topic. You live in a part of the country where turkey vultures habitate. You notice that vultures seem to be circling your home for the past several days. You become alarmed by this and carefully search through the house, but find no dead animals around that might account for vultures nosing in on you. The issue is, what might have triggered these birds' interest in your property?

Many people today do not think that birds have working noses, and biologists often assume that the sense of smell does not matter much in avian lifestyles. Decades of studies, however, have shown that birds do have a sense of smell, sometimes as fine as or even more fine than the mammal. Take homing pigeons, for example. It has been proposed that pigeons memorize patterns of odors in the wind—a pine-forest tang here, a seashore saltiness there, etc. In otherwise unfamiliar landscapes, homing pigeons may very well use their memories of these odors much as a person uses a map. In fact, it has been shown that if a pigeon is sabotaged by altering its smell capability, such birds are less likely than unimpaired pigeons to find their way home from an unfamiliar place. So what does this have to do with turkey vultures? Some 60 years ago, a report noted that it was possible for California gas-company repair crews to find leaks in their lines by watching for circling turkey vultures attracted to the carrion-like scent added to the gas as a safety alert. Thus it is, if you see a vulture circling over head, take your pulse first to see if you are alive. Check then to be sure that you have not passed any gas. Last, be sure that there are no gas leaks around.[1]

J. A. Stockman III, MD

Reference

1. Milius S: Myth of the bad-nose birds: Study of avian sense of smell recovers from Audubon's blunder. *Sci News* 168:120-123, 2005.

Does Crying Turn Tympanic Membranes Red?

Yamamoto LG, Sumida RN, Yano SS, et al (Univ of Hawaii, Honolulu)
Clin Pediatr (Phila) 44:693-697, 2005
5–7

Summary.—The diagnosis of acute otitis media is based on several clinical factors. One of these factors is the color of the tympanic membrane (TM). Crying can cause flushing and hyperemia of the face. The purpose of this study is to determine whether crying affects the color of tympanic membranes. Infants and toddlers (age 30 months or less) evaluated in an outpatient clinic or primary care pediatrician's office for routine well-baby checks who received at least 2 parenteral immunizations were enrolled on a convenience basis. Ill children were excluded. The initial physician assessed crying and TM color/visibility. Following immunizations, a second physician assessed crying and the TM color/visibility. Color differences were stratified by the degree of crying. One hundred twenty-one study subjects received 2–5 parenteral immunizations. TM colors were most often in the pink range or less. Only 2 TMs were assessed as light red and none were assessed as red. Twenty-eight percent of the TMs with greater crying on the second exam were noted to be redder on the second exam compared to the first exam versus 11% for the comparison group (p=0.0007); 19% of the TMs with greater crying on the second exam were noted to be redder by 2 or more increment levels compared to the first exam versus 5% for the comparison group (p=0.0004); 31% of the TMs with greater crying on the second exam at the 3+ and 4+ level were noted to be redder on the second exam compared to the first exam versus 14% for the comparison group (p=0.003). Our data indicate that, in some instances, crying can result in an increase in pinkness of the TM. Crying in well children does not result in a red tympanic membrane.

▶ Who would have believed that it has taken so long for someone to do a study to determine whether crying produces red TMs? This study, done in well children, shows that some children who cry excessively during a physical examination will develop some pinkness to their TMs. That is about all that this study really tells us. The usefulness of this article is limited because those youngsters in whom we really want to know if crying produces a red TM are those youngsters who are ill and in whom we are trying to exclude or make a diagnosis of otitis media. Presumably, sick youngsters will also have colored TMs as a result of fever as well as crying. We all know, however, that a red TM is hardly the only sign we should be looking for to make a diagnosis of otitis media.

One additional comment about the tympanic membrane and that is that it is a good barometer of the seriousness of trauma induced by an explosive blast. Primary blast injuries are caused by barotrauma, either overpressurization or underpressurization relative to atmospheric pressure. Primary blast injuries most commonly involve air-filled organs and air-fluid interfaces. Organs are damaged by dynamic pressure changes at tissue-density (eg, air fluid) interfaces due to the interaction of a high-frequency stress wave and a lower-frequency shear wave. The most important primary forms of blast injury are rupture of the tympanic membranes, pulmonary damage and air embolization, and rupture of hollow viscera. It is the tympanic membrane that is the structure injured most frequently as a result of barotrauma. It is also the organ that is damaged by the least pressure from blasts. The eardrum thus represents a sentinel site for detecting primary effects of blasts. An increase in pressure of as little as 5 psi above atmospheric pressure (1atm is equivalent to 14.7 psi or 760 mm Hg) can rupture the human eardrum. Even if the tympanic membrane is not ruptured, blast injury can cause temporary neuropraxia in the receptor organs of the ear, manifested by deafness, tinnitus, and vertigo. If dynamic overpressurization is sufficiently high enough, the ossicles of the middle ear can be dislocated. Traumatic disruption of the oval or round window can cause permanent hearing loss. In contrast, pressure gradients of 56 psi to 76 psi (3.6 to 5.2 atm) are needed to cause damage to other organs. It should be noted that ruptured tympanic membranes and lung injuries (the cause of death) were found at the autopsy of Al Zarkowi, the Jordanian terrorist killed in Iraq by a 500-pound bomb blast.

Thus, the ear is a good place to look at after initially stabilizing a patient with a blast injury. If there is no rupture of the tympanic membrane, then primary effects of blasts on other air-containing organs is significantly much less likely.[1]

J. A. Stockman III, MD

Reference

1. DePalma RG, Burris DG, Champion HR, et al: Blast injuries. *N Engl J Med* 352:1335-1342, 2005.

Delayed Prescription May Reduce the Use of Antibiotics for Acute Otitis Media: A Prospective Observational Study in Primary Care
Marchetti F, for the Italian Study Group on Acute Otitis Media (IRCCS Burlo Garofolo, Trieste, Italy; et al)
Arch Pediatr Adolesc Med 159:679-684, 2005   5–8

Objectives.—To evaluate the applicability and the effectiveness of practice guidelines based on a wait-and-see strategy for children with acute otitis media (AOM).

Population.—Children from 1 to 14 years old having AOM who were referred to primary care pediatric practices.

Study Design.—Prospective observational study.

Main Outcome Measure.—Proportion of children having a diagnosis of AOM and eligible for symptomatic treatment who, at 72 hours from enrollment, recovered from their symptoms (fever and earache) without receiving antibiotic treatment.

Results.—One hundred sixty-nine pediatricians participated in the study and enrolled 1672 children. One thousand two hundred seventy-seven children were included in the analysis. One hundred seventy-eight children received antibiotic treatment at first contact according to the practice guidelines criteria (presence of otorrhea or recurrent AOM). Of the 1099 children who were eligible for symptomatic treatment only, 743 (67.6%) recovered without antibiotic treatment at 3 days and 716 (65.1%) at 30 days. No complications were observed. Coexistence of a high fever (temperature ≥38.4°C) and red and bulging tympanic membrane as well as male sex were significantly associated with antibiotic use.

Conclusions.—Practice guidelines based on a wait-and-see strategy for children with AOM are applicable and effective in primary care. This strategy was able to avoid the administration of antibiotic treatment in 2 of 3 children.

▶ We have said it before in the YEAR BOOK OF PEDIATRICS, and it will be said again. Those in Europe seem to be light years ahead of us here in the United States with respect to reduced antibiotic use as part of the management of AOM. We see in this report that if one writes a prescription, but tells a patient not to fill it and "wait-and-see" after a diagnosis of AOM is made, two thirds of the children will never need the antibiotic. If one looks at Great Britain, for example, the use of antibiotics by children with upper respiratory tract infections has been halved in the last decade.[1] This decline is as a result of a reduction in prescribing by general practitioners in Great Britain. This follows the publication of a randomized trial in that country in 1997.[2] The trick, as found in Great Britain, is delayed prescribing of antibiotics. Specifically, this means giving a prescription to a patient and either telling them not to fill it for a day or 2 or to return to pick up the prescription if they are not well in a day or 2. The latter does work in reducing antibiotic use, the former may not.

The approach in Great Britain that is used to manage AOM is to advise parents to watch and wait for no longer than 72 hours after a child is first seen with fever and ear pain with a diagnosis of AOM having been made. After 2 to 3 days, a return to pick up a prescription is advised if symptoms have not improved. Studies have suggested that in AOM, such delays are unlikely to lead to complications. The only significant complication of AOM, the development of mastoiditis, is sufficiently uncommon to necessarily warrant universal administration of antibiotics, because 1 study demonstrated a single case of mastoiditis occurring in a cohort of 5000 patients being treated for AOM with the delayed antibiotic approach. That 1 patient waited nearly a week after being seen before returning for further evaluation.

If you want to read more about how antibiotics are prescribed on the other side of the pond for respiratory tract infections, including AOM, see the excellent editorial by Little.[3] Also, see the report which follows. This study performed here in the United States also shows that 2 of 3 children with AOM who are managed with watchful waiting will never require antibiotic use.[4] This year's YEAR BOOK OF PEDIATRICS also includes an article asking the question whether parents are really ready for the watchful waiting approach for AOM.[5] The answer to the question of whether parents are ready for the wait-and-see approach may be summed up by analyzing the analogy to the national flower of the radiologist: the hedge—"maybe yes/maybe no."

J. A. Stockman III, MD

References

1. Charland M, Kendall H, Yeates D, et al: Antibiotic prescribing in general practice and hospital admissions for peritonsillar abscess, mastoiditis and rheumatic fever in children: Time-trend analysis. *BMJ* 330:328-329, 2005.
2. Little PS, Williamson I, Warner G, et al: An open randomized trial of prescribing strategies for sore throat. *BMJ* 314:722-727, 1997.
3. Little P: Delayed prescribing of antibiotics for upper respiratory tract infection. *BMJ* 331:301-302, 2005.

4. McCormick DP, Chonmaitree T, Pittman C, et al: Nonsevere acute otitis media: A clinical trial comparing outcomes of watchful waiting versus immediate antibiotic treatment. *Pediatrics* 115:1455-1465, 2005.
5. Finkelstein JA, Stille CJ, Rifas-Shiman SL, et al: Watchful waiting for acute otitis media: Are parents and physicians ready. *Pediatrics* 115:1466-1473, 2005.

Nonsevere Acute Otitis Media: A Clinical Trial Comparing Outcomes of Watchful Waiting Versus Immediate Antibiotic Treatment

McCormick DP, Chonmaitree T, Pittman C, et al (Univ of Texas, Galveston; Univ of Colorado, Denver)

Pediatrics 115:1455-1465, 2005   5–9

Objective.—The widespread use of antibiotics for treatment of acute otitis media (AOM) has resulted in the emergence of multidrug-resistant pathogens that are difficult to treat. However, it has been shown that most children with nonsevere AOM recover without ABX. The objective of this study was to evaluate the safety, efficacy, acceptability, and costs of a non-ABX intervention for children with nonsevere AOM.

Methodology.—Children 6 months to 12 years old with AOM were screened by using a novel AOM-severity screening index. Parents of children with nonsevere AOM received an educational intervention, and their children were randomized to receive either immediate antibiotics (ABX; amoxicillin plus symptom medication) or watchful waiting (WW; symptom medication only). The investigators, but not the parents, were blinded to enrollment status. Primary outcomes included parent satisfaction with AOM care, resolution of symptoms, AOM failure/recurrence, and nasopharyngeal carriage of *Streptococcus pneumoniae* strains resistant to ABX. Secondary outcomes included medication-related adverse events, serious adverse events, unanticipated AOM-related office and emergency department visits and telephone calls, the child's absence from day care or school resulting from AOM, the parent's absence from school or work because of their child's AOM, and costs of treatment. Subjects were defined as failing (days 0-12) or recurring (days 13-30) if they experienced a higher AOM-severity score on reexamination.

Results.—A total of 223 subjects were recruited: 73% were nonwhite, 57% were <2 years old, 47% attended day care, 82% had experienced prior AOM, and 83% had not been fully immunized with heptavalent pneumococcal vaccine. One hundred twelve were randomized to ABX, and 111 were randomized to WW. Ninety-four percent of the subjects were followed to the 30-day end point. Parent satisfaction with AOM care was not different between the 2 treatment groups at either day 12 or 30. Compared with WW, symptom scores on days 1 to 10 resolved faster in subjects treated with immediate ABX. At day 12, among the immediate-ABX group, 69% of tympanic membranes and 25% of tympanograms were normal, compared with 51% of normal tympanic membranes and 10% of normal tympanograms in the WW group. Parents of children in the ABX group gave their children fewer doses of pain medication than did parents of children in the WW group. Subjects in the ABX group experienced 16% fewer failures than subjects in the WW group. Of the children in the WW group, 66% completed the study without needing ABX. Immediate ABX resulted in eradication of *S pneumoniae* carriage in the majority of children, but *S pneumoniae* strains cultured from children in the ABX group at day 12 were more likely to be multidrug-resistant than strains from children in the WW group. More ABX-related adverse events were noted in the ABX group, compared with the WW group. No serious AOM-related adverse events were observed in either group. Office and emergency department visits, phone calls, and days of work/school missed were not different between groups. Prescriptions for ABX were reduced by 73% in the WW group compared with the ABX group. Costs of ABX averaged $47.41 per subject in the ABX group and $11.43 in the WW group.

Conclusions.—Sixty-six percent of subjects in the WW group completed the study without ABX. Parent satisfaction was the same between groups regardless of treatment. Compared with WW, immediate ABX treatment was associated with decreased numbers of treatment failures and improved symptom control but increased ABX-related adverse events and a higher percent carriage of multidrug-resistant *S pneumoniae* strains in the nasopharynx at the day-12 visit. Key factors in implementing a WW strategy were (*a*) a method to classify AOM severity; (*b*) parent education; (*c*) management of AOM symptoms; (*d*) access to follow-up care; and (*e*) use of an effective ABX regimen, when needed. When these caveats are observed, WW may be an acceptable alternative to immediate ABX for some children with nonsevere AOM.

Watchful Waiting for Acute Otitis Media: Are Parents and Physicians Ready?
Finkelstein JA, Stille CJ, Rifas-Shiman SL, et al (Harvard Med School, Boston; Children's Hosp Boston; Univ of Massachusetts, Worcester)
Pediatrics 115:1466-1472, 2005   5–10

Objective.—To assess the current use of initial observation ("watchful waiting") of acute otitis media among community physicians and the acceptability of this option to parents of young children.

Setting.—Sixteen nonoverlapping Massachusetts communities enrolled in a community intervention study on appropriate antibiotic use.

Design.—Pediatricians, family physicians, and a random sample of parents of children <6 years old were surveyed. Parents predicted what their satisfaction would be with initial observation of an ear infection without antibiotics if suggested by their physician and concerns they would have regarding this watchful-waiting approach. Physicians reported the frequency with which they use this approach in children ≥2 years and those <2 years old. Separate multivariable models identified factors independently associated with parental satisfaction and with frequency of self-reported use by physicians. All models accounted for clustering of responses within communities.

Results.—Two thousand fifty-four (40%) parents and 160 (58%) physicians responded. Of the parents, 34% would be somewhat or extremely satisfied if initial observation was recommended, another 26% would be neutral, and the remaining 40% would be somewhat or extremely dissatisfied. The multivariable model showed lower parental education (odds ratio [OR]: 0.50; 95% confidence interval [CI]: 0.35, 0.71, for high school education or less compared with college graduation) and Medicaid enrollment (OR: 0.77; CI: 0.57, 1.0) was associated with lower predicted satisfaction. Higher antibiotic-related knowledge (OR: 1.2; CI: 1.1, 1.3, per question correct), belief that antibiotic resistance is a serious problem (OR: 2.3; CI: 1.8, 2.8), and reporting feeling included in medical decisions (OR: 1.4; CI: 1.1, 1.7) all were independently associated with higher predicted satisfaction. Thirty-eight percent of physicians treating children ≥2 years old never or almost never reported using initial observation, 39% reported use occasionally, 17% sometimes, and 6% most of the time. In a multivariable model, only more years in practice (OR: 0.96; CI: 0.93, 0.99) was associated with a decreased likelihood of occasional or more-frequent use of watchful waiting (compared with those who never use initial observation). However, a secondary model that combined occasional users with nonusers (compared with those reporting use sometimes or more often) identified several correlates of use of observation: years in practice (OR: 0.95; CI: 0.91, 0.99), family medicine specialization (OR: 4.5; CI: 1.9, 11), belief that antibiotic resistance is a significant problem (OR: 4.3; CI: 1.3, 14.5), and practice in a community receiving a judicious antibiotic-use intervention (OR: 3.5; CI: 1.3, 9.1).

Conclusions.—A majority of physicians reported at least occasionally using initial observation, but few use it frequently. Many parents have concerns regarding this option, but acceptability is increased among those with more education and those who feel included in medical decisions. Substantial change in both parental and provider views would be needed to make initial observation a widely used alternative for acute otitis media.

Large Dosage Amoxicillin/Clavulanate, Compared With Azithromycin, for the Treatment of Bacterial Acute Otitis Media in Children
Hoberman A, Dagan R, Leibovitz E, et al (Children's Hosp of Pittsburgh, Pa; Ben Gurion Univ, Beer Sheva, Israel; Hosp Santiago del Rio, Chile; et al)
Pediatr Infect Dis J 24:525-532, 2005   5–11

Background.—A large dosage pediatric formulation of amoxicillin/clavulanate with an improved pharmacokinetic/pharmacodynamic profile was developed to eradicate many penicillin-resistant strains of *Streptococ-*

cus pneumoniae and *Haemophilus influenzae* (including β-lactamase-producing strains).

Methods.—This randomized, investigator-blinded, multicenter trial examined treatment of bacterial acute otitis media (AOM) in children 6-30 months of age with amoxicillin/clavulanate (90/6.4 mg/kg/d in 2 divided doses for 10 days) versus azithromycin (10 mg/kg for 1 day followed by 5 mg/kg/d for 4 days). Tympanocentesis was performed at entry for bacteriologic assessment, at the on-therapy visit (day 4–6) to determine bacterial eradication and at any time before the end-of-therapy visit (day 12–14) if the child was categorized as experiencing clinical failure. Clinical assessments were performed at the on-therapy, end-of-therapy and follow-up (day 21–25) visits.

Results.—We enrolled 730 children; AOM pathogens were isolated at baseline for 249 of the amoxicillin/clavulanate group and 245 of the azithromycin group. For children with AOM pathogens at baseline, clinical success rates at the end-of-therapy visit were 90.5% for amoxicillin/clavulanate versus 80.9% for azithromycin ($P < 0.01$), and those at the on-therapy and follow-up visits were 94.9% versus 88.0% and 80.3% versus 71.1%, respectively (all $P < 0.05$). At the on-therapy visit, pretherapy pathogens were eradicated for 94.2% of children receiving amoxicillin/clavulanate versus 70.3% of those receiving azithromycin ($P < 0.001$). Amoxicillin/clavulanate eradicated 96.0% of *S. pneumoniae* (92.0% of fully penicillin-resistant *S. pneumoniae*) and 89.7% of *H. influenzae* (85.7% [6 of 7 cases] of β-lactamase-positive *H. influenzae*). Corresponding rates for azithromycin were 80.4% (54.5%) for *S. pneumoniae* and 49.1% (100% [1 of 1 case]) for *H. influenzae* (all $P < 0.01$ for between-drug comparisons).

Conclusion.—Amoxicillin/clavulanate was clinically and bacteriologically more effective than azithromycin among children with bacterial AOM, including cases caused by penicillin-resistant *S. pneumoniae* and β-lactamase-positive *H. influenzae*.

▶ A large-dose amoxicillin/clavulanate formulation (90/6.4 mg/kg/d; Augmentin ES-600; Glaxo-Smith-Kline, Durham, NC) was approved in the United States for the treatment of children with recurrent and persistent cases of AOM, particularly for those for whom resistant *S pneumoniae* was prevalent. Because this formulation and azithromycin are frequently prescribed for the treatment of children with this condition, the investigators from Pittsburgh, Israel, and Chile decided to evaluate the efficacy of amoxicillin/clavulanate in comparison with azithromycin for the treatment of bacterial AOM in children. We see that amoxicillin/clavulanate, while not a perfect drug, fared far better than azithromycin in this regard.

It has been a few years since the American Academy of Pediatrics Subcommittee on Management of Acute Otitis Media produced its recommendations and guidelines for the diagnosis and management of AOM.[1] Every pediatrician should be familiar with these guidelines. Recommendation 1 reads: "The clinician should confirm a history of acute onset, identify signs of middle ear effusion, and evaluate for signs and symptoms of middle ear inflammation as part of the history and physical examination of the child with acute otitis media." Recommendation 2 reads: "An assessment for pain should be completed and, if pain is present, the clinician should recommend treatment to reduce pain." Recommendation 3A reads: "Observation without the use of antibacterial agents in a child with uncomplicated acute otitis media is an option for selected children based on diagnostic certainty, age, severity of illness, and assurance of followup." The latter option includes watchful waiting for 48 to 72 hours in selected children with pain management only. Appropriate patients for this option include those otherwise healthy children aged 6 months to 2 years with nonsevere symptoms and an uncertain diagnosis, and those children aged 2 to 12 years who have nonsevere symptoms or an uncertain diagnosis. If this option is chosen, the patient and family must have reliable access to the clinician for the purposes of consultation, reevaluation, and obtaining medication. If there is any concern about impending or obvious complications, if the child has an underlying medical condition that would make this option potentially problematic, or if the family does not have ready access to follow-up medical care for any reason, then this may not be an appropriate management strategy for the child.

Recommendation 3B of the American Academy of Pediatrics Subcommittee reads: "If a decision is made to treat with an antibacterial agent, the clinician should prescribe amoxicillin for most children. When amoxicillin is used, the dose should be 80 mg/kg to 90 mg/kg per day." Recommendation 4 reads: "If the patient fails to respond to the initial management option within 48 to 72 hours, the clinician must reassess the patient to confirm acute otitis media and exclude other causes of illness. If acute otitis media is confirmed in the patient initially managed with observation, the clinician should begin antibacterial therapy. If the patient was initially managed with an antibacterial agent, the clinician should change the antibacterial agent." The alternative antibiotic recommended is amoxicillin/clavulanate (90 mg/kg/d of amoxicillin with 6.4 mg/kg/d of clavulanate in 2 divided doses)."

Recommendation 5 deals with the prevention of AOM and reads: "Clinicians should encourage the prevention of acute otitis media through reduction of risk factors." This would include breast-feeding during infancy, avoiding supine bottle feeding, reducing or eliminating pacifier use, minimizing child care use, eliminating exposure to tobacco smoke, etc. This recommendation also includes the use of appropriate vaccines, recognizing that they are not a panacea. It should be noted that the American Academy of Pediatric guidelines make no specific recommendations regarding the use of complementary or alternative medicine in the management of AOM, a recommendation based on lack of evidence of the efficacy or effectiveness of any alternative medicine in comparison with the natural history of AOM.

If you want to read more about otitis media and new guidelines from the otolaryngologist's point of view, see the excellent commentary on this topic by Kenna.[2]

J. A. Stockman III, MD

References

1. American Academy of Pediatrics Subcommittee on Management of Acute Otitis Media: Diagnosis and management of acute otitis media. *Pediatrics* 113:1451-1465, 2004.
2. Kenna MA: Otitis media and the new guidelines. *J Otolaryngol* 34:S24-S32, 2005.

Acute Otitis Media Due to Penicillin-Nonsusceptible *Streptococcus pneumoniae* Before and After the Introduction of the Pneumoccal Conjugate Vaccine

McEllistrem MC, Adams JM, Patel K, et al (Univ of Pittsburgh, Pa; Baylor College of Medicine, Houston; Children's Hosp and Health Ctr, San Diego, Calif; et al)

Clin Infect Dis 40:1738-1744, 2005   5–12

Background.—The impact of the 7-valent pneumococcal conjugate vaccine (PCV7 [Prevnar]) on penicillin-nonsusceptible *Streptococcus pneumoniae* (PNSP) recovered from children with acute otitis media (AOM) is unclear.

Methods.—At 5 hospitals, 505 pneumococcal isolates were collected from children with AOM between 1 January 1999 and 31 December 2002. Molecular subtyping was performed on 158 isolates.

Results.—Overall, the percentage of AOM cases due to non-PCV7 serogroups (including serotype 3) increased over time (from 12% in 1999 to 32% in 2002; $P < .01$) and according to the number of PCV7 doses received (18% [$\leq$1 dose] vs. 35% [2–4 doses]; $P < .01$). The percentage of cases due to vaccine-related serotypes (including serotype 19A) increased according to the number of PCV7 doses received (10% [$\leq$1 dose] vs. 19% [2–4 doses]; $P = .05$) but not over time, whereas the percentage of cases due to serotype 19F remained unchanged both over time and according to the number of PCV7 doses received. The frequency of penicillin nonsusceptibility among PCV7 serotypes (range, 65%–75%) and non-PCV7 serogroups (range, 11%–27%) did not significantly change overall. Although no change was detected among isolates collected from children with spontaneous drainage, the percentage of pneumococci recovered at the time of myringotomy and/or tympanostomy tube placement that were nonresistant to penicillin decreased over time (from 73% in 1999 to 53% in 2002; $P = .03$). All of the serotype 3 strains were genetically related, whereas 88% of the isolates that were either serotype 19F or serotype 23F were related to 1 of 3 international clones.

Conclusions.—Among children with AOM, the proportion of cases due to non-PCV7 serogroups increased, vaccine-related serotypes increased, and serotype 19F remained unchanged. Although a decrease in the proportion of cases due to PNSP occurred among children who required myringotomy and/or tympanostomy tube placement, the proportion of PNSP remained unchanged overall and among children with spontaneous drainage. Because future trends in the susceptibility patterns of pneumococcal isolates recovered from children with AOM are not easy to predict, continued surveillance is essential.

▶ This report gives us information about the change in the prevalence of AOM secondary to PNSP before and after the introduction of the pneumococcal conjugate vaccine. One would think that there would be a decrease in the incidence of AOM resulting from the use of vaccines against relevant bacteria and viruses. Most of us had hoped that the introduction of Prevnar to young infants would reduce the incidence of AOM. This hope has been tempered by evidence that this reduction has turned out not to be large, ranging somewhere between 10% and 30% in terms of a decreased rate of AOM. Ten percent to 30% is not 0%, so we are at least grateful for whatever benefit the pneumococcal vaccine has afforded children here in the United States. More specifically, among 37,868 infants randomly assigned to receive either the pneumococcal vaccine or the meningococcus type C conjugate vaccine in California, those receiving the pneumococcal vaccine experienced just a 7.8% relative reduction in clinically diagnosed cases of AOM, and a 20% relative reduction in the placement of ventilatory tubes.[1]

Thus, the pneumococcal vaccine has not turned out to be a panacea against AOM. A number of questions remain. Will the incidence of AOM caused by *S pneumoniae* strains not contained in the vaccine increase because the strains substitute for those reduced in prevalence by the vaccine? Will the net result be no change or even an increase in the incidence of AOM? Will other bacteria, such as *Moraxella catarrhalis*, non–group B *H influenzae*, or *Streptococcus pyogenes*, substitute for the *S pneumoniae* serotypes in children who have received the vaccine?

In the United States, we do not routinely tap the tympanic membranes of patients with AOM and culture the contents. We must rely on information provided from cultures of fluid from spontaneously ruptured tympanic membranes or fluid obtained during surgical drainage procedures. Unfortunately, these sources may not have the same distribution of bacteria as fluid directly collected from the middle ear in children with AOM. This is why the study of McEllistrem is so important, since it includes data from children who have had direct ear cultures.

See the excellent review by Regelmann[2] of the benefits of the pneumococcal vaccine vis-à-vis its effect on AOM.

J. A. Stockman III, MD

References

1. Black S, Shinefeld H, Fireman B, et al: Efficacy, safety and immunogenicity of heptavalent pneumococcal conjugate vaccine in children. Northern California Kaiser Permanente Vaccine Study Center Group. *Pediatr Infect Dis J* 19:187-195, 2000.
2. Regelmann WE: A pain in the ear: What has the 7-valent conjugated pneumococcal vaccine done to reduce the incidence of acute otitis media? *Clin Infect Dis* 40:1745-1747, 2005.

Effect of Combined Pneumococcal Conjugate and Polysaccharide Vaccination on Recurrent Otitis Media With Effusion

van Heerbeek N, Straetemans M, Wiertsema SP, et al (Radboud Univ, Nijmegen, The Netherlands; Wilhelmina Children's Hosp, Utrecht, The Netherlands)

Pediatrics 117:603-608, 2006   5-13

Background.—Otitis media with effusion (OME) is very common during childhood. Because *Streptococcus pneumoniae* is one of the most common bacterial pathogens involved in OME, pneumococcal vaccines may have a role in the prevention of recurrent OME.

Objective.—We sought to assess the effect of combined pneumococcal conjugate and polysaccharide vaccinations on the recurrence of OME.

Methods.—A randomized, controlled trial was performed with 161 children, 2 to 8 years of age, with documented persistent bilateral OME. All subjects were treated with tympanostomy tubes (TTs). One half of the subjects were assigned randomly to additional vaccination with a 7-valent pneumococcal conjugate vaccine 3 to 4 weeks before and a 23-valent pneumococcal polysaccharide vaccine 3 months after tube insertion. Blood samples were drawn at the first vaccination, at the time of TT placement, and 1 and 3 months after the second vaccination. Levels of IgA and IgG serum antibody against the 7-valent pneumococcal conjugate vaccine serotypes 4, 6B, 9V, 14, 18C, 19F, and 23F were measured with enzyme-linked immunosorbent assays. All children were monitored for recurrence of OME for 6 months after spontaneous extrusion of the TTs.

Results.—The overall recurrence rate of bilateral OME was 50%. Pneumococcal vaccinations induced significant 4.6- to 24.4-fold increases in the geometric means of all conjugate vaccine serotype antibody titers but did not affect recurrence of OME.

Conclusions.—Combined pneumococcal conjugate and polysaccharide vaccination does not prevent recurrence of OME among children 2 to 8 years of age previously known to have persistent OME. Therefore, pneumococcal vaccines are not indicated for the treatment of children suffering from recurrent OME.

▶ It is pretty clear that the pneumococcal vaccine cannot work miracles. Without question, *S pneumoniae* is the most common bacterial pathogen causing middle ear effusion. One might think that vaccination against this pathogen for children prone to OME may be effective in preventing additional recurrences. Before the study abstracted, no studies had been published on the effectiveness of vaccination among children who are at most risk to develop long-term sequelae (ie, children with recurrent OME). The report abstracted represents a clinical trial that attempted to establish the effect of combined pneumococcal conjugate and polysaccharide vaccine among children 2 to 8 years of age who were already known to be prone to recurrent OME and therefore most at risk to develop long-term sequelae such as speech delay and hearing problems. What we learn is that such children with prior episodes of OME do not have any decrease in subsequent episodes of otitis media just because they have received the vaccine. Win one for OME, and score one loss for the vaccine.

This report does not mean that many other direct and indirect effects of pneumococcal vaccine administration do not occur. Clearly, as a result of the vaccine, there has been a remarkable reduction in infection caused by vaccine strains in vaccine recipients. In studies involving children in a Kaiser Permanente Health System, the administration of Prevnar nearly eliminated meningitis and bacteremic pneumonia caused by vaccine serotypes. Not surprisingly, a lesser impact was observed for diseases in which the cause was less specifically determined.[1] The Kaiser Permanente Group showed that the overall reduction in acute otitis media was less than 10%, however.

We should be aware of one additional significant effect, albeit an indirect one, of the use of pneumococcal vaccine in children. In a closed environment, such as a child care center, the rate of colonization by vaccine serotypes is inversely proportional to the number of attendees who have been vaccinated, up to a certain threshold. Once a certain proportion of children have received the vaccine, pneumococci will not spread successfully throughout the center. This is a typical "herd effect." Those who are not vaccinated will benefit from those who are. Recognize, of course, that the herd effect, although important from an epidemiologic perspective, is much less strongly protective than is the direct effect of vaccination. The herd effect cannot be counted on to protect unvaccinated children, and parents should be aware of this. One should also recognize an unwanted effect of vaccination, namely, the emergence of what are called "replacement strains." Whereas disease caused by the bacterial serotypes in the vaccines has tremendously declined, there has been a substantial increase in nonvaccine serotypes such as 11, 15, and 19A. One must conclude that the prognosis for a lasting suppression of pneumococcal disease as a result of the vaccine is somewhat guarded.

To read more about the pneumococcal vaccine and its direct and indirect effects, see the superb review by Musher.[2]

J. A. Stockman III, MD

References

1. Black S, Shinefeld H, Fireman B, et al: Efficacy, safety and immunogenicity of heptavalent pneumococcal conjugate vaccine in children. Northern California Kaiser Permanente Vaccine Study Center Group. *Pediatr Infect Dis J* 19:187-195, 2000.
2. Musher DM: Pneumococcal vaccines: Direct and indirect "herd" effects. *N Engl J Med* 354:1522-1524, 2006.

Ultrasonic Detection of Middle Ear Effusion: A Preliminary Study

Discolo CM, Byrd MC, Bates T, et al (Cleveland Clinic Found, Ohio; Case Western Reserve Univ, Cleveland, Ohio)
Arch Otolaryngol Head Neck Surg 130:1407-1410, 2004   5–14

Objective.—To assess the ability to detect and characterize middle ear effusion in children using A-mode ultrasonography.

Design.—Prospective nonblinded comparison study.

Setting.—Tertiary children's hospital.

Patients.—Forty children (74 ears) scheduled to undergo bilateral myringotomy with pressure equalization tube placement.

Interventions.—Before myringotomy, ultrasound examination of the tympanic membrane and middle ear space was performed on each ear. Afterward, myringotomy was performed and the type of effusion (serous, mucoid, or purulent) was recorded. Pressure equalization tubes were then placed.

Main Outcome Measure.—Comparison of ultrasound findings with the visual assessment of the type of middle ear effusion present.

Results.—Of the 74 ears tested, 45 (61%) had effusion on direct inspection. The effusion was purulent in 8 ears (18%), serous in 9 ears (20%), and mucoid in 28 ears (62%). Ultrasound identified the presence or absence of effusion in 71 cases (96%) ($P = .04$). Ultrasound distinguished between serous and mucoid effusion with 100% accuracy ($P = .04$). The probe did not distinguish between mucoid and purulent effusion.

Conclusions.—Ultrasonography is an accurate method of diagnosing middle ear effusion in children. Moreover, it can distinguish thin from mucoid fluid. Further refinements in probe design may further improve the sensitivity of fluid detection and allow differentiation of sterile vs infectious effusion.

▶ Elsewhere in this chapter of the YEAR BOOK OF PEDIATRICS (see Abstract 5–16), we learn about the long-term consequences of placement of tympanostomy tubes to manage middle ear effusions. Clearly, there are consequences to the placement of such tubes. Given these consequences, we all should be absolutely sure that a child does, in fact, have a middle ear effusion before drawing any conclusions about how to manage the problem. As we see from this article by Discolo et al, US is an accurate method of diagnosing middle ear effusion in children. Moreover, it seems capable of distinguishing thin from thick middle ear fluid. It is far better than otoscopy.

Currently, tympanometry is the diagnostic test most commonly used to determine the presence of middle ear effusion. It provides a graphic representation of the compliance of the tympanic membrane; however, as we see from this article, tympanometry fails to detect many cases that can be diagnosed with the use of US. Unlike tympanometry, which indirectly infers the presence of effusion, US gives a direct image of the middle ear space.

It is hard to say when US probes to detect middle ear effusions might enter the office practice setting of the generalist pediatrician because these are not inexpensive devices. When one thinks about it, however, middle ear effusion is so prevalent these days, anything that would add to our diagnostic accuracy of such a common problem should be thought about seriously when creating an equipment budget for one's practice.

J. A. Stockman III, MD

Developmental Outcomes After Early or Delayed Insertion of Tympanostomy Tubes

Paradise JL, Campbell TF, Dollaghan CA, et al (Univ of Pittsburgh, Pa; Children's Hosp of Pittsburgh, Pa)
N Engl J Med 353:576-586, 2005   5–15

Background.—To prevent later developmental impairments, myringotomy with the insertion of tympanostomy tubes has often been undertaken in young children who have persistent otitis media with effusion. We previously reported that prompt as compared with delayed insertion of tympanostomy tubes in children with persistent effusion who were younger than three years of age did not result in improved developmental outcomes at three or four years of age. However, the effect on the outcomes of school-age children is unknown.

Methods.—We enrolled 6350 healthy infants younger than 62 days of age and evaluated them regularly for middle-ear effusion. Before three years of age, 429 children with persistent middle-ear effusion were randomly assigned to have tympanostomy tubes inserted either promptly or up to nine months later if effusion persisted. We assessed developmental outcomes in 395 of these children at six years of age.

Results.—At six years of age, 85 percent of children in the early-treatment group and 41 percent in the delayed-treatment group had received tympanostomy tubes. There were no significant differences in mean (±SD) scores favoring early versus delayed treatment on any of 30 measures, including the Wechsler Full-Scale Intelligence Quotient (98±13 vs. 98±14); Number of Different Words test, a measure of word diversity (183±36 vs. 175±36); Percentage of Consonants Correct-Revised test, a measure of speech-sound production (96±2 vs. 96±3); the SCAN test, a measure of central auditory processing (95±15 vs. 96±14); and several measures of behavior and emotion.

Conclusions.—In otherwise healthy children younger than three years of age who have persistent middle-ear effusion within the duration of effusion that we studied, prompt insertion of tympanostomy tubes does not improve developmental outcomes at six years of age.

▶ This article is a wonderful follow-up, and an extremely important one, to earlier studies that have shown that, at 3 to 4 years of age, the insertion of tympanostomy tubes conveys no particular benefit on developmental outcomes when these children are looked at a somewhat older age. The authors found no significant differences in developmental outcome scores favoring early-treatment groups over delayed-treatment groups for those who had persistent fluid in the middle ear.

The findings from this article reinforce recent clinical practice guidelines from the American Academy of Family Physicians, American Academy of Otolaryngology-Head and Neck Surgery, and the American Academy of Pediatrics, all of which recommend that otherwise healthy children with persistent otitis media with effusion, instead of undergoing tube insertion, should be re-examined at 3- to 6-month intervals until the effusion is no longer present, significant hearing loss is identified, or structural abnormalities of the eardrum or middle ear are suspected.[1] Thus, it is that simple persistent effusion does not equal tube placement as a matter of routine.

Please note, however, that the authors of this article are very careful to point out that the findings from their study cannot be generalized (1) to children who are not otherwise healthy or who have handicapping conditions such as sensorineural hearing loss, cleft palate, or Down syndrome, (2) to children with periods of effusion lasting longer than the children who were involved in this study, or (3) to children whose effusion is consistently accompanied by moderately severe (rather than the more usual mild to moderate) hearing loss.

Thus, we should all accept that the data are clear: the insertion of tympanostomy tubes for persistent otitis media with effusion in the first year of life should, in fact, not be a matter of routine. This procedure does not improve developmental outcomes of children when studied at varying ages. Given the fact that placement of such tubes is not without risk, there just does not seem to be any reason for performing this procedure any longer if the indication has been solely for persistence of fluid without other complicating factors.

J. A. Stockman III, MD

Reference

1. The American Academy of Family Physicians, American Academy of Otolaryngology-Head and Neck Surgery, American Academy of Pediatrics Subcommittee on Otitis Media with Effusion: Otitis media with effusion. *Pediatrics* 113:1412-1429, 2004.

Hearing Thresholds and Tympanic Membrane Sequelae in Children Managed Medically or Surgically for Otitis Media With Effusion

Stenstrom R, Pless IB, Bernard P (Univ of British Columbia, Vancouver, Canada; McGill Univ, Montreal; Univ of Ottawa, Ontario, Canada)
Arch Pediatr Adolesc Med 159:1151-1156, 2005   5–16

Objective.—To determine the long-term effects of ventilation tube insertion on hearing thresholds and tympanic membrane pathologic abnormalities in children with otitis media with effusion.

Design.—Prospective cohort study.

Setting.—Tertiary care children's hospital, otorhinolaryngology and audiology service.

Participants.—Patients aged 8 to 16 years who participated in a randomized controlled trial of medical vs surgical (ventilation tube [VT]) treatment for recurrent otitis media with effusion at ages 2.5 to 7 years.

Main Outcome Measures.—Hearing thresholds and tympanic membrane sequelae.

Methods.—One hundred thirteen of 125 children who had participated in the trial underwent blinded audiometric, tympanometric, otomicroscopic, and parental questionnaire evaluation 6 to 10 years following the trial. Thirty of 56 medical subjects received ventilation tubes and 18 of 57 VT subjects received more than 1 set of tubes. To evaluate sequelae risk associated with ventilation tubes independent of disease severity, we compared 27 medical subjects who never received ventilation tubes and 38 subjects randomized to VT who only received 1 set of tubes.

Results.—Tympanic membrane pathologic abnormalities were present in 81% of VT subjects and 19% of medical subjects (relative risk, 4.4; 95% confidence interval, 2.2-9.9). Hearing thresholds were 2.1 to 8.1 dB higher in subjects treated with tubes ($P = .005$).

Conclusions.—In children who were candidates for ventilation tube insertion randomly assigned to receive medical or VT treatment for otitis media with effusion, elevated hearing thresholds and tympanic membrane pathologic abnormalities were more common in VT subjects 6 to 10 years after insertion.

▶ The shine, at least a bit, seems to have gone off the insertion of VTs for the treatment of chronic and recurrent otitis media with effusion (OME). The authors of this article point out that as many as 700,000 children annually still undergo myringotomy and the insertion of VTs for the management of OME in the United States.

Stenstrom et al significantly add to our understanding of the long-term adverse effects of VTs for OME. This Canadian study looked at youngsters 6 to 9 years after tube placement and found some very interesting results. The study found that children who had received VTs had higher average mean hearing thresholds at all of the threshold frequencies tested and had a relative risk of having a hearing threshold greater than 15 dB that was 3.3 times greater than in those who were medically treated. These findings are consistent with other articles that show that surgical VT insertion is associated with more future tympanic membrane pathologic abnormalities and elevated hearing thresholds. It is likely that these effects are additive to the age-related sensorineural hearing loss and noise-induced hearing loss that we all experience over time as we age.

The American Academy of Pediatrics' recommendations for VT placement include the following indications: when OME has lasted for 4 months or longer with persistent hearing loss or other signs and symptoms, if OME is recurrent or persistent in children at risk regardless of hearing status, and if OME has caused structural damage to the tympanic membrane.[1] One might think that this is an overly generous set of recommendations in light of the knowledge that we have gained in recent years about the long-term sequelae of VT placement.

For full airing of the pros and cons of VT placement for OME, see the superb editorial by Berman.[2]

J. A. Stockman III, MD

References

1. American Academy of Family Physicians; American Academy of Otolaryngology, Head and Neck Surgery; American Academy of Pediatrics Subcommittee on Otitis Media with Effusion: Clinical practice guidelines: Otitis media with effusion. *Pediatrics* 113:1412-1429, 2004.
2. Berman S: Long-term sequelae of ventilating tubes. Implications for management of otitis media with effusion. *Arch Pediatr Adolesc Med* 159:1183-1185, 2005.

Bacterial Meningitis Among Children With Cochlear Implants Beyond 24 Months After Implantation

Biernath KR, Reefhuis J, Whitney CG, et al (Centers for Disease Control and Prevention, Atlanta, Ga; Food and Drug Administration, Rockville, Md)
Pediatrics 117:284-289, 2006   5–17

Background.—More than 11 000 children in the United States with severe-to-profound hearing loss have cochlear implants. A 2002 investigation involving pediatric cochlear implant recipients identified meningitis episodes from January 1, 1997, through September 15, 2002. The incidence of pneumococcal meningitis in the cohort was 138.2 cases per 100 000 person-years, >30 times higher than that for children in the general US population. Children with implants with positioners were at higher risk than children with other implant models. This higher risk of bacterial meningitis continued for up to 24 months after implantation.

Objective.—To evaluate additional reported cases to determine whether the increased rate of bacterial meningitis among children with cochlear implants extended beyond 24 months after implantation.

Methods.—Our study population consisted of the cohort of children identified through the 2002 investigation; it included 4265 children who received cochlear implants in the United States between January 1, 1997, and August 6, 2002, and who were <6 years of age at the time of implantation. We calculated updated incidence rates and incidence according to time since implantation.

Results.—We identified 12 new episodes of meningitis for 12 children. Eleven of the children had implants with positioners; 2 children died. Six episodes occurred >24 months after implantation. When cases identified in the 2002 and 2004 investigations were combined, the incidence rate of ≥24-months postimplantation bacterial meningitis among children with positioners was 450 cases per 100 000 person-years, compared with no cases among children without positioners.

Conclusions.—Our updated findings support continued monitoring and prompt treatment of bacterial infections by health care providers and parents of children with cochlear implants. This vigilance remains important beyond 2 years after implantation, particularly among children with positioners. The vaccination recommendations for all children with implants, with and without positioners, and all potential recipients of implants continue to apply.

▶ Children with severe-to-profound hearing loss more and more frequently are undergoing cochlear implant procedures. It is estimated that more than 11,000 children in the United States have had such a surgery, which involves the placement of an electrode that is inserted into the cochlea. It was in 2002 that the US Food and Drug Administration first received reports of bacterial meningitis among children and adults who had undergone a cochlear implant procedure. In an investigation that identified meningitis episodes from early 1997 through late 2002, it was observed that the incidence of pneumococcal meningitis in those receiving cochlear implants was 30 times higher than in the US population. These were mostly children.[1] The children at highest risk were those who had implants with a positioner. A positioner is a small Silastic wedge inserted next to the implanted electrode in certain earlier device models, to facilitate transmission of electrical signals by pushing the electrode against the medial wall of the cochlea. These positioner models were available from 1999 through July 2002, at which time they were voluntarily removed from the market by the manufacturer. The 2002 investigation found that the rate of bacterial meningitis decreased rapidly in the first few months after implantation for children with the cochlear implants that did not include positioner placement.

What we see in this report is a continued high rate of meningitis among children with cochlear implants who received these during the era in which positioners were being used. The rate of pneumococcal meningitis among children with implants with positioners 24 to 47 months after implantation was 214 cases per 100,000 person-years, compared with the rate among children aged 24 to 59 months in the general population of just 0.3 cases per 100,000 population. While a more accurate comparison would be the incidence of bacterial meningitis in the population of deaf or hard-of-hearing children without cochlear implants, such data are currently unavailable.

One of the current puzzles regarding cochlear implants is whether those who had these placed with a positioner should have the positioner removed. At the time of publication of the first results from the 2002 study looking at the rates of meningitis, explantation (removal) of the positioner was not recommended as a means of preventing meningitis. If the increased risk of meningitis stems from cochlear trauma produced by the positioner, then the potential benefit of elective removal is not entirely clear. Furthermore, the meningitis risk associated with reopening the cochleostomy and adequately resealing the void created by the positioner at the cochleostomy site must be considered in any decision related to elective removal of the positioner. In fact, one child who underwent removal of a positioner developed meningitis 40 days after the surgical procedure.

So what does all this mean for pediatricians? Clearly, those children for whom we provide care who had a cochlear implant before 2002 remain at a somewhat increased risk of meningitis. We also must be vigilant about those who have had surgical procedures since that time. The authors of this article suggest continued vigilance for symptoms of meningitis, as well as acute otitis media, by health care providers and parents of all children with cochlear implants. This vigilance is important, particularly during the 2-year period after implantation and even for a longer period after implantation if the implant procedure used a positioner. Clearly, all children who have received a cochlear implant should have received the benefits of both the pneumococcal and *Haemophilus influenzae* type b vaccinations. These recommendations should be taken quite seriously.

J. A. Stockman III, MD

Reference

1. Reefhuis J, Honein MA, Whitney CG, et al: Risk of bacterial meningitis in children with cochlear implants. *N Engl J Med* 349:435-445, 2003.

Universal Newborn Screening for Permanent Childhood Hearing Impairment: An 8-Year Follow-up of a Controlled Trial

Kennedy C, McCann D, Campbell MJ, et al (Univ of Southampton, England; Univ of Sheffield, England; MRC Inst of Hearing Research, Southampton, England)
Lancet 366:660-662, 2005   5-18

Background.—Bilateral permanent childhood hearing impairment (PCHI) of 40 decibels (dB) or more hearing level that is congenital, or not known to be acquired, affects 112 per 100,000 population. Less than half of the cases occur in children at high risk. The benefits of universal newborn screening have been disputed, but preliminary evidence has suggested that enrollment in an intervention program before 8 months of age could reduce the resulting deficit of verbal relative to nonverbal intelligence quotient by up to 19 months. The findings of an 8-year follow-up study of the birth cohort of babies enrolled in the Wessex controlled trial of universal newborn screening for PCHI are described. Whether universal newborn screening would increase the proportion of all true cases of PCHI in children ages 7 to 9 years who are enrolled early was established.

Methods.—All infants born in 4 participating hospitals between October 1, 1993 and October 31, 1996 were included. Screening of all infants for hearing impairment at 7 to 8 months of age with the distraction test continued throughout the trial. Over 10 years, a series of visits were conducted, and the investigators received regular updates from the 4 local audiology services participating in the study.

Results.—There were 53,781 live births in the 4 participating hospitals in the 3 years of the study. Of these, 25,609 were born during periods of universal screening, and 83% of these newborns received screening. Of those who received screening, 392 (2%) screened positive. In September 2003, 66 children with bilateral PCHI of 40 dB or more were identified from the trial birth cohort. Seven children with an early diagnosis were reported as having progressed in severity since the time of their first assessment. Of 31 cases of PCHI in September 2003, among children born during periods with universal newborn screening, a positive screening with universal screening was confirmed in 22 patients (71%). Of 35 children with PCHI in September 2003 who were born in periods without universal screening, 12 (34%) were referred after failing the distraction test screen, and 6 (17%) had false-negative findings and had passed the distraction test screen. The 2-stage method of universal newborn screening appeared to be effective in increasing the percentage of all cases of bilateral PCHI of 40 dB or greater in children ages 7 to 9 years referred for hearing assessment before age 6 months from 31% to 74%.

Conclusions.—These findings are the strongest evidence to date for the added benefit of universal newborn screening in the early detection of PCHI.

▶ This article provides a timely follow-up to the 1993-1996 Wessex birth cohort trial, which evaluated the effectiveness of neonatal hearing screening for detecting deafness in babies compared with the effectiveness of detecting deafness at a later date in Great Britain. Clearly, the data favor newborn screening. Unfortunately, at least in that country, it is obvious that, despite the big increase achieved by early identification of deaf infants, the management (usually involving the fitting of hearing aids and the start of early intervention) is not occurring in roughly half the cases until a baby is 18 months of age or older. Hopefully, the dismal snapshot from almost 10 years ago has improved.

The concern of any neonatal screening program is the substantial number of deaf babies who "pass" neonatal screening but who emerge later on and might be given a diagnosis very late because of a false sense of security generated in their families and their care providers by the apparently normal neonatal screening result. No neonatal screening program is perfect. Are false-negatives due to a problem in the instrumentation or the screener? Is deafness possibly acquired after the screen? The article by Kennedy et al looked at these issues and found that about one quarter of deafness that is undetected in neonatal screening programs turns out to be the result of acquired hearing loss.

Why do substantial numbers of children subsequently have hearing loss in childhood after neonatal screening results have been normal? It has been suggested that major causes contributing to this, other than middle ear infections, are intrauterine infection with cytomegalovirus, inner ear malformations, such as large vestibular aqueduct syndrome, and genetic hearing losses that become progressive with time.

To read more about neonatal hearing screens, their strengths, and weaknesses, see the excellent review by Mutton and Peacock.[1]

J. A. Stockman III, MD

Reference

1. Mutton P, Peacock K: Neonatal hearing screens: Wessex re-visited. *Lancet* 366:612-613, 2005.

A Multicenter Evaluation of How Many Infants With Permanent Hearing Loss Pass a Two-Stage Otoacoustic Emissions/Automated Auditory Brainstem Response Newborn Hearing Screening Protocol

Johnson JL, White KR, Widen JE, et al (Univ of Hawaii, Honolulu; Utah State Univ, Logan; Univ of Kansas, Kansas City; et al)
Pediatrics 116:663-672, 2005   5-19

Objective.—Ninety percent of all newborns in the United States are now screened for hearing loss before they leave the hospital. Many hospitals use a 2-stage protocol for newborn hearing screening in which all infants are screened first with otoacoustic emissions (OAE). No additional testing is done with infants who pass the OAE, but infants who fail the OAE next are screened with automated auditory brainstem response (A-ABR). Infants who fail the A-ABR screening are referred for diagnostic testing to determine whether they have permanent hearing loss (PHL). Those who pass the A-ABR are considered at low risk for hearing loss and are not tested further. The objective of this multicenter study was to determine whether a substantial number of infants who fail the initial OAE and pass the A-ABR have PHL at approximately 9 months of age.

Methods.—Seven birthing centers with successful newborn hearing screening programs using a 2-stage OAE/A-ABR screening protocol participated. During the study period, 86,634 infants were screened for hearing loss at these sites. Of those infants who failed the OAE but passed the A-ABR in at least 1 ear, 1524 were enrolled in the study. Data about prenatal, neonatal, and socioeconomic factors, plus hearing loss risk indicators, were collected for all enrolled infants. When the infants were an average of 9.7 months of age, diagnostic audiologic evaluations were done for 64% of the enrolled infants (1432 ears from 973 infants).

Results.—Twenty-one infants (30 ears) who had failed the OAE but passed the A-ABR during the newborn hearing screening were identified with permanent bilateral or unilateral hearing loss. Twenty-three (77%) of the ears had mild hearing loss (average of 1 kHz, 2 kHz, and 4 kHz ≤40-decibel hearing level). Nine (43%) infants had bilateral as opposed to unilateral loss, and 18 (86%) infants had sensorineural as opposed to permanent conductive hearing loss.

Conclusions.—If all infants were screened for hearing loss using the 2-stage OAE/A-ABR newborn hearing screening protocol currently used in many hospitals, then ~23% of those with PHL at ~9 months of age would have passed the A-ABR. This happens in part because much of the A-ABR screening equipment in current use was designed to identify infants with moderate or greater hearing loss. Thus, program administrators should be certain that the screening program, equipment, and protocols are designed to identify the type of hearing loss targeted by their program. The results also show the need for continued surveillance of hearing status during childhood.

▶ In a short 10-year period, the percentage of infants here in the United States who have undergone neonatal hearing screening has increased from less than 5% to over 90%. The major breakthrough in this regard came with the application of the revolutionary work of Dr David Kemp and the development of the OAE technology that could be applied to screening of hearing in infants, and the development of automated procedures and equipment to do ABR testing. It took Surgeon General C. Everett Koop, however, to set the challenge that by the year 2000, 90% of all infants with significant hearing loss would be identified within the first year of life, and most of these, hopefully, at birth.

The first demonstration of the adequacy of the technology for newborn hearing screening came with a project begun in 1989, a large-scale newborn hearing screening program that showed that 6 per 1000 infants were being identified with congenital hearing loss. By March 1993, the NIH held a consensus conference about early identification of hearing loss and recommended that all infants be screened for hearing loss during the first 6 months of life using a 2-stage screening protocol. This report stated that the preferred model for screening should begin with an evoked OAE test and should be followed by an ABR test for all infants who fail the evoked OAE test.[1] This recommendation was later modified to say that universal detection of hearing loss should be performed by no later than 3 months of age, with interventions beginning by no later than 6 months of age. Within 2 years, it became obvious that the way to do this screening would be in the nursery setting. Automated equipment was developed for this purpose, allowing virtually 100% of infants to be checked before discharge.

The report of Johnson et al adds further insights into the value, and limitations, of newborn hearing programs. Some infants, particularly those with mild hearing loss, may be missed by 1 part of the 2-stage screening test. For this reason, screening for PHL should be extended into early childhood. Likely settings for this screening include physicians' offices and early childhood programs. Such additional hearing screening is important because even a perfect newborn hearing screening program will never uncover late-onset PHL or identify fluctuating hearing loss caused by otitis media. In addition, mild cases of PHL can be missed in the nursery. For this reason, it is critically important to continue to emphasize to families and physicians that passing a hospital-based hearing screening test does not eliminate the need to monitor systematically and consistently language development and to conduct additional hearing screening. This report also reminds us that it is important for hearing screening programs to use equipment that is designed specifically for the level of hearing loss targeted for identification by the program. Programs that aim to identify infants with mild and unilateral hearing loss must use different stimulus levels (which may require different equipment) than they would use if their aim was to identify only moderate or greater hearing loss.

Just because we are now able to pick up most cases of congenital PHL, we should not lower our guard with respect to cases that are missed, or hearing loss that is acquired during infancy. Delayed language development is usually the tip-off to a significant problem, and a hearing test should be part of the early evaluation of any child with delayed speech.

See the report that follows by Halloran et al (Abstract 5–20), who tell us how good (or unfortunately bad) we are as pediatric care providers in following up on hearing screening tests.

J. A. Stockman III, MD

Reference

1. Early identification of hearing impairment in infants and young children. *NIH Consens Statement* 11:1-24, 1993.

Hearing Screening at Well-Child Visits
Halloran DR, Wall TC, Evans HH, et al (Univ of Alabama, Birmingham; Univ of Alabama at Tuscaloosa)
Arch Pediatr Adolesc Med 159:949-955, 2005   5–20

Objectives.—To determine hearing screening failure rates in primary care settings and to examine the referral practices in response to an abnormal screening test.

Methods.—We enrolled a convenience sample of children between 3 and 19 years of age who were undergoing hearing screening during a well-child visit. A failure was defined as missing any frequency (1000, 2000, or 4000 Hz) in either ear at 20-dB hearing level. The pediatrician made the decision of whether to refer the patient for further evaluation.

Results.—Three academic and 5 private practices enrolled 1061 children. Sixty-seven children (7%) were unable to complete the screening. Of the 948 children who completed the screen, a total of 852 children (90%) passed the screening and 96 children (10%) failed. After multivariable logistic regression analysis, the only statistically significant factor predictive of a failed screen was developmental delay ($P = .02$). Of the 96 children who failed the hearing screening, 57 (59%) had no further evaluation, 12 (13%) were rechecked, and 27 (28%) were referred. Similar percentages were seen with children who could not be screened.

Conclusions.—Although 10% of the children failed hearing screening, pediatricians neither rechecked nor referred more than half of these children. Screening that does not result in action for those failing the screening wastes resources and fails to properly identify hearing impairment in children.

▶ The Joint Commission on Infant Hearing not only advocates universal newborn screening, but also recommends periodic hearing screening throughout childhood as an important means of detecting acquired hearing loss as well as congenital cases missed by inadequate or inaccurate newborn screening.[1] At a minimum, the American Academy of Pediatrics advocates hearing screening at 4, 5, and 6 years of age as well as at 8, 10, 12, 15, and 18 years of age, regardless of the presence or absence of risk factors for hearing loss.[2] Earlier recommendations had indicated that hearing screening should be done for

3-year-old children, but current standards have changed to periodic screening to begin at 4 years of age.

The study from Alabama examined outcomes of hearing screening in children in pediatric practices. Unfortunately, almost 60% of children with abnormal hearing screening tests received no further evaluation. This is like the compulsive person who checks the air in his tires, but has no means to ever inflate the ones that do not come up to snuff.

We need to determine why pediatricians do not always act on the information they are provided when they order tests. Recommendations on follow-up are clearly stated by the American Academy of Pediatrics.[3]

This is the final commentary in the Dentistry and Otolaryngology chapter, which has contained much information having to do with the ears. We close with 2 questions: (1) have you ever wondered why some have ear wax that is dry and others have moist sticky ear wax and (2) if you have to have your ears pierced, what is the best age to do so?

The answers to these questions are as follows: Whether your ear wax is wet or dry seems to depend on your genes. The dry variety is found more commonly in East Asian populations and the wet stuff is more common in African and European populations. We also know why this is true. The gene responsible for determining ear wax type is known as ABCC11, which was identified by examining a Japanese population with both types of ear wax.[4]

As far as when to have your ears pierced, it may be better to do so before the age of 11 than after the age of 11, particularly if you have a family history of keloids. In a study of patients with keloids resulting from ear piercing, 80% of the 17 who had their ears pierced after the age of 11 developed keloids, compared with 24% of the 15 who had ear piercings before the age of 11.[5] Some facts never fail to amaze!

J. A. Stockman III, MD

References

1. Joint Commission on Infant Hearing, American Academy of Audiology, American Academy of Pediatrics, American Speech-Language Hearing Association, Directors of Speech and Hearing Programs in State Health and Welfare Agencies: Year 2000 position statement: Principles and guidelines for early hearing detection and intervention programs. *Pediatrics* 106:798-817, 2000.
2. American Academy of Pediatrics, Committee on Practice and Ambulatory Medicine: Recommendations for preventive pediatric health care. *Pediatrics* 105:645-646, 2000.
3. Cunningham M, Cox EO, Committee on Practice and Ambulatory Medicine and the Section on Otolaryngology and Bronchoesophagology: Hearing assessment in infants and children: Recommendations beyond neonatal screening. *Pediatrics* 111:436-440, 2003.
4. Yoshiura K, Kinoshita A, Ishida T, et al: A SNP in the ABCC11 gene is the determinant of human earwax type. *Nat Genet* 38:324-330, 2006.
5. Lane JE, Waller JL, Davis LS: Relationship between age of ear piercing and keloid formation. *Pediatrics* 115:1312-1314, 2005.

6 Endocrinology

Microalbuminuria and Abnormal Ambulatory Blood Pressure in Adolescents With Type 2 Diabetes Mellitus
Ettinger LM, Freeman K, DiMartino-Nardi JR, et al (Children's Hosp at Montefiore, Bronx, NY; Albert Einstein College of Medicine, Bronx, NY; Montefiore Med Ctr, Bronx, NY)
J Pediatr 147:67-73, 2005   6–1

Objective.—To determine whether risk factors for cardiovascular disease and diabetic nephropathy, as evidenced by abnormalities of ambulatory blood pressure (ABP), dyslipidemia, and microalbuminuria (MA), are present in adolescents with type 2 diabetes mellitus (T2DM).

Study Design.—We enrolled 26 minority adolescents recently diagnosed with T2DM and 13 obese control subjects without diabetes mellitus. ABP monitoring was performed, and a 24-hour urine, a fasting lipid profile, blood urea nitrogen, creatinine, homocysteine, and hemoglobin A_1c levels were obtained. The patients with T2DM underwent echocardiograms.

Results.—Forty percent of the patients with T2DM had MA ($\geq$30 mg of microalbumin/day), compared with none of the control subjects ($P < .05$). There were no significant differences between patients with T2DM who had MA and patients with T2DM who didn't have MA in demographics, characteristics, casual BP, echocardiographic findings, and hemoglobin A_1c levels. Average daytime systolic BP was greater in patients with T2DM with MA than patients without MA (129 versus 121 mm Hg, $P = .03$) and compared with the control subjects (113 mm Hg, $P = .01$). Patients with MA had an average daytime systolic BP load that was higher than patients without MA (37.1 versus 5.1%, $P = .008$) and compared with the control subjects (2.6%, $P < .001$).

Conclusion.—As in adults, adolescents with T2DM exhibit abnormalities of ABP, dyslipidemia, and microalbuminuria.

▶ This article is from a children's service in a hospital in New York City, where the number of children in whom T2DM has been diagnosed has increased some 10-fold in a recent 10-year period. This rise is directly correlated with the changing prevalence of obesity. As bad as this problem is, we now learn that childhood T2DM is associated with the presence of MA and abnormalities in ABP monitoring, both of which are harbingers of doom if the underlying source of the problem is not dealt with in a relatively quick and systematic manner.

The MA presumably relates to renal hyperfiltration, which is an early functional renal change in patients with diabetes. Hyperfiltration causes structural changes leading to MA, which is followed by proteinuria, then renal insufficiency, and, finally, end-stage renal disease. Renal hyperfiltration is seen in 30% to 40% of patients with newly diagnosed T2DM. In this article, 40% of young patients with diabetes already had MA, which suggests that they may be on the pathway of the continuum to frank nephropathy. High blood pressure only complicates this pathophysiology.

The authors of this article previously studied what happens to children with a diagnosis of T2DM when followed up 15 years into the course of their disease. Of 79 children who were recontacted a decade and a half after the diagnosis of T2DM, 9% had already died. Some 6.3% were currently receiving dialysis, and 38% of subsequent pregnancies of these diabetic patients were lost.[1]

What we have learned in the last year or two about obesity in children is chilling. Obesity is more than simply a matter of putting on a few more pounds. One can develop serious liver disease. When type 2 diabetes occurs, it can quickly lead to compromised renal functioning and even death in young adulthood. This is, indeed, serious stuff.

We need to look for ways to minimize the prevalence of diabetes. Improvements in fitness, body composition and insulin sensitivity have been observed in overweight children who engage in school-based exercise programs.[2] Even something as simple as breast feeding seems to lower the incidence of type 2 diabetes. For example, in the Nurses Health Study, some 5145 cases of type 2 diabetes were diagnosed among approximately 1.2 million person years of follow up between 1986 and 2002. Women in that study who breast fed for extended periods of time had a significantly reduced risk of type 2 diabetes. Each 12-month period of lactation reduced the risk of diabetes by some 15%! Follow up is now being done to see if in this study breast feeding also reduced the risk of diabetes in the offspring.[3]

J. A. Stockman III, MD

References

1. Dean H, Flett V: Natural history of the type 2 diabetes diagnosed in childhood: Long-term followup in young adults. *Diabetes* 51:24A, 2002.
2. Carrel AL, Clark RR, Peterson SE, et al: Improvement of fitness, body composition and insulin sensitivity in overweight children in a school-based exercise program. *Arch Pediatr Adolesc Med* 159:963-967, 2005.
3. Stuebe AM, Rich-Edwards JW, Willett WC, et al: Duration of lactation in incidence of type 2 diabetes. *JAMA* 294:2601-2610, 2005.

Insulin Needs After CD3-Antibody Therapy in New-Onset Type 1 Diabetes
Keymeulen B, Vandemeulbroucke E, Ziegler AG, et al (Brussels Free Univ-VUB, Belgium; Hosp München-Schwabing, Munich; Katholieke Universiteit Leuven, Belgium; et al)
N Engl J Med 352:2598-2608, 2005   6–2

Background.—Type 1 diabetes mellitus is a T-cell–mediated autoimmune disease that leads to a major loss of insulin-secreting beta cells. The further decline of beta-cell function after clinical onset might be prevented by treatment with CD3 monoclonal antibodies, as suggested by the results of a phase 1 study. To provide proof of this therapeutic principle at the metabolic level, we initiated a phase 2 placebo-controlled trial with a humanized antibody, an aglycosylated human IgG1 antibody directed against CD3 (ChAglyCD3).

Methods.—In a multicenter study, 80 patients with new-onset type 1 diabetes were randomly assigned to receive placebo or ChAglyCD3 for six consecutive days. Patients were followed for 18 months, during which their daily insulin needs and residual beta-cell function were assessed according to glucose-clamp–induced C-peptide release before and after the administration of glucagon.

Results.—At 6, 12, and 18 months, residual beta-cell function was better maintained with ChAglyCD3 than with placebo. The insulin dose increased in the placebo group but not in the ChAglyCD3 group. This effect of ChAglyCD3 was most pronounced among patients with initial residual beta-cell function at or above the 50th percentile of the 80 patients. In this subgroup, the mean insulin dose at 18 months was 0.22 IU per kilogram of body weight per day with ChAglyCD3, as compared with 0.61 IU per kilogram with placebo (P<0.001). In this subgroup, 12 of 16 patients who received ChAglyCD3 (75 percent) received minimal doses of insulin (≤0.25 IU per kilogram per day) as compared with none of the 21 patients who received placebo. Administration of ChAglyCD3 was associated with a moderate "flu-like" syndrome and transient symptoms of Epstein–Barr viral mononucleosis.

Conclusions.—Short-term treatment with CD3 antibody preserves residual beta-cell function for at least 18 months in patients with recent-onset type 1 diabetes.

▶ No one any longer questions the fact that type 1 diabetes mellitus begins as an autoimmune process. As an autoimmune process, one might think rather simplistically that it would be possible to interfere in some way with the progression of the disease by applying principles that we have learned from other disorders that are manageable with immunosuppressants. As pointed out in a commentary by Lernmark,[1] the development of type 1 diabetes is actually a 2-step process. In the first step, presumed environmental triggers cause the destruction of beta cells. It is assumed that pancreatic antigen-presenting cells engulf dead beta cells. The antigen-presenting cells are thought to migrate to lymph nodes that drain the pancreas and in which islet-beta-cell–

specific antigen presentation takes place. A variety of T lymphocytes recognize beta-cell peptides, which initiate an islet autoimmune reaction. Islet cell autoimmunity is best detected with the use of standardized tests for autoantibodies to insulin. These autoantibodies sometimes present for more than a decade before the onset of clinical diabetes, and a number of studies have documented that they can predict type 1 diabetes. After autoantibodies have developed, there is a second step, in which genetic as well as environmental factors seem to aggravate the islet cell autoimmunity. Cytotoxic T cells are induced and lead a rapid onslaught on beta cells. High blood sugar levels ensue when 80% to 90% of beta cells have been destroyed. Sadly, the disease is more aggressive in young children, and type 1 diabetes is being diagnosed at progressively younger ages, even though the total incidence may not be increasing.

Immunosuppressive or immunomodulating agents have been used in an increasing number of clinical studies because there is growing evidence that type 1 diabetes is, indeed, an autoimmune disease. Most studies have been poorly designed or have had inadequate numbers of patients. Cyclosporine was the first immunosuppressive agent that was used in important, well-designed, placebo-controlled, double-blind clinical trials. With the use of cyclosporine, beta-cell functioning has been preserved, although rarely beyond 12 months. Unfortunately, nephrotoxicity precludes cyclosporine's routine clinical application in new-onset diabetes or in the prevention of diabetes in high-risk patients. In the article from Brussels, the supposition was that CD3 monoclonal antibodies might affect the course of autoimmune diabetes. The study clearly shows that short-term treatment with CD3 autoantibodies is capable of preserving residual beta-cell functioning for at least 18 months in patients with recent-onset diabetes. A careful reading of this article, however, shows the disclaimers. The most important is the fact that those patients who respond to monoclonal antibodies are those who have the most residual beta-cell functioning at the initiation of their diabetes. The antibody was effective only in a subgroup of patients who initially had increased residual beta-cell functioning at or above the 50% percentile. This finding, if validated, suggests that CD3 antibodies will have limited applicability because injecting the CD3 monoclonal antibody serves no purpose if the beta-cell killing has gone too far. Furthermore, a significant subset of patients did develop flu-like symptoms, which is not uncommon with the administration of monoclonal antibodies.

Provided that monoclonal antibody treatment proves to be safe (see other articles on this topic in this year's YEAR BOOK OF PEDIATRICS), it may be reasonable to consider therapy with CD3 monoclonal antibodies for patients with a genetic risk of type 1 diabetes who test positive for islet cell autoantibodies. Screening to detect such patients is carried out by the TrialNet Network (www.diabetestrialnet.org/hindex.html), sponsored by the National Institutes of Health. If CD3 monoclonal antibodies do not prove to be the magic bullet for preventing the onset of clinical diabetes, perhaps their use in combination with other immunosuppressive agents will prove more effective.

J. A. Stockman III, MD

Reference

1. Lernmark A: Type 1-diabetes: Does suppressing T-cells increase insulin? *N Engl J Med* 352:2642-2644, 2005.

The Phenotype of Short Stature Homeobox Gene (SHOX) Deficiency in Childhood: Contrasting Children With Leri-Weill Dyschondrosteosis and Turner Syndrome

Ross JK, Kowal K, Quigley CA, et al (Thomas Jefferson Univ, Philadelphia; Al duPont Hosp for Children, Wilmington, Del; Eli Lilly and Company, Indianapolis, Ind; et al)
J Pediatr 147:499-507, 2005   6–3

Objective.—To evaluate the growth disorder and phenotype in prepubertal children with Leri-Weill dyschondrosteosis (LWD), a dominantly inherited skeletal dysplasia, and to compare the findings from girls with Turner syndrome (TS).

Study Design.—We studied the auxologic and phenotypic characteristics in 34 prepubertal LWD subjects (ages 1 to 10 years; 20 girls, 14 boys) with confirmed short stature homeobox-containing gene (*SHOX*) abnormalities. For comparative purposes, we evaluated similar physical and growth parameters in 76 girls with TS (ages 1 to 19 years) and 24 girls with LWD (ages

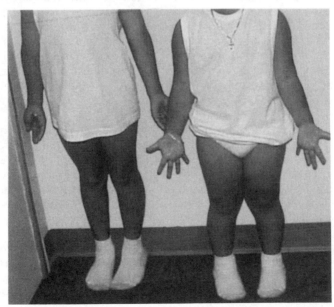

FIGURE 6.—Apparent muscle hypertrophy in a boy with LWD (**right**) compared with his unaffected older brother (**left**). (Courtesy of Ross JL, Kowal K, Quigley CA, et al: The phenotype of short stature homeobox gene (SHOX) deficiency in childhood: Contrasting children with Leri-Weill dyschondrosteosis and Turner syndrome. *J Pediatr* 147:499-507. Copyright 2005 by Elsevier.)

1 to 15 years) by using data collected from the postmarketing observational study, GeNeSIS.

Results.—In the clinic sample LWD subjects, height standard deviation score ranged from −5.5 to +0.1 (−2.3 ± 1.3, girls and −1.8 ± 0.6, boys). Wrist changes related to Madelung deformity were present in 18 of 34 (53%) LWD subjects. In comparing the LWD and TS populations in the GeNeSIS sample, Madelung deformity, increased carrying angle, and scoliosis were more prevalent in the LWD population, whereas high arched palate was similarly prevalent in the two populations.

Conclusions.—Short stature is common in both LWD (girls and boys) and TS (girls). Clinical clues to the diagnosis of SHOX haploinsufficiency in childhood include short stature, short limbs, wrist changes, and tibial bowing (Fig 6).

▶ From time to time, the YEAR BOOK OF PEDIATRICS includes reports having to do with uncommon disorders to make us more aware of such entities. One such disorder is LWD. This is a dominantly inherited skeletal dysplasia first described in 1929. The disorder affects both sexes and causes short stature, mesomelia, and wrist deformities. The presentation of the disorder is more severe in girls than in boys, likely because of sex differences and estrogen levels. The molecular basis for LWD is haploinsufficiency for the gene *SHOX* (short stature homeobox-containing gene), which is located on the distal part of the X-chromosome pseudoautosomal region. Deletions or mutations in *SHOX* have been detected in up to 100% of patients with LWD. The mutations ultimately result in a disorder that affects bone growth and development in early childhood, before the onset of puberty. It is one of the causes of short stature, and LWD should be considered in a young child with any 1 or more of the following findings: short stature, a high-arch palate, an increased upper-to-lower segment ratio for age (ie, shorter legs than trunk), a reduced arm span for age and also relative to height, an increased carrying angle of the elbow, wrist deformity, tibial bowing, and the appearance of muscular hypertrophy of the calf.

Before leaving the topic of unusual presentations of genetic disorders, what would you do, if anything, to further evaluate a 6-year-old girl you are seeing who presents with an inguinal hernia? Inguinal hernias, of course, are quite common in boys, but not so common in girls. Should you see one, you might consider a further evaluation. One study has shown that more than half of patients, for example, with complete androgen insensitivity syndrome will in fact present with inguinal hernia of which half will be bilateral and one-third will contain gonads. A survey of endocrinologists in Great Britain found that virtually all would consider the possibility of complete androgen insensitivity syndrome in any girl presenting with a hernia.[1] Girls with inguinal hernia, particularly presenting early in life, should have a sex chromosome analysis.

J. A. Stockman III, MD

Reference

1. Deeb A, Hughes IA: Inguinal hernia in a female infant: a clue to check sex chromosomes. *Brit J Urol* 96:401-403, 2005.

Multiplier Method for Prediction of Adult Height in Patients With Achondroplasia
Paley D, Matz AL, Kurland DB, et al (Sinai Hosp of Baltimore, Md)
J Pediatr Orthop 25:539-542, 2005   6–4

Abstract.—To date, the only way to predict adult height in achondroplastic dwarves has been to consult a growth chart. The purpose of this study was to ascertain whether the multiplier method of predicting adult height at skeletal maturity in healthy persons can be applied to persons with achondroplasia. Previous studies have shown that the multiplier method can be applied to lower limb length, upper limb length, total height, foot length, and foot height. It is therefore reasonable to suggest that the growth pattern for total height in achondroplastic dwarves might also be characterized by a multiplier. Total height multipliers for achondroplastic dwarves ("achondroplasia height multipliers") were calculated from two separate databases by dividing height at maturity by height at each respective age for both genders. Little variability was found among multipliers for each age and among multipliers calculated from different databases. Upper torso (sitting height) multipliers and lower limb multipliers were also derived for achondroplastic dwarves. Lower limb and total height growth rates were slower in achondroplastic dwarves compared with healthy persons. However, sitting height multipliers for achondroplastic dwarves were closely related to sitting height multipliers for healthy persons. Because these findings showed that the multiplier values were independent of population and percentile, the multiplier method may be a valid method for quickly predicting height at any age for achondroplastic dwarves.

▶ Very little has been written about growth patterns in children with achondroplasia. In fact, only 2 such studies exist,[1,2] the first of which appeared when I was a junior faculty person back in the late 1970s. The most commonly used database for achondroplastic dwarfs was compiled by Horton et al[1] in a study of 403 affected individuals. The Horton database contains total measurements for each age from birth to 18 years, presented as a mean ± 1 or 2 SD. The authors of the current article use the now 30-year-old Horton database to calculate achondroplasia height multipliers for each centile at each age by dividing height for boys and girls at skeletal maturity by the corresponding height at each year of age from birth to skeletal maturity. This converted every data point from the graphs presented by Horton et al into a multiplier (M) for height at skeletal maturity: $M = H_m/H$. This allows a fairly accurate prediction of what the adult height will be in patients with achondroplasia.

If you are not familiar with the multiplier method for prediction of adult height, it determines the length or height at skeletal maturity by the use of an age- and gender-specific coefficient multiplied by the current height or length at that age.[3] Normal growth multipliers for each percentile are the same; therefore, short and tall individuals have the same multiplier for each age. Multipliers have been found to be similar among different populations. The multiplier method is a concise way to characterize growth patterns and predict lengths and heights of normal individuals at maturity. Interestingly, multipliers are different for each anatomical location, which indicates that the growth pattern for each body segment is different. Lower limb length, upper limb length, total height, foot length, and foot height have been characterized by the multiplier method.

Height prediction in youngsters with achondroplasia is important because most of us are not familiar with what the normal growth pattern is for these youngsters. Any major discrepancy between an achondroplastic individual's growth (as is true of anyone) and normal growth should be a warning sign of infection, disease, malnutrition, or other congenital or developmental disorders. The multiplier method for predicting height in these youngsters will greatly benefit achondroplastic dwarfs and their families as well as physicians. Predicting maturity height for achondroplastic dwarfs also helps families to decide about stature-increasing methods, such as limb-lengthening procedures and growth hormone treatment. The study by Paley et al shows that the achondroplasia height multiplier is both population and percentile independent. These multipliers appear to be unique for achondroplastic dwarfs and are distinct from healthy individuals. This is largely the result of differences in long-bone growth because length multipliers for sitting height are essentially the same for achondroplastic and healthy individuals.

If you have any patients with achondroplasia in your practice, it may very well be worth your while to read this article in some detail.

J. A. Stockman III, MD

References

1. Horton WA, Rotter JI, Rimoin DL, et al: Standard growth curves for achondroplasia. *J Pediatr* 93:435-438, 1978.
2. Nehme AM, Riseborough EJ, Tredwell SJ: Scale of the growth and development of the achondroplastic dwarf. *Clin Orthop* 116:8-25, 1976.
3. Paley D, Behave A, Herzemberg JE, et al: Multiplier method for predicting limb-length discrepancy. *J Bone Joint Surg Am* 82:1432-1446, 2000.

Safety of Growth Hormone Treatment in Pediatric Patients With Idiopathic Short Stature

Quigley CA, Gill AM, Crowe BJ, et al (Eli Lilly and Co, Indianapolis, Ind; Univ of Cincinnati, Ohio; Thomas Jefferson Univ, Philadelphia; et al)
J Clin Endocrinol Metab 90:5188-5196, 2005   6–5

Context.—Recombinant human GH was approved by the United States Food and Drug Administration in 2003 for the treatment of idiopathic short stature (ISS). However, to date, the safety of GH in this patient population has not been rigorously studied.

Objective.—The objective of this study was to address the safety of GH treatment in children with ISS compared with GH safety in patient populations for which GH has been approved previously: Turner syndrome (TS) and GH deficiency (GHD).

Design/Setting.—The rates of serious adverse events (SAEs) and adverse events (AEs) of particular relevance to GH-treated populations were compared across the three patient populations among five multicenter GH registration studies.

Patients.—Children with ISS, TS, or GHD were studied.

Intervention.—Treatment consisted of GH doses ranging from 0.18–0.37 mg/kg·wk.

Main Outcome Measures.—The main outcome measures were rates of SAEs and AEs of special relevance to patients receiving GH. Laboratory measures of carbohydrate metabolism were used as outcome measures for the ISS studies.

Results.—Within the ISS studies, comprising one double-blind, placebo-controlled study and one open-label, dose-response study, SAEs (mainly hospitalizations for accidental injury or acute illness unrelated to GH exposure) were reported for 13–14% of GH-treated patients. Overall AE rates (serious and nonserious) as well as rates of potentially GH-related AEs were similar in the GHD, TS, and ISS studies (for ISS studies combined: otitis media, 8%; scoliosis, 3%; hypothyroidism, 0.7%; changes in carbohydrate metabolism, 0.7%; hypertension, 0.4%). Measures of carbohydrate metabolism were not affected by GH treatment in patients with ISS. There was no significant GH effect on fasting blood glucose in either study (GH dose range, 0.22–0.37 mg/kg·wk) or on insulin sensitivity (placebo-controlled study only).

Conclusion.—GH appears safe in ISS; however, the studies were not powered to assess the frequency of rare GH-related events, and longer-term follow-up studies of GH-treated patients with ISS are warranted.

▶ Thus it is that growth hormone treatments are probably safe. To date, there seems to be virtually no evidence that such treatments are unsafe. Just because something is safe, however, does not mean that it should be used. This is discussed in detail by Gill in a review of the use of growth hormone.[1] Most pediatricians entered our field of medicine in order to make children better, but does making small normal children bigger also make them better? Gill points out that this is the fundamental and simplistic question underpinning the use of growth hormone in "idiopathic" short stature. He also notes that some simple truisms about growth are worth stating. Most children, especially boys, would like to be bigger than they are. Being bigger is perceived as being stronger, better, more successful. Tallness often leads to success in sports. Is the opposite true, however? Is short stature a disability? What is the evidence for the hypothesis that "bigger is better"? Do any of the studies performed to date truly show that making children bigger makes them truly happier?

Without answers to these types of questions, it seems hard to understand what the cost effective benefit is of growth hormone for children with idiopathic short stature. A recent report by Lee et al tells us that in order to grow an inch, you will have to buy $52,634 worth of growth hormone with a maximum growth benefit peaking at 1.9 inches for the average treatment ($99,959 per treatment).[2] The latter is about the cost of college tuition for a 4-year university these days, not that someone with deep pockets could not be both educated and 2 inches taller. Nonetheless, very little else in this world has a price tag so high per millimeter.

J. A. Stockman III, MD

References

1. Gill DG: "Anything you can do, I can do bigger?": The ethics and equity of growth hormone for small children. *Arch Dis Child* 91:270-272, 2006.
2. Lee JM, Davis MM, Clark SJ, et al: Estimated cost-effectiveness of growth hormone therapy for idiopathic short stature. *Arch Pediatr Adolesc Med* 160:263-269, 2006.

Efficacy and Safety Results of Long-term Growth Hormone Treatment of Idiopathic Short Stature

Kemp SF, Kuntze J, Attie KM, et al (Univ of Arkansas, Little Rock; Burfordville, Mo; Rio de Janeiro, Brazil; et al)
J Clin Endocrinol Metab 90:5247-5253, 2005   6–6

Context.—Small clinical trials of GH treatment of idiopathic short stature (ISS) show variable efficacy.

Objective.—The study was an analysis of a large GH registry for efficacy and safety of GH treatment of ISS. There was also a comparison with a specific clinical trial.

Design.—Up to 7 yr of GH treatment of ISS was evaluated for efficacy and safety in the National Cooperative Growth Study (NCGS).

Setting.—The NCGS study was conducted at Genentech, Inc. and included 47,226 patients.

Patients.—The ISS group included maximum stimulated GH 10 ng/ml or more and/or a report of ISS by investigator (n = 8018; all included for safety). Cohort 1 (n = 2520) was similar to the clinical trial, cohort 2 (n = 283) included subjects younger than 5 yr of age, and cohort 3 (n = 940) was pubertal at GH start.

Intervention.—GH, approximately 0.30 mg/kg·wk, was given.

Main Outcome Measures.—These included growth velocities and height SD (HtSDS).

Results.—Mean first-year growth velocities in cohorts 1, 2, and 3 increased 4.6, 3.9, and 4.4 cm/yr over pretreatment, respectively. Measures included: baseline mean HtSDS, −2.9, −3.2, and −2.8; mean HtSDS at 1 yr, −2.4, −2.3, and −2.3, respectively. Mean HtSDS after 7 yr in cohorts 1 (n = 303) and 2 (n = 85) and 5 yr in cohort 3 (n = 58) were: −1.2, −1.0, and −1.5, respectively. Cohort 3 shorter treatment time was due to advanced baseline age (mean 13.8 yr) and puberty. Mean HtSDS gain in cohort 1 was comparable with the clinical trial. No new safety signals specific to the NCGS ISS population were observed.

Conclusion.—ISS patients in the GH registry demonstrate a significant increase in HtSDS with the safety profile similar to GH-deficient patients. Results were similar to the clinical trial.

▶ Recombinant human GH was first approved by the US Food and Drug Administration in 1985. This approval was for children with growth failure due to GH deficiency. Since then, GH has been approved for children with short stature or growth failure in 5 other disorders that are generally not associated with deficiency of endogenous GH production: chronic renal insufficiency, Turner syndrome, Prader-Willi syndrome, small-for-gestational-age birth, and, most recently, ISS or non–growth hormone–deficient short stature. Since its initial Food and Drug Administration approval, an estimated 200,000 individuals have been managed with GH therapy, representing more than half a million patient-years of exposure. Thus, ample time has evolved to accumulate a set of adverse effects that result from the use of GH. These have ranged from relatively common minor problems such as edema and injection site reactions to more significant but, fortunately, rare events such as benign intracranial hypertension and slipped capital femoral epiphysis. In general, however, GH has been considered to be safe.

Safety is always a relative issue, no matter how "safe" a therapy may be. Risks must be weighed against benefits. Thus, even small risks when the indications for treatment are so-so mean that the relative benefit to risk ratio may be marginal in certain circumstances. This has been a concern with GH for the treatment of ISS. About 9000 patients have been treated in this way, representing about 27,000 patient years of GH exposure. To date, overall adverse reaction rates for these patients have been similar to or, in some cases, lower than those for patients with other GH-treated conditions. The current article and one other (see Abstract 6–5) have recently examined the safety of GH therapy using data from national registries. In the study abstracted here, the registry used was the NCGS. This is a North American, multicenter, postmarketing surveillance study established in 1985. It is designed to follow-up the use, safety, and effectiveness of recombinant DNA biosynthetic GH. The present article demonstrates a safety profile for GH treatment in patients with ISS similar to that seen in clinical trials of similar duration in patients with GH deficiency or Turner syndrome, both of which are disorders for which synthetic GH has been used for more than 20 years. Specifically, rates of otitis media, scoliosis, slipped capital femoral epiphysis, hypothyroidism, disturbances of carbohydrate metabolism, and hypertension in patients were similar to or lower than the rates of these conditions in patients with GH deficiency or Turner syndrome, and no case of benign intracranial hypertension, edema, pancreatitis, or prepubertal gynecomastia has been reported in youngsters treated for ISS.

All of this is good news when it come to the benefit–risk ratio for children with ISS who are being treated with synthetic GH. Unlike some children with other forms of non–GH short stature, children with ISS have no underlying risk of disturbances of carbohydrate metabolism and, thus, are probably at lesser risk of complications from GH therapy.

One final comment about the management of short stature. If your pockets are not deep enough to afford recombinant growth hormone and if you are treating idiopathic short stature, you might consider the use of tamoxifen. It might prove to be a lot cheaper and if further studies bear out its effectiveness, it just might add some height to those with idiopathic short stature. Historically, the alternative to growth hormone has been long-acting gonadotropin-releasing hormone analogs, which have been used in pubertal growth hormone deficient and non-growth hormone deficient patients as a way of delaying epiphyseal fusion and increasing adult height. However, new discoveries highlighting the importance of estrogen in mediating the closure of growth plates has led to the evaluation of novel alternative therapies aimed at decreasing estrogen synthesis or blocking estrogen effects. These therapies have included the use of antiestrogens in the form of aromatase inhibitors and selective estrogen receptor modulators such as tamoxifen. A recent report of 7 pubertal boys who were treated with tamoxifen was conducted to determine the effects of this therapy on skeletal maturation and predicted adult height.[1] It was observed that tamoxifen significantly decreased the rate of skeletal maturation and increased the predicted adult height of these boys without negative effects on sexual maturation. If the tamoxifen saga plays itself out in a favorable manner, you can be guaranteed that popping a pill is better than taking a series of expensive injections when the latter turns out not to be an affordable form of therapy.

J. A. Stockman III, MD

Reference

1. Kreher NC, Eugster EA, Shankar RR: The use of tamoxifen to improve adult height potential in short pubertal boys. *Pediatrics* 116:1513-1515, 2005.

Interpreting the Continued Decline in the Average Age at Menarche: Results From Two Nationally Representative Surveys of US Girls Studied 10 Years Apart

Anderson SE, Must A (Tufts Univ, Boston)
J Pediatr 147:753-760, 2005   6–7

Objectives.—To determine whether average age at menarche declined in the United States during the past decade, and whether associations between menarcheal timing, weight status, and race/ethnicity changed.

Study Design.—Relative weight, race/ethnicity, and menarcheal status of girls (n = 1577) in the National Health and Nutrition Examination Survey (NHANES) III (1988-1994) were compared with those of girls (n = 1720) in NHANES 1999-2002. Probit analysis estimated average age at menarche overall and also by race/ethnicity. Logistic regression assessed associations of relative weight and race/ethnicity with menarcheal status.

Results.—In the United States, average age at menarche declined from 12.53 years (95% confidence interval [CI] = 12.43 to 12.63 years) in 1988-1994 to 12.34 years (95% CI = 12.24 to 12.45 years) in 1999-2002. By race/ethnicity, average age at menarche estimates were as follows: non-Hispanic whites, 12.57 years (95% CI = 12.45 to 12.69 years) and 12.52 years (95% CI = 12.38 to 12.67 years); non-Hispanic blacks, 12.09 years (95% CI = 11.82 to 12.36 years) and 12.06 years (95% CI = 11.81 to 12.32 years); and Mexican Americans, 12.24 years (95% CI = 11.88 to 12.59 years) and 12.09 years (95% CI = 11.81 to 12.37 years). Higher relative weight was consistently associated with increased likelihood of having reached menarche.

Conclusions.—Average age at menarche in the United States declined by 2.3 months between 1988-1994 and 1999-2002; by race/ethnicity, declines were considerably smaller. Changes in the population distribution of race/ethnicity and relative weight should be considered when interpreting trends in age at menarche.

▶ More than 30 years ago, during the 1970s, a secular decrease in age at menarche was noted.[1] More recently, some European researchers have noted that, although the age at menarche has decreased over the last several decades, the latest cohorts of children followed up have shown the rate of decrease has declined.[2]

The data presented by Anderson and Must are consistent with the data published by our European colleagues and may prove to be a harbinger of future findings in the United States. They show that during a recent decade, the average age at menarche declined from 12.53 years to 12.34 years. A few months here or there and a few decades from now, one wonders if menarche will be occurring in kindergartners. There is also some suggestion that there is a correlation between adiposity and this earlier onset of menarche.

J. A. Stockman III, MD

References

1. Wyshak G, Frisch RE: Evidence for a secular trend in age of menarche. *N Engl J Med* 306:1033-1035, 1982.
2. Fredriks AM, van Buuren S, Burgmeijer RJF, et al: Continuing positive secular growth change in the Netherlands, 1955-1997. *Pediatr Res* 47:316-323, 2000.

Is Sexual Maturity Occurring Earlier Among US Children?

Sun SS, Schubert CM, Liang R, et al (Wright State Univ, Dayton, Ohio; Pennsylvania State Univ, Hershey; Univ of Minnesota, Minneapolis)

J Adolesc Health 37:345-355, 2005   6–8

Purpose.—To compare the onset and completion of sexual maturation among U.S. children between 1966 and 1994.

Methods.—Tanner stages were from 3042 non-Hispanic white boys, 478 black boys, 2625 white girls, and 505 black girls (NHES 1966–70), from 717 Mexican-American boys and 712 Mexican-American girls (HHANES 1982–84) and from 259 non-Hispanic white boys, 411 black boys, 291 white girls, 415 black girls, 576 Mexican-American boys and 512 Mexican-American girls (NHANES III 1988–1994). Proportions of entry into a stage, probit analysis estimated medians and selected percentiles for ages at entry were calculated using SUDAAN.

Results.—NHANES III (1988-1994) non-Hispanic white boys entered stage 2, 3, and 4 genital development and stages 3 and 4 pubic hair earlier than NHES (1966–1970) white boys, but they entered stage 5 genital development significantly later. NHANES III (1988–1994) Mexican-American boys were in stage 2, 3 and 4 genital development earlier than HHANES (1982–1984) boys, but entry into stage 5 genital and pubic hair development was not significant. NHANES III (1988–1994) white girls entered stage 5 pubic hair later than NHES (1966–1970) white girls. NHANES III (1988–1994) Mexican-American girls entered stage 2 breast and pubic hair development earlier than HHANES (1982–1984) girls, entered stage 4 breast and pubic hair development earlier but entered stage 5 pubic hair later than the HHANES (1982–1984) girls.

Conclusion.—Persuasive evidence of a secular trend toward early maturation is not found between 1966 and 1994 in non-Hispanic black boys and non-Hispanic black and white girls. Some evidence of this trend is found in non-Hispanic white boys between 1966 and 1994 and in Mexican-American boys and girls between 1982 and 1994.

▶ Are children today experiencing puberty at an earlier age than their parents, and if so, why? The answer to the first question is straightforward. The answer to the second question, not so. The earlier onset of puberty here in the United States was first reported by Herman-Giddens et al[1] in the late 1990s. This cross-sectional study demonstrated that the prevalence of Tanner stage 2 breast and pubic hair development at the age of 8 years was 15% for white girls and 48% for black girls, representing a significant increase in the percentage of children entering puberty at an earlier age than previously reported in national cross-sectional studies. However, in spite of earlier entry into puberty by girls in the latter study, the timing of menarche for white girls remained relatively stable. The situation was different for black girls, however, with an earlier onset of menses clearly documented. This report set off a firestorm of controversy about whether girls were, in fact, entering puberty earlier. If so, some have suggested that better nutrition is the reason why.

In the report of Sun et al, the evidence of a trend toward earlier pubertal maturation was not as clear. There was some evidence to suggest that country of origin and immigrant status might contribute to undernutrition and, therefore, affected pubertal timing. The authors unequivocally have stated that childhood obesity does not account for an earlier onset of puberty, despite recent evidence regarding the causal mechanism of earlier entry into puberty with a higher body mass index.[2]

It is hard to say whether this report examining the National Health and Nutrition Examination Survey data will settle the question of whether youngsters in the United States are entering puberty earlier. The authors conclude that there is no persuasive evidence that sexual maturation for US children as a whole has begun earlier, but some evidence of earlier sexual maturation was found in non-Hispanic white boys and Mexican-American boys and girls. The report concludes that there is insufficient evidence and data to support a secular trend towards early maturation in the United States when looking at the period 1966-1994, but there is some suggestion of a secular trend toward early maturation in non-Hispanic white boys between 1966 and 1994 and Mexican-American boys between 1982 and 1994.

Stay tuned for further debate on this topic. The report that follows (Abstract 6–9), from Denmark, gives us detailed information about the prevalence of precocious puberty in that nation. This has some relevance to what we might expect to see here in the United States in the white population, given the demographics of our country and similarities between the 2 countries.

J. A. Stockman III, MD

References

1. Herman-Giddens ME, Slora EJ, Wasserman RC, et al: Secondary sexual characteristics and menses in young girls seen in office practice: A study from the Pediatric Research in Office Settings Network. *Pediatrics* 99:505-512, 1997.
2. Biro FM, Lucky AW, Simbartl LA, et al: Pubertal maturation in girls and the relationship to anthropomorphic changes: Pathways through puberty. *J Pediatr* 142:643-646, 2003.

Prevalence and Incidence of Precocious Pubertal Development in Denmark: An Epidemiologic Study Based on National Registries

Teilmann G, Pedersen CB, Jensen TK, et al (Univ of Copenhagen; Univ of Aarhus, Denmark)

Pediatrics 116:1323-1328, 2005

6–9

Objective.—To our knowledge, no population-based epidemiologic studies on the incidence and prevalence of precocious pubertal development have been published. Danish national registries provide sufficient data for estimating the prevalence and incidence of this condition. The aim of this study was to estimate the prevalence and incidence of precocious pubertal development in Denmark in a 9-year period.

Methods.—The age- and gender-specific incidence rates as well as prevalence rates of precocious pubertal development in Denmark were estimated using data from the Danish National Patient Registry and Statistics Denmark from 1993 to 2001.

Results.—Overall, 670 children with precocious pubertal development were registered with a diagnosis of precocious puberty (PP) from 1993 to 2001, corresponding to 50 to 70 new cases of PP per year in Denmark. The incidence of PP was constant during the study period from 1993 to 2001. The incidence of PP subdivided by gender and age at diagnosis was ~0.5 per 10,000 in girls who were younger than 2 years, decreasing to levels below 0.05 per 10,000 in girls aged 2 to 4 years, thereafter gradually rising to 8 per 10,000 for girls aged 5 to 9 years. For boys who were younger than 8 years, the incidence was very low (<1 per 10,000) and increased only slightly to 1 to 2 per 10,000 in boys aged 8 to 10 years. The prevalence of PP was ~20 to 23 per 10,000 in girls, whereas the prevalence was fivefold lower for boys (<5 per 10,000).

Conclusions.—From this first epidemiologic study based on national registries, we estimated that 0.2% of all Danish girls and <0.05% of Danish boys had some form of precocious pubertal development.

▶ Despite the previous report (Abstract 6–8), which suggested that there was no unequivocal evidence for earlier onset of puberty here in the United States, during the past 2 centuries, an earlier sexual maturation, indicated by an earlier age at menarche, has been observed in European countries, although this downward trend in age of onset of puberty seems to have leveled off in the last few decades. The suggestion that age of puberty has declined prompted the Lawson Wilkins Pediatric Endocrine Society to review the current guidelines for ages at which the causes of PP should be searched for, and it has recommended lowering the prevailing standards from 8 to 7 years for white girls and to 6 years for black girls, whereas no changes in the current guidelines for evaluating boys have been suggested. Europe has taken a different stance. European endocrinologists are concerned about overlooking serious endocrine pathology as a potential consequence of lowering the age limit for defining PP. In Europe, the definitions of PP and diagnostic guidelines have remained unchanged, as no major changes in the onset of puberty have been shown in recent times. In addition, it was noted recently that the suggested American guidelines if applied to a European child population would not be safe in selecting girls with central PP who require brain imaging.[1] Too much pathology would be missed.

In the report abstracted, we see the first nationwide register-based epidemiologic study on the incidence and prevalence of precocious pubertal development, based on a well-defined background population. The prevalence of PP was found to be 20 to 23 per 10,000 girls. The incidence was 8 per 10,000 for girls aged 5 to 9 years and much lower for boys at the same ages (1 to 2 per 10,000). In Denmark, at least, one can estimate that just 0.2% of all Danish girls develop some form of PP between birth and 9 years of age. The authors found an incidence of 8 per 10,000 among 5- to 9-year-old girls that did not change over a 10-year period of observation. In boys, the condition appears to be very rare, with a prevalence as low as 1 to 2 per 10,000.

So what do we learn from this report? We learn that if you look at one country, you have looked at one country. Even the authors of this report suggest that the results cannot be applied directly to other countries, particularly those with populations of different ethnic and racial compositions. Nonetheless, the report does provide us with excellent data about a highly characterized population and sets a standard for investigation for us to replicate here in the United States.

The report abstracted was from Denmark. See how you might answer the following question about sexual maturity of girls in Thailand. Three girls are born into a family in Thailand. The question is, if one of these girls is to become a prostitute, one is to stay at home to assist the family with its daily tasks, and one is to go off to be educated, which one is likely to become the prostitute: the first born, the second born, or the third born?

It is the middle child. It is unclear precisely how many child prostitutes Thailand has produced. The United Nations International Labor Organization estimates that 100,000 to 200,000 Thai women and girls work in a variety of overseas venues where sex is sold. The Protection Project, a human rights research institute in Washington, DC, places the number of Thai females participating in Japan's commercial sex market alone at between 50,000 and 70,000. It seems that neither poverty nor lack of education are the driving forces behind trafficking of northern Thai children. Daughters from both poor and relatively well-off families become prostitutes in roughly equal proportions. Many Thai girls, particularly in the north, find prostitution as a bearable choice because they feel obligated to repay their parents for past sacrifices and to improve the family's financial standing. This obligation stands even if the parents own farmland and make a decent living. In a setting devoid of other well-paying job opportunities, the oldest profession represents the only way for a girl to make enough money to maintain or enhance their family's property and status in the village. Even in landowning families, middle-born daughters are the most likely to become prostitutes. In Thailand, first-born girls typically stay at home to assist their parents in daily tasks and rarely enter the sex trade. Middle-born girls are traditionally regarded as the family's financial helpers. Thanks to the labor of their older sisters, last-born girls typically receive more schooling than their sisters. It is not uncommon for one female sibling to be working in the fields alongside the parents, another to be working in a bar in Bangkok, and a third child getting a secondary education. In contrast, parents do not expect much pay back from sons, who traditionally move into the homes of their wives' families after marriage.[2]

In an interesting twist, Buddhist beliefs in northern Thailand contribute to the community acceptance of former prostitutes, who often marry local men. Thai Buddhists hold that each person's soul inhabits many physical bodies over time, with the quality of each life influenced by the soul's store of merit. Prostitution performed out of need to aid one's family is considered a process that builds up merit (although not necessarily desirable) despite the nature of the job itself.

J. A. Stockman III, MD

References

1. Chalumeau M, Hadjiathanasiou CG, Ng SM, et al: Selecting girls with precocious puberty for brain imaging: Validation of European evidence-based diagnosis rule. *J Pediatr* 143:445-450, 2003.
2. Bower B: Childhood's end: In Thailand, poverty isn't the primary reason that girls become prostitutes. *Science News* 168:200-201, 2005.

Ovarian Transplantation Between Monozygotic Twins Discordant for Premature Ovarian Failure

Silber SJ, Lenahan KM, Levine DJ, et al (St Luke's Hosp, St Louis; Paternity Testing, Columbia, Md; Greenwood Genetic Ctr, SC; et al)
N Engl J Med 353:58-63, 2005

6–10

Abstract.—Monozygotic 24-year-old twins presented with discordant ovarian function. One had had premature ovarian failure at the age of 14 years, whereas her sister had normal ovaries and three naturally conceived children. After unsuccessful egg-donation therapy, the sterile twin received a transplant of ovarian cortical tissue from her sister by means of a mini-laparotomy. Within three months after transplantation, the recipient's cycles resumed and serum gonadotropin levels fell to the normal range. During the second cycle, she conceived, and her pregnancy progressed uneventfully. At 38 weeks' gestation, she delivered a healthy-appearing female infant.

▶ This article is included in the YEAR BOOK OF PEDIATRICS for 2 reasons. First, although none of us are likely to ever care for a child born after ovarian transplantation between monozygotic twins discordant for premature ovarian failure, most pediatricians will be caring for the offspring of pregnancies in which novel fertility procedures have been used. Second, this article, as unique as it is, exemplifies for us all the relatively vast array of technologies that are capable of being used to improve fertility.

In this article from St Louis, we learn of 24-year-old twin sisters, confirmed to be monozygotic by means of genetic fingerprinting, one of whom developed premature ovarian failure. The sister who had no problems with prior conceptions was willing to donate an ovary to her twin sister. More specifically, she donated the cortex of 1 ovary, which was engrafted onto the medulla of the twin who had experienced ovarian failure. The transplanted twin had her first postoperative menses 80 days after transplantation (and her first menses in many years). It lasted just a day, but it did occur. After her second menstrual period, the recipient became pregnant, and at 38 weeks' gestation delivered, in an uneventful way, a 3600 g baby who did fine.

You may be wondering why the entire ovary was not transplanted in this patient. The grafting of ovarian cortex turns out to be significantly more minimally invasive and involves substantially less risk and recovery time than a full vascular graft of a complete ovary. One simply has to sew the cortex onto the medulla and let time heal everything up. There is a risk of ischemia, but this risk is fairly small.

Well worth your reading is an editorial by Lobo[1] that appeared in the *New England Journal of Medicine* dealing with potential options for preservation of fertility in women. Adult women have a number of options available to preserve fertility, including cryopreservation of embryos and oocytes. Children are different. Children being treated for cancer with agents that are likely to cause infertility really have only 1 option, and that is cryopreservation of ovarian tissue. As of now, it is not exactly clear how effective this approach is because, as of this writing, just a single pregnancy has been reported after orthotopic transplantation of a frozen ovary.[2]

J. A. Stockman III, MD

References

1. Lobo RA: Potential option for preservation of fertility in women. *N Engl J Med* 353:64-73, 2005.
2. Donnez J, Dolmans MM, Demylle D, et al: Live birth after orthotopic transplantation of cryopreserved ovarian tissue. *Lancet* 364:1405-1410, 2004.

Neurodevelopmental Outcomes in Congenital Hypothyroidism: Comparison of Initial T$_4$ Dose and Time to Reach Target T$_4$ and TSH
Selva KA, Harper A, Downs A, et al (Legacy Emanuel Hosp, Portland, Ore; Oregon Health Science Univ, Portland)
J Pediatr 147:775-780, 2005   6-11

Objectives.—To compare neurodevelopmental outcomes in severe and moderate congenital hypothyroidism (CH) among 3 different initial L-thyroxine doses and to examine the effect of the time to thyroid function normalization on neurodevelopmental outcomes.

Study Design.—Neurodevelopmental assessments of 31 subjects included the Mullen Scales of Early Learning, Wechsler Preschool and Primary Scale of Intelligence-Revised, Wechsler Intelligence Scale for Children, Wide-Range Achievement Test, and Child Behavioral Checklist.

Results.—Subjects started on higher initial L-thyroxine doses (50 µg) had full-scale IQ scores 11 points higher than those started on lower (37.5 µg) initial doses. However, verbal IQ, performance IQ, and achievement scores did not differ among the 3 treatment cohorts. Subjects with moderate CH had higher full-scale IQ scores than subjects with severe CH, regardless of the initial treatment dose. Subjects who took longer than 2 weeks to normalize thyroid function had significantly lower cognitive, attention, and achievement scores than those who achieved normal thyroid function at 1 or 2 weeks of therapy.

Conclusions.—Initial L-thyroxine dose and faster time to normalization of thyroid function are important to optimal neurodevelopmental outcome. In severe CH, it is important to choose an initial dose at the higher end of the recommended range to achieve these goals.

▶ No one will argue that some schoolchildren who have received early treatment for CH have subnormal IQs combined with behavioral problems (mostly attentional) and subtle defects in language, memory, and visuospatial skills. To date, most articles have focused on the negative effect of undertreatment after birth in patients with CH. The article by Selva et al tells us a great deal about the need to get on top of the problem quickly. These investigators studied the time interval to achieve normal thyroid studies from the point of initial treatment. Back in 2002,[1] the group reported the results of a treatment study that examined 3 initial doses of L-thyroxine and the pattern of thyroid function normalization over 12 weeks. They used 3 treatment doses (37.5 µg, 50 µg, and a loading dose of 62.5 µg for 3 days, followed by 37.5 µg). A dose of 50 µg/d led to the most rapid normalization of TSH by 2 weeks of therapy. It was recommended that one consider a slightly higher increased target of T_4 (10 µg/dL-18 µg/dL) and free T_4 (1.6 ng/dL-2.5 ng/dL) during the first month of therapy to quickly normalize T_4 and TSH, followed by frequent monitoring and adjustment of thyroid doses thereafter to maintain normal thyroid functioning. In the current article, these same investigators have now examined the relationship between a faster time to normalization of thyroid functioning and later neurodevelopmental outcomes.

So, does quickly gaining control of thyroid functioning in an infant with CH really make a difference? It turns out that babies started with higher initial thyroxine doses (50 µg) have a full-scale IQ score that is 11 points higher than those starting with modestly lower doses (37.5 µg T_4). Despite the full-scale IQ score improvement, verbal IQ, performance IQ, and achievement scores did not differ among treatment groups. Patients whose thyroid functioning took longer than 2 weeks to normalize did have significantly lower cognitive, attention, and achievement scores than did those whose thyroid functioning normalized more quickly.

See the article that follows (Abstract 6–12) for additional information about how important it is to gain control of thyroid functioning as quickly as possible in those with CH. Please note, however, that a theoretical risk of overtreatment might be associated with a subsequent higher prevalence of attention deficit disorder.

J. A. Stockman III, MD

Reference

1. Selva KA, Mandel SH, Rien L, et al: Initial treatment dose of L-thyroxine in congenital hypothyroidism. *J Pediatr* 141:786-792, 2002.

Influence of Timing and Dose of Thyroid Hormone Replacement on Mental, Psychomotor, and Behavioral Development in Children With Congenital Hypothyroidism

Bongers-Schokking JJ, de Muinck Keizer-Schrama SMPF (Erasmus Med Ctr, Rotterdam, The Netherlands)
J Pediatr 147:768-774, 2005
6–12

Objectives.—To evaluate the influence of initial and postinitial treatment factors on cognitive, psychomotor, and psychological outcome in schoolchildren with congenital hypothyroidism (CH).

Study Design.—We studied 45 patients (19 with severe CH and 26 with mild CH) and 37 control children by correlating initial and postinitial treatment factors (free thyroxine and thyroid-stimulating hormone [TSH] concentrations, and the percentage of overtreatment and undertreatment periods) with the results of neuropsychological tests and behavior (as reported on the Teacher Report Form [TRF]).

Results.—The global IQ of the children with CH was comparable to that of the controls; visuomotor and verbal scores were lower, and total TRF scores were higher. Ethnic group, previous development, and overtreatment predicted IQ and verbal scores, with higher scores seen for the overtreated patients than for the control children and those patients who had not been overtreated. As initial treatment was less satisfactory, total TRF scores were higher.

Conclusions.—Our study suggests that initial and postinitial suboptimal treatment of CH leads to abnormalities in IQ and specific fields. Overtreatment may advance cognitive development in 5-1/2- to 7-year-olds. Suboptimal initial treatment may lead to behavioral problems. We recommend that TSH concentrations be maintained within the normal range in patients with CH.

7 Gastroenterology

Clinical Features of Pathologic Childhood Aerophagia: Early Recognition and Essential Diagnostic Criteria
Hwang J-B, Choi WJ, Kim JS, et al (Keimyung Univ School of Medicine, Daegu, Korea; Daegu Catholic Univ School of Medicine, Korea; Kyungpook Natl Univ School of Medicine, Daegu, Korea)
J Pediatr Gastroenterol Nutr 41:612-616, 2005   7–1

Objective.—This study investigated the early recognition and diagnosis of pathologic childhood aerophagia to avoid unnecessary diagnostic approaches and serious complications.

Methods.—Between 1995 and 2003, data from 42 consecutive patients with pathologic childhood aerophagia, aged 2 to 16 years, were reviewed. An esophageal air sign was defined as an abnormal air shadow on the proximal esophagus adjacent to the trachea on a full-inflated chest radiograph.

Results.—Of the 42 patients, the chief complaints were abdominal distention (52.4%), recurrent abdominal pain syndrome (21.4%), chronic diarrhea (11.9%), acute abdominal pain (7.1%) and others (7.2%). Mean symptom duration before diagnosis was 10.6 months (range, 1 to 60 months), and it exceeded 12 months for 16 (38.1%) patients. The clinical features common to all patients were abdominal distention that increased progressively during the day, increased flatus on sleep, increased bowel sound on auscultation and an air-distended stomach with increased gas in the small and large bowel by radiography. Visible or audible air swallowing (26.2%) and repetitive belching (9.5%) were also noted. Esophageal air sign was observed in 76.2% of the patients and in 9.7% of the controls ($P = 0.0001$). The subgroups of pathologic childhood aerophagia divided by underlying associations were pathologic childhood aerophagia without severe mental retardation (76.2%), which consisted of psychological stresses and uncertain condition, and pathologic childhood aerophagia with severe mental retardation (23.8%).

Conclusions.—The common manifestations of pathologic childhood aerophagia may be its essential diagnostic criteria, and esophageal air sign may be useful for the early recognition of pathologic childhood aerophagia. Our observations show that the diagnostic clinical profiles suggested by

Rome II criteria should be detailed and made clearer if they are to serve as diagnostic criteria for pathologic childhood aerophagia.

▶ Although we all know that aerophagia exists, I have to be frank about the fact that this is the first comprehensive article I have seen on the study of childhood aerophagia. I was surprised to learn that criteria exist for the precise diagnosis of pathologic childhood aerophagia. These are the Rome II criteria.[1] The Rome II criteria tell us that to make a diagnosis, children must have at least 2 of the following signs and symptoms for a minimum period of 12 weeks (which need not be consecutive) in the preceding 12 months: air swallowing, abdominal distention from intraluminal air, and repetitive belching and/or increased flatus. Most of the flatus, by the way, as this article notes, occurs during sleep. Increased flatus during sleep is suspected to occur as a result of increased sleep associated parasympathomimetic activity resulting in increased gastrointestinal motility. Thus, these kids often have a distended abdomen during the day and evening but one that is flat on awakening in the morning.

This study on pediatric childhood aerophagia adds a bit more understanding to the Rome II criteria. The findings from the study show that the following manifestations of pathologic childhood aerophagia constitute a more satisfactory set of diagnostic criteria than do the Rome criteria: abdominal distention that progressively increases during the course of the day (minimal in the early morning and maximal in the late evening), increased flatus during sleep, increased bowel sounds on auscultation of a distended abdomen, and an abdominal radiograph—if taken in late afternoon—that shows an air-distended stomach and increased gas in the small and large bowel without signs of obstruction. Also, if one sees air in the esophagus on a chest radiograph, it is a good sign that the child has been swallowing air. It is likely to be a helpful sign for the early diagnosis of pathologic childhood aerophagia, although it is not specific without other signs being present. Belching after having drunk a carbonated drink will produce exactly the same sign.

Pathologic childhood aerophagia is often more of a nuisance problem than anything else, but it can cause abdominal discomfort and irritability. It is a common disorder in the mentally retarded population for reasons that are not well understood. In patients with severe mental retardation, excessive degrees of aerophagia can cause massive distention of the bowel, possibly leading to surgical emergencies such as ileus, volvulus, and even intestinal necrosis or perforation. In an emergency situation, one can decompress the stomach either by placement of a nasogastric tube or a percutaneous endoscopic gastrostomy catheter.

While on the topic of "gas" in the gastrointenstinal tract, here is a bit more information on the subject. In many parts of the world, beans are a very stable staple component of the diet of humans. Pythagorus was among the first to recognize complications resulting from the eating of beans when he advised his pupils to abstain from beans, probably to avoid the consequences of favism from glucose-6-phosphate dehydrogenase deficiency. Beans, red or otherwise, are a good source of nutrition and are high in protein (one cup = about 16 grams protein), unsaturated fats, fiber, vitamins, and minerals while being low in cholesterol. A certain legendary prince is supposed to have deflowered numerous virgins in a single night while taking no other nourishment other than chickpeas. Most physicians are not aware of why many humans cannot eat beans without "breaking wind." Why is this?

Humans cannot digest the oligosaccharides originating from beans because they lack the enzyme alpha-galactosidase. Instead, humans break oligosaccharides down to hydrogen, carbon dioxide, and certain malodorous gases. Attempts to produce a "low flatulence" bean have been largely unsuccessful to date and maneuvers such as soaking beans in water to leach out the oligosaccharides are equally unsuccessful. The only major serious side effect that has been reported in association with the flatulence resulting from bean ingestion is as reported a quarter of a century ago by Dr Michael Levett, who references a case of a dramatic explosion occurring during cautery of the colon in a patient who had eaten beans prior to the procedure. Presumably, the ratio of methane to hydrogen reached an incendiary range causing a frightening blast.[2]

To read more about beans, beans, good for the heart, etc, read the overview by Dunea.[3]

J. A. Stockman III, MD

References

1. Rasquine-Webber A, Hyman PE, Cucchiara S, et al: Childhood functional gastrointestinal disorders. *Gut* 45:(suppl 2)1160-1168, 1999.
2. Levett M: An explosive situation. *N Engl J Med* 302:1474, 1980.
3. Dunea G: Beans. *BMJ* 331:973, 2005.

A Randomised Clinical Trial of the Management of Esophageal Coins in Children

Waltzman ML, Baskin M, Wypij D, et al (Children's Hosp of Boston)
Pediatrics 116:614-619, 2005   7–2

Context.—Children frequently ingest coins. When lodged in the esophagus, the coin may cause complications and must either be removed or observed to pass spontaneously.

Objectives.—(1) To compare relatively immediate endoscopic removal to a period of observation followed by removal when necessary and (2) to evaluate the relationship between select clinical features and spontaneous passage.

Design/Setting.—Randomized, prospective study of children <21 years old who presented to an emergency department with esophageal coins in the esophagus. Exclusion criteria were (1) history of tracheal or esophageal surgery, (2) showing symptoms, or (3) swallowing the coin >24 hours earlier. Children were randomized to either endoscopic removal (surgery) or admission for observation, with repeat radiographs ~16 hours after the initial image.

Outcome Measures.—Proportion of patients requiring endoscopic removal, length of hospital stay, and the number of complications observed.

Thus, a key challenge for children and their care providers is to combat this nutritional failure.

Poustie et al present us with an important, well-planned, and carefully executed randomized, multicenter study of oral supplements in patients with cystic fibrosis. The trial was conducted to detect a 10-point difference in centile for body mass index within 1 year of the intervention, comparing patients receiving dietary advice with patients who were also prescribed oral protein energy supplements. The design of the study was able to detect a weight gain of as little as 2 kg at the age of 9 years in patients with cystic fibrosis. Unfortunately, the study showed that the prescription of extra oral supplements failed to improve the nutritional status of cystic fibrosis patients.

Studies such as this one by Poustie et al document how difficult it is to maintain good nutrition in the face of chronic disease. Mealtimes can be a psychological battlefield for any family but particularly for a family with a child who has cystic fibrosis. Treatments for cystic fibrosis are time-consuming, generally unpleasant, and potentially anxiety provoking. Most kids with cystic fibrosis feel well most of the time, so getting them to comply with treatment, including eating better, may not be an easy task.

J. A. Stockman III, MD

The Metabolic Syndrome as a Predictor of Nonalcoholic Fatty Liver Disease

Hamaguchi M, Kojima T, Takeda N, et al (Asahi Univ, Gifu, Japan)
Ann Intern Med 143:722-728, 2005   7–4

Background.—The frequent association of nonalcoholic fatty liver disease with components of the metabolic syndrome such as obesity, hyperglycemia, dyslipidemia, and hypertension is well known. However, no prospective study has examined the role of the metabolic syndrome in the development of this disease.

Objective.—To characterize the longitudinal relationship between the metabolic syndrome and nonalcoholic fatty liver disease.

Design.—A prospective observational study.

Setting.—A medical health checkup program in a general hospital.

Participants.—4401 apparently healthy Japanese men and women, 21 to 80 years of age, with a mean body mass index (BMI) of 22.6 kg/m² (SD, 3.0).

Measurements.—Alcohol intake was assessed by using a questionnaire. Biochemical tests for liver and metabolic function and abdominal ultrasonography were done. Modified criteria of the National Cholesterol Education Program Adult Treatment Panel III were used to characterize the metabolic syndrome.

Results.—At baseline, 812 of 4401 (18%) participants had nonalcoholic fatty liver disease. During the mean follow-up period of 414 days (SD, 128), the authors observed 308 new cases (10%) of nonalcoholic fatty liver disease among 3147 participants who were disease-free at baseline and who completed a second examination. Regression of nonalcoholic fatty liver disease was found in 113 (16%) of 704 participants who had the disease at baseline and who completed a second examination. Men and women who met the criteria for the metabolic syndrome at baseline were more likely to develop the disease during follow-up (adjusted odds ratio, 4.00 [95% CI, 2.63 to 6.08] and 11.20 [CI, 4.85 to 25.87], respectively). Nonalcoholic fatty liver disease was less likely to regress in those participants with the metabolic syndrome at baseline.

Limitations.—Ultrasonography may lead to an incorrect diagnosis of nonalcoholic fatty liver disease in 10% to 30% of cases and cannot distinguish steatohepatitis from simple steatosis. Self-reported alcohol intake may cause bias. Because all of the participants were Japanese, generalizability to non-Japanese populations is uncertain.

Conclusions.—The metabolic syndrome is a strong predictor of nonalcoholic fatty liver disease.

▶ This report from Japan deals only with adults, many of them young adults, but it is a good predictor of what will happen to obese children who are at risk for the metabolic syndrome as far as their probability of developing liver disease is concerned. Nonalcoholic fatty liver disease is an underrecognized manifestation of the metabolic syndrome and refers to a spectrum of fatty liver disease that occurs in the absence of significant alcohol consumption. At the benign end of the spectrum, most patients with nonalcoholic fatty liver disease have only fatty liver (simple steatosis). A small proportion (thought to be about 10%) also have features of liver cell injury or fibrosis, referred to as nonalcoholic steatohepatitis. This distinction between simple steatosis and nonalcoholic steatohepatitis is important because the natural history of these 2 entities differs substantially. Persons with simple steatosis usually have a benign prognosis from the point of view of liver disease. In contrast, as many as 1 in 5 persons with nonalcoholic steatohepatitis will ultimately develop advanced liver disease. The liver disease includes cirrhosis, and its prognosis is poor. Hepatocellular cancer is also a recently recognized complication of nonalcoholic steatohepatitis–related cirrhosis.

Although only a minority of patients with nonalcoholic fatty liver disease will develop advanced liver disease, the condition is extremely worrisome because of its increasing prevalence. A recent large population study done here in the United States found a prevalence of hepatic steatosis that is currently running about 34%.[1]

The data provided from the Japanese study clearly demonstrate the very strong relationship between nonalcoholic fatty liver disease and the metabolic syndrome. About 1 in 3 patients with nonalcoholic fatty liver disease fulfill the current criteria for metabolic syndrome. Those patients with the metabolic syndrome who were followed up prospectively showed an 11 times greater risk for the development of nonalcoholic fatty liver disease.

This report from Japan uses abdominal US to diagnose nonalcoholic fatty liver disease. The problem with abdominal US is that it is an imperfect tool to diagnose this liver disorder. Newer methods such as MR spectroscopy perform much better. MRI, however, cannot easily distinguish between nonalcoholic fatty liver disease and nonalcoholic steatohepatitis. If elevated liver enzymes are present, the patient is more likely to fall into the latter category, although liver enzymes are not a precise instrument either. Liver biopsy remains the gold standard for diagnosis but, of course, is largely unfeasible for large population-based studies.

See the report that follows (Abstract 7–5), which tells us about the relationship of abdominal fat distribution and hepatic steatosis in a pediatric population.

J. A. Stockman III, MD

Reference

1. Browning JD, Szczepaniak LS, Dobbins R, et al: Prevalence of hepatic steatosis in an urban population in the United States: Impact of ethnicity. *Hepatology* 40:1387-1395, 2004.

Relationship of Hepatic Steatosis to Adipose Tissue Distribution in Pediatric Nonalcoholic Fatty Liver Disease

Fishbein MH, Mogren C, Gleason T, et al (SIU, Springfield, Ill)
J Pediatr Gastroenterol Nutr 42:83-88, 2006   7–5

Objective.—Central adiposity, a component of insulin resistance syndrome, is a risk factor for nonalcoholic fatty liver disease (NAFLD) in adults. To determine whether a similar relationship occurs in children, hepatic fat content and adipose tissue distribution were assessed in obese children at risk for NAFLD.

Methods.—We reviewed the charts of obese children undergoing evaluation for NAFLD because of hepatomegaly or elevated serum alanine aminotransferase (ALT) without obvious etiology. Hepatic fat fraction and adipose tissue distribution were obtained by rapid magnetic resonance imaging (MRI) techniques. Hepatic fat content was determined by a modification of the Dixon method that involves fast gradient echo. Body fat distribution was assessed by using heavily T1-weighted fast gradient echo technique on a single slice at the level of the umbilicus, and regions of interest were demarcated based upon pixel intensity threshold value including visceral adipose tissue (VAT) and subcutaneous adipose tissue content (SAT).

Results.—Ten children underwent hepatic MRI only. Twenty-nine children underwent hepatic and adipose tissue distribution MRI. There was a correlation between hepatic fat fraction and VAT (r = 0.37, P < 0.05) but not body mass index or SAT. Elevated serum ALT was associated with a higher hepatic fat fraction (P < 0.001) and VAT (P = 0.06).

Conclusion.—Visceral adiposity is a risk factor for pediatric NAFLD.

▶ The preceding report (Abstract 7–4) showed us how common liver abnormalities are in persons with the metabolic syndrome. We now recognize in pediatric patients that NAFLD is also a component of the insulin-resistant syndrome. It is also clear that visceral fat may be a major contributor to fatty liver disease in insulin-resistant states. In fact, there is some suggestion that visceral adiposity is more influential than body mass itself in predicting fatty liver. The report from Illinois is critical in understanding the problem since it uses the best noninvasive tool to tell us about visceral adiposity and hepatic steatosis—MRI. MRI is far better than US in discerning what is fat and what is not fat, and determining just how much fat is present in a specific geographic area of the body.

We see in this report a very strong correlation between the amount of visceral fat we have and the amount of fat that is deposited in the liver. Exactly why children and adults who have visceral fat adiposity appear to be at greater risk for fatty liver remains speculative, but it is suspected that this is a result of their ability to transport free fatty acids directly into the portal vein for conversion to triglycerides within the liver. Unfortunately, in children, correlations between anthropometric measures and visceral adiposity are poor. CT scanning and MRI are far better techniques in determining whether someone has too much fat within their abdomen. A single scanning slice of the liver and a single slice across the abdomen are all that are needed if one is simply trying to determine the presence of hepatic steatosis and visceral adiposity. Obviously, not every overweight child will be a candidate for such studies given the cost significance and prevalence of such a common problem, but scanning is useful in the study of this and related problems.

J. A. Stockman III, MD

Positive Association of Macrophage Migration Inhibitory Factor Gene-173G/C Polymorphism With Biliary Atresia
Arikan C, Berdeli A, Ozgenc F, et al (Ege Univ, Izmir, Turkey)
J Pediatr Gastroenterol Nutr 42:77-82, 2006   7–6

Background.—Macrophage migration inhibitory factor (MIF) is a pleiotrophic lymphocyte and macrophage cytokine; it is likely to play an important role in innate immunity. Its expression was increased in several inflammatory diseases, and MIF gene polymorphisms have an effect on disease outcome and response to glucocorticoid treatment.

Aim.—To investigate the role of the 173G/C polymorphism of the MIF gene for susceptibility to biliary atresia (BA).

Method.—Between February 2002 and November 2004, 18 patients (mean age 1 ± 0.4 years) diagnosed as having BA were studied. After informed consent, blood was collected, and DNA was obtained. MIF 173C/G polymorphism was detected using the polymerase chain reaction-restriction fragment length polymorphism based method. BA patients were compared with a group of chronic liver disease patients (CLD) (n = 36) and a group of unrelated healthy controls (n = 103).

Results.—MIF-173C allele frequency was significantly higher than both the CLD and healthy control groups ($P = 0.03$, odds ratio [OR] 4.4, 95% confidence interval [CI] 1.3-15.1; $P = 0.000$, OR 4.1, 95% CI 2.3-7.6, respectively). Univariate analysis showed that MIF-173G/C polymorphism was significantly associated with BA (for GC genotype, OR = 6, 95% CI

2.8-11.5, $P = 0.000$). There was no significant correlation between pediatric end stage liver disease score and MIF genotypes both in BA and CLD groups.

Conclusion.—Our results suggest that the -173C allele of the MIF gene might be associated with the susceptibility to BA.

▶ The last 10 years or so has witnessed a tremendous increase in our understanding of the molecular basis of cholestatic liver disease in children. Initial studies of children with severe genetic defects have provided clear-cut evidence of the role of specific genes in fundamental biological processes. We are now at the point where an understanding of these genes helps us to see how they act as modifiers of previously "well-described" disease processes. The article by Arikan et al reports an increased prevalence of a polymorphism in the *MIF* gene in children with BA. Because genetic polymorphisms are frequent throughout the genome, determination of true associations with biological processes such as cholestasis often requires a large patient population. For example, a sample size of approximately 100 subjects is minimally necessary to detect a 2-fold difference in the frequency of a genetic polymorphism in infants with cholestasis when a 0.30 minor allele frequency is estimated in the control population. You can imagine how hard it is putting together 100 or more cases of a relatively uncommon problem such as described here.

The cause and pathogenetic mechanisms of BA largely remain unknown. One part of the process, however, is clear; it involves an ongoing inflammatory and fibrosing obstruction of the biliary system. *MIF* is clearly involved with this process. *MIF* is a lymphocyte and macrophage cytokine. An individual's capacity for cytokine production mainly depends on genetics, and the variation in this regard between individuals can be quite striking. Clearly, our genes regulate some of this and put some infants at increased risk of more rapidly progressive disease.

Please recognize that inflammation is a major part of BA progression. Studies have shown that the administration of steroids after the Kasai procedure has improved overall survival rates, again documenting the role of cytokines such as *MIF*. To achieve *MIF* suppression, one must use high-dose steroids. *MIF* is biphasically regulated by steroids, with suppression at high concentrations of steroids and induction at lower concentrations.

The report by Arikan et al documents that we now have evidence for the importance of the *MIF* gene and the pathology of BA. This finding is important. Humanized anti-*MIF* antibodies have been developed and may very well ultimately be used to mitigate the pathogenesis of BA.

For more on the topic of gene modifiers in BA, see the article by Hermeziu et al.[1]

J. A. Stockman III, MD

Reference

1. Hermeziu B, Sanlaville D, Gerard M, et al: Heterozygous bile salt export pump deficiency: A possible genetic predisposition to transient neonatal cholestasis. *J Pediatr Gastroenterol Nutr* 42:114-116, 2005.

Peginterferon Alfa-2a, Lamivudine, and the Combination for HBeAg-Positive Chronic Hepatitis B

Lau GKK, for the Peginterferon Alfa-2a HBeAg-Positive Chronic Hepatitis B Study Group (Univ of Hong Kong, China; Songklanakarin Hosp, Thailand; Nangfang Hosp, Guangzhou, China; et al)

N Engl J Med 352:2682-2695, 2005   7–7

Background.—Current treatments for chronic hepatitis B are suboptimal. In the search for improved therapies, we compared the efficacy and safety of pegylated interferon alfa plus lamivudine, pegylated interferon alfa without lamivudine, and lamivudine alone for the treatment of hepatitis B e antigen (HBeAg)–positive chronic hepatitis B.

Methods.—A total of 814 patients with HBeAg-positive chronic hepatitis B received either peginterferon alfa-2a (180 µg once weekly) plus oral placebo, peginterferon alfa-2a plus lamivudine (100 mg daily), or lamivudine alone. The majority of patients in the study were Asian (87 percent). Most patients were infected with hepatitis B virus (HBV) genotype B or C. Patients were treated for 48 weeks and followed for an additional 24 weeks.

Results.—After 24 weeks of follow-up, significantly more patients who received peginterferon alfa-2a monotherapy or peginterferon alfa-2a plus lamivudine than those who received lamivudine monotherapy had HBeAg seroconversion (32 percent vs. 19 percent [$P<0.001$] and 27 percent vs. 19 percent [$P=0.02$], respectively) or HBV DNA levels below 100,000 copies per milliliter (32 percent vs. 22 percent [$P=0.01$] and 34 percent vs. 22 percent [$P=0.003$], respectively). Sixteen patients receiving peginterferon alfa-2a (alone or in combination) had hepatitis B surface antigen (HBsAg) seroconversion, as compared with 0 in the group receiving lamivudine alone ($P=0.001$). The most common adverse events were those known to occur with therapies based on interferon alfa. Serious adverse events occurred in 4 percent, 6 percent, and 2 percent of patients receiving peginterferon alfa-2a monotherapy, combination therapy, and lamivudine monotherapy, respectively. Two patients receiving lamivudine monotherapy had irreversible liver failure after the cessation of treatment—one underwent liver transplantation, and the other died.

Conclusions.—In patients with HBeAg-positive chronic hepatitis B, peginterferon alfa-2a offers superior efficacy over lamivudine, on the basis of HBeAg seroconversion, HBV DNA suppression, and HBsAg seroconversion.

Long-Term Therapy With Adefovir Dipivoxil for HBeAg-Negative Chronic Hepatitis B

Hadziyannis SJ, for the Adefovir Dipivoxil 438 Study Group (Henry Dunant Hosp, Athens, Greece; Western Attica Gen Hosp, Athens, Greece; Univ of Toronto; et al)
N Engl J Med 352:2673-2681, 2005   7–8

Background.—Treatment with adefovir dipivoxil for 48 weeks resulted in histologic, virologic, and biochemical improvement in patients with hepatitis B e antigen (HBeAg)–negative chronic hepatitis B. We evaluated the effect of continued therapy as compared with cessation of therapy.

Methods.—One hundred eighty-five HBeAg-negative patients with chronic hepatitis B were assigned to receive 10 mg of adefovir dipivoxil or placebo once daily for 48 weeks (ratio, 2:1). After week 48, patients receiving adefovir dipivoxil were again randomly assigned either to receive an additional 48 weeks of the drug or to switch to placebo. Patients originally assigned to placebo were switched to adefovir dipivoxil. Patients treated with adefovir dipivoxil during weeks 49 through 96 were subsequently offered continued therapy. The primary end points were changes in hepatitis B virus (HBV) DNA and alanine aminotransferase levels.

Results.—Treatment with adefovir dipivoxil resulted in a median decrease in serum HBV DNA of 3.47 log copies per milliliter (on a base-10 scale) at 96 weeks and 3.63 log copies per milliliter at 144 weeks. HBV DNA levels were less than 1000 copies per milliliter in 71 percent of patients at week 96 and 79 percent at week 144. In the majority of patients who were switched from adefovir dipivoxil to placebo, the benefit of treatment was lost (median change in HBV DNA levels from baseline, − 1.09 log copies per milliliter; only 8 percent of patients had levels below 1000 copies per milliliter at week 96). Side effects during weeks 49 through 144 were similar to those during the initial 48 weeks. Resistance mutations rtN236T and rtA181V were identified in 5.9 percent of patients after 144 weeks.

Conclusions.—In patients with HBeAg-negative chronic hepatitis B, the benefits achieved from 48 weeks of adefovir dipivoxil were lost when treatment was discontinued. In patients treated for 144 weeks, benefits were maintained, with infrequent emergence of viral resistance.

▶ This article and the one by Lau et al (see Abstract 7–7) provide us with insights on newer ways to manage chronic hepatitis B infection. Worldwide, there are approximately 350 million carriers of HBV, of whom half a million to 1 million die of liver disease every year. Once somebody is detected as having chronic HBV, the goal is to prevent the onset of cirrhosis, liver failure, and hepatocellular carcinoma. This is best accomplished by eradicating HBV before serious damage to the liver has occurred. The difficulty is that HBV resides in numerous extrahepatic reservoirs and that this virus is capable of replicating itself without the need for reinfection. Therefore, when antiviral therapies are administered, they often can control the spreading of the virus and its replication. When therapy is stopped, rapid viral rebound usually occurs.

A handful of treatments have now been approved by the US Food and Drug Administration for the treatment of chronic hepatitis B here in the United States. These are interferon alpha-2b, lamivudine, adefovir, entecavir, and pegylated interferon (peg interferon) alpha-2a. The average patient will consume $5,000 to $15,000 a year in pharmaceuticals geared to directly attacking HBV.

In the study by Lau et al (Abstract 7–7), we see a report that combination peg interferon and lamivudine produces the greatest degree of virus suppression, followed by lamivudine therapy or peg interferon alone. Lamivudine is a pure antiviral agent whereas interferon has both immunomodulatory and antiviral effects. The study reported by Hadziyannis et al shows the benefits of adefovir dipivoxil in patients with HBeAg-negative chronic hepatitis B. As effective as this agent is in suppressing viral replication, once it is stopped, it has no lasting effects. These disappointing results confirm that current treatments suppress but do not eradicate HBV. Thus, once treatment with these agents is started, one is in for the long haul, if not a lifetime of treatment.

The treatment of HBV is not without its complications. Of foremost importance is drug resistance. Also, resistance to 1 antiviral agent may confer resistance to other agents and may limit future treatment options.

So what are we left with? Given multiple treatment options that are less than ideal, the remaining open issues are who should be treated, with what, and when can treatment be stopped. As tough as it is to answer these questions for adults, the answers are virtually impossible to find for children. The decision to treat or not to treat and the choice of treatment involve a complex discussion between the care provider and the patient and deals with the balance of benefits and risks. Such a discussion is usually well above the heads of most of us; thank goodness for our colleagues who work in the field of hepatology. While we can agree that substantial progress has been made in the treatment of hepatitis B, the maze of new therapies remains a challenge for the average practitioner, who will need backup in most instances.

For more on this topic, see the excellent editorial dealing with hepatitis B by Lok.[1]

J. A. Stockman III, MD

Reference

1. Lok AS-F: The maze of treatments for hepatitis B. *N Engl J Med* 325:2743-2745, 2005.

Peginterferon Alfa-2b and Ribavirin for 12 vs 24 weeks in HCV Genotype 2 or 3

Mangia A, Santoro R, Minerva N, et al (IRCCS Casa Sollievo della Sofferenza Hosp, San Giovanni Rotondo, Italy; Hosp Canosa, Italy; Univ La Sapienza, Rome; et al)

N Engl J Med 352:2609-2617, 2005   7–9

Background.—We hypothesized that in patients with hepatitis C virus (HCV) genotype 2 or 3 in whom HCV RNA is not detectable after 4 weeks of therapy, 12 weeks of treatment is as effective as 24 weeks.

Methods.—A total of 283 patients were randomly assigned to a standard 24-week regimen of peginterferon alfa-2b at a dose of 1.0 µg per kilogram weekly plus ribavirin at a dose of 1000 mg or 1200 mg daily, on the basis of body weight. Of these, 70 patients were assigned to the 24-week regimen (standard-duration group) and 213 patients to a variable regimen (variable-duration group) of 12 or 24 weeks, depending on whether tests for HCV RNA were negative or positive at week 4. The primary end point was HCV that was not detectable by polymerase-chain-reaction (PCR) assay 24 weeks after the completion of therapy.

Results.—In the standard-duration group, 45 (64 percent) patients had HCV that was not detectable by PCR assay at week 4, as compared with 133 (62 percent) in the variable-duration group (difference [the rate in the standard-duration group minus that in the variable-duration group], 2 percent; 95 percent confidence interval, -11 to 15 percent). Fifty-three patients (76 percent) in the standard-duration group and 164 patients (77 percent) in the variable-duration group had a sustained virologic response (difference, -1 percent; 95 percent confidence interval, -13 to 10 percent). Fewer patients in the variable-duration group receiving the 12-week regimen had adverse events and withdrew than in the group receiving the 24-week regimen (P=0.045). The rate of relapse (defined as HCV not detectable at the end of treatment but detectable at the end of follow-up) was 3.6 percent in the standard-duration group and 8.9 percent in the variable-duration group (P=0.16). Overall, the rate of sustained virologic response was 80 percent among patients with HCV genotype 2 and 66 percent among those with genotype 3 (P<0.001).

Conclusions.—A shorter course of therapy over 12 weeks with peginterferon alfa-2b and ribavirin is as effective as a 24-week course for patients with HCV genotype 2 or 3 who have a response to treatment at 4 weeks.

▶ The articles by Hadziyannis et al (Abstract 7–8) and Lau et al (Abstract 7–7) dealt with hepatitis B infection and ways of limiting the consequence of this infection. This article from Italy tells us about agents similar to those used in hepatitis B treatment applied to the management of HCV. As noted in the commentary dealing with hepatitis B virus, there are a number of immunomodulatory agents and antiviral agents that can be used to help manage patients with hepatitis these days. With hepatitis B virus, a relapse is very common once drug therapy is stopped. The long-term risks of such failure with respect to the development of cirrhosis and hepatocellular carcinoma are monumental. As the article from Rome points out, with respect to HCV, shorter term therapy (as short as 12 weeks) seems to produce excellent responses, and such an approach, if validated, would forestall much of the overtreatment of some patients with chronic HCV infection that is true now.

Trying to navigate the literature on how best to manage patients with HCV infection is a monumental task for most of us and is one that is probably best left to our subspecialty colleagues.

J. A. Stockman III, MD

Risk of Celiac Disease Autoimmunity and Timing of Gluten Introduction in the Diet of Infants at Increased Risk of Disease

Norris JM, Barriga K, Hoffenberg EJ, et al (Univ of Colorado at Denver; Roche Molecular Systems, Inc, Alameda, Calif)
JAMA 293:2343-2351, 2005   7–10

Context.—While gluten ingestion is responsible for the signs and symptoms of celiac disease, it is not known what factors are associated with initial appearance of the disease.

Objective.—To examine whether the timing of gluten exposure in the infant diet was associated with the development of celiac disease autoimmunity (CDA).

Design, Setting, and Patients.—Prospective observational study conducted in Denver, Colo, from 1994-2004 of 1560 children at increased risk for celiac disease or type 1 diabetes, as defined by possession of either HLA-DR3 or DR4 alleles, or having a first-degree relative with type 1 diabetes. The mean follow-up was 4.8 years.

Main Outcome Measure.—Risk of CDA defined as being positive for tissue transglutaminase (tTG) autoantibody on 2 or more consecutive visits or being positive for tTG once and having a positive small bowel biopsy for celiac disease, by timing of introduction of gluten-containing foods into the diet.

Results.—Fifty-one children developed CDA. Findings adjusted for HLA-DR3 status indicated that children exposed to foods containing wheat, barley, or rye (gluten-containing foods) in the first 3 months of life (3 [6%] CDA positive vs 40 [3%] CDA negative) had a 5-fold increased risk of CDA compared with children exposed to gluten-containing foods at 4 to 6 months (12 [23%] CDA positive vs 574 [38%] CDA negative) (hazard ratio [HR], 5.17; 95% confidence interval [CI], 1.44-18.57). Children not exposed to gluten until the seventh month or later (36 [71%] CDA positive vs 895 [59%] CDA negative) had a marginally increased risk of CDA compared with those exposed at 4 to 6 months (HR, 1.87; 95% CI, 0.97-3.60). After restricting our case group to only the 25 CDA-positive children who had biopsy-diagnosed celiac disease, initial exposure to wheat, barley, or rye in the first 3 months (3 [12%] CDA positive vs 40 [3%] CDA negative) or in the seventh month or later (19 [76%] CDA positive vs 912 [59%] CDA negative) significantly increased risk of CDA compared with exposure at 4 to 6 months (3 [12%] CDA positive vs 583 [38%] CDA negative) (HR, 22.97; 95% CI, 4.55-115.93; P = .001; and HR, 3.98; 95% CI, 1.18-13.46; P = .04, respectively).

Conclusion.—Timing of introduction of gluten into the infant diet is associated with the appearance of CDA in children at increased risk for the disease.

▶ The YEAR BOOK OF PEDIATRICS comments fairly frequently on the topic of celiac disease in children. This is because it is such a common health problem. It is estimated that at least 1% of youngsters and adults in North America and Western Europe have gluten-sensitive enteropathy. Although the cause of celiac disease is not fully understood, most do consider it to be an autoimmune-type disease, and tissue transglutaminase has been suggested as a major autoantigen. The process is triggered in individuals who carry either HLA-DQ2 or HLA-DQ8 genes by the presence in the diet of wheat gluten and similar proteins from rye and barley. However, the fact that only a few genetically susceptible individuals actually develop celiac disease, even though virtually all individuals are exposed to gluten, has long suggested that the etiology of celiac disease is actually multifactorial and that other genetic and environmental factors must play a role in the occurrence of the clinical manifestations of the disease. Because autoimmunity resulting in celiac disease typically develops between the ages of 4 and 24 months after weaning, when cereals are first introduced into the diet, many have suspected an environmental influence of infant diet on disease risk and presentation. Indeed, evidence for the influence of infant feeding patterns on the disease process has been accumulating in recent years. Termination of breast-feeding before the introduction of gluten, high consumption of gluten, and early introduction of cow's milk or gluten-containing foods have been hypothesized as environmental risk factors.

It was more than half a century ago that it was suggested that breast-fed infants have a later onset of celiac disease. This view was later supported by a number of European case-controlled studies, but the true influence of infant feeding on the etiology of celiac disease has remained controversial. Exactly how breast-feeding might be protective is also controversial. It remains unclear whether the association of celiac disease and breast milk is direct and causal, that is, breast milk may reduce the risk of celiac disease in childhood through its immunomodulating potential and its numerous protective immune components including secretory IgA. It is also possible that the protective effect of breast milk may be totally indirect in that it merely modulates the timing of gluten introduction, resulting in a less abrupt, a postponed, or a reduced amount of dietary gluten in the infant diet and, thereby, fewer symptoms of the disease.

This article is the first study that attempts to outline the link between early infant diet and the development of celiac disease examined in a prospective manner. The study examined whether early gluten exposure in infants is associated with the development of celiac disease–related autoimmunity as defined by the presence of autoantibodies or small bowel biopsy evidence of celiac disease in some 1560 children at increased risk of type 1 diabetes and celiac disease. These were youngsters who had a first-degree relative with type 1 diabetes or the presence of genes associated with an increased risk of celiac disease. It turns out that children initially exposed to gluten in the first 3 months of life have a 5-fold increased risk of the development of celiac disease–related autoimmune problems in comparison with babies who are exposed to gluten only after 4 months of age. Early exposure to rice or oats was not associated with this problem. It is clear that long-term follow-up of these children will be needed to help clarify whether early exposure to gluten actually results in a real increase in the risk of celiac disease itself, an earlier presentation of the disorder, or neither. Nonetheless, it is clear that breast-feeding—exclusive breast-feeding (or at least for the first 4 months of life)—is best. The data are somewhat reassuring that one can introduce cereals at 4 to 6 months without any undue increase in the risk of the development of celiac disease later in life.

The article by Kalayci et al (Abstract 7–11) reminds us that many children with celiac disease have iron deficiency and iron deficiency anemia. Most iron deficiency here in the United States is due to dietary depravation. Nonetheless, failure to absorb iron or iron loss can result from as common a disorder as celiac disease. Think of celiac disease any time you see iron deficiency in a child who should not have it on the basis of poor diet.

J. A. Stockman III, MD

The Prevalence of Coeliac Disease as Detected by Screening in Children With Iron Deficiency Anaemia

Kalayci AG, Kanber Y, Birinci A, et al (Ondokuz Mayis Univ, Samsun, Turkey)
Acta Paediatr 94:678-681, 2005   7–11

Aim.—Iron deficiency anaemia is a frequent finding seen in coeliac disease, which can be diagnosed alone or with other findings. In this study, our aim was to determine the prevalence of coeliac disease in children with iron deficiency anaemia without significant gastrointestinal symptoms.

Methods.—There were 135 children with iron deficiency anaemia in the patient group (group 1), and 223 healthy children without iron deficiency anaemia in the control group (group 2) in this study. Antiendomysial antibody (EMA) IgA test was given to both groups. Antiendomysial antibody-positive patients underwent small intestine biopsy.

Results.—The mean age was 7.2 ± 4.6 (2-16) y in the patient group (group 1) and 8.2 ± 3.8 (2-16) y in the control group (group 2), and no significant difference between the two groups was detected. In terms of gender, there was a significant difference between groups 1 and 2 (M/F: 74/61 and 98/125, respectively) ($p<0.05$). EMA was positive in six cases in group 1 (4.4%), and villous atrophy and/or inflammation in the lamina propria with increased intraepithelial lymphocytes was seen on small intestine biopsy in these patients. In the control group, EMA was negative in all children. In detailed histories of patients with coeliac disease diagnosis, recurrent iron deficiency anaemia/pica was found in four patients (66.7%) and occasionally foul-smelling or watery stool attacks were seen in four patients (66.7%). Three of these six patients (50%) had short stature.

Conclusion.—The prevalence of coeliac disease was high in patients with iron deficiency anaemia; therefore, gastrointestinal findings should be further examined for coeliac disease, and the possibility of coeliac disease should be investigated in patients with recurrent iron deficiency anaemia and short stature. no comment

Progressive Multifocal Leukoencephalopathy After Natalizumab Therapy for Crohn's Disease

Van Assche G, Van Ranst M, Sciot R, et al (Univ of Leuven, Belgium)
N Engl J Med 353:362-368, 2005   7–12

Background.—Natalizumab has shown much promise as a treatment for both multiple sclerosis and inflammatory bowel disease. However, 2 cases of progressive multifocal leukoencephalopathy (PML) have been reported in patients who were treated with a humanized monoclonal antibody against α_4 integrins, natalizumab, in combination with interferon beta-1a. A third case of PML in a patient with Crohn disease who received 300 mg of open-label natalizumab as part of a clinical trial was reported.

Case Report.—Man, 60, with long-standing ileal Crohn disease was seen in the emergency department with severe confusion and disorientation. He had been treated with natalizumab for approximately 17 months before presentation. The patient had initially received 3 monthly infusions of 300 mg of natalizumab IV during a clinical trial, followed by 300 mg IV every 4 weeks after a relapse of Crohn disease. The patient was mentally slow on admission, but with normal arousal. No focal signs were found on neurologic examination. There were no remarkable physical findings. Routine hematologic and biochemical measurements showed mild iron-deficiency anemia. Levels of C-reactive protein were normal, as were the findings on ECG and chest radiography. CT of the brain showed a nonenhancing hypodense lesion in the right frontal lobe. Because the patient's condition progressively deteriorated, a decisison to perform surgery was made quickly, and a spinal tap was not done. Trephination was performed, and the right frontal lesion was partially resected. Histologically, the resected lesion contained primarily abnormalities of the white matter, consisting of a mixture of astrocytes with large and atypical nuclei, lymphocytes, and foamy macrophages. A diagnosis of astrocytoma of World Health Organization grade III was made based on the large size of the frontal lesion, the atypical aspect of the nuclei, and the increase in Ki67-MIB1 proliferation index. Postoperatively, the patient experienced prolonged confusion, somnolence, and seizures, which were treated with phenytoin. There was a temporary improvement in the patient's condition, followed by a return of somnolence and confusion. MRI performed 6 weeks after surgery showed enlargement of the lesions in the right temporal and left front lobes, and postoperative changes in the right frontal lobe. Corticosteroid treatment was initiated, and radiotherapy was planned, but the patient died 3 months after the start of corticosteroid therapy. Included in the pathologic findings was a finding of JC virus DNA detected in a serum sample obtained 2 months before admission, when the patient was receiving monthly infusions of natalizumab.

Conclusions.—This case report and the 2 previously reported cases suggest that natalizumab therapy can result in JC virus–induced PML.

▶ This report shows us the advantages and disadvantages of using innovative therapies to manage immune-mediated disorders. Natalizumab is a humanized monoclonal antibody against α_4 integrins. The latter monoclonal antibody is being increasingly studied for the treatment of inflammatory bowel disease and multiple sclerosis. It is being used in children, largely on an experimental basis. The more we learn about immunomodulatory agents to manage such disorders, the more we learn that they can have serious complications associated with them, warranting their use only in refractory cases.

The patients reported in this year's YEAR BOOK OF PEDIATRICS were among 3000 that had participated in clinical trials of natalizumab for the treatment of multiple sclerosis or Crohn disease. The reports describe in detail the onset of PML. This is a deadly opportunistic infection of the CNS for which there is no specific treatment. It is caused by reactivation of a clinically latent JC polyomavirus infection. This virus infects and destroys oligodendrocytes, leading to multifocal areas of demyelination and associated neurologic dysfunction. The occurrence of PML as a consequence of this form of therapy was totally unexpected, since it almost invariably occurs in the context of profoundly impaired cell-mediated immunity in patients with AIDS or leukemia or in the post–organ transplant situation.

Not much is known about the JC virus itself. We do know that seropositivity rates for JC virus increase with age and vary in different populations. After the initial infection, from which one normally recovers, the virus remains quiescent in the kidneys and in lymphoid organs of people who are immunologically competent. The virus is often present in urine but rarely is recovered from blood. However, JC viremia is detectable in patients with immunosuppression, and hematogenous dissemination is the likely source of entry into the CNS.

The logical question that is raised is whether it is possible to predict and prevent the occurrence of PML in those who must receive α_4-integrin blockers. Only individuals who have been previously infected with JC virus are at risk for PML, and it could be worthwhile seroscreening for this virus, but one should anticipate high seropositivity rates. There are few data yet telling us what the seropositivity is at varying ages within the pediatric population, but the seropositivity of healthy adults in varying studies runs from 50% to 86%. Thus, adults would seem to be poor candidates, in general, for α_4-integrin blockers since only a minority are seronegative for the JC virus.

While on the topic of transmissible forms of encephalopathy, do you know how long scrapie, the transmissible spongiform encephalopathy found in sheep, has been around? It is generally held that scrapie can be traced back only to the early 18th century based on records in the United Kingdom, France, and Germany. More recent research, however, suggests that it may have existed 2000 years or more ago and had its origins in China.[1] If you are not aware, the English name "scrapie" is derived in the English language from the fact that afflicted sheep suffer pruritus and wind up scraping off much of their coats. So what does this have to do with China? If you look at the way Chinese is written, Chinese word characters are often composed of 2 or more parts. One component may hint at the meaning, while another gives the sound, or both may contribute to the meaning. The word character for "pruritus" or "itchy" is composed of 2 parts, an outer wrapper meaning "disease" and an inner component meaning "sheep." The supposition is that the Chinese saw a lot of itchy sheep and ascribed the term pruritus to the phenomenon they saw in sheep.

See the Neurology and Psychiatry chapter for 2 additional reports (Abstracts 13–3 and 13–4) of PML complicating the management of neurologic diseases being treated with natalizumab.

J. A. Stockman III, MD

Reference

1. Winckner RB: Scrapie in ancient China? *Science* 309:874, 2005.

Sargramostim for Active Crohn's Disease

Korzenik JR, for the Sargramostim in Crohn's Disease Study Group (Harvard Med School; et al)

N Engl J Med 352:2193-2201, 2005   7–13

Background.—Sargramostim, granulocyte–macrophage colony-stimulating factor, a hematopoietic growth factor, stimulates cells of the intestinal innate immune system. Preliminary studies suggest sargramostim may have activity in Crohn's disease. To evaluate this novel therapeutic approach, we conducted a randomized, placebo-controlled trial.

Methods.—Using a 2:1 ratio, we randomly assigned 124 patients with moderate-to-severe active Crohn's disease to receive 6 µg of sargramostim per kilogram per day or placebo subcutaneously for 56 days. Antibiotics and aminosalicylates were allowed; immunosuppressants and glucocorticoids were prohibited. The primary end point was a clinical response, defined by a decrease from baseline of at least 70 points in the Crohn's Disease Activity Index (CDAI) at the end of treatment (day 57). Other end points included changes in disease severity and the health-related quality of life and adverse events.

Results.—There was no significant difference in the rate of the primary end point of a clinical response defined by a decrease of at least 70 points in the CDAI score on day 57 between the sargramostim and placebo groups (54 percent vs. 44 percent, P=0.28). However, significantly more patients in the sargramostim group than in the placebo group reached the secondary end points of a clinical response defined by a decrease from baseline of at least 100 points in the CDAI score on day 57 (48 percent vs. 26 percent, P=0.01) and of remission, defined by a CDAI score of 150 points or less on day 57 (40 percent vs. 19 percent, P=0.01). The rates of either type of clinical response and of remission were significantly higher in the sargramostim group than in the placebo group on day 29 of treatment and 30 days after treatment. The sargramostim group also had significant improvements in the quality of life. Mild-to-moderate injection-site reactions and bone pain were more common in the sargramostim group, and three patients in this group had serious adverse events possibly or probably related to treatment.

Conclusions.—This study was negative for the primary end point, but findings for the secondary end points suggest that sargramostim therapy decreased disease severity and improved the quality of life in patients with active Crohn's disease.

▶ This article includes young adults 18 years or older as well as older adults. Nonetheless, because precious few data exist regarding innovative therapies for children with active Crohn's disease, we should pay attention to articles such as this.

The pathophysiology of Crohn's disease is being better understood with time. The disease results from defective functioning of the intestinal innate immune system. This compromises intestinal epithelium and phagocytic cells of the lamina propria, including neutrophils and macrophages. Breakdown of this defensive barrier may permit persistent exposure of the lamina propria cells to microbes in the lumina of the gut, resulting in a chronic inflammatory process mediated by T cells. One can conceive of therapies augmenting the intestinal innate immune defense as well as suppressing a secondary inflammatory response in active Crohn's disease. Most therapies, to date, have been immunomodulatory and designed to suppress inflammatory responses. Granulocyte–macrophage colony-stimulating factor (GM-CSF), a myeloid growth factor, is geared toward enhancing the bowel's defense mechanisms rather than suppressing immunity.

GM-CSF functions in the development of phagocytic cells. It also has some effect on T cells; therefore, it can augment host defenses while ameliorating the inflammation associated with Crohn's disease. Sargramostim is a yeast-derived recombinant human GM-CSF. The most common application of this agent is for prompt recovery of myeloid cell functioning after a round of chemotherapy. Early pilot studies suggested a high rate of clinical response and minimal adverse side effects when it was used to treat active Crohn's disease. We see in this article that the rates of clinical response and remission are, in fact, higher with sargramostim treatment.

A betting person would place favorable odds on the newer agents that have appeared in recent times making their way into the therapeutic armamentarium utilized for the treatment of inflammatory bowel disease. The odds do seem to favor GM-CSF. See the article by Feagan et al (Abstract 7–15) telling us about the role of antibodies to integrin and the role they play in the management of inflammatory bowel disease. As you will see elsewhere in this year's YEAR BOOK OF PEDIATRICS, there is a price to pay for using such humanized antibodies—a price that involves serious neurologic consequences.

On a totally unrelated topic, are you aware that chewing gum has some medical advantages and some medical disadvantages? Can you name one in each category? In the category of medical advantages, if the digestive system can be "woken up" earlier after abdominal surgery, an individual may be able to leave the hospital faster. It turns out that chewing gum acts as a form of "sham feeding," where chewing and swallowing stimulate hormones involved in making the gastrointestinal tract begin to work after abdominal surgery. A study of the chewing of gum after surgery has shown that subjects who chewed gum after laparoscopic procedures went home a day earlier than patients who did not chew gum. Chewing gum was not able to overcome, however, the lazy bowel that is seen following open abdominal surgery (www.usatoday.com/news/health/2005-12-14-gum-colon-patients_x.htm, accessed on July 19, 2006).

So the above is the good news. The not so good news is the fact that children who chew gum before surgery may in fact present a higher anesthetic risk than those who do not. A comparison of children not chewing gum before arriving in the OR with children who were told to chew gum found that those who had chewed gum had a significantly greater gastric fluid volume than the non-chewers. Whether this actually translates into an adverse clinical situation remains to be investigated.[1]

J. A. Stockman III, MD

Reference

1. Schoenfelder RC, Ponnamma CM, Freyle D, et al: Residual gastric fluid volume and chewing gum before surgery. *Anesth Analg* 102:415-417, 2006.

Natalizumab Induction and Maintenance Therapy for Crohn's Disease
Sandborn WJ, for the International Efficacy of Natalizumab as Active Crohn's Therapy (ENACT-1) and the Evaluation of Natalizumab as Continuous Therapy (ENACT-2) Trial Groups (Mayo Clinic, Rochester, Minn; et al)
N Engl J Med 353:1912-1925, 2005   7–14

Background.—Natalizumab, a humanized monoclonal antibody against α_4 integrin, inhibits leukocyte adhesion and migration into inflamed tissue.

Methods.—We conducted two controlled trials to evaluate natalizumab as induction and maintenance therapy in patients with active Crohn's disease. In the first trial, 905 patients were randomly assigned to receive 300 mg of natalizumab or placebo at weeks 0, 4, and 8. The primary outcome was response, defined by a decrease in the Crohn's Disease Activity Index (CDAI) score of at least 70 points, at week 10. In the second trial, 339 patients who had a response to natalizumab in the first trial were randomly reassigned to receive 300 mg of natalizumab or placebo every four weeks through week 56. The primary outcome was a sustained response through week 36. A secondary outcome in both trials was disease remission (a CDAI score of less than 150).

Results.—In the first trial, the natalizumab and placebo groups had similar rates of response (56 percent and 49 percent, respectively; P=0.05) and remission (37 percent and 30 percent, respectively; P=0.12) at 10 weeks. Continuing natalizumab in the second trial resulted in higher rates of sustained response (61 percent vs. 28 percent, P<0.001) and remission (44 percent vs. 26 percent, P=0.003) through week 36 than did switching to placebo. Serious adverse events occurred in 7 percent of each group in the first trial and in 10 percent of the placebo group and 8 percent of the natalizumab group in the second trial. In an open-label extension study, a patient treated with natalizumab died from progressive multifocal leukoencephalopathy, associated with the JC virus, a human polyomavirus.

Conclusions.—Induction therapy with natalizumab for Crohn's disease resulted in small, nonsignificant improvements in response and remission rates. Patients who had a response had significantly increased rates of sustained response and remission if natalizumab was continued every four weeks. The benefit of natalizumab will need to be weighed against the risk of serious adverse events, including progressive multifocal leukoencephalopathy.

▶ Over the past few years, we have learned more and more about the pathophysiologic mechanisms that are involved with the evolution of inflammatory bowel disease. It would appear that a key feature of the disease is the recruitment of white blood cells into gut tissue, which results in inflammation. Natalizumab, a humanized IgG monoclonal antibody that blocks the adhesion and subsequent migration of white blood cells into the gut by binding α_4 integrin, is a relatively new agent representing a class of molecules referred to as selective adhesion-molecule inhibitors. This class of drug has already been used and approved for the treatment of patients with multiple sclerosis. It is now being actively studied as part of the potential treatment of inflammatory bowel disease. We learn from this cooperative trial that natalizumab is not a great drug at inducing a remission in patients with inflammatory bowel disease but that it does significantly assist in maintaining a remission.

Agents such as natalizumab, when effective, come at a price. That price is the unintended consequence of a secondary immunodeficiency induced by such powerful agents. Progressive multifocal leukoencephalopathy developed in at least 3 patients who received natalizumab, including 1 patient with Crohn's disease. Two of the 3 patients died. Progressive multifocal leukoencephalopathy is caused by the nearly ubiquitous JC virus, a human polyomavirus that is present in about 80% of the adult population. The virus is likely encountered in childhood and persists in a latent form within the epithelium of the gastrointestinal tract and kidney throughout life. Activation of latent virus and subsequent dissemination have been causally linked to the development of progressive multifocal leukoencephalopathy. Such activation can occur when powerful immunosuppressants are given.

As far as natalizumab is concerned, is the benefit worth the risk? Unfortunately, there is no answer to this question yet; it is just too early to know. For now, natalizumab is best given only to those who have not responded to other forms of therapy, and recent studies have suggested that close surveillance for the earliest signs of progressive multifocal leukoencephalopathy with brain MRI is in order.

To read more about selective adhesion-molecule therapy and inflammatory bowel disease, see the superb editorial by Podolsky.[1]

J. A. Stockman III, MD

Reference

1. Podolsky DK: Selective adhesion molecule therapy and inflammatory bowel disease: A tale of Janus? *N Engl J Med* 353:1965-1968, 2005.

Treatment of Ulcerative Colitis With a Humanized Antibody to the $\alpha_4\beta_7$ Integrin

Feagan BG, Greenberg GR, Wild G, et al (Robarts Research Inst, London, Ontario, Canada; Univ of Western Ontario, London, Canada; Univ of Toronto; et al)
N Engl J Med 352:2499-3507, 2005   7–15

Background.—Selective blockade of interactions between leukocytes and vascular endothelium in the gut is a promising strategy for the treatment of inflammatory bowel diseases.

Methods.—We conducted a multicenter, double-blind, placebo-controlled trial of MLN02, a humanized antibody to the $\alpha_4\beta_7$ integrin, in patients with active ulcerative colitis. We randomly assigned 181 patients to receive 0.5 mg of MLN02 per kilogram of body weight, 2.0 mg per kilogram, or an identical-appearing placebo intravenously on day 1 and day 29. Eligible patients also received concomitant mesalamine or no other treatment for colitis. Ulcerative colitis clinical scores and sigmoidoscopic assessments were evaluated six weeks after randomization.

Results.—Clinical remission rates at week 6 were 33 percent, 32 percent, and 14 percent for the group receiving 0.5 mg of MLN02 per kilogram, the group receiving 2.0 mg per kilogram, and the placebo group, respectively (P=0.03). The corresponding proportions of patients who improved by at least 3 points on the ulcerative colitis clinical score were 66 percent, 53 percent, and 33 percent (P=0.002). Twenty-eight percent of patients receiving 0.5 mg per kilogram and 12 percent of those receiving 2.0 mg per kilogram had endoscopically evident remission, as compared with 8 percent of those receiving placebo (P=0.007). For the minority of patients in whom an MLN02 antibody titer greater than 1:125 developed, incomplete saturation of the $\alpha_4\beta_7$ receptor on circulating lymphocytes was observed and no benefit of treatment was identifiable.

Conclusions.—In this short-term study, MLN02 was more effective than placebo for the induction of clinical and endoscopic remission in patients with active ulcerative colitis.

► We have been hearing more and more about the use of monoclonal antibodies as part of the management of diseases that are immunologically based. One such humanized monoclonal antibody is an agent that has been developed against integrin. Integrins are heterodimeric proteins that regulate cellular movement. They function as cellular adhesion molecules. $\alpha_4\beta7$ integrin, which is primarily involved in the recruitment of leukocytes to the gut, is present on the cell surface of a small population of circulating T lymphocytes. Its administration produces a blockade of the interaction between T cells and the endothelium of the intestinal vasculature as well as attachment to inflamed tissue. This is a potentially highly effective therapy for inflammatory bowel diseases.

We see from this article that patients with ulcerative colitis who receive humanized monoclonal antibody against integrins have a 2-fold greater probability of achieving remission as opposed to those receiving a placebo. This finding is highly clinically meaningful.

In the series of patients treated in this article, no important differences in the occurrence of adverse effects were identified among treatment groups. No deaths, cancers, or opportunistic infections were observed. Note, however, that a different anti-integrin has been associated with the development of a progressive multifocal leukoencephalopathy (see Abstract 7–12).

The authors of this article are wise to point out that, although a short-term study of this type has identified an effective treatment for patients with active inflammatory bowel disease, the role of such therapies in clinical practice remains largely unknown, and additional long-term studies are badly needed.

This is the last entry in the Gastroenterology chapter, so we will close with a question having to do with bowel preps. The pediatric gastroenterologists that you refer your patients to for colonoscopy evaluation complain that the prep that you order is frequently inadequate to allow a good visualization of the colon. In the older pediatric age population (as well as the adult population), what simple maneuver can you recommend to complement the use of bowel prep that will markedly increase the quality of that prep?

The answer is fairly simple: light gentle exercise. Yes, patients who walk intermittently while taking bowel preparation solution have cleaner bowels than patients who sit still. If you do not believe this is true, see the recent study on this topic by Kim et al.[1] Investigators in South Korea studied 383 outpatients undergoing colonoscopy following standard bowel preparations. All the participants had a liquid dinner the night before their colonoscopy and 5 mg of bisacodyl as a premedication followed by 2.5 to 3.0 liters of polyethylene glycol. Those randomized to exercise took the solution and 250 mL doses and walked around for at least 5 minutes after each dose. Control patients took 250 mL of polyethylene glycol every 10 minutes and rested between doses. The interval between bowel preparation and colonoscopy averaged 4.5 hours. All patients had the same endoscopist, who rated the quality of the bowel preparation on a 4-point scale (excellent, good, fair, or poor). The endoscopist was totally unaware of the randomization used. So what did the endoscopist find? He found that patients who had walked around during their bowel preparation had significantly cleaner bowels (50% cleaner than the control group) as judged by having good or excellent bowel preps.

The report of walking exercise improving bowel prep before colonoscopy turns out to be the one and only reason to ever exercise. The report itself constitutes the best article of 2005. If you have a patient who still believes that you are born with a finite number of heartbeats and they should not be expended on exercise, you can probably achieve the same benefits of a better bowel prep by telling the patient to drink the bowel prep solution in the basement and restrict the use of the toilet to the one on the second floor. That should be exercise enough.

J. A. Stockman III, MD

Reference

1. Kim HS, Park DH, Kim JW, et al: Effectiveness of walking exercise as a bowel preparation for colonoscopy: A randomized control trial. *Am J Gastroenterol* 100:1964-1969, 2005.

8 Genitourinary Tract

Clinical and Demographic Factors Associated With Urinary Tract Infection in Young Febrile Infants
Zorc JJ, for the Multicenter RSV-SBI Study Group of the Pediatric Emergency Medicine Collaborative Research Committee of the American Academy of Pediatrics (Univ of Pennsylvania, Philadelphia; et al)
Pediatrics 116:644-648, 2005   8–1

Objective.—Previous research has identified clinical predictors for urinary tract infection (UTI) to guide urine screening in febrile children <24 months of age. These studies have been limited to single centers, and few have focused on young infants who may be most at risk for complications if a UTI is missed. The objective of this study was to identify clinical and demographic factors associated with UTI in febrile infants who are ≤60 days of age using a prospective multicenter cohort.

Methods.—We conducted a multicenter, prospective, cross-sectional study during consecutive bronchiolitis seasons. All febrile (≥38°C) infants who were ≤60 days of age and seen at any of 8 pediatric emergency departments from October through March 1999-2001 were eligible. Clinical appearance was evaluated using the Yale Observation Scale. UTI was defined as growth of a known bacterial pathogen from a catheterized specimen at a level of (1) ≥50,000 cfu/mL or (2) ≥10,000 cfu/mL in association with a positive dipstick test or urinalysis. We used bivariate tests and multiple logistic regression to identify demographic and clinical factors that were associated with the likelihood of UTI.

Results.—A total of 1025 (67%) of 1513 eligible patients were enrolled; 9.0% of enrolled infants received a diagnosis of UTI. Uncircumcised male infants had a higher rate of UTI (21.3%) compared with female (5.0%) and circumcised male (2.3%) infants. Infants with maximum recorded temperature of ≥39°C had a higher rate of UTI (16.3%) than other infants (7.2%). After multivariable adjustment, UTI was associated with being uncircumcised (odds ratio: 10.4; bias-corrected 95% confidence interval: 4.7-31.4) and maximum temperature (odds ratio: 2.4 per °C; 95% confidence interval: 1.5-3.6). Factors that were reported previously to be associated with risk for UTI in infants and toddlers, such as white race and ill appearance, were not significantly associated with risk for UTI in this cohort of young infants.

Conclusions.—Being uncircumcised and height of fever were associated with UTI in febrile infants who were ≤60 days of age. Uncircumcised male infants were at particularly high risk and may warrant a different approach to screening and management.

► The findings of this report have great impact on the way in which we practice pediatrics. The findings should influence our decision making with respect to risk criteria for the evaluation of fever in young infants. Circumcision status is frequently not considered in the management decision of a febrile male infant. If one looks at large numbers of patient charts from little boys being evaluated for a UTI, you will find that circumcision status is often undocumented. We see in this report that there is a 10-fold greater risk of UTI if an infant male has not been circumcised.

Surely the debate around the pros and cons of circumcision will rage on for both medical and social reasons. If, for any reason, you have been a naysayer about the link between UTI and the uncircumcised state, please read the report of Zorc et al in detail. You may be convinced that the foreskin, like the umbilical cord, should be shed after birth if you want to minimize the risk of a subsequent UTI.

J. A. Stockman III, MD

Choice of Urine Collection Methods for the Diagnosis of Urinary Tract Infection in Young, Febrile Infants
Schroeder AR, Newman TB, Wasserman RC, et al (Univ of California, San Francisco; Amercian Academy of Pediatrics, Elk Grove Village, Ill; Univ of Vermont, Burlington)
Arch Pediatr Adolesc Med 159:915-922, 2005   8–2

Background.—The optimal method of urine collection in febrile infants is debatable; catheterization, considered more accurate, is technically difficult and invasive.

Objectives.—To determine predictors of urethral catheterization in febrile infants and to compare bag and catheterized urine test performance characteristics.

Design.—Prospective analysis of infants enrolled in the Pediatric Research in Office Settings' Febrile Infant Study.

Setting.—A total of 219 practices from within the Pediatric Research in Office Settings' network, including 44 states, the District of Columbia, and Puerto Rico.

Patients.—A total of 3066 infants aged 0 to 3 months with temperatures of 38°C or higher.

Main Outcome Measures.—We calculated adjusted odds ratios for predictors of catheterization. Diagnostic test characteristics were compared between bag and catheterization. Urinary tract infection was defined as pure growth of 100,000 CFU/mL or more (bag) and 20,000 CFU/mL or more (catheterization).

Results.—Seventy percent of urine samples were obtained by catheterization. Predictors of catheterization included female sex, practitioner older than 40 years, Medicaid, Hispanic ethnicity, nighttime evaluation, and severe dehydration. For leukocyte esterase levels, bag specimens demonstrated no difference in sensitivity but somewhat lower specificity (84% [bag] vs 94% [catheterization], $P<.001$) and a lower area under the receiver operating characteristic curve for white blood cells (0.71 [bag] vs 0.86 [catheterization], $P=.01$). Infection rates were similar in bag and catheterized specimens (8.5% vs 10.8%). Ambiguous cultures were more common in bag specimens (7.4% vs 2.7%, $P<.001$), but 21 catheterized specimens are needed to avoid each ambiguous bag result.

Conclusions.—Most practitioners obtain urine from febrile infants via catheterization, but choice of method is not related to the risk of urinary tract infection. Although both urine cultures and urinalyses are more accurate in catheterized specimens, the magnitude of difference is small but should be factored into clinical decision making.

► This study from the Pediatric Research in the Office Setting (PROS) provides critical new information about what we as pediatricians do in the collection of urine specimens as part of the evaluation of young, febrile infants. The study asked a number of questions: (1) Which urine collection techniques do practitioners use to diagnose urinary tract infections in young, febrile infants? (2) What are the infant and practitioner characteristics that predict the choice of urine collection method used? (3) Do the diagnostic test characteristics of urinalysis differ between bag and catheterized methods? (4) Do the rates of positive culture results and ambiguous urine culture results differ between methods of collection?

What we learn from this report is that the significant majority of practitioners who feel that a young, febrile infant should be evaluated for a possible urinary tract infection obtain a urine sample by catheterization. The older the care provider, the more likely it was that a catheter specimen will be obtained as opposed to a bag specimen. Girl babies more frequently had catheter specimens than boy babies.

As one might suspect, the PROS febrile infant study yields important information. Among this information is the observation that only 54% of febrile infants aged 0 to 93 days in fact had their urine tested. Bag specimens seem to be, by and large, adequate for most purposes, although it was more likely that more than one organism may be found in a bag specimen. Thus, if critical decision making is needed (such as administering antibiotics, hospitalizing a baby, or both), it would seem that catheterization should be favored. That having been said, see the report that follows by McGillivray et al (Abstract 8–3), who does a head-to-head comparison of "clean-void" bag versus catheter urinalysis in the diagnosis of urinary tract infection in young infants.

J. A. Stockman III, MD

A Head-to-Head Comparison: "Clean-Void" Bag Versus Catheter Urinalysis in the Diagnosis of Urinary Tract Infection in Young Children
McGillivray D, Mok E, Mulrooney E, et al (McGill Univ, Montreal)
J Pediatr 147:451-456, 2005   8–3

Objective.—To compare the validity of the urinalysis on clean-voided bag versus catheter urine specimens using the catheter culture as the "gold" standard.

Study Design.—This is a cross-sectional study of 303 nontoilet-trained children under age 3 years at risk for urinary tract infection (UTI) who presented to a children's hospital emergency department. Paired bag and catheter specimens were obtained from each child and sent for dipstick and microscopic urinalysis. Sensitivity and specificity were compared using McNemar's χ^2 test for paired specimens and the ordinary χ^2 test for unpaired comparisons.

Results.—The bag dipstick was more sensitive than the catheter dipstick for the entire study sample: 0.85 (95% confidence interval [CI] = 0.78 to 0.93) versus 0.71 (95% CI = 0.61 to 0.81), respectively. Both bag and catheter dipstick sensitivities were lower in infants ≤90 days old (0.69 [95% CI = 0.44 to 0.94] and 0.46 [95% CI = 0.19 to 0.73], respectively) than in infants >90 days old (0.88 [95% CI = 0.81 to 0.96] and 0.75 [95% CI = 0.65 to 0.86], respectively). Specificity was consistently lower for the bag specimens than for the catheter specimens: 0.62 (95% CI = 0.56 to 0.69) versus 0.97 (95% CI = 0.95 to 0.99), respectively (Table 2).

Conclusions.—Urine collection methods alter the diagnostic validity of urinalysis. These differences have important implications for the diagnostic and therapeutic management of children with suspected UTI.

▶ The preceding study by Schroeder et al (Abstract 8–2) was undertaken by the Pediatric Research in the Office Setting (PROS) group. PROS examined the characteristics of various urine tests, including bag- and catheter-collected specimens. The urinalysis from catheter specimens was found to be more

TABLE 2.—Comparison of Combined Dipstick and Microscopic
Sensitivity and Specificity in Paired Bag Versus Catheter Urine Specimens,
Overall and in 2 Age Groups

	Bag	Catheter	P Value
Sensitivity			
Overall (n = 287)	0.95 (0.90 to 1.00)	0.83 (0.74 to 0.91)	.004
≤90 days (n = 52)	0.77 (0.54 to 1.00)	0.62 (0.35 to 0.88)	.480
>90 days (n = 235)	0.99 (0.96 to 1.00)	0.87 (0.78 to 0.95)	.013
Specificity			
Overall (n = 287)	0.45 (0.38 to 0.52)	0.95 (0.92 to 0.98)	<.001
≤90 days (n = 52)	0.54 (0.38 to 0.69)	1.00 (0.92 to 1.00)	<.001
>90 days (n = 235)	0.43 (0.35 to 0.50)	0.94 (0.90 to 0.98)	<.001

(Courtesy of McGillivray D, Mok E, Mulrooney E, et al: A head-to-head comparison: "Clean-void" bag versus catheter urinalysis in the diagnosis of urinary tract infection in young children. *J Pediatr* 147:451-456. Copyright 2005 by Elsevier.)

sensitive and more specific than the bag urinalysis, although urine specimens were not paired. The authors of the report clearly indicated that it would be necessary to undertake a paired urine study (ie, both types of specimens from the same child at the same visit) to address this deficiency. The report of McGillivray et al accepted the challenge and did a head-to-head comparison of catheterized specimens and bag specimens from the same children. Why was this study necessary?

Urine cultures by catheterization or suprapubic aspiration are necessary to unequivocally detect UTI in infants. The American Academy of Pediatrics practice parameter for the diagnosis, treatment, and evaluation of the initial UTI in febrile infants and young children suggests 2 options for managing the infant or young child (age 2 months to 2 years) with unexplained fever who is assessed as not being so ill as to require immediate antibiotic therapy. One option is the "catheterize all" approach; the other is to "obtain a urine specimen by the most convenient means and perform a urinalysis. If the urinalysis suggests a UTI, obtain and culture a urine specimen, collected by suprapubic or transurethral catheterization."[1] If the urinalysis is negative, then the Academy suggests that it is "reasonable to follow the clinical course without initiating antibiotic therapy, recognizing that a negative urinalysis does not rule out a urinary tract infection."

What was found in this report was a higher bag versus catheter dipstick sensitivity for the detection of UTI. This most likely resulted from the presence of white cells or bacteria in the urethra or introitus in girls and under the foreskin of boys. For the very same reason, the presence of white blood cells in the perineal skin, vaginal introitus, or urethra would likely explain the lower specificity of the bag urine in girls. However, the finding of a higher sensitivity of the bag urine from boys despite circumcision status suggests that the presence of periurethral white blood cells or bacteria is less common in boys. There was a lower sensitivity of the bagged urine in infants younger than 3 months. This could be caused by either a decreased inflammatory response or the frequent voiding and low bladder "dwell" time in newborns and young infants versus older infants.

The authors of this report suggest that not every non–toilet-trained child truly at high risk for UTI should be catheterized to obtain both a urinalysis and culture. In children with a fever without a source and at low risk for UTI (no previous history of UTI, no anatomic abnormalities, not immunosuppressed, no urinary symptoms), a "selective catheterization" strategy that is outlined in the American Academy of Pediatrics practice parameter appears reasonable, based on the findings of the report. Recognize, however, that using a dipstick screening strategy for UTI in infants older than 90 days will miss somewhere between 4% and 12% of UTIs, in the subsequent catheterized specimen, depending on the threshold chosen for colony counts. Such a miss rate probably is acceptable in low-risk children, since serious consequences of infection are far less likely and the risk of missing a UTI is likely to be outweighed by the risks of catheterization, including pain, false-positive results, trauma, or even the introduction of infection. Thus, the physician may choose to use a bag screening strategy to reduce the number of unnecessary catheterizations. The consequences of insisting on a "catheterize all" strategy for all non–toxic-appearing children with fever without a source may also have the potential to lead to test resistance by nurses, physicians, and parents who are concerned about painful procedures and the unknown risk of introducing infection.

For more on the topic about pediatricians' screening urinalysis preferences, see the report that follows (Abstract 8–4).

J. A. Stockman III, MD

Reference

1. Roberts K, Downs S, Hellerstein S, et al: Practice parameter: The diagnosis, treatment, and evaluation of the initial urinary tract infection in febrile infants and young children. *Pediatrics* 103:843-852, 1999.

Pediatricians' Screening Urinalysis Practices
Sox CM, Christakis DA (Harvard Med School, Boston; Univ of Washington, Seattle)
J Pediatr 147:362-365, 2005   8–4

Objective.—To determine pediatricians' routine screening urinalysis practices.

Study Design.—This was a survey of a nationally representative sample of pediatricians practicing in the U.S. regarding their screening urinalysis practices in childhood.

Results.—Of the 1502 pediatricians sampled, 653 eligible subjects participated, for an estimated response rate of 49.5%. The vast majority of participants (78%) routinely screen asymptomatic children with urinalysis in at least 1 age group. Pediatricians' screening urinalysis practice varies based on age group: 9% screen during infancy (<1 year), 60% screen during early childhood (1 up to 5 years), 55% screen during late childhood (5 to 12 years), and 58% screen during adolescence (13 to 20 years). The majority of pediatricians (58%) routinely screen more than 1 age group. Some 38% of the pediatricians surveyed believe that the overall health of children is improved by screening all asymptomatic children with urinalysis.

Conclusions.—Many pediatricians routinely conduct screening urinalysis during childhood, frequently at ages not recommended by the American Academy of Pediatrics.

▶ The preceding 2 studies (Abstracts 8–2 and 8–3) tell us a great deal about the best way to collect urine for culture, and this report reminds us about guidelines for routine screening urinalysis at varying ages. Enough said, but see how you would handle the following case. You are seeing a 9-year-old girl who was referred to you for evaluation of persistent microscopic hematuria, abdominal pain, and chronic fatigue. These findings have been present for 18 months. The physical examination is normal. A urinary dipstick shows 4+ blood. There are 40 red blood cells per high power field with no peculiar shapes to the red cells. There is no protein in the urine, the osmolality is 1.010, and the pH is 6. Repeated urinary cultures are negative. Renal function studies are normal. There is no evidence of orthostatic proteinuria. A broad battery of laboratory studies for blood disorders, such as sickle cell disease, systemic infections, autoimmune diseases, malignancy, and metabolic disorders are all negative. Iron studies are normal. A renal biopsy is performed and shows 35 glomeruli with mild increase in cellularity. There are no other abnormal findings at the time of renal biopsy although red blood cells are seen in the tubular lumens. Immunofluorescence is negative, and electron microscopy does not show evidence of thin basement membrane disease or Alport syndrome.

Having found little to explain what is going on, you follow the child, and after a year her findings remain the same, although her abdominal pain and fatigue have increased somewhat, leading to absenteeism from school. As a last ditch effort, you perform a CT scan with angiography. What do you think the findings would be?

This is a real case.[1] The CT scan showed compression of the left renal vein between the aorta and the superior mesenteric artery, characteristic of what is known as the "Nutcracker syndrome." The youngster was sent to the OR for translocation of the renal vein to a lower site on the inferior vena cava. Four months later, all of her signs and symptoms, including the hematuria, had completely resolved.

If you are not familiar with the Nutcracker syndrome, it is reported to be an important cause, often missed, of hematuria. The syndrome is characterized by left-sided renal bleeding caused by compression of the left renal vein between the aorta and the superior mesenteric artery, leading to an elevation of the left renal vein pressure, renal hilar varices, and the development of collateral veins. Typical clinical features of this syndrome are microscopic hematuria associated with mild to moderate proteinuria that may in fact be orthostatic, or the sudden onset of dark urine. The condition has also been associated with the chronic fatigue syndrome. Exactly why hematuria occurs in the Nutcracker syndrome remains unclear. It has been suggested that compression of the left renal vein results in left renal vein hypertension, leading to the development of collaterals with intrarenal and perirenal varicosities, which bleed, causing the hematuria.

Most patients with the Nutcracker syndrome can be managed the way this 9-year-old was managed. Some require nephrectomy. Other management has included autotransplantation of the left kidney. Those who are really good at placing stents have done so intravascularly and some have been cured with this maneuver.

J. A. Stockman III, MD

Reference

1. Bhimma R, Robbs J: Nutcracker. *Lancet* 365:1280, 2005.

Kluyvera Urinary Tract Infection: Case Report and Review of the Literature

Narchi H (Sandwell Gen Hosp, West Bromwich, England)
Pediatr Infect Dis J 24:570-572, 2005   8–5

Background.—A case of *Kluyvera ascorbata* urinary tract infection that presented as acute pyelonephritis is reported in a 19-month-old girl. The literature is reviewed with regard to infections with this uncommon organism, and pediatric urinary tract infections are particularly emphasized.

> *Case Report.*—Female infant, 19 months, presented with a 4-day history of fever, abdominal pain, chills, and lethargy. Her growth measures were normal on admission, and her temperature was 40.2°C. The patient was normotensive and did not appear toxic. The physical examination was unremarkable. Blood tests showed a peripheral white blood cell count of 17.1×10^9/L, normal platelet count and a C-reactive protein level of 90 µg/mL. She was febrile for 3 days. Two clean catch urine specimens showed many leukocytes, a positive nitrite reaction, and a pure growth of >105 colonies of *K ascorbata*, susceptible to first and second-generation cephalosporins, trimethoprim, and nitrofurantoin but resistant to amoxicillin. Intravenous cefuroxime was initiated, followed by defervescence within 24 hours. Treatment was changed to oral cephalexin after 3 days of defervescence, and the patient received antibiotic treatment for 2 weeks. Trimethoprim antibiotic prophylaxis was initiated and continued for 6 months. The patient remained well over a follow-up period of 15 months, and antibiotic prophylaxis was discontinued.

Conclusions.—Little information is available regarding antibiotic susceptibilities and the clinical effectiveness of antibiotics in *Kluyvera* infections, and definitive recommendations cannot be made as to the choice of the most appropriate antibiotic therapy because of the small sample size of the analyzed strains. *Kluyvera* infection is more common in female patients, regardless of age, and is more often seen as acute pyelonephritis in children younger than 5 years; an underlying uropathy is seen in only 1 of 3 children. In all cases reported, the patients have responded rapidly to appropriate antibiotic therapy. Identification of *Kluyvera* may be difficult because its biochemical identification patterns are similar to those of other enteric bacteria. Increased awareness and thorough evaluation of the growth and susceptibility patterns of *Kluyvera* would allow proper identification and appropriate antibiotic therapy.

▶ Pay attention to *K ascorbata*. Several reports have recently appeared, confirming its potential to cause urinary tract infection in children. *Kluyvera* is a gram-negative bacillus in the family of *Enterobacteriaceae*. The organism was initially considered to be a benign saprophyte predominantly colonizing the respiratory, gastrointestinal, and urinary tracts. Recently, however, serious infections occurring in immunocompromised as well as immunocompetent hosts have been reported as the result of infection with *Kluyvera*. These infections have primarily involved the gastrointestinal tract; however, more recently, reports of infection in the urinary tract have appeared. *Kluyvera* has been implicated in central venous catheter infection, mediastinitis, sepsis, enteritis, biliary tract infections, intra-abdominal abscesses, peritonitis, and post-traumatic urethrorectal fistula. Infection with this organism has caused fatalities.

Little information is available regarding antibiotic susceptibilities and the clinical effectiveness of antibiotics in *Kluyvera* urinary tract infections. Most individuals attempting to treat such infections use third-generation cephalosporins, fluoroquinolones, aminoglycosides, imipenem, and, when all else fails, chloramphenicol. Most strains of this organism are resistant to ampicillin, first- and second-generation cephalosporins, and ticarcillin.

Remember *Kluyvera*. Chances are, you are going to be hearing a great deal more about this class of bacteria in the future.

J. A. Stockman III, MD

Antibiotic Resistance Patterns in Children Hospitalized for Urinary Tract Infections
Lutter SA, Currie ML, Mitz LB, et al (Med College of Wisconsin, Milwaukee)
Arch Pediatr Adolesc Med 159:924-928, 2005   8–6

Background.—Children admitted to the hospital with urinary tract infections (UTIs) receive empirical antibiotic therapy. There is limited information on bacterial resistance to commonly prescribed intravenous antibiotics or on the risk factors for increased resistance in these patients.

Objectives.—To determine the antibiotic resistance pattern in children admitted to the hospital with UTIs, and to determine if history of UTI, antibiotic prophylaxis, or vesicoureteral reflux increases the risk of resistant organisms.

Design/Methods.—We reviewed all of the cases of UTI in children up to 18 years of age who were admitted during a 5-year period to Children's Hospital of Wisconsin, Milwaukee. We recorded age, sex, culture and sensitivity results, imaging that was performed, and past medical history.

Results.—We identified 361 patients with UTIs. *Escherichia coli* caused 87% of the infections, although *E coli* was significantly less common in children receiving prophylactic antibiotics (58%; $P<.001$) or in children with a history of UTI (74%; $P<.001$). Resistance to cefotaxime sodium was 3% in the patients not receiving antibiotic prophylaxis, but was 27% in the children receiving prophylactic antibiotics (relative risk, 9.9; 95% confidence interval, 4.0-24.5; $P<.001$). Resistance to aminoglycoside antibiotics was 1% in the children not receiving prophylaxis and 5% in the children receiving prophylactic antibiotics.

Conclusions.—Children who are receiving prophylactic antibiotics and are admitted to the hospital for a UTI are often infected with an organism that is resistant to third-generation cephalosporins. These children are more appropriately treated with an aminoglycoside antibiotic.

▶ It should come as no surprise that infants and children who have been managed with prophylactic antibiotics, who wind up being admitted to the hospital for treatment of a UTI are frequently diagnosed with an organism that is resistant to powerful third-generation cephalosporins. It was only a decade ago that highly febrile children with a UTI were routinely admitted to the hospital for parenteral antibiotic management. Such children with presumed pyelonephritis were treated parenterally with ampicillin and gentamicin. In the interval period, aminoglycosides have largely fallen into disfavor because of their potential nephrotoxicity and ototoxicity, and the requirement to carefully monitor blood levels in the absence of oral forms of the antibiotic that would permit patients to go home on the same or very similar antibiotic. It is for these reasons that third-generation cephalosporins were a welcome addition to the therapeutic armamentarium. These have been great drugs because of their long half-life and efficacy against gram-negative bacteria. Third-generation cephalosporins also have a very favorable safety profile and can be readily transitioned to oral agents. Third-generation cephalosporin-related drugs have been so effective that UTIs and pyelonephritis in children are often managed entirely as outpatient disorders or disorders that require a very short hospitalization.

The rub with the current management of pyelonephritis is the emergence of antimicrobial resistance to third-generation cephalosporins now seen in almost one third of children with UTIs who have been receiving prophylactic antibiotics. The report abstracted shows us how common the problem of antibiotic resistance is in children who have been receiving outpatient antibiotics as a prophylactic tool. Thus, we are faced with the dilemma of whether to use a "reasonable" starter antibiotic in someone who has been receiving prophylaxis recognizing, however, that there is some risk of failure, or to start a broad-spectrum antibiotic that would contribute to "antibiotic pressure" and increasing antibiotic resistance. Many are unable to wait the 24 hours for laboratory results and wind up starting with the "big guns" when big guns are actually not needed.

There are several messages to be learned from the report of Lutter et al. The first is that one should follow clear guidelines in administering prophylactic antibiotics. All too often, children with first UTIs wind up getting prophylactic antibiotics when they should not. Prophylactic antibiotics for UTIs are reserved for children who have urologic anomalies, including ureterovesical reflux after an episode of pyelonephritis (at least for a period of time), or recurrent episodes of cystitis, even in the absence of underlying anomalies. The second message is that previous antibiotic use should alert a care provider to the possibility of an antibiotic-resistant pathogen in a child with previous UTIs who presents with fever.

An excellent editorial that accompanied this report suggests that once cultures and sensitivity data are available, therapy should be quickly modified to use the antibiotic with the narrowest spectrum, lowest cost, and best safety profile.[1] Pediatricians should thoroughly reexamine their practice of prescribing prophylactic antibiotics, given that this practice further contributes to anti-biotic pressure and resistance.

J. A. Stockman III, MD

Reference

1. Yared A, Edwards KM: Re-evaluating antibiotic therapy for urinary tract infections in children (editorial). *Arch Pediatr Adolesc Med* 159:992-993, 2005.

Non-*Escherichia coli* Versus *Escherichia coli* Community-Acquired Urinary Tract Infections in Children Hospitalized in a Tertiary Center: Relative Frequency, Risk Factors, Antimicrobial Resistance and Outcome

Marcus N, Ashkenazi S, Yaari A, et al (Schneider Children's Med Ctr, Petach Tikva, Israel; Tel Aviv Univ, Israel)

Pediatr Infect Dis J 24:581-585, 2005   8–7

Background.—Currently hospitalization for children with urinary tract infections (UTIs) is reserved for severe or complicated cases. Changes may have taken place in the characteristics and causative uropathogens of hospital-treated community-acquired UTI.

Objectives.—To study children hospitalized in a tertiary center with community-acquired UTI, compare *Escherichia coli* and non-*E. coli* UTI, define predictors for non-*E. coli* UTI and elucidate the appropriate therapeutic approach.

Patients and Methods.—A prospective clinical and laboratory study from 2001 through 2002 in a tertiary pediatric medical center. Patients were divided by results of the urine culture into *E. coli* and non-*E. coli* UTI groups, which were compared.

Results.—Of 175 episodes of culture-proved UTI, 70 (40%) were caused by non-*E. coli* pathogens. Non-*E. coli* UTI was more commonly found in children who were male ($P = 0.005$), who had underlying renal abnormalities ($P = 0.0085$) and who had received antibiotic therapy in the prior month ($P = 0.0009$). Non-*E. coli* uropathogens were often resistant to antibiotics usually recommended for initial therapy for UTI, including cephalosporins and aminoglycosides; 19% were initially treated with inappropriate empiric intravenous antibiotics (compared with 2% for *E. coli* UTI, $P = 0.0001$), with a longer hospitalization.

Conclusions.—Current treatment routines are often inappropriate for hospitalized children with non-*E. coli* UTI, which is relatively common in this population. The defined risk factors associated with non-*E. coli* UTIs and its antimicrobial resistance patterns should be considered to improve empiric antibiotic therapy for these infections.

▶ UTIs remain a common cause of fever and a very frequent reason for a generalist to refer to emergency departments and for hospitalization. This is particularly true when the UTI occurs in infancy. Most babies will do well, but the early introduction of an appropriate antibiotic remains key to the therapeutic outcome. *E coli* remains the most frequent cause of UTIs, accounting for as many as 90% of all infections, depending on which study one reads. For most UTIs, outpatient management is adequate, but young babies and those patients who may have questionable compliance are the ones that frequently wind up in hospitals. Current guidelines of the American Academy of Pediatrics[1] recommend that infants and toddlers should be hospitalized if they appear to have toxemia, are dehydrated, may possibly have bacteremia, are vomiting, or are unable to retain oral intake, including their medications.

The really big question to ask when hospitalizing a youngster for a UTI is which antibiotic should be initiated. This article goes a long way to helping us in this regard. We see that the prevalence of *E coli* infection is not as common as one might suspect in hospitalized infants with culture-proven UTIs. Some 40% of infections appear to be caused by non-*E coli* pathogens. The authors of the article suggest that the relative prevalence of non-*E coli* UTIs may actually be increasing. Certainly, that is their experience. It is in this subset of infants infected with non-*E coli* UTIs that it is more likely that the wrong antibiotic will be chosen. For example, with non-*E coli* uropathogens, some 40% were shown to be resistant to cefuroxime, cefotaxime, or ceftriaxone, and some 17% were resistant to gentamicin.

If the information from this article is correct, and it likely is, then current guidelines for the initial treatment of children hospitalized with suspected UTIs must be improved, particularly when a non-*E coli* UTI is strongly suspected. We should all be aware of the risk factors for non-*E coli* UTIs. These include antibiotic therapy during the preceding 30 days, male gender, and an underlying renal pathologic condition. Any such risk factors should strongly increase our index of suspicion for the possibility of a non-*E coli* UTI and should stimulate us to start more appropriate therapy from the get-go.

The management of young infants who are hospitalized with UTIs obviously is not always a straightforward affair. This article helps us a great deal in understanding how to deal with the roadblocks that seem to occur from time to time in the management of such babies.

J. A. Stockman III, MD

Reference

1. Committee on Quality Improvement, Subcommittee on Urinary Tract Infection: Practice parameter: The diagnosis, treatment and evaluation of the initial UTI in febrile infants and young children. *Pediatrics* 103:843-852, 1999.

Compliance With Guidelines for the Medical Care of First Urinary Tract Infections in Infants: A Population-Based Study

Cohen AL, Rivara FP, Davis R, et al (Univ of Washington, Seattle)
Pediatrics 115:1474-1478, 2005   8–8

Background.—No population-based studies have examined the degree to which practice parameters are followed for urinary tract infections in infants.

Objective.—To describe the medical care of children in their first year of life after a first urinary tract infection.

Methods.—Using Washington State Medicaid data, we conducted a retrospective cohort study of children with a urinary tract infection during their first year of life to determine how many of these children received recommended care based on the most recent guidelines from the American Academy of Pediatrics. Recommended care included timely anatomic imaging, timely imaging for reflux, and adequate antimicrobial prophylaxis. Multivariate logistic-regression models were used to evaluate if hospitalization for first urinary tract infection, young age at time of diagnosis, gender, race, primary language of parents, having a managed care plan, and rural location of household residence were associated with recommended care.

Results.—Less than half of all children diagnosed with a urinary tract infection in their first year of life received the recommended medical care. Children who were hospitalized for their first urinary tract infection were significantly more likely than children who were not hospitalized to receive anatomic imaging (relative risk [RR]: 1.38; 95% confidence interval [CI]: 1.20-1.57) and imaging for reflux (RR: 1.62; 95% CI: 1.34-1.90).

Conclusions.—There is poor compliance with guideline-recommended care for first urinary tract infections in infants in a Medicaid population. Given the trend toward increased outpatient management of urinary tract infections, increased attention to outpatient imaging may be warranted.

▶ The recommendations of the American Academy of Pediatrics (AAP) for the evaluation of young children with a first urinary tract infection (UTI) are pretty straightforward. These recommendations include imaging studies (both renal US and either voiding cystourography or radionuclide cystourography) and antimicrobial prophylaxis for children with known vesicoureteral reflux. These recommendations apply to children younger than 2 years presenting with a UTI. Either voiding cystourography or radionuclide cystourography can be considered the gold standard for diagnosing reflux; antibiotic prophylaxis has been clearly documented to be associated with fewer recurrent UTI episodes and renal scarring.

UTIs are one of the most common disorders seen in pediatric practice. It has been estimated that as many as 6.5% of girls and 3.3% of boys will have a UTI during the first year of life.[1] Despite the presence of clear guidelines from the AAP, recent studies have questioned the currently recommended imaging studies, as well as the necessity of prophylactic antibiotics. Nonetheless, current practice parameters are accepted as recommended care. Thus, this article is important because it tells us just how carefully we follow these parameters. The punch line is straightforward: in most instances, we do not. Fewer than half of all children given a diagnosis of a UTI in the first year of life will receive the complete recommended medical care in terms of study and therapy.

So why are the majority of young children not treated according to the AAP protocol? The answer probably has to do with the fact that most of us accept practice parameters as guidelines, not mandates that must be tailored to individual patient circumstances. This statement most likely is a cop-out. It may well be that most of us do not believe that the guidelines are correct or do not apply in most instances. It may also be that some just have an aversion to being directed, believing that the "art of medicine" based on one's experience overrides dictum. In fact, many studies have found less than complete compliance with national guidelines for a variety of conditions, including pediatric asthma care, vision screening, sexually transmitted infection treatment in adolescents, treatment of otitis media, hyperbilirubinemia, and fevers in the young infant.

It is true that there is an art to the practice of medicine. Please recognize, however, that this art complements treatment guidelines. More children are likely harmed by clinicians not following the guidelines than are benefited by individualized approaches.

J. A. Stockman III, MD

Reference

1. American Academy of Pediatrics, Committee on Quality Improvement, Subcommittee on Urinary Tract Infections: Practice parameter: The diagnosis, treatment and evaluation of the initial urinary tract infection in febrile infants and young children. *Pediatrics* 103:843-852, 1999.

Clinical Significance of Primary Vesicoureteral Reflux and Urinary Antibiotic Prophylaxis After Acute Pyelonephritis: A Multicenter, Randomized, Controlled Study

Garin EH, Olavarria F, Nieto VG, et al (Univ of South Florida, Tampa; Universidad Austral, Valdivia, Chile; Hosp Nuestra Senora de la Candelaira, Tenerife, Spain; et al)

Pediatrics 117:626-632, 2006   8–9

Objectives.—To evaluate the role of primary vesicoureteral reflux (VUR) in increasing the frequency and severity of urinary tract infections (UTIs) and renal parenchymal damage among patients with acute pyelonephritis and to determine whether urinary antibiotic prophylaxis reduces the frequency and/or severity of UTIs and/or prevents renal parenchymal damage among patients with mild/moderate VUR.

Methods.—Patients 3 months to 18 years of age with acute pyelonephritis, with or without VUR, were assigned randomly to receive urinary antibiotic prophylaxis or not. Patients were monitored every 3 months for 1 year. Dimercaptosuccinic acid renal scans were repeated at 6 months or if there was a recurrence of febrile UTI. Urinalysis and urine culture were performed at each clinic visit. Renal ultrasound scans and voiding cystourethrograms were repeated at the end of 1 year of follow-up monitoring.

Results.—Of the 236 patients enrolled in the study, 218 completed the 1-year follow-up monitoring. Groups were similar with respect to age, gender, and reflux grade distribution for those with VUR. No statistically significant differences were found among the groups with respect to rate of recurrent UTI, type of recurrence, rate of subsequent pyelonephritis, and development of renal parenchymal scars.

Conclusions.—After 1 year of follow-up monitoring, mild/moderate VUR does not increase the incidence of UTI, pyelonephritis, or renal scarring after acute pyelonephritis. Moreover, a role for urinary antibiotic prophylaxis in preventing the recurrence of infection and the development of renal scars is not supported by this study.

▶ The principal finding of this report has monumental significance. The recurrence rate for UTI seen among children with VUR not receiving antibiotic prophylaxis was similar to that observed among patients without VUR. This finding, if confirmed by others, will be highly clinically significant, because the aim of urinary antibiotic prophylaxis has been to prevent a postulated increase in risk of UTI recurrence among patients with VUR.

Currently, the therapeutic options considered for patients with VUR are either surgery to correct the reflux or the use of urinary antibiotic prophylaxis. The purpose of prolonged administration of antibiotics for patients with VUR is to keep the urinary tract sterile, preventing the development of acute pyelonephritis and the formation of renal scars. Before this report appeared, however, the clinical significance of VUR has remained questionable, since there have been no controlled studies among children that support the role of VUR in recurrence of UTI, pyelonephritis, or the formation of renal scars. In fact, a systematic review of the available data on the use of primary antibiotic prophylaxis or surgery to correct VUR has shown that "it is not clear whether any intervention does more good than harm" for such children.[1] Until the report of Garin et al appeared, there were no controlled, randomized studies to tell us whether antibiotic prophylaxis after a UTI in a child with VUR was worthwhile. We will need more studies, hopefully with more patients included in them, to convince the world of the ineffectiveness of antibiotics in such circumstances. It is critical that we see these studies. We are hearing more and more about problems with *Clostridium difficile* in children (and adults) being treated with prophylactic antibiotics.

J. A. Stockman III, MD

Reference

1. Wheeler D, Vimalachandra D, Hodson EM, et al: Antibiotics and surgery for vesicoureteral reflux. *Arch Dis Child* 88:688-694, 2003.

Messenger RNA for *FOXP3* in the Urine of Renal-Allograft Recipients
Muthukumar T, Dadhania D, Ding R, et al (Weill Medical College of Cornell Univ, New York; New York Presbyterian Hosp–Weill Cornell Med Ctr, New York; Univ of Pennsylvania, Philadelphia; et al)
N Engl J Med 353:2342-2351, 2005
8–10

Background.—The outcome of renal transplantation after an episode of acute rejection is difficult to predict, even with an allograft biopsy.

Methods.—We studied urine specimens from 36 subjects with acute rejection, 18 subjects with chronic allograft nephropathy, and 29 subjects with normal biopsy results. Levels of messenger RNA (mRNA) for *FOXP3*, a specification and functional factor for regulatory T lymphocytes, and mRNA for CD25, CD3ε, perforin, and 18S ribosomal RNA (rRNA) were measured with a kinetic, quantitative polymerase-chain-reaction assay. We examined associations of mRNA levels with acute rejection, rejection reversal, and graft failure.

Results.—The log-transformed mean (±SE) ratio of *FOXP3* mRNA copies to 18S ribosomal RNA copies was higher in urine from the group with acute rejection (3.8±0.5) than in the group with chronic allograft nephropathy (1.3±0.7) or the group with normal biopsy results (1.6±0.4) (P<0.001 by the Kruskal–Wallis test). *FOXP3* mRNA levels were inversely correlated with serum creatinine levels measured at the time of biopsy in the acute-rejection group (Spearman's correlation coefficient = −0.38, P=0.02) but not in the group with chronic allograft nephropathy or the group with normal biopsy results. Analyses of receiver-operating-characteristic curves demonstrated that reversal of acute rejection can be predicted with 90 percent sensitivity and 73 percent specificity with use of the optimal identified cutoff for *FOXP3* mRNA of 3.46 (P=0.001). *FOXP3* mRNA levels identified subjects at risk for graft failure within six months after the incident episode of acute rejection (relative risk for the lowest third of *FOXP3* mRNA levels, 6; P=0.02). None of the other mRNA levels were predictive of reversal of acute rejection or graft failure.

Conclusions.—Measurement of *FOXP3* mRNA in urine may offer a noninvasive means of improving the prediction of outcome of acute rejection of renal transplants.

▶ This is a powerful article. While there have been major improvements in preventing organ rejection that have involved the evolution of new therapeutic agents, there has been little in the way of diagnostic improvements to detect organ rejection, at least until this article and similar ones have begun to appear. One of the most common problems nephrologists face is the patient who has decreasing renal functioning after transplantation. Is this the result of complications of immunosuppressive therapy or does it represent organ rejection? To aid in the resolution of this difficult differential diagnosis, US and renal biopsy are often performed. These are often done too little too late. The advent of reverse transcriptase polymerase chain reaction and DNA microarray technology has begun to allow for sensitive, accurate, and quantitative detection of transcriptional profiles of tissue samples from recipients and donors, therefore enabling the discovery of a molecular signature for acute cellular rejection. Acute allograft rejection is characterized by infiltration of the transplanted tissues by activated T cells. Accordingly, expression of T-cell-activation genes is evident in renal transplant biopsy specimens obtained from patients who are undergoing transplant rejection. Given that activated donor-specific cytotoxic T lymphocytes infiltrate organs that are being rejected, the expression of T-cell-activation genes that control this process can be detected in renal transplant biopsy specimens, and now, as we see, the urine begins to reflect rejection along similar lines. The article shows how cleverly we can look at urine sediment cells for transcriptional profiling studies.

The potential for molecular diagnostic techniques to predict renal transplant rejection, the safety of drug withdrawal, and other long-term and short-term outcomes is phenomenal. The hope is that the molecular biology laboratory will allow us to detect the very earliest stages of kidney rejection, which, in turn, would allow a more titrated approach to the individual patient; it would, perhaps, allow less therapy to be given when it is safe and more therapy to be given when it is clearly needed.

J. A. Stockman III, MD

Circumcision for the Prevention of Urinary Tract Infection in Boys: A Systematic Review of Randomised Trials and Observational Studies

Singh-Grewal D, Macdessi J, Craig J (Children's Hosp at Westmead, Sydney)
Arch Dis Child 90:853-858, 2005   8–11

Objective.—To undertake a meta-analysis of published data on the effect of circumcision on the risk of urinary tract infection (UTI) in boys.

Data Sources.—Randomised controlled trials and observational studies comparing the frequency of UTI in circumcised and uncircumcised boys were identified from the Cochrane controlled trials register, MEDLINE, EMBASE, reference lists of retrieved articles, and contact with known investigators.

Methods.—Two of the authors independently assessed study quality using the guidelines provided by the MOOSE statement for quality of observational studies. A random effects model was used to estimate a summary odds ratio (OR) with 95% confidence intervals (CI).

Results.—Data on 402,908 children were identified from 12 studies (one randomised controlled trial, four cohort studies, and seven case–control studies). Circumcision was associated with a significantly reduced risk of UTI (OR = 0.13; 95% CI, 0.08 to 0.20; p<0.001) with the same odds ratio (0.13) for all three types of study design.

Conclusions.—Circumcision reduces the risk of UTI. Given a risk in normal boys of about 1%, the number-needed-to-treat to prevent one UTI is 111. In boys with recurrent UTI or high grade vesicoureteric reflux, the risk of UTI recurrence is 10% and 30% and the numbers-needed-to-treat are 11 and 4, respectively. Haemorrhage and infection are the commonest complications of circumcision, occurring at rate of about 2%. Assuming equal utility of benefits and harms, net clinical benefit is likely only in boys at high risk of UTI.

▶ Some of us were wondering whether it was time once again for a scientific review of the value of circumcision in the prevention of UTIs in boys. Apparently, the time has come, given the publication of this large systematic review of randomized trials on this topic.

Circumcision remains the most common surgical procedure carried out, at least in boys, throughout the world. If you look carefully back through history, you will see that the "operation" originated some 15,000 years ago.[1] Early on, it was done for religious, ritualistic, and cultural reasons. It was not until the 19th century that the procedure was "medicalized." The original therapeutic circumcision was for phimosis, and since then, indications for the procedure have altered with the trends du jour. In some countries, these trends simply relate to dogma, resulting in the virtual routine circumcision of all boys. Here in the United States, it was estimated that more than 60% of all boys were circumcised by the late 1980s. Such trends tend to be infectious. For example, traditionally, Koreans did not circumcise their boys until their exposure to many thousands of American troops during the Korean War. Now, Korea is the only country in the Orient practicing routine circumcision.

It was in 1999 that the American Academy of Pediatrics issued a rather specific circumcision policy statement indicating that "existing scientific evidence demonstrates potential benefits of newborn male circumcision; however, these data are not sufficient to recommend routine neonatal circumcision."[2] It is the prevention of UTIs that remains the most interesting and, perhaps, the most persuasive relative indication for male circumcision and one that continues to provoke controversy; however, the question remains as to whether the prevention of UTIs is a strong enough argument to justify the continuation of the lucrative practice of routine circumcision and whether it is even a truly medical benefit.

The association between UTIs and the uncircumcised state was first recognized in the early 1980s when it was shown that uncircumcised infant boys had a 10-fold greater likelihood of having a UTI in the first year of life in comparison with boys who had been circumcised in the immediate newborn period.[3] Other studies have shown a 3- to 7-fold increased risk of UTIs in uncircumcised compared with circumcised infants, and the greatest risk was for an infant younger than 1 year of age. Unfortunately, over the years, there have been many methodological problems with studies trying to show a link between the uncircumcised state and the presence of UTIs; thus, the relevance of these studies has been difficult to assess. This is what prompted Singh-Grewal et al to undertake a meta-analysis of 12 studies assessing the association between UTIs and circumcision. They applied very stringent criteria before accepting any study into their analysis. The authors of this article conclude that slightly more than 100 circumcisions are required to prevent 1 UTI. When looked at from the prospective of the United Kingdom, this procedure costs the national health system approximately £55,000 per 1 UTI prevented (the author's math, not this editor's). On this basis alone, it would be doubtful that a cost–benefit analysis could ever justify routine circumcision for the prevention of UTIs. However, the same study estimated that only 11 circumcisions would be required in boys with recurrent UTIs and only 4 circumcisions would be needed in boys with grade 3 or more reflux to prevent a single UTI, which makes the cost–benefit analysis much more acceptable and attractive. In parts of the world where circumcision is not routinely performed for all males, many urologists do recommend circumcision for boys who have had 1 UTI or in whom reflux has been documented.

So, is the pendulum swinging away from routine circumcision again? It might be worthwhile reading an editorial of Malone[4] on this topic. Malone provides us with a note of caution before completely dismissing the role of circumcision in reducing the risk of UTIs. The cost–benefit of preventing a single UTI may be questionable, but he raises the issue about the cost–benefit of preventing renal scarring. Data suggest that as many as 20% of boys who have a single UTI may, in fact, have the development of some degree of renal scarring. Is it possible that a more complicated problem such as this might be able to be prevented by a neonatal circumcision? It's time for another meta-analysis of the literature. Certainly, the review of Singh-Grewal in no way unequivocally answers the question about whether a newborn circumcision should or should not be performed as a matter of routine.

One final comment, a study in South Africa has shown for the first time that circumcising adult men can dramatically lower their risk of becoming infected with HIV through heterosexual sex. Indeed, for the past 20 years, observational studies have suggested that circumcision protects men from HIV infection, but until recently there was no prospective evidence to support the conclusion. A study was reported of 3,000 uncircumcised men, 18 to 24 years of age, living in the Orange Farm Township near Johannesburg. Half of the men were circumcised at the onset of a clinical trial. The data from the study were so conclusive that the study code was broken early. The investigators found that "the protective effect of male circumcision was so high that it would have been unethical to continue the study." It turns out that 18 men in the circumcised group acquired HIV infections as opposed to 51 in the uncircumcised group. This was despite the fact that in the circumcised group, the men reported 18% more sexual contacts than controls. These data suggest that circumcision can offer 65% greater protection against HIV infection.[5]

The study linking male circumcision to a lower risk of HIV infection must be viewed with caution in terms of any recommendation for widespread circumcision of men in parts of the world where HIV infection has a high prevalence. Adult circumcision carries serious risks, especially when performed by traditional healers who do not have proper training. Since circumcision clearly does not provide complete protection against HIV infection, recommending circumcision could easily backfire if it encouraged men to have more unprotected sex. This would also greatly raise the risk for women. There are now several trials underway in Uganda and Kenya to determine whether circumcision will confirm the findings from South Africa. If the data hold up, someone will be fully occupied removing foreskins.

J. A. Stockman III, MD

References

1. Dunsmuir WD, Gordon EM: The history of circumcision. *BJU Int* 83(Suppl 1):1-12, 1999.
2. American Academy of Pediatrics: Circumcision policy statement. *Pediatrics* 103:686-693, 1999.
3. Ginsberg CM, McCracken GH: Urinary tract infection in young infants. *Pediatrics* 69:409-412, 1982.

4. Malone PSJ: Circumcision for preventing urinary tract infection in boys: European view. *Arch Dis Child* 90:773-774, 2005.
5. Cohen J: Male circumcision thwarts HIV infection. *Science* 309:860, 2005.

Desmopressin Associated Symptomatic Hyponatremic Hypervolemia in Children: Are There Predictive Factors?

Thumfart J, Roehr C-C, Kapelari K, et al (Charité Children's Hosp, Berlin; Univ Children's Hosp, Kiel (PE), Germany; Univ Children's Hosp, Innsbruck, Austria)
J Urol 174:294-298, 2005   8–12

Purpose.—Desmopressin is widely used in primary nocturnal enuresis, bleeding disorders, central diabetes insipidus and diagnostic urine concentration testing. Hyponatremic hypervolemia leading to seizures has been reported as a rare but potentially life threatening side effect of desmopressin therapy. We sought to identify factors that predispose patients to hyponatremia and to find predictive factors associated with increased risk of water intoxication.

Materials and Methods.—We report 13 novel cases of desmopressin associated water intoxication and review the literature. A total of 93 instances of symptomatic hyponatremia during desmopressin treatment in children were identified. Specific data were reported in 58 of 93 cases. These 58 cases, in addition to our 13 novel cases, were further analyzed.

Results.—All children were treated with intranasal or intravenous desmopressin. No patient received oral desmopressin. Younger children are at greater risk for water intoxication than older children. The risk is particularly high at the beginning of desmopressin therapy. A total of 45 patients (63%) had prodromal symptoms, eg nausea, vomiting and headache. In 10 cases (14%) desmopressin was prescribed without an evident need.

Conclusions.—Based on this analysis, we conclude that the use of desmopressin should be cautiously considered, careful monitoring should be performed during the initiation of therapy, and particular care should be taken when treating young children and when prodromal symptoms such as nausea, vomiting and headaches occur.

▶ No one likes to see water intoxication and hyponatremia that develops as part of the management for a simple problem like nocturnal enuresis. This does occur. See the Blood chapter (Abstract 3–12) to see how common the problem actually is when DDAVP is used to manage bleeding associated with vWD. The only thing we know for sure about what causes hyponatremia that is induced by DDAVP is that it is more likely to occur in young children and in those who are allowed liberal access to fluids. If you do use DDAVP as part of the management of nocturnal enuresis, be sure to let parents know that if their youngster becomes irritable or acts strangely, the child should be seen, evaluated, and have electrolyte determinations.

This is the last entry in the Genitourinary Tract chapter, so we will close with a question to challenge your knowledge: what is the risk to a newborn that undergoes a Metzitzah b'peh? In early 2006, a huge controversy developed in

New York City when there was consideration of a ban on Metzitzah b'peh ("suction by mouth"). In Metzitzah b'peh the practitioner is a mohel performing a circumcision accompanied by a sucking of the blood from the wound to clean it. This ritual form of circumcision is still practiced in some ultra-orthodox Jewish communities. Health department officials in New York State said the practice led to the death of one newborn boy from herpes simplex type 1 infection and caused brain damage in another. In fact, over the last 9 years, 7 cases of herpes have been linked to this practice. Three of the 5 most recent cases were traced to a single practitioner.

It is not known what the frequency is of infectious complications resulting from circumcisions involving Metzitzah b'peh. Because religious circumcisions are usually done 8 days after the birth in the parents' home, there is no way to know how often Metzitzah b'peh is performed. Rough estimates say that in New York City, the frequency of such types of circumcision runs from 2000 to 4000 each year. Obviously, even if this form of circumcision were banned, it would be impossible to enforce the ban.[1]

(P.S. My compliments to the first author of the desmopressin report for having the courage to retain her last name.)

J. A. Stockman III, MD

Reference:

1. Tann EJH: Ultra-orthodox Jews criticized over circumcision practice. *BMJ* 332:137, 2006.

9 Heart and Blood Vessels

Combined Influence of Body Mass Index and Waist Circumference on Coronary Artery Disease Risk Factors Among Children and Adolescents
Janssen I, Katzmarzyk PT, Srinivasan SR, et al (Queen's Univ, Kingston, Ontario, Canada; Tulane Univ, New Orleans, La; Tarleton State Univ, Stephenville, Tex; et al)
Pediatrics 115:1623-1630, 2005   9–1

Objectives.—In adult populations, it is recognized widely that waist circumference (WC) predicts health risk beyond that predicted by BMI alone; current recommendations for adults are that a combination of BMI and WC be used to classify obesity-related health risk. For children and adolescents, however, little is known about the combined influence of BMI and WC on health outcomes. The objectives of this study were to determine whether BMI and WC predict coronary artery disease (CAD) risk factors independently for children and adolescents and to assess the clinical utility of using WC in combination with BMI to identify CAD risk.

Methods.—Subjects included 2597 black and white, 5- to 18-year-old, male and female youths. Outcome measures included 7 CAD risk factors. In the first analysis step, BMI and WC were used as continuous variables to predict CAD risk factors. In the second analysis step, participants were placed into normal-weight, overweight, and obese BMI categories and, within each BMI category, CAD risk factors were compared for groups with low and high WC values.

Results.—When BMI and WC were included in the same regression model to predict CAD risk factors, the added variance above that predicted by BMI or WC alone was minimal, which indicated that BMI and WC did not have independent effects on the risk factors. For example, for systolic blood pressure, BMI alone explained 7.3% of the variance, WC alone explained 7.7% of the variance, and the combination of BMI and WC explained 8.1% of the variance. When BMI and WC values were categorized with a threshold approach, WC provided information on CAD risk beyond that provided by BMI alone, particularly when the categories were used to predict elevated CAD risk factor levels. For instance, in the overweight BMI category, the high-WC group was approximately 2 times more likely to have high triglyceride levels, high insulin levels, and the metabolic syndrome, compared with the low-WC group.

Conclusion.—These findings provide some evidence that a combination of BMI and WC should be used in clinical settings to evaluate the presence of elevated health risk among children and adolescents.

▶ This is another article on BMI showing us how important it is as a predictor of CAD risk factors in children and adolescents. Previous studies from the International Obesity Task Force along with the task force recommendations of the Centers for Disease Control and Prevention have cutoffs for the upper limit of normal (actually acceptable) BMI. These cutoffs are tied to adult overweight (25 kg/m^2) and obesity (30 kg/m^2) thresholds.[1] These cutoffs roughly represent the 85th and 95th centiles of the child and adolescent population. As important as BMI, WC is now accepted as a significant predictor of CAD risk factors among all people, including children and adolescents. Whereas BMI is thought to be an indicator of overall adiposity, WC is an additional indicator of abdominal fat content that many relate to the risk of type 2 diabetes. Currently, WC is not routinely measured in the pediatric office setting. There have been no firm endorsements of WC as part of a routine examination. Part of the issue with WC has been the "firmness" of WC cutoffs. The current article is important because it is among the first that attempts to correlate WC when added to BMI to predict CAD in children and adolescents. If you believe the adult data, evidence indicates that WC predicts adult risks beyond that predicted by BMI alone. The same should be true for children, and this is what this article shows.

This article is worth reading in detail because it does provide some new evidence that could incline us all to add a WC measurement to our routine measurement of BMI. Taken individually, both measurements provide important information for understanding problems that kids will run into on the long haul; taken together, they add even more information.

We close this first commentary in the Heart and Blood Vessels chapter recognizing that it contains no entries on blood vessels, so we will pose a question to the readers on a common blood vessel problem: bad veins. You are a consultant to your local high school and frequently meet with groups of students to advise them regarding various health issues and to answer their questions. One 15-year-old young lady asks you for your advice about how to prevent the onset of the development of varicose veins. Specifically, she wishes to know whether there are any occupations that she might go into that would increase her risk of the development of varicose veins. How would you answer this young lady's query?

A 12-year prospective study confirms that prolonged standing at work results in an increased risk of hospital admissions for varicose veins of the legs. A follow-up study of some 8600 Danish adults showed that people with jobs that required them to stand or to walk for long periods had a relative increase in risk of the development of varicose veins of 75% for men and 82% for women with occupational risk counting for more than one-fifth of all cases of varicose veins in people of working age, at least in Denmark.[2] Needless to say that if you were recommending against certain occupations for this teen, high on the list would be that of female postal worker.

J. A. Stockman III, MD

References

1. Cole TJ, Bellizzi MC, Flegal KM, et al: Establishing a standard for childhood overweight and obesity worldwide: International survey. *BMJ* 320:1240-1243, 2000.
2. Tuchsen F, Hannerz H, Burr H, et al: Prolonged standing at work and hospitalization due to varicose veins: A 12 year prospective study of the Danish population. *Occup Environ Med* 62:847-850, 2005.

Longitudinal Study of Birth Weight and Adult Body Mass Index in Predicting Risk of Coronary Heart Disease and Stroke in Women
Rich-Edwards JW, Kleinman K, Michels KB, et al (Harvard Med School, Boston; Harvard School of Public Health, Boston)
BMJ 330:1115-1118, 2005   9–2

Objectives.—To determine whether birth weight and adult body size interact to predict coronary heart disease in women, as has been observed for men. To determine whether birth weight and adult body size interact to predict risk of stroke.

Design.—Longitudinal cohort study.

Setting and Participants.—66,111 female nurses followed since 1976 who were born of singleton, term pregnancies and reported their birth weight in 1992.

Main Outcome Measures.—1504 events of coronary heart disease (myocardial infarction or sudden cardiac death) and 1164 strokes.

Results.—For each kilogram of higher birth weight, age adjusted hazard ratios from prospective analysis were 0.77 (95% confidence interval 0.69 to 0.87) for coronary heart disease and 0.89 (0.78 to 1.01) for total stroke. In combined prospective and retrospective analysis, hazard ratios were 0.84 (0.76 to 0.93) for total stroke, 0.83 (0.71 to 0.96) for ischaemic stroke, and 0.86 (0.66 to 1.11) for haemorrhagic stroke. Exclusion of macrosomic infants (>4536 g) yielded stronger estimates. Risk of coronary heart disease was especially high for women who crossed from a low centile of weight at birth to a high centile of body mass index in adulthood. The association of lower birth weight with increased risk of stroke was apparent across categories of body mass index in adults and was not especially strong among heavier women.

Conclusions.—Higher body mass index in adulthood is an especially strong risk factor for coronary heart disease among women who were small at birth. In this large cohort of women, size at birth and adiposity in adult-

fetal undernutrition. Babies who are thin or short at birth lack muscle, which is a deficiency that will persist into childhood because not much muscle cell replication occurs after birth. The authors of this article suggest that rapid weight gain in such children could lead to a disproportionately high fat mass in relation to muscle mass. This may underlie the strong associations between this path of growth and insulin resistance, as observed in this article, and may offer one explanation of why this pattern of growth leads to later coronary heart disease.

Thus, folks who have coronary events as adults may have been small at birth as well as thin in the first couple years of life.

One additional comment about cardiac risk factors: data over the last decade and a half have suggested that moderate drinking actually can reduce your risk of cardiovascular disease. Is this really true? Researchers from New Zealand now report that drinking is unlikely to be good for you, ever. The popular notion that 1 or 2 units of alcohol a day protects you from heart disease seems to have been well supported by observational data in the literature. It now seems that people who never drink are simply too different from people who drink sensibly to sort out any impact of alcohol on heart disease. In one recent study, 27 out of 30 possible cardiovascular risk factors turn out to be more common among abstainers than among moderate drinkers.[1] This makes drinkers look good, even though their lower cardiovascular risk has nothing to do with the occasional glass of wine.

J. A. Stockman III, MD

Reference

1. Naimi TS, Brown DW, Brewer RD, et al: Cardiovascular risk factors and confounders among nondrinking and moderate-drinking U.S. adults. *Am J Prev Med* 28:369-373, 2005.

Cardiovascular Health After Maternal Placental Syndromes (CHAMPS): Population-Based Retrospective Cohort Study
Ray JG, Vermeulen MJ, Schull MJ, et al (Univ of Toronto)
Lancet 366:1797-1803, 2005   9–4

Background.—Maternal placental syndromes, including the hypertensive disorders of pregnancy and abruption or infarction of the placenta, probably originate from diseased placental vessels. The syndromes arise most often in women who have metabolic risk factors for cardiovascular disease, including obesity, pre-pregnancy hypertension, diabetes mellitus, and dyslipidaemia. Our aim was to assess the risk of premature vascular disease in women who had had a pregnancy affected by maternal placental syndromes.

Methods.—We did a population-based retrospective cohort study in Ontario, Canada, of 1.03 million women who were free from cardiovascular disease before their first documented delivery. We defined the following as maternal placental syndromes: pre-eclampsia, gestational hypertension, placental abruption, and placental infarction. Our primary endpoint was a composite of cardiovascular disease, defined as hospital admission or revascularisation for coronary artery, cerebrovascular, or peripheral artery disease at least 90 days after the delivery discharge date.

Findings.—The mean (SD) age of participants was 28.2 (5.5) years at the index delivery, and 75,380 (7%) women were diagnosed with a maternal placental syndrome. The incidence of cardiovascular disease was 500 per million person-years in women who had had a maternal placental syndrome compared with 200 per million in women who had not (adjusted hazard ratio [HR] 2.0, 95 CI 1.7–2.2). This risk was higher in the combined presence of a maternal placental syndrome and poor fetal growth (3.1, 2.2–4.5) or a maternal placental syndrome and intrauterine fetal death (4.4, 2.4–7.9), relative to neither.

Interpretation.—The risk of premature cardiovascular disease is higher after a maternal placental syndrome, especially in the presence of fetal compromise. Affected women should have their blood pressure and weight assessed about 6 months postpartum, and a healthy lifestyle should be emphasised.

▶ Maternal placental syndromes include preeclampsia, gestational hypertension, placental abruption, and placental infarction. These conditions are most common in women with metabolic risk factors for cardiovascular disease, such as obesity, pre-pregnancy hypertension, diabetes mellitus, and dyslipidemia. These syndromes have been the subject of an ongoing study known as the Cardiovascular Health After Maternal Placental Syndromes (CHAMPS) study. In the CHAMPS trial, Ray et al have found that the risk of developing premature cardiovascular disease is doubled in women who have had a pregnancy affected by maternal placental syndromes, and further increased in those with fetal compromise or preexisting risk factors for cardiovascular disease.

All too often, young women who have delivered a baby fall through the medical cracks of care providers. As tough as a pregnancy may be on a woman who suffers from pregnancy-related maternal placental syndrome, once the pregnancy is over and done with, these women frequently seem quite normal when, in fact, they have a doubling of the risk of premature cardiovascular disease when compared with women who have undergone a pregnancy without the syndrome. The syndrome should be a signal to internists and family physicians to keep a careful eye on these women in order to manage problems that may ultimately lead to the onset of the metabolic syndrome.

It is important for us pediatricians to be aware of the maternal placental syndrome. It is we who take care of the products of such affected pregnancies and who should be aware of the recurrence of these problems with subsequent pregnancies. In addition, we are probably seeing more mothers in the postpartum period who are at risk for cardiovascular disease than the obstetrician, family physician, or internist. This does not mean that we need to take care of a mother's health care needs, but we should be reasonably certain that care is being provided in some fashion. Sometimes, care of a child means looking out for the mother.

On a different note, for years this editor has said that exercising 30 minutes a day in 1 clip is way overboard for what an individual really needs or most are interested in doing. He has now been vindicated by a recent report. For those of us who struggle to get into the routine of regular exercise, there is some good news. A study of young men in the *American Journal of Clinical Nutrition* reports that accumulating multiple short bouts of exercise throughout the day (10 three-minute episodes to be exact) is as effective in reducing postprandial blood fat concentrations as a single 30-minute exercise session.[1] All forms of exercise are a waste of the fixed number of heartbeats we are each born with, but if one must exercise, tiny frequent sessions seem infinitely more tolerable, at least to this editor.

Last, so what is the real skinny on chocolate these days? Does it or does it not improve one's cardiovascular risk factors? It seems that dark chocolate induces a rapid improvement in endothelial and platelet function in healthy smokers. White chocolate has no such effect. Twenty male smokers volunteered for measurement of flow mediated dilatation by ultrasonography of the brachial artery and of sheer stress dependent platelet function. After abstaining from polyphenol-rich foods for 24 hours, the subjects ate 40g of either dark or white chocolate and measurements were repeated. Flow mediated dilatation increased by 7% after dark chocolate, versus 4.4% at baseline, and the effect lasted about 8 hours. White chocolate had no effect on flow-mediated dilatation. Within 2 hours, platelet function decreased by one third, but only after dark chocolate. The total antioxidant status increased, again only after dark chocolate.

Thus it is, if there is not an apple a day accessible to you, a small daily treat of dark chocolate is a great substitute. Indeed, dark chocolate is the food of love, perhaps; there's nothing like a dark chocolate Hershey's Kiss.[2]

J. A. Stockman III, MD

References

1. Miyashita M, Burns SF, Stensel DJ: Exercise and postprandial lipemia: effect of continuous compared with intermittent activity patterns. *Am J Clin Nutr* 83:24-29, 2006.
2. Hermann F, Spieker LE, Ruschitzka K, et al: Dark chocolate improves endothelial and platelet function. *Heart* 92:119-120, 2006.

Efficacy of Bystander Cardiopulmonary Resuscitation and Out-of-Hospital Automated External Defibrillation as Life-Saving Therapy in Commotio Cordis

Salib EA, Cyran SE, Cilley RE, et al (Pennsylvania State Univ, Hershey; Minneapolis Heart Inst Found)
J Pediatr 147:863-866, 2005   9–5

Background.—Sudden death during participation in competitive sports is commonly due to cardiovascular causes, most often undiagnosed structural or electrical cardiac abnormalities such as hypertrophic cardiomyopathy, coronary artery anomalies, myocarditis, and congenital prolongation of the QTc interval. However, sudden death can also occur in individuals with no underlying cardiac disease if they are struck by a projectile over the anterior left hemithorax. This phenomenon is known as commotio cordis. In this situation, ventricular tachycardia or fibrillation is triggered by the impact of the projectile, which results in cardiac arrest. The survival rate of commotio cordis is only 16%, but survival is more likely when bystander CPR and the use of an external automated defibrillator (AED) is initiated within 3 minutes of the cardiac arrest. A case in which a child developed commotio cordis and was rescued by bystander CPR and the use of an AED is reported.

> *Case Report.*—Boy, 13 years, with a past medical history of an "innocent" murmur and a structurally normal heart sustained a blow to the lateral chest wall from a pitch while participating in a Little League baseball game. He collapsed after taking a few steps away from the batter's box. Bystander CPR, with chest compressions and mouth-to-mouth resuscitation, was immediately started by his coaching staff, and the emergency medical system was activated. Paramedics arrived within 6 to 8 minutes of the event and immediately used an AED monitor on the child. The child was determined to be in ventricular fibrillation, and the AED recommended defibrillation, which was then delivered. The child converted to sinus rhythm, and his rhythm strip showed him to be in normal sinus rhythm with ST depression. He was transported to a local emergency department because of continued unresponsiveness. In the emergency department, he initially demonstrated decerebrate posturing and so was transferred to the pediatric ICU. Within an hour, he was awake and following commands. His left lateral chest wall had an area of ecchymosis measuring approximately 4 cm in diameter. He continued to progress and was discharged on hospital day 3.

Discussion.—The general survival rate of commotio cordis is 16%; however, this figure rises to 25% when resuscitative measures are initiated within 3 minutes of the event. The fact that survival is only 3% in cases in which resuscitative efforts are delayed for more than 3 minutes is evidence of the need for more effective first-responder therapy to improve survival in these previously healthy athletes. It is suggested that communities and school districts examine the need for accessible AEDs and CPR-trained coaches and instructors at organized sporting events for children.

▶ Not one among us has not heard something about commotio cordis. Sudden death in athletes is usually due to cardiovascular causes, most often related to undiagnosed structural or electrical cardiac abnormalities such as hypertrophic cardiomyopathy, coronary artery abnormalities, myocarditis, and congenital prolongation of the QT interval. One must add to this list commotio cordis, an event usually triggered by a projectile that strikes the chest and triggers an episode of ventricular tachycardia or fibrillation and subsequent cardiac arrest. The survival rate for commotio cordis is only 16%, but if resuscitative measures are initiated within 3 minutes of the event, survival rates approach 25%. These dismal rates demonstrate that more effective first-responder therapy is needed to improve survival rates in these otherwise healthy athletes.

So what can improve the survival rate? It is the presence of a readily available AED. In the case reported, a 13-year-old healthy boy with no history of any significant medical problems collapsed after being hit in the chest by a pitched baseball. Fortunately, bystanders administered CPR, and paramedics arrived within 6 to 8 minutes using an AED to convert the patient's ventricular fibrillation. After a few rocky hours, the teen came around after his cardiac arrest and appears to have suffered no long-term damage. This case report suggests that AEDs might best be available at all sporting events, even those relatively innocent ones involving sandlot functions. The wearing of chest protectors by batters does not eliminate the risk of commotio cordis because 1 study[1] has shown that 28% of reported cases of this problem occurred despite the use of chest protectors. Animal models also seem to suggest that commercially available chest protectors may not reduce the likelihood of ventricular fibrillation. Some have suggested using softer "safety" baseballs in Little League, as the risk of sudden cardiac death appears to be reduced, at least in 1 animal model study.[2]

Please note that AEDs are not the whole solution to sudden cardiac arrest in children. Ventricular fibrillation (as opposed to asystole) remediable by defibrillation is not as common as in adults as a cause of sudden arrest.

See the article by Nadkarni et al (Abstract 9–6), which tells us more about pediatric resuscitation and the differences between kids and adults in this regard.

J. A. Stockman III, MD

References

1. Maron BJ, Gohman TE, Kyle SB, et al: Clinical profile and spectrum of commotio cordis. *JAMA* 287:1142-1146, 2002.
2. Link MS, Maron BJ, Wang PJ, et al: Reduced risk of sudden death from chest blows (commotio cordis) with safety baseballs. *Pediatrics* 109:873-877, 2002.

First Documented Rhythm and Clinical Outcome From In-Hospital Cardiac Arrest Among Children and Adults
Nadkarni VM, for the National Registry of Cardiopulmonary Resuscitation Investigators (Univ of Pennsylvania School of Medicine, Philadelphia; Univ of Texas Southwestern Med Ctr, Dallas; Virginia Commonwealth Univ Health Systems, Richmond; et al)
JAMA 295:50-57, 2006   9–6

Context.—Cardiac arrests in adults are often due to ventricular fibrillation (VF) or pulseless ventricular tachycardia (VT), which are associated with better outcomes than asystole or pulseless electrical activity (PEA). Cardiac arrests in children are typically asystole or PEA.

Objective.—To test the hypothesis that children have relatively fewer in-hospital cardiac arrests associated with VF or pulseless VT compared with adults and, therefore, worse survival outcomes.

Design, Setting, and Patients.—A prospective observational study from a multicenter registry (National Registry of Cardiopulmonary Resuscitation) of cardiac arrests in 253 US and Canadian hospitals between January 1, 2000, and March 30, 2004. A total of 36,902 adults ($\geq$18 years) and 880 children (<18 years) with pulseless cardiac arrests requiring chest compressions, defibrillation, or both were assessed. Cardiac arrests occurring in the delivery department, neonatal intensive care unit, and in the out-of-hospital setting were excluded.

Main Outcome Measure.—Survival to hospital discharge.

Results.—The rate of survival to hospital discharge following pulseless cardiac arrest was higher in children than adults (27% [236/880] vs 18% [6485/36,902]; adjusted odds ratio [OR], 2.29; 95% confidence interval [CI], 1.95-2.68). Of these survivors, 65% (154/236) of children and 73% (4737/6485) of adults had good neurological outcome. The prevalence of VF or pulseless VT as the first documented pulseless rhythm was 14% (120/880) in children and 23% (8361/36,902) in adults (OR, 0.54; 95% CI, 0.44-0.65; P<.001). The prevalence of asystole was 40% (350) in children and 35% (13,024) in adults (OR, 1.20; 95% CI, 1.10-1.40; P = .006), whereas the prevalence of PEA was 24% (213) in children and 32% (11,963) in adults (OR, 0.67; 95% CI, 0.57-0.78; P<.001). After adjustment for differences in preexisting conditions, interventions in place at time of arrest, witnessed and/or monitored status, time to defibrillation of VF or pulseless VT, intensive care unit location of arrest, and duration of cardiopulmonary resuscitation, only first documented pulseless arrest rhythm remained significantly associated with differential survival to discharge (24% [135/563] in children vs 11% [2719/24,987] in adults with asystole and PEA; adjusted OR, 2.73; 95% CI, 2.23-3.32).

Conclusions.—In this multicenter registry of in-hospital cardiac arrest, the first documented pulseless arrest rhythm was typically asystole or PEA in both children and adults. Because of better survival after asystole and PEA, children had better outcomes than adults despite fewer cardiac arrests due to VF or pulseless VT.

▶ The authors of this article remind us about the differences between children and adults when it comes to sudden cardiac arrest. Adults with cardiac arrest typically have sudden unexpected VF and often have underlying coronary artery disease with myocardial ischemia. The focus, therefore, of adult-oriented treatments is prompt defibrillation. Outcomes from witnessed VF are often excellent in adults, but outcomes from asystole and PEA are generally poor. In contrast, children who experience cardiac arrest rarely have coronary artery disease. Instead, cardiac arrest generally results from progressive tissue hypoxia and acidosis due to respiratory failure, circulatory shock, or both. Electrocardiographic rhythms of cardiac arrest in children usually progress through bradyarrhythmias to asystole or PEA rather than to VF. Although the outcomes from respiratory arrest or shock in children are generally good, the outcomes from pulseless cardiac arrest in children are usually quite poor.

The authors of this article do us a great service by characterizing the type of in-hospital cardiac arrest that occurs in children. We see that the first documented pulseless arrest rhythm is typically asystole or PEA. This cannot be managed by a defibrillator. Just what are the current American Heart Association CPR guidelines these days? According to these guidelines (relatively new ones), a lone resuscitator must decide if the unresponsive patient, regardless of age, has had a VF arrest or an asphyxial arrest. For any age individual who collapses suddenly, the lone rescuer should call first for an automated external defibrillator (AED) and then initiate CPR. For the unresponsive individual of any age with an asphyxial arrest, the rescuer should provide 5 cycles of CPR before calling emergency services. No longer is there an adult or pediatric chain but a chain with 2 branches (1 for the unresponsive patient whose arrest was most likely respiratory and 1 for the patient who is in arrest who most likely has VF). AEDs certainly help. Studies have shown that the use of an AED significantly decreases the time it takes to recognize VF by almost 90% and the actual time to defibrillation by more than 75% in comparison with access to an EKG only.[1]

To read more about adult and pediatric resuscitation, see the superb review by Quan.[2] We are reminded that the 2 pillars of resuscitation, CPR and defibrillation, are intertwined, interlocked, and, now, ageless. The pediatric and adult in-hospital and out-of-hospital chain of survival appear to be one and the same. Those involved in resuscitation care, regardless of the arrest, patient's age, and setting, should approach the problem in a similar way, recognizing that only differences in placement of paddles and AED energy-dosing vary between adults and children. As Dr Quan points out, the differences between children and adults are minor in this regard and that "what is good for the goose is also good for the gosling."

This commentary closes with an interesting fictitious case scenario that teaches some important points about tests for cardiac disease. You have been experiencing some chest pain. Your symptoms seem to be most compatible with gastroesophageal reflux, but your internist insists that you have an exercise treadmill test. You hurry to have this done since you are scheduled to leave town in a few days on an overseas flight to an international meeting. Fortunately, the exercise treadmill test, one that included a thallium[201] myocardial perfusion scintigram, was completely normal. The question is, just how likely is it that you will be able to complete your international trip without encountering significant difficulty?

This question is best answered by the experience of a 55-year-old commercial pilot who had been referred to a cardiologist for further evaluation after a routine medical examination suggested that he might have mitral valve prolapse. Although never complaining of chest pain or breathlessness or having a significant cardiac history, an exercise treadmill test showed ECG changes suggestive of coronary artery disease. This exercise test was done in association with a thallium[201] myocardial perfusion scintigram, which was normal. Two days after the scan, the pilot traveled to Moscow as a crewmember. While passing through customs, a radiation detector alarm was triggered and the pilot was detained by airport security officers for a number of hours while he attempted to explain why he was radioactive. On leaving the country 4 days later, he again set off the security alarms.

Most of us do not think of ourselves, or our patients, as being radioactive after certain diagnostic procedures involving the use of radioisotopes, but we are. Here in the US, more than 18 million diagnostic and therapeutic procedures using such substances are carried out each year. The most common of these studies are thyroid, bone scans, myocardial profusion scans, and radioactive iodine therapy. Each of these is capable of setting off radiation detector alarms in high security areas. It was almost 20 years ago that the first report of this occurrence appeared when a patient was documented to have triggered a radiation detector at a bank vault 3 days after undergoing a thallium stress test.[3] Two other individuals were detained by the US Secret Service after setting off radiation detectors during visits to the White House, a few days after thallium stress testing.[4]

If you must undergo a thallium stress test and might be near a radiation detector, realize that the half-life of thallium[201] is 73 hours and that the usual IV dose of radioactivity is 80 MBq. Because it generally takes 5 half-lives for radioactivity to fall to insignificant levels, anyone undergoing such a stress test would trigger a radiation detector for at least 2 weeks. It would not be unusual with that to have some radiation detectable for as long as 30 days. Individuals being treated for thyroid cancer with I[131] are radioactive for at least 3 months.

Many of us are not familiar with the fact that radiation detectors are now ubiquitous not only in airports, but also in many other areas that are at risk for terrorist attacks. In certain parts of the world, radiation detectors have been placed in areas where people congregate such as subway concourses.[5]

J. A. Stockman III, MD

References

1. American Heart Association: 2005 American Heart Association Guidelines for Cardiopulmonary Resuscitation and Emergency Cardiovascular Care: Overview of CPR. *Circulation* 112:12S-18S, 2005.
2. Quan L: Adult and pediatric resuscitation: Finding common ground. *JAMA* 295:96-98, 2006.
3. Levin ME, Fischer KC: Thallium stress test and bank vaults. *N Engl J Med* 319:587, 1988.
4. Toltzis RJ, Morton DJ, Gerson MC: Problems on Pennsylvania Avenue. *N Engl J Med* 315:836-837, 1986.
5. Iqbal MB, Sharma R, Underwood SR, et al: Radioisotopes and airport security. *Lancet* 366:342, 2005.

Acquired QT Prolongation Associated With Esophagitis and Acute Weight Loss: How to Evaluate a Prolonged QT Interval

Koch JJ, Porter CJ, Ackerman MJ (Mayo Eugenio Litta Children's Hosp, Rochester, Minn; Mayo Clinic College of Medicine, Rochester, Minn)
Pediatr Cardiol 26:646-650, 2005   9–7

Abstract.—When the physician is confronted with a patient having significant QT prolongation, it is critical to determine whether the patient harbors a genetic defect and a transmissible form of long QT syndrome (LQTS) or whether the QT prolongation has an acquired cause. The distinction has profound ramifications for the type of care provided to the patient and family. We report the case of a previously healthy 14-year-old boy who presented with a 10-day history of painful swallowing, a 10-lb weight loss, and chest pain. A 12-lead electrocardiogram (ECG) showed marked QT prolongation. Endoscopy and culture identified a *Herpes simplex* esophageal ulcer. After treatment with acyclovir, the patient recovered completely. Three weeks after the resolution of his symptoms and recovery from his acute weight loss, a follow-up ECG showed complete normalization of the QT interval. This case illustrates yet another potential mechanism for acquired QT prolongation. We also provide a diagnostic algorithm for the careful evaluation of a prolonged QT interval.

▶ This article reminds us that you cannot always make a diagnosis of prolonged QT interval syndrome solely on the basis of ECG. In human beings, genetic testing is needed because a large overlap exists between normal ranges for QT intervals and the prolongation sometimes seen in patients with LQTS. The causes of QT prolongation are divided into 2 groups: inherited/familial and acquired QT. Inherited forms of LQTS include rare genetic problems such as the Jervell and Lange–Nielsen syndrome (sensorineural hearing loss in association with a prolonged QT interval) and the autosomal dominant genetic disorder known as Romano–Ward syndrome. Autosomal dominant LQTS is actually more common than most of us appreciate: its incidence approaches 1 in 5000. The disorder is due to genetic abnormalities producing defective cardiac ion channels.

Acquired forms of QT prolongation are usually caused by drugs, but electrolyte abnormalities and certain medical conditions can also cause QT prolongation. Acquired QT prolongation can also set one up for a lethal arrhythmia.

If you find that a patient has a significant QT prolongation, it is incumbent on you to determine whether this has a genetic basis or is due to an acquired cause. Genetic causes obviously result in the need to follow-up family members and to outline a course of management that can be quite complex for the patient. On the other hand, if the patient has acquired QT prolongation, management of the reason for the problem usually totally eradicates the potential for a fatal arrhythmia.

We learn in this article that we need to add acute weight loss associated with esophagitis to the list of causes of acquired QT prolongation. Although acute weight loss has not been previously reported as a cause of QT interval prolongations, chronic malnutrition, starvation, and chronic weight loss such as commonly seen in patients with anorexia nervosa can prolong the QT interval. Even when you see what appears to be an apparently secondary cause for the problem, it is still incumbent on you to think about the genetic causes. The patient described in this article was an elite athlete at the junior high school level, and his father was the school coach. Having inherited LQTS was not a desirable diagnosis and, fortunately, was able to be excluded in this teenager.

On an unrelated cardiac topic, Laënnec named his invention that allowed him to listen to breath and heart sounds the stethoscope. What is the origin of the word stethoscope? Fast fact: "Stethoscope" is derived from the Greek stethos, meaning chest, and kopein, meaning to observe. To read more about the stethoscope and the art of listening, see the superb historical review by Markel.[1]

J. A. Stockman III, MD

Reference

1. Markel H: The stethoscope and the art of listening. *N Engl J Med* 354:551-553, 2006.

Genetic Testing in the Long QT Syndrome: Development and Validation of an Efficient Approach to Genotyping in Clinical Practice
Napolitano C, Priori SG, Schwartz PJ, et al (IRCCS Fondazione S Maugeri Found, Pavia, Italy; Univ of Pavia, Italy; IRCCS Policlinico S Matteo, Pavia, Italy)
JAMA 294:2975-2980, 2005   9–8

Context.—In long QT syndrome (LQTS), disease severity and response to therapy vary according to the genetic loci. There exists a critical need to devise strategies to expedite genetic analysis.

Objective.—To perform genetic screening in patients with LQTS to determine the yield of genetic testing, as well as the type and the prevalence of mutations.

Design, Patients, and Setting.—We investigated whether the detection of a set of frequently mutated codons in the *KCNQ1, KCNH2,* and *SCN5A* genes may translate in a novel strategy for rapid efficient genetic testing of 430 consecutive patients referred to our center between June 1996 and June 2004. The entire coding regions of *KCNQ1, KCNH2, SCN5A, KCNE1,* and *KCNE2* were screened by denaturing high-performance liquid chromatography and DNA sequencing. The frequency and the type of mutations were defined to identify a set of recurring mutations. A separate cohort of 75 consecutive probands was used as a validation group to quantify prospectively the prevalence of the recurring mutations identified in the primary LQTS population.

Main Outcome Measures.—Development of a novel approach to LQTS genotyping.

Results.—We identified 235 different mutations, 138 of which were novel, in 310 (72%) of 430 probands (49% *KCNQ1*, 39% *KCNH2*, 10%

SCN5A, 1.7% *KCNE1*, and 0.7% *KCNE2*). Fifty-eight percent of probands carried nonprivate mutations in 64 codons of *KCNQ1*, *KCNH2*, and *SCN5A* genes. A similar occurrence of mutations at these codons (52%) was confirmed in the prospective cohort of 75 probands and in previously published LQTS cohorts.

Conclusions.—We have developed an approach to improve the efficiency of genetic screening for LQTS. This novel method may facilitate wider access to genotyping resulting in better risk stratification and treatment of LQTS patients.

▶ We now know that multiple LQTSs exist. The genetic bases for all of these have now been elucidated. These syndromes include QT1, in which mutations in the gene *KCNQ1* lead to a slow delayed-rectifier potassium current. QT2 produces mutations in a rapid delayed-rectifier potassium current-related gene. QT3 produces mutations in a gene that regulates a sodium channel current. Once genetic testing became available for LQTSs, it became clear that clinical evaluation based on resting electrocardiograms was inadequate to detect many cases of LQTS. Genetic testing, therefore, is now considered mandatory in cases in which the disorder is suspected.

The availability of genetic testing has led to an understanding of important clinical differences between the individual genetic disorders (QT1 vs QT2 vs QT3). Patients with QT1 are at particularly high risk of cardiac events during physical exercise, especially swimming. Patients with QT2 are susceptible to cardiac events during emotional or auditory stimuli and during the postpartum period. Patients with QT3 may have cardiac events during rest or sleep. These differences in LQTS types have implications for risk assessment and for clinical treatment decisions. Knowledge of a patient's genotype is important because it can guide a clinician's decision whether to give a patient a diagnosis of LQTS (especially when the electrocardiographic findings are borderline), whether to restrict activity in a young athlete, whether to treat with medication or consider implantable cardioverter–defibrillator therapy, and how to counsel patients about the risks of LQTS in potential offspring. Once an abnormal genotype has been identified in a family, it is relatively easy then to screen additional family members for the specific mutation. This is important because negative genotypes in the face of borderline–normal QT intervals on EKGs mean that individuals do not have LQTS, which then allows them to rest assured that they will not get into trouble.

So how much does genotyping cost if one is trying to detect LQTS with a high degree of accuracy? Screening for all the long QT genotypes can be completed with a turnaround time of about 6 weeks but at a cost of approximately $5400 for the comprehensive testing of an index patient. If a mutation is found, the cost for each additional family member runs about $900 because it is only necessary to look for the specific genotype. Insurance often does not cover the cost of genotyping, which makes such testing out of reach for many families. To remedy this situation, Napolitano et al propose a streamlined process for genetic testing in LQTS, designed to reduce cost and to make genetic testing more widely available. The authors have proposed an efficient strategy for screening LQTS mutations: first, test the 64 most commonly repeated codons; if no mutations are found, test the entire codon region of the 2 most common gene abnormalities. In addition, if no positive results are found, then screen for the mutations in the remaining potential genes. Such an approach could make genetic analysis much more efficient, affordable, and accessible because of a more tailored testing process. The rub with the approach is that about 5% of individuals with LQTS may, in fact, have 2 or more mutations; thus, stopping with the first one found could give some false reassurance. Nonetheless, the data provided by Napolitano et al do provide important new information about the yield of genetic testing and about the distribution of mutations causing the syndrome.

Hopefully, the problem of the cost of complete testing for LQTS, as well as many other genetic disorders, will be minimized with novel technologies for rapid efficient DNA sequencing. Such techniques are on the horizon.[1] Once these technologies are in place, the medical community and patients will have much more affordable and accessible means of genetic testing.

One final comment on something that can cause an irregular heartbeat, caffeine. Caffeine is metabolized by the enzyme CYP1A2, which has a fast and a slow variant. People homozygous for the fast variant (1A) metabolize caffeine remarkably faster than people carrying the slow variant (1F). Investigators have actually determined that caffeine is more risky for slow metabolizers with respect to the onset of heart disease. A study was carried out in Costa Rico that recruited and genotyped 2014 men and women with non-fatal heart attacks and the same number of healthy matched controls. The study interviewed these individuals using food frequency questionnaires. The study concluded that drinking 2 or more cups of coffee a day was associated with a significant increase in the odds of having a heart attack, but only among adults with the slow metabolizing genotype. Coffee did not seem to harm the others. Among the slow metabolizers, the odds ratio for heart attack was increased to 1.36 for adults drinking 2 to 3 cups of coffee a day, and were increased to 1.64 for those drinking 4 cups of coffee or more a day. Corresponding odds ratios for fast metabolizers were 0.78 and 0.99, respectively.

The linkage between caffeine metabolizing rates and coffee drinking does appear to be a strong one, particularly in younger people (under the age of 50) and is not influenced by other risk factors such as smoking.[2]

J. A. Stockman III, MD

Reference

1. Margulies M, Engholm M, Altman WE, et al: Genome sequencing in micro-fabricated high-density picoliter reactors. *Nature* 437:376-380, 2005.
2. Cornelis MC, El-Sohemy A, Kabagambe EK, et al: Coffee, CYP1A2 genotype, and risk of myocardial infarction. *JAMA* 295:1135-1141, 2006.

Daclizumab to Prevent Rejection After Cardiac Transplantation

Hershberger RE, Starling RC, Eisen HJ, et al (Oregon Health and Science Univ, Portland; Cleveland Clinic Found, Ohio; Temple Univ, Philadelphia; et al)
N Engl J Med 352:2705-2713, 2005   9–9

Background.—Daclizumab, a humanized monoclonal antibody against the interleukin-2 receptor, reduced the risk of rejection without increasing the risk of infection among renal-transplant recipients and, in a single-center trial, among cardiac-transplant recipients. We conducted a multicenter, placebo-controlled, double-blind study to confirm these results in cardiac-transplant patients.

Methods.—We randomly assigned 434 recipients of a first cardiac transplant treated with standard immunosuppression (cyclosporine, mycophenolate mofetil, and corticosteroids) to receive five doses of daclizumab or placebo. The primary end point was a composite of moderate or severe cellular rejection, hemodynamically significant graft dysfunction, a second transplantation, or death or loss to follow-up within six months.

Results.—By six months, 104 of 218 patients in the placebo group had reached the primary end point, as compared with 77 of the 216 patients in the daclizumab group (47.7 percent vs. 35.6 percent, P=0.007), a 12.1 percent absolute risk reduction and a 25 percent relative reduction. The rate of rejection was lower in the daclizumab group than in the placebo group (41.3 percent vs. 25.5 percent). Among patients reaching the primary end point, the median time to the end point was almost three times as long in the daclizumab group as in the placebo group during the first 6 months (61 vs. 21 days) and at 1 year (96 vs. 26 days). More patients in the daclizumab group than in the placebo group died of infection (6 vs. 0) when they received concomitant cytolytic therapy.

Conclusions.—Daclizumab was efficacious as prophylaxis against acute cellular rejection after cardiac transplantation. Because of the excess risk of death, concurrent or anticipated use of cytolytic therapy with daclizumab should be avoided.

▶ This decade seems to be the decade of the use of monoclonal antibodies to treat or prevent just about every immune-mediated disorder. Daclizumab is one such monoclonal antibody, directed against interleukin-2 receptors. We see in this article its effectiveness in preventing the rejection of transplanted hearts. The first human-to-human cardiac transplantation was performed in 1967. The results of the first randomized controlled clinical trial[1] of immunosuppression among heart transplant recipients were not published, however, until 30 years later. A few other clinical trials of immunosuppression among heart transplant recipients have been reported since then, including the one from Oregon. The paucity of data from clinical trials is largely because of the relatively small number of cardiac transplantations performed here in the United States each year. The number has been running about 2500 and has not increased appreciably in the last 15 years. Approximately 150 heart transplantation centers perform this small number of operations each year. Most studies of immunosuppressives come from large cardiac transplantation centers. Among this group of 150, all are sure that their particular immunosuppressive cocktail is the best. Trying to get centers together, therefore, to agree on a common protocol is no easy task. Another problem with studying the role of immunosuppression is the fact that, if one simply looks at survival rates, 1-year survival rates are so high (85%) that death is hardly a good end point because it yields too few patients in any 1 study. Biopsy evidence of rejection is probably a more accurate measurement of the quality of immunosuppression. Unfortunately, or fortunately, most patients with histologic evidence of rejection have absolutely no change in the functioning of their heart, and the histologic findings are usually easily reversed with more aggressive immunosuppressive therapy. On the other hand, many patients with cardiac function abnormalities do not have the classic findings of acute rejection on biopsy. Currently, rejection as a documented cause of death primarily in the first year after transplantation is now a rarity. In one recent study, such rejection as a cause of death in the first year after transplantation ran only 2%. This is in contrast to the incidence of histologic rejection, which runs 50% to 75% in some studies.

So what do the data of Hershberger et al show? They show that the risk of a primary composite end point of histologic rejection, graft dysfunction, a second transplantation, or death within 6 months after an initial transplant was reduced by treatment with the monoclonal antibody daclizumab. If one looks carefully at the data, however, one sees the worrisome finding that the overall mortality rate with daclizumab is actually higher at 6 months, even though other composite variables are favorable.

Read the excellent editorial by Hosenpud[2] to fully understand the current status of immunosuppression after cardiac transplantation. Dr Hosenpud closes his editorial with the statement, "I am certain that I would not be willing to trade even the small increase in the risk of death from infection for a reduction in the risk of histologic rejection." He makes this statement largely on the basis that transplant cardiologists now have good tools available to manage early rejection without taking on the added risk of highly potent immunosuppressives, which likely should be reserved for patients who do not seem to be responding to more simple measures.

J. A. Stockman III, MD

References

1. Kobashigawa J, Miller L, Renlund D, et al: A randomized active-controlled trial of mycophenolate mofetil in heart transplant recipients. *Transplantation* 66:507-515, 1998.
2. Hosenpud JD: Immunosuppression in cardiac transplantation. *N Engl J Med* 352:2749-2750, 2005.

Disparities in Outcome for Black Patients After Pediatric Heart Transplantation

Mahle WT, Kanter KR, Vincent RN (Emory Univ School of Medicine, Atlanta, Ga)
J Pediatr 147:739-743, 2005

9–10

Objective.—To examine the relationship of black race to graft survival after heart transplantation in children.

Study Design.—United Network for Organ Sharing records of heart transplantation for subjects <18 years of age from 1987 to 2004 were reviewed. Analysis was performed using proportional hazards regression controlling for other potential risk factors.

Results.—Of the 4227 pediatric heart transplant recipients, 717 (17%) were black. The 1-year graft survival rate did not differ among groups; however, the 5-year graft survival rate was significantly lower for black recipients, 51% versus 69%, $P < .001$. The median graft survival for black recipients was 5.3 years as compared with 11.0 years for other recipients. Black recipients had a greater number of human leukocyte antigen mismatches, lower median household income, and a greater percentage with Medicaid as primary insurance, $P < .001$, $P < .001$, and $P < .001$. After adjusting for economic disparities, black race remained significantly associated with graft failure, odds ratio = 1.67 (95% CI 1.47 to 1.87), $P < .001$.

Conclusions.—Median graft survival after pediatric heart transplantation for black recipients is less than half that of other racial groups. These differences do not appear to be related primarily to economic disparities.

▶ There is more to organ rejection than the eye can see. Much has been written about race and ethnicity and survival of kidney transplants in the United States. We have known for more than a third of a century that dissimilar results occur across ethnic backgrounds with respect to survival of organ transplants. Minority groups, primarily African Americans but also Native Americans and others, are not only at greater risk of end-stage renal disease but also less likely to receive optimal transplantation therapy once end-stage renal disease develops. Those who receive a transplant seem to reject their organs more frequently. The article by Mahle et al documents this. The article also documents what has long been suspected to be a cause: socioeconomic disadvantage; however, socioeconomic disadvantage is hardly the only cause and probably not the principle cause of organ rejection failure rates.

The study of Mahle et al looks at outcomes from a national registry of pediatric cardiac organ recipients. Once again, we see that African American children fare substantially worse than do white children. It is true that the black youngsters were at substantial socioeconomic disadvantage. Nonetheless, socioeconomic factors did not seem to account for the differential outcomes, which led the authors to the reason that physiologic differences play a significant role in explaining the relationship between ethnicity and outcomes. The disparity could be discerned only in African Americans and not among other ethnic or minority groups. These data suggest that organ rejection seems to be a common phenomenon across all organs that are transplanted.

So what do these data really mean? They suggest that even if we eliminate the socioeconomic disadvantage seen in some populations, say, by providing universal health coverage to allow access to medical care, we will still face major organ rejection differences among populations who undergo transplantation. We need better methods to both detect and to manage rejection. See the article by Muthukumar et al (Abstract 8–10), which shows us one new technique for detecting early rejection. Hopefully, this will help those who are at greatest risk of this problem.

J. A. Stockman III, MD

Characteristics of Kawasaki Disease in Infants Younger Than Six Months of Age
Chang F-Y, Hwang B, Chen S-J, et al (Natl Yang-Ming Univ, Taipei, Taiwan)
Pediatr Infect Dis J 25:241-244, 2006   9–11

Background.—Kawasaki disease is the leading cause of acquired heart disease in childhood. However, there are only a few reports in infants younger than 6 months. The objective of this study is to investigate the clinical and laboratory characteristics of Kawasaki disease in infants younger than 6 months.

Methods.—From 1994 to 2003, 120 patients with Kawasaki disease diagnosed at our institution were included. Group 1 consisted of 20 (17%) patients younger than 6 months, and group 2 consisted of 100 (83%) patients older than 6 months. Clinical manifestations, laboratory results, echocardiographic findings, treatment and outcome were compared between these 2 groups.

Results.—Clinical manifestations (hydrops of gallbladder: 0% versus 16%, $P < 0.001$) and laboratory results (white blood cell count 21,740 ± 11,706 versus 11,830 ± 4390/mm^3, $P < 0.001$; hemoglobin 9.98 ± 1.25 versus 10.8 ± 1.37 g/dL, $P = 0.015$; platelet 483 ± 393 versus 355 ± 138 × 1000/mm^3, $P = 0.011$; triglyceride 138 ± 77.5 versus 107 ± 17 mg/dL, $P < 0.001$) were different between patients with Kawasaki disease younger and older than 6 months, respectively. Younger infants were more likely to have incomplete presentation (35% versus 12%, $P = 0.025$), coronary involvement (65% versus 19%, $P < 0.001$), late intravenous immunoglobulin treatment and relatively poor outcome.

Conclusions.—Infants younger than 6 months with prolonged unexplained febrile illnesses should be suspected as having Kawasaki disease, despite the incomplete clinical presentation. Because early diagnosis and timely treatment are difficult in younger infants with Kawasaki disease because of delayed and incomplete clinical presentations, echocardiogram becomes an important implement for diagnosis. Early intravenous immunoglobulin treatment is required in view of the highest risk of coronary involvement in them.

▶ The more we learn about Kawasaki disease, the more we learn how Kawasaki disease can be atypical, particularly in younger children. The criteria for the diagnosis of Kawasaki disease were developed by the American Heart Association and are based on the existence of high fever for greater than 5 days and 4 or 5 of the following: (1) bilateral bulbar conjunctival injection, generally nonpurulent; (2) changes in the mucosa of the oropharynx, including injected pharynx, injected and/or dry fissured lips, and strawberry tongue; (3) changes in the extremities, such as edema and/or erythema of the hands or feet in the acute phase or periungual desquamation in the subacute phase; (4) rash, primarily truncal, polymorphous, but nonvesicular; and (5) cervical lymphadenopathy with at least one lymph node with a diameter of 1.5 cm or greater and usually unilateral. Incomplete Kawasaki disease is defined as high fever and fewer than 4 criteria, but with coronary involvement.

Kawasaki disease is generally a disease of children younger than 4 years. It can affect adults, and it does affect infants younger than 6 months. What we learn from this report is that several clinical manifestations and laboratory findings are different in these young patients. Generally speaking, the outlook for younger patients is poorer. In some cases, this relates to the late diagnosis that is made in these patients along with the delayed treatment with IV immune globulin (IVIG). Curiously in this report, we also find that the male-to-female ratio in very young patients with Kawasaki disease is an astounding 9:1, different than that reported in an overall series of patients with Kawasaki disease in which the ratio is 1.5:1. Cervical lymphadenopathy tends to occur less frequently in the young child. On the other hand, the incidence of sterile pyuria seems to be higher in younger patients, so misdiagnosis of a urinary tract infection could delay the correct diagnosis. Higher white blood cell counts are also found in younger infants.

The most significant problem for patients with Kawasaki disease is the occurrence of coronary artery involvement. This report indicates that patients with Kawasaki disease in the younger age group can be expected to have a significantly higher frequency of coronary involvement.

It is a shame that younger children are being treated later than they should be with IVIG for a diagnosis of Kawasaki disease. We need to think about this diagnosis even in the youngest of children. See the report that follows (Abstract 9–12), which gives us information about the risk of development of coronary artery disease in patients with Kawasaki syndrome.

J. A. Stockman III, MD

Kawasaki Syndrome and Risk Factors for Coronary Artery Abnormalities: United States, 1994-2003
Belay ED, Maddox RA, Holman RC, et al (Ctrs for Disease Control and Prevention, Atlanta, Ga)
Pediatr Infect Dis J 25:245-249, 2006   9–12

Background.—Kawasaki syndrome (KS) causes significant morbidity among children in the United States and other countries and can result in a range of cardiac and noncardiac complications.

Methods.—To describe the occurrence of KS in the United States and risk factors for the development of coronary artery abnormalities (CAA), national KS surveillance data were analyzed for patients with KS onset during 1994–2003. The surveillance is a passive system, and information is collected on a standardized case report form.

Results.—During 1994 through 2003, 3115 patients who met the KS case definition were reported to the national KS surveillance system. The median age of KS patients was 32 months; the male-female ratio was 1.5:1. Nearly one-third (31.8%) of the cumulative number of KS cases occurred during January through March. During the study period, 362 (12.9%) of 2798 KS patients had CAA. The proportion of patients with CAA increased from 10.0% in 1994 to 17.8% in 2003. Age younger than 1 year and 9–17 years, male sex, Asian and Pacific Islander race and Hispanic ethnicity (a previously unidentified risk factor) were significantly associated with the development of CAA.

Conclusions.—The increase in CAA was attributed to widespread use of the criteria of de Zorzi et al, resulting in increased recognition of coronary artery dilatations. The factors contributing to a higher risk of CAA, such as delayed treatment, particularly among Hispanics, need to be investigated.

▶ There have been a couple of new observations in the past year or two about Kawasaki syndrome that are worth mentioning. The first is that we now know that a familial occurrence of Kawasaki syndrome can happen. A retrospective record review at 2 medical centers in California and Texas uncovered 18 families with multiple affected members. If one runs the math, about 1% of Kawasaki syndrome occurs in families where another sibling has been affected.[1]

As far as the management of Kawasaki disease is concerned, IVIG and aspirin remain the standard of therapy. A recent review of the literature, however, demonstrates that when combined with aspirin-containing regimens as initial therapy, corticosteroids significantly reduce the incidence of coronary artery aneurisms. There is an active study underway now to address the use of steroids in combination with IVIG and aspirin as an initial therapy for Kawasaki disease.[2]

Finally, until a report recently appeared, this editor was comfortable naming only Kawasaki disease as a cause of coronary aneurysms. It turns out, however, that regular cocaine users are about 4 times as likely as nonusers to have coronary artery aneurysms. This could, in fact, be a partial explanation as to why some cocaine users have a heightened risk of heart attack. Investigators at the Minneapolis Heart Foundation match 112 cocaine users with 79 nonusers. All were being hospitalized because of the occurrence of myocardial infarction. It turns out that more than 30% of the cocaine users actually had coronary artery aneurysms that were contributing to the myocardial infarction compared with 8% of nonusers who had idiopathic coronary aneurysms.[3] What is interesting in this report is the fact that coronary artery aneurysms were found in individuals who had used cocaine many, many years previously and had not been using the drug in recent times.

J. A. Stockman III, MD

References

1. Dergun M, Kao N, Hauger S, et al: Familial occurrence of Kawasaki syndrome in North America. *Arch Pediatr Adolesc Med* 159:876-881, 2005.
2. Wooditch AC, Aronoff SC: Effect of initial corticosteroid therapy on coronary artery aneurysm formation in Kawasaki disease: A meta-analysis of 862 children. *Pediatrics* 116:989-995, 2005.
3. Satran A, Bart BA, Henry CR, et al: Increased prevalence of coronary artery aneurysms among cocaine users. *Circulation* 111:2424-2449, 2005.

Cardiac Changes Associated With Growth Hormone Therapy Among Children Treated With Anthracyclines

Lipschultz SE, Vlach SA, Lipsitz SR, et al (Univ of Miami, Fla; Children's Hosp, Boston; Med Univ of South Carolina, Charleston; et al)
Pediatrics 115:1613-1622, 2005   9–13

Objective.—The objective was to assess the cardiac effects of growth hormone (GH) therapy. Anthracycline-treated childhood cancer survivors frequently have reduced left ventricular (LV) wall thickness and contractility, and GH therapy may affect these factors.

Methods.—We examined serial cardiac findings for 34 anthracycline-treated childhood cancer survivors with several years of GH therapy and baseline cardiac z scores similar to those of a comparison group (86 similar cancer survivors without GH therapy).

Results.—LV contractility was decreased among GH-treated patients before, during, and after GH therapy (-1.08 SD below the age-adjusted population mean before therapy and -1.88 SD 4 years after therapy ceased, with each value depressed below normal). Contractility was higher in the control group than in the GH-treated group, with this difference being nearly significant. The GH-treated children had thinner LV walls before GH therapy (-1.38 SD). Wall thickness increased during GH therapy (from -1.38 SD to -1.09 SD after 3 years of GH therapy), but the effect was lost shortly after GH therapy ended and thickness diminished over time (-1.50 SD at 1 year after therapy and -1.96 SD at 4 years). During GH therapy, the wall thickness for the GH-treated group was greater than that for the control group; however, by 4 years after therapy, there was no difference between the GH-treated group and the control group.

Conclusions.—GH therapy among anthracycline-treated survivors of childhood cancer increased LV wall thickness, but the effect was lost after therapy was discontinued. The therapy did not affect the progressive LV dysfunction.

▶ Anthracyclines are potent anticancer agents currently used in the treatment of many childhood malignancies and, as a result, a growing number of children have survived childhood cancer with the consequent effects of anthracyclines on their heart. Cardiac damage after anthracycline chemotherapy is a serious problem among young childhood cancer survivors who generally have a long life expectancy after successful cancer treatment. The frequency of asymptomatic anthracycline chemotherapy-induced cardiac damage is reported to be as high as 60% and the long-term risk of heart failure remains a real threat to these youngsters as they grow older. This problem is sufficiently bad that guidelines now advise indefinite monitoring of cardiac function of children treated with anthracyclines. The management of childhood cancer survivors with asymptomatic anthracycline-associated cardiac damage remains unclear. Many are thinking about using angiotensin converting enzyme (ACE) inhibitors and/or β-blockers with the thought that afterload-reducing agents might relieve the stress these patients are experiencing on their LV myocardium. There are no studies that yet document whether this might be effective. This is the topic for the study which follows from the Netherlands (Abstract 9–14).

The study by Lipschultz et al from Boston Children's Hospital gives us a clue about whether GH therapy might produce advantageous or disadvantageous consequences to pediatric cancer patients who have been treated with anthracyclines. It is well known that part of the anthracycline-induced cardiomyopathy problem relates to excess afterload attributable to LV wall thickness. The authors of this report have previously noted that LV wall thickness decreases over time in cancer patients treated with anthracyclines and does so most rapidly among youngsters who had substantial growth induced by GH therapy for radiation- or chemotherapy-induced GH insufficiency—a common endocrine effect of oncology therapy among long-term survivors of childhood cancer. On the other hand, the use of GH has actually been proposed as a possible therapy for some types of LV dysfunction because GH may enhance contractility. GH, either directly or through insulin-like growth factor-1, also appears to induce LV hypertrophy and theoretically, thereby, might improve LV performance by decreasing systolic wall stress. In fact, it has been shown that adults with GH insufficiency do have LV structural and functional abnormalities, which improve with GH replacement therapy. It is for these reasons that the authors of this report decided to more carefully study whether GH might be of benefit (or harm) to those who have been treated with anthracyclines.

The results of the studies in Boston using GH to treat anthracycline-induced cardiomyopathy were a good news-bad news story. GH, when administered to these cancer patients, did increase LV wall thickness, but once GH therapy was stopped, several years later, no difference was seen in the GH-treated group and the control group.

Unfortunately, when it comes to cardiac damage from cancer therapy, the more we learn, the less we know. I hope youngsters so treated will not grow up to be adults who need heart transplants. These children deserve better.

J. A. Stockman III, MD

Management of Asymptomatic Anthracycline-induced Cardiac Damage After Treatment for Childhood Cancer: A Postal Survey Among Dutch Adult and Pediatric Cardiologists

van Dalen EC, van der Pal HJH, Reitsma JB, et al (Academic Med Ctr, Amsterdam; Sophia Children's Hosp, Rotterdam, the Netherlands; Ctr for Congenital Anomalies of the Heart Amsterdam/Leiden)
J Pediatr Hematol Oncol 27:319-322, 2005   9–14

Summary.—Asymptomatic anthracycline-induced cardiac damage (A-CD) is a serious problem among young childhood cancer survivors. The aim of this survey was to assess the current treatment policy in these patients in the Netherlands. A questionnaire was sent to all 136 departments of adult or pediatric cardiology in the Netherlands. It was returned by 61% of the departments. Sixty-six percent of the respondents started medical treatment (ie, an ACE inhibitor and/or a beta-blocker) in childhood cancer survivors with asymptomatic A-CD. Fifty-eight percent of the respondents indicated that their treatment decision was based on published findings in the literature, but none of them referred to studies evaluating the treatment of asymptomatic A-CD. A majority of adult and pediatric cardiologists started medical treatment in childhood cancer survivors with asymptomatic A-CD without knowledge of the benefits and risks of treatment in this patient group. Before ACE inhibitors and/or beta-blockers can be recommended as routine practice in childhood cancer survivors with asymptomatic A-CD, randomized controlled trials should be performed. Until then, the authors recommend centralizing the treatment of childhood cancer survivors with asymptomatic A-CD in a specialized center to cluster the available knowledge and experience.

▶ The preceding commentary related all this editor knows about this topic, so this commentary relates a bit of history related to the heart. Even before Hippocrates (ca. 460-380 BC) taught the importance of listening to breath sounds, references to its usefulness appeared in the Ebers Papyrus (ca. 1500 BC) and the Hindu Vedas (ca. 1500-1200 BC). Nonetheless, it was not until the early 19th century that physicians began to explore in a systematic way the precise clinical meanings of both breath and heart sounds by correlating data gathered during patient examinations with what was ultimately discovered on the autopsy table. This was the period when Paris reigned as the international center for all things medical. Drawings from a system of hospitals affording limitless access to what then was referred to as "clinical material," the Paris Medical School boasted a talented faculty that represented the vanguard of medicine.

One of the brightest stars in the European firmament was the man credited with creating the stethoscope, René Théophile Hyacinthe Laënnec (1781-1826). Substantially before he assumed the position of Chief of Service at the Necker Hospital in 1816, Laënnec became adept at a technique we call percussion, striking the chest with one's fingertips in search of pathologic processes. Leopold Auenbrugger, the Physician-in-Chief of Vienna's Holy Trinity Hospital, first described the method in his 1761 treatise *Inventum novum*, but it was largely ignored until 1808, when Laënnec's professor and Napoleon's favorite physician, Jean Nicolas Corvisart, translated Auenbrugger's text into French and began teaching percussion to his students and colleagues. By this point in the history of medicine, physicians were listening to breath sounds by placing an ear against a patient's chest, a technique that Laënnec found disgusting in view of some of his patients' hygiene.

It was in the fall of 1816 that, while running through a courtyard in the Louvre, Laënnec observed a group of laughing children playing atop a pile of old timber. A pair of youngsters were toying with a long, narrow wooden beam. While one child held the beam to his ear, the other tapped nails against the opposite end and all enjoyed a jolly good time transmitting sound. This led Laënnec to ask for a quire of paper, which he rolled into a cylinder and applied it to a young woman's chest that had been suffering from heart disease. Between 1816 and 1819, Laënnec experimented with a series of hollow tubes that he fashioned out of clear cedar or ebony, arriving at a model approximately 1 foot in length and 1.5 inches in diameter with a ¼-inch central channel. Laënnec became the first physician to reliably distinguish among bronchiectasis, emphysema, pneumothorax, lung abscess, hemorrhagic pleurisy, and pulmonary infarcts.

Although medical historians consider the golden age of the stethoscope to have run from the publication of Laënnec's treatise on the use of the stethoscope and the death of Sir William Osler in 1919, the stethoscope continues to be of great clinical value to those who take the time to use it properly. Most studies show that the average resident out of training has less than a 50% probability of detecting what otherwise are readily detectable murmurs to the trained ear.

The story is told that Laënnec frequently auscultated himself since he had tuberculosis and ultimately hung up his stethoscope shortly before his death from this same disease.

J. A. Stockman III, MD

10 Infectious Diseases/ Immunology

Effectiveness of a Parental Educational Intervention in Reducing Antibiotic Use in Children: A Randomized Controlled Trial
Taylor JA, Kwan-Gett TSC, McMahon EM Jr (Univ of Washington, Seattle; Virginia Mason Sand Point Pediatrics, Seattle; Ballard Pediatric Clinic, Seattle)
Pediatr Infect Dis J 24:489-493, 2005   10–1

Objective.—To determine whether an educational intervention aimed at parents leads to fewer antibiotic prescriptions for their children.

Design.—Placebo-controlled, randomized controlled trial.

Setting.—Offices of primary care pediatricians who are members of a regional practice-based research network.

Participants.—Healthy children younger than 24 months old enrolled at the time of an office visit.

Interventions.—Parents of study children were randomized to receive either a pamphlet and videotape (featuring one of their child's pediatricians) promoting the judicious use of antibiotics (intervention group) or brochures about injury prevention (control group). A total of 499 eligible children were enrolled, and data on outpatient visits during a 12-month observation period were collected.

Main Outcome Measures.—We compared the number of visits for upper-respiratory tract infections (URIs), number of diagnoses and antibiotic prescriptions for otitis media and/or sinusitis and total number of antibiotics per patient among children in the intervention and control groups using Poisson regression analysis, adjusted for clustering into different practices.

Results.—Data on 4924 visits were reviewed; 28.8% of these visits were because of URI symptoms. The mean number of visits per study patient for URI symptoms was 2.8. Including all visits, the mean number of diagnoses of otitis media in study children was 2.1, mean number of diagnoses of otitis media and/or sinusitis was 2.3 and mean number of antibiotic prescriptions was 2.4; there were no significant differences between children in the intervention and control groups for any of these outcomes. Overall physicians prescribed 1 or more antibiotics during 45.9% of visits for a chief complaint of URI symptoms; 92% of antibiotic usage in children presenting with URI symptoms was for a diagnosis of otitis media and/or sinusitis.

Conclusions.—An educational intervention aimed at parents did not result in a decrease in the number of antibiotic prescriptions in their children. The use of antibiotics among children with URI symptoms was common; other interventions promoting the judicious use of these medications are needed.

▶ It would be easier to move mountains than to convince parents, and perhaps some care providers, that it would be better not to use antibiotics in certain circumstances than to prescribe them. We see in this report that, even after intensive parent education, overall, pediatric-care providers prescribe 1 or more antibiotics during 45.9% of visits for a chief complaint of a URI problem. Overall, 92% of antibiotic use in children seen with cold symptoms was for the diagnosis of otitis media and/or sinusitis.

The data of Taylor et al are virtually identical to the data of Little et al, showing the benefits (or lack of benefits) of teaching adults about antibiotic prescribing.[1] Specifically, these investigators looked at prescribing trends in adults seen with a chief complaint of cough. Here in the United States, more than 30 million visits a year to physicians are made for a chief complaint of cough, at least 10 million of which are made by otherwise healthy adults diagnosed with acute bronchitis. The significant majority of such patients receive an antibiotic prescription, often for a broad-spectrum macrolide or quinolone, a prescription costing from $50 to $100. At best, the literature suggests that if there is any benefit to prescribing antibiotics for common bronchitis in adults, this shortens the duration of cough by at most half a day. This benefit, if indeed at all present, must be balanced by all the adverse side effects associated with antibiotic prescribing, including the emergence of antibiotic resistance. The study of Little et al enrolled more than 800 adults and children who were seen with cough by their primary-care physician and at least 1 symptom referable to the lower respiratory tract (colored sputum, chest pain, shortness of breath, or wheezing). In this series, patients were randomly assigned to receive immediate antibiotic treatment, no antibiotics, or an offer of delayed antibiotics if symptoms had not resolved after 10 days. The delayed prescription could be picked up from the receptionist without having to actually visit the physician. The patients in this report were typical of those diagnosed with acute bronchitis in a primary care practice: two of 3 patients had fever and more than 40% reported production of green sputum. The patients who were in this study had their symptoms monitored for 3 weeks. The findings of this study will probably surprise most patients but perhaps not their doctors. There was no significant difference in any of the primary outcomes between patients receiving antibiotics and those receiving placebo. It should be noted that neither children nor adults with colored sputum benefited from antibiotic use, and elderly patients were actually less likely to benefit from antibiotics.

The punch-line from all of this is that when a patient is seen with a respiratory tract infection, one consistent with bronchitis, the age-old dictum holds: if you see your doctor and get a prescription, you will be better in 7 days. If you do not, you will be better in a week.

J. A. Stockman III, MD

Reference

1. Little P, Rumsby K, Kelly J, et al: Information leaflet and antibiotic prescribing strategies for acute lower respiratory tract infection: A randomized control trial. *JAMA* 293:3029-3035, 2005.

Significance of Extreme Leukocytosis in the Evaluation of Febrile Children

Shah SS, Shofer FS, Seidel JS, et al (Univ of Pennsylvania, Philadelphia; Harbor-UCLA Med Ctr, Torrance)
Pediatr Infect Dis J 24:627-630, 2005   10–2

Background.—Emergency department evaluation of young febrile children often includes a white blood cell count. Although a high white blood cell count is associated with an increased likelihood of infection, the clinical significance of extreme leukocytosis (EL), defined as a white blood cell count of $\geq 25,000/mm^3$, has not been well-studied.

Objective.—To determine diagnoses associated with EL in febrile children evaluated in a pediatric emergency department and to compare rates of serious bacterial infection in those with EL and in those with more modest leukocytosis (LK) ($15,000-24,999/mm^3$).

Methods.—A retrospective case-control study of children 2–24 months of age was performed. Those with EL were frequency age- and gender-matched to controls with LK.

Results.—Sixty-nine patients with EL and 94 patients with LK were included. The mean age was 9.9 months, and 91 (56%) patients were male. The diagnoses were similar between the 2 groups, with otitis media, viral syndrome and pneumonia being the most common. The rates of proven serious bacterial infection were similar between EL (25%; 95% confidence interval, 15–36%) and LK (17%; 95% confidence interval, 10–26%) patients. Using different white blood cell cutoff points did not distinguish between patients with and without serious bacterial infection.

Conclusion.—Young febrile children whose emergency department evaluation revealed EL had diagnoses and rates of serious bacterial infection similar to those of children with LK.

▶ Previous studies have looked at the significance of extreme leukocytosis (defined as a white blood cell count of $25,000/mm^3$) as an indicator of severe bacterial infection. These studies, however, were largely undertaken in the pre-*Haemophilus influenzae* type b immunization era. This report attempts to modernize our understanding of what a very high white count means in a child with fever. What we learn from this report is that a white count greater than $25,000/mm^3$ is no more meaningful than is a white count of 15,000 to 25,000/mm^3, at least in the post-*H influenzae* type b immunization era.

It is important to understand the implications of this report. Historically, patients with very elevated white blood cell counts have been thought to be more at risk for serious bacterial infection. Indeed, in this report, patients in the former category in this study were, in fact, hospitalized at higher rates than patients with lower white blood cell counts. The trigger point for concern, if the data from this report are to be believed, occurs at 15,000/mm³ rather than at 25,000/mm³ with higher white blood cell counts adding no greater discrimination with respect to risk for serious bacterial infection.

J. A. Stockman III, MD

Combined Tetanus, Diphtheria, and 5-Component Pertussis Vaccine for Use in Adolescents and Adults
Pichichero ME, Rennels MB, Edwards KM, et al (Univ of Rochester, NY; Univ of Maryland, Baltimore; Vanderbilt Univ, Nashville, Tenn; et al)
JAMA 293:3003-3011, 2005   10–3

Context.—Increasing reports of pertussis among US adolescents, adults, and their infant contacts have stimulated vaccine development for older age groups.

Objective.—To assess the immunogenicity and reactogenicity of a tetanus-diphtheria 5-component (pertussis toxoid, filamentous hemagglutinin, pertactin, and fimbriae types 2 and 3) acellular pertussis vaccine (Tdap) in adolescents and adults.

Design, Setting, and Participants.—A prospective, randomized, modified double-blind, comparative trial was conducted in healthy adolescents and adults aged 11 through 64 years from August 2001 to August 2002 at 39 US clinical centers.

Interventions.—A single 0.5-mL intramuscular dose of either Tdap or tetanus-diphtheria vaccine (Td).

Main Outcome Measures.—Antibody titers to diphtheria and tetanus toxoids for Tdap and Td were measured in sera collected from subsets of adolescents and adults, before and 28 days after vaccination. For pertussis antigens, titers in sera from Tdap vaccinees were assessed vs those from infants who received analogous pediatric diphtheria-tetanus-acellular pertussis vaccine (DTaP) in a previous efficacy trial. Safety was assessed via solicited local and systemic reactions for 14 days and adverse events for 6 months following vaccination.

Results.—A total of 4480 participants were enrolled. For both Tdap and Td, more than 94% and nearly 100% of vaccinees had protective antibody concentrations of at least 0.1 IU/mL for diphtheria and tetanus, respectively. Geometric mean antibody titers to pertussis toxoid, filamentous hemagglutinin, pertactin, and fimbriae types 2 and 3 exceeded (by 2.1 to 5.4 times) levels in infants following immunization at 2, 4, and 6 months with DTaP. The incidence of solicited local and systemic reactions and adverse events was generally similar between the Tdap and Td groups.

Conclusions.—This Tdap vaccine elicited robust immune responses in adolescents and adults to pertussis, tetanus, and diphtheria antigens, while exhibiting an overall safety profile similar to that of a licensed Td vaccine.

These data support the potential routine use of this Tdap vaccine in adolescents and adults.

▶ This is another article showing that it not only is feasible to administer tetanus–diphtheria–pertussis vaccine to adolescents and adults, but the vaccine actually produces good immune responses. The findings are especially important, particularly when it comes to the prevention of adult pertussis. Pertussis in teenagers and adults is a seriously unrecognized disease. Complications from infection are extremely high and include pneumonia, urinary incontinence, and a cough that lasts for an average of 3 months. Sinusitis, vomiting, fractured ribs, fatigue, encephalitis, and disturbed sleep are frequent sequelae of the infection. Transmission of this disease from an infected teenager or an adult to an unimmunized or underimmunized infant leads to even worse morbidity and mortality. Unfortunately, the diagnosis of pertussis is rarely, if ever, considered by internists, despite clear data about its incidence and significance among adults and knowledge that adults are, in fact, the reservoir of infection for susceptible children. Studies have suggested that adults seen with one or more weeks of a cough will have a likelihood of 10% to 15% of meeting the serologic criteria for pertussis infection.[1]

Until recently, internists have had nothing in their armamentarium to prevent pertussis in folks like us. The only pertussis vaccine licensed in the United States has been for children up to the age of 7 years because of significant local and systemic reactions when used in adults. Immunization in childhood is not long lasting. It takes about 10 years for immunity to essentially fully wane in someone who has been immunized with pertussis.

The article by Pichichero et al demonstrates the immunogenicity and safety of acellular pertussis vaccines in adults. The study reports the results of a randomized, double-blind, comparative clinical trial. This study, conducted across 39 centers in the United States, answered several previously raised questions on acellular pertussis vaccine. Overall, 4480 healthy individuals 11 to 64 years of age were enrolled and received a single 0.5-mL IM dose of either a licensed Td vaccine or a Tdap vaccine. The pertussis combination vaccine was both safe and immunogenic in this diverse population.

Why should internists adopt pertussis immunization? The answer is pretty clear. First, the disease is increasingly being diagnosed in adults, and immunization would reduce the burden of disease in this population. Second, because adults form the reservoir of infection for underimmunized or unimmunized infants and children, vaccinating adults should reduce disease transmission to this high-risk age group. The Tdap vaccine is now licensed by the US Food and Drug Administration for 1-dose use in adolescents and adults aged 11 to 64 years. Physicians who administer pertussis vaccines to adults should take care to avoid using the pediatric formulation, DTaP (Boostrix). This vaccine is licensed for use only in the pediatric population.

If you are uncertain whether the study reported by Pichichero et al is a valid one, a virtually similar report appeared from the Adult Pertussis Trial (APERT).[2] The APERT trial found that in adolescents and adults vaccine protection with the acellular pertussis vaccine was 92%. The incidence of pertussis in the control group not receiving the vaccine ranged from 307 to 450 cases per 100,000 person years. The vaccine does, in fact, work!

J. A. Stockman III, MD

References

1. Wright SW, Edwards KM, Decker MD, et al: Pertussis infection in adults with persistent cough. *JAMA* 273:1044-1046, 1995.
2. Ward JI, Cherry JD, Chan WS-J, et al: Efficacy of an acellular pertussis vaccine among adolescents and adults. *N Engl J Med* 353:1555-1563, 2005.

Invasive Pneumococcal Disease Among Infants Before and After Introduction of Pneumococcal Conjugate Vaccine

Poehling KA, Talbot TR, Griffin MR, et al (Vanderbilt Univ, Nashville, Tenn; Tennessee Dept of Health, Nashville; Centers for Disease Control and Prevention, Atlanta, Ga; et al)
JAMA 295:1668-1674, 2006

10–4

Context.—*Streptococcus pneumoniae* is a serious infection in young infants. A heptavalent pneumococcal conjugate vaccine (PCV7) was licensed in 2000 and recommended for all children aged 2 to 23 months.

Objective.—To determine the rates of invasive pneumococcal disease (IPD) in young infants before and after PCV7 was incorporated into the childhood immunization schedule in June 2000.

Design, Setting, and Participants.—A prospective, population-based study of infants aged 0 to 90 days who resided in areas in 8 US states with active laboratory surveillance for invasive *S pneumoniae* infections from July 1, 1997, to June 30, 2004.

Main Outcome Measures.—Rates of laboratory-confirmed IPD before (July 1, 1997-June 30, 2000) and after (July 1, 2001-June 30, 2004) PCV7 introduction, excluding a transition year (July 1, 2000-June 30, 2001).

Results.—There were 146 cases of IPD, 89 before and 57 after PCV7 introduction. Isolated bacteremia occurred in 94 cases (64%), pneumonia in 27 (18%), meningitis in 22 (15%), and septic arthritis and/or osteomyelitis in 3 (2%). Mean rates of IPD for infants aged 0 to 90 days decreased 40% from 11.8 (95% confidence interval [CI], 9.6-14.5) to 7.2 (95% CI, 5.6-9.4; $P=.004$) per 100 000 live births following PCV7 introduction. Among black infants, mean rates of IPD decreased significantly from 17.1 (95% CI, 11.9-24.6) to 5.3 (95% CI, 2.8-10.1; $P=.001$) per 100 000 live births, with a nonsignificant decrease from 9.6 (95% CI, 7.3-12.7) to 6.8 (95% CI, 4.9-9.4) per 100 000 live births for white infants. Rates of PCV7-serotype isolates decreased significantly from 7.3 (95% CI, 5.3-10.1) to 2.4 (95% CI, 1.6-3.8; $P<.001$) per 100 000 live births, while rates of non-PCV7 serotypes remained stable ($P=.55$).

Conclusions.—Since PCV7 introduction, rates of IPD in young infants have decreased significantly, providing evidence that vaccinating children aged 2 to 23 months has led to changes in pneumococcal carriage in infants too young to receive PCV7. With a significant decrease in rates of IPD among black infants, the previous racial difference has been eliminated.

▶ Another report of a "spin" effect of using PCV7 in children aged 2 months and older. The world is full of unintended consequences of vaccine use. One of the consequences, perhaps unintended, of use of PCV7 is that it does seem to decrease the rate of pneumococcal disease even in those who have not been immunized. Before this report appeared, it was unclear whether this vaccine, when used to immunize children aged 2 months and older, would protect neonates and very young infants by changing pneumococcal carriage in those too young to receive the vaccine, similar to the effects reported after *Haemophilus influenzae* type b vaccination. This report hypothesized that the rates of IPD in very young infants would decline from the period 1997-1999 to the period 2001-2004, periods that coincided temporally with a period before and coincident with the introduction of PCV7 (in the year 2000).

What we learn from this report is that since the introduction of PCV7, there has been a truly remarkable decline in IPD in young infants who have not yet received the vaccine. This is a true example of herd immunity. Studies such as this do not conclusively prove that the introduction of PCV7 was responsible for this effect, but it is hard to ignore the probable relationship. Continued surveillance of IPD in this young age group (as well as in older children) is critical to determine whether this downward trend continues or whether serotypes not included in PCV7 will emerge as an important cause of IPD in infants and young children. The spread effect of administration of pneumococcal conjugate vaccine to children also extends to older adults. Lexau et al showed that among adults age 50 years or older, the incidence of disease caused by the 7 conjugate vaccine serotypes, even in those not immunized, declined 55% from 22.4 to 10.2 cases per 100,000 population.[1] These findings indicate that the use of the conjugate vaccine in children has substantially benefited older adults. Unfortunately, persons with certain comorbid conditions (such as HIV infection) seem to benefit less than healthier persons from the indirect effects of the new vaccine.

J. A. Stockman III, MD

Reference

1. Lexau CA, Lynfield R, Danila R, et al: Changing epidemiology of invasive pneumococcal disease among older adults in the era of pediatric pneumococcal conjugate vaccine. *JAMA* 294:2043-2051, 2005.

Childhood Vaccination and Nontargeted Infectious Disease Hospitalization
Hviid A, Wohlfahrt J, Stellfeld M, et al (Statens Serum Institut, Copenhagen)
JAMA 294:699-705, 2005   10–5

Context.—It has been hypothesized that multiple-antigen vaccines, such as measles-mumps-rubella vaccine, or aggregated vaccine exposure could lead to immune dysfunction, resulting in nontargeted infectious diseases as a result of an "overload" mechanism.

Objective.—To evaluate the relationship between routinely administered childhood vaccines (*Haemophilus influenzae* type b; diphtheria-tetanus-inactivated poliovirus; diphtheria-tetanus-acellular pertussis-inactivated poliovirus; whole-cell pertussis; measles-mumps-rubella; oral poliovirus) and hospitalization for nontargeted infectious diseases.

Design, Setting, and Participants.—Population-based cohort comprising all children born in Denmark from 1990 through 2001 (N = 805 206). Longitudinal information was collected on type and number of vaccine doses received and hospitalization with infectious diseases, specifically acute upper respiratory tract infection, viral and bacterial pneumonia, septicemia, viral central nervous system infection, bacterial meningitis, and diarrhea.

Main Outcome Measures.—Rate ratios for each type of infectious disease according to vaccination status.

Results.—During 2 900 463 person-years of follow-up, 84 317 cases of infectious disease hospitalization were identified. Out of 42 possible associations (6 vaccines and 7 infectious disease categories), the only adverse association was for *Haemophilus influenzae* type b vaccine and acute upper respiratory tract infection (rate ratio, 1.05; 95% confidence interval, 1.01-1.08 comparing vaccinated participants with unvaccinated participants). This one adverse association of 42 possible outcomes was within the limits of what would be expected by chance alone and the effect was not temporal or dose-response. When considering aggregated vaccine exposure, we found no adverse associations between an increasing number of vaccinations and infectious diseases.

Conclusion.—These results do not support the hypotheses that multiple-antigen vaccines or aggregated vaccine exposure increase the risk of nontargeted infectious disease hospitalization.

▶ This article answers a question that naysayers of vaccinations and vaccines have posed for a long time. The question is whether multiple-antigen vaccines such as the mumps–rubella vaccine or other combination vaccines so overload the immune system that the incidence of nontargeted infectious diseases is increased as a result. The data from this article speak for themselves. Chance alone explains any possible increase in nontargeted infectious diseases. The punch line is straightforward. Vaccines work for the diseases against which they are targeted. The incidence of other types of infections does not increase as a consequence of the use of targeted vaccines.

J. A. Stockman III, MD

Household Based Treatment of Drinking Water With Flocculant-Disinfectant for Preventing Diarrhoea in Areas With Turbid Source Water in Rural Western Kenya: Cluster Randomised Controlled Trial

Crump JA, Otieno PO, Slutsker L, et al (Ctrs for Disease Control and Prevention, Atlanta, Ga; Ctrs for Disease Control and Prevention, Kisumu, Kenya; Procter & Gamble Health Sciences Inst, Mason, Ohio)
BMJ 331:478-481, 2005   10–6

Objective.—To compare the effect on prevalence of diarrhoea and mortality of household based treatment of drinking water with flocculant-disinfectant, sodium hypochlorite, and standard practices in areas with turbid water source in Africa.

Design.—Cluster randomised controlled trial over 20 weeks.

Setting.—Family compounds, each containing several houses, in rural western Kenya.

Participants.—6650 people in 605 family compounds.

Intervention.—Water treatment: flocculant-disinfectant, sodium hypochlorite, and usual practice (control).

Main Outcome Measures.—Prevalence of diarrhoea and all cause mortality. *Escherichia coli* concentration, free residual chlorine concentration, and turbidity in household drinking water as surrogates for effectiveness of water treatment.

Results.—In children <2 years old, compared with those in the control compounds, the absolute difference in prevalence of diarrhoea was −25% in the flocculant-disinfectant arm (95% confidence interval −40 to −5) and −17% in the sodium hypochlorite arm (−34 to 4). In all age groups compared with control, the absolute difference in prevalence was −19% in the flocculant-disinfectant arm (−34 to −2) and −26% in the sodium hypochlorite arm (−39 to −9). There were significantly fewer deaths in the intervention compounds than in the control compounds (relative risk of death 0.58, P = 0.036). Fourteen per cent of water samples from control compounds had *E coli* concentrations <1 CFU/100 ml compared with 82% in flocculant-disinfectant and 78% in sodium hypochlorite compounds. The mean turbidity of drinking water was 8 nephelometric turbidity units (NTU) in flocculant-disinfectant households, compared with 55 NTU in the two other compounds (P < 0.001).

Conclusions.—In areas of turbid water, flocculant-disinfectant was associated with a significant reduction in diarrhoea among children <2 years. This health benefit, combined with a significant reduction in turbidity, suggests that the flocculant-disinfectant is well suited to areas with highly contaminated and turbid water.

▶ We do not tend to think about the risk of infection from drinking water much here in the United States, but it is a problem worldwide and occasionally is a problem here as well. Several organizations have adopted a 3-pronged approach for treating water at the point of use. This includes using simple household bleach (sodium hypochlorite) to disinfect the water, using narrow-mouthed storage vessels, and working with communities to educate people about the causes and prevention of diarrhea. It has proved difficult to convince individuals in certain parts of the world to add bleach to drinking water because it affects the taste. Furthermore, bleach may not be effective in water that is turbid or that contains chlorine-resistant organisms such as *Cyclospora cayetanensis* or *Cryptosporidium parvum*.

If one does not use chlorination to provide safe drinking water, one can also obviously boil water. The problem with boiling water, particularly in undeveloped parts of the world, is that it consumes a lot of energy. It takes about 1 kg of wood to boil 1 L of water. That is a lot of combustible material. So what are the other alternatives? Various interventions have recently involved the promotion of removal of particles and microbes from water. Although cloth has been found to remove zooplankton and phytoplankton containing *Vibrio cholerae* and is used extensively for the eradication of guinea worm, cloth is not recommended for routine treatment of water in the home because its pores are too large to remove bacteria and viruses. Chemical precipitation (coagulation and flocculation) removes particles and microbes. It can be used in households to reduce transmission of diarrheal disease, but its use in developing countries has been limited by issues of safety, effectiveness, cost, and sustainability. This is why the findings in the article by Crump et al represent an important advance in treating water in households.

In a randomized trial, Crump et al compared the standard practice of using sodium hypochlorite (bleach) with flocculant-disinfectant treatment of drinking water in homes in a rural area of western Kenya where the water is highly turbid and contaminated with fecal bacteria. The treatment lowered the turbidity of drinking water, improved the acceptability of water treatment at home, and reduced the prevalence of diarrhea by some 25% among participants. The authors also reported fewer deaths in the intervention group.

In third-world countries, it is hoped that flocculant-disinfectant will become an acceptable alternative to bleach with its poor aftertaste in disinfecting household water. Bleach also does nothing to reduce the turbidity of drinking water, whereas flocculant-disinfectant not only purifies the water, but makes it look clear. Hopefully, the latter improvement will make the technique more acceptable to families.

Before ending this comment, it seems important to note certain similarities between what occurs in underdeveloped parts of the world and the situation in the United States post Hurricane Katrina. In the wake of Hurricane Katrina, open wounds exposed to brackish seawater along the Gulf coast led to 6 deaths and 24 other severe infections from Vibrio bacteria. It should be recognized that 19 varieties of Vibrio bacteria are found naturally in warm seawater; the CDC tells us that some 400 infections here in the US occur each year from exposure to Vibrio organisms, with most of these infections resulting from Vibrio microbes ingested by people eating raw shellfish. These cases are rarely fatal. On the other hand, about one-fourth of Vibrio infections arise from subspecies that pass through the skin via scratches, cuts, or abrasions. Among these, infections caused by Vibrio vulnificus are the most serious.

The spate of Vibrio infections occurring soon after Hurricane Katrina is probably attributable to people's increased contact with brackish seawater.

Prompt treatment within a day or two of such exposure is uniformly curative. All those who died post Katrina as a result of Vibrio infections or who lost limbs were not hospitalized until 2 or more days after redness had appeared.

If you are a beach lover who has contact with ocean water and if you notice any wounds that become red and angry for more than a day, see a healthcare provider![1]

J. A. Stockman III, MD

Reference

1. Exposure to seawater proves deadly (editorial). *Sci News* 168:270, 2005.

A Predominantly Clonal Multi-Institutional Outbreak of *Clostridium difficile*-Associated Diarrhea With High Morbidity and Mortality

Loo VG, Poirier L, Miller MA, et al (McGill Univ, Montreal; Université de Montréal; Hôpital Jean Talon, Montreal; et al)
N Engl J Med 353:2442-2449, 2005   10–7

Background.—In March 2003, several hospitals in Quebec, Canada, noted a marked increase in the incidence of *Clostridium difficile*–associated diarrhea.

Methods.—In 2004 we conducted a prospective study at 12 Quebec hospitals to determine the incidence of nosocomial C. *difficile*–associated diarrhea and its complications and a case–control study to identify risk factors for the disease. Isolates of C. *difficile* were typed by pulsed-field gel electrophoresis and analyzed for binary toxin genes and partial deletions in the toxin A and B repressor gene *tcdC*. Antimicrobial susceptibility was evaluated in a subgroup of isolates.

Results.—A total of 1703 patients with 1719 episodes of nosocomial C. *difficile*–associated diarrhea were identified. The incidence was 22.5 per 1000 admissions. The 30-day attributable mortality rate was 6.9 percent. Case patients were more likely than matched controls to have received fluoroquinolones (odds ratio, 3.9; 95 percent confidence interval, 2.3 to 6.6) or cephalosporins (odds ratio, 3.8; 95 percent confidence interval, 2.2 to 6.6). A predominant strain, resistant to fluoroquinolones, was found in 129 of 157 isolates (82.2 percent), and the binary toxin genes and partial deletions in the *tcdC* gene were present in 132 isolates (84.1 percent).

Conclusions.—A strain of C. *difficile* that was resistant to fluoroquinolones and had binary toxin and a partial deletion of the *tcdC* gene was responsible for this outbreak of C. *difficile*–associated diarrhea. Exposure to fluoroquinolones or cephalosporins was a risk factor.

An Epidemic, Toxin Gene–Variant Strain of *Clostridium difficile*

McDonald LC, Killgore GE, Thompson A, et al (Centers for Disease Control and Prevention, Atlanta, Ga; Univ of Vermont, Burlington; Loyola Univ, Hines, Ill)
N Engl J Med 353:2433-2441, 2005   10–8

Background.—Recent reports suggest that the rate and severity of *Clostridium difficile*–associated disease in the United States are increasing and that the increase may be associated with the emergence of a new strain of *C. difficile* with increased virulence, resistance, or both.

Methods.—A total of 187 *C. difficile* isolates were collected from eight health care facilities in six states (Georgia, Illinois, Maine, New Jersey, Oregon, and Pennsylvania) in which outbreaks of *C. difficile*-associated disease had occurred between 2000 and 2003. The isolates were characterized by restriction-endonuclease analysis (REA), pulsed-field gel electrophoresis (PFGE), and toxinotyping, and the results were compared with those from a database of more than 6000 isolates obtained before 2001. The polymerase chain reaction was used to detect the recently described binary toxin CDT and a deletion in the pathogenicity locus gene, *tcdC*, that might result in increased production of toxins A and B.

Results.—Isolates that belonged to one REA group (BI) and had the same PFGE type (NAP1) were identified in specimens collected from patients at all eight facilities and accounted for at least half of the isolates from five facilities. REA group BI, which was first identified in 1984, was uncommon among isolates from the historic database (14 cases). Both historic and current (obtained since 2001) BI/NAP1 isolates were of toxinotype III, were positive for the binary toxin CDT, and contained an 18-bp *tcdC* deletion. Resistance to gatifloxacin and moxifloxacin was more common in current BI/NAP1 isolates than in non-BI/NAP1 isolates (100 percent vs. 42 percent, P<0.001), whereas the rate of resistance to clindamycin was the same in the two groups (79 percent). All of the current but none of the historic BI/NAP1 isolates were resistant to gatifloxacin and moxifloxacin (P<0.001).

Conclusions.—A previously uncommon strain of *C. difficile* with variations in toxin genes has become more resistant to fluoroquinolones and has emerged as a cause of geographically dispersed outbreaks of *C. difficile*–associated disease.

▶ This article and the one by Loo et al (see Abstract 10–7) are truly scary. The emergence of *C difficile* that is resistant to fluoroquinolones should shake us to the core. It is clear that old pathogens, including influenza, avian influenza, and community-acquired methicillin-resistant *Staphylococcus aureus* are capable of emerging with increased virulence. An equal challenge seems to be provided by *C difficile*. This organism is a bad actor: it is associated with a disease that is almost exclusively seen in the presence of exposure to antibiotics, it is the only anaerobe that poses a nosocomial risk, and it is the only anaerobe that produces a toxin in vivo (in the colon).

It has been estimated that about 3% of healthy individuals harbor *C difficile*. This percentage increases to somewhere between 20% and 40% for hospitalized patients. In healthy folks, this organism is metabolically inactive in the spore form, but when there is something that disturbs competing flora in the gut, the spore is converted to a vegetative form that replicates and produces toxins, which results in the characteristic watery diarrhea with cramps and the finding of a pseudomembranous colitis. Over the past 2 decades, *C difficile* has become the most frequently recognized microbial cause of nosocomial diarrhea, reflecting high rates of colonization in hospitalized patients and the frequent use of antimicrobial agents. The most frequently implicated agent in the 1970s, you may recall, was clindamycin. By the 1980s, it was cephalosporins. The recent surge of cases suggests that fluoroquinolones may now play a major role.

The articles by McDonald et al and Loo et al describe a new strain of *C difficile* and implicate a possible role of fluoroquinolones in driving its emergence. The article by McDonald et al represents an extensive analysis of 187 isolates obtained from patients with *C difficile*–associated enteric disease from 8 outbreaks in health facilities in the United States during the period 2000 through 2003. The article by Loo et al provides a similar microbial analysis accompanied with important clinical data. Loo et al report on a review of *C difficile*–associated disease in almost 2000 patients in 12 hospitals in Canada over a period of just 5.5 months back in 2004. They report an incidence of this problem of 22.5 per 1000 admissions, and the mortality rate was an astounding 6.9%. The incidence among individuals increases substantially with age. For example, if you are 90 years old and admitted to hospital, you have a 10% chance of developing a *C difficile*–associated disease with a mortality rate of almost 15%.

We need to be very cognizant of this problem of *C difficile*–associated disease in children. Treatment basics consist of the prompt discontinuation of the implicated antibiotic and the administration of oral metronidazole. For older patients and those who do not have a prompt response, oral vancomycin should be considered. Patients should be isolated, and the environment should be carefully cleaned with agents effective against *C difficile*. Obviously, fastidious hand washing is critical. Please recognize that alcohol-based sanitizers do not eradicate *C difficile*. Good old soap and water is best on one's hands. Lastly, be very parsimonious in your use of second- and third-generation cephalosporins, clindamycin, and fluoroquinolones or any combination of these drugs.

Fast fact: What is the origin of the word "gangrene?" Few medical words strike as much terror in a clinician and the public as gangrene with all of its associations of rotting, corruption, and putrefaction. The word is of Greek origin and comes to English by way of Latin and French. It has always had an indivisible meaning, in its literal sense: modification of a part of a body. Gangrene seems to have first appeared in English use in the British Isles in the 16th century as a noun. It was used most often by surgeons whose domain was the cure of external conditions. By the 17th century, it had passed into common speech, although it was usually used in a narrow pathological sense. Shakespeare begins to give it metaphorical wings in Coriolanus: "*The Service of the Foote Being Once Gangren'd Is Not Been Respected For What it Was Before."*

J. A. Stockman III, MD

Supplemental Perioperative Oxygen and the Risk of Surgical Wound Infection: A Randomized Controlled Trial
Belda FJ, for the Spanish Reduccion de la Tasa de Infeccion Quirurgica Group (Hosp Clínico Universitario, Valencia, Spain; Hosp de Galdakao, Bizkaia, Spain; Hosp Universitario de La Princesa, Madrid; et al)
JAMA 294:2035-2042, 2005   10–9

Context.—Supplemental perioperative oxygen has been variously reported to halve or double the risk of surgical wound infection.

Objective.—To test the hypothesis that supplemental oxygen reduces infection risk in patients following colorectal surgery.

Design, Setting, and Patients.—A double-blind, randomized controlled trial of 300 patients aged 18 to 80 years who underwent elective colorectal surgery in 14 Spanish hospitals from March 1, 2003, to October 31, 2004. Wound infections were diagnosed by blinded investigators using Centers for Disease Control and Prevention criteria. Baseline patient characteristics, anesthetic treatment, and potential confounding factors were recorded.

Interventions.—Patients were randomly assigned to either 30% or 80% fraction of inspired oxygen (FIO_2) intraoperatively and for 6 hours after surgery. Anesthetic treatment and antibiotic administration were standardized.

Main Outcome Measures.—Any surgical site infection (SSI); secondary outcomes included return of bowel function and ability to tolerate solid food, ambulation, suture removal, and duration of hospitalization.

Results.—A total of 143 patients received 30% perioperative oxygen and 148 received 80% perioperative oxygen. Surgical site infection occurred in 35 patients (24.4%) administered 30% FIO_2 and in 22 patients (14.9%) administered 80% FIO_2 ($P=.04$). The risk of SSI was 39% lower in the 80% FIO_2 group (relative risk [RR], 0.61; 95% confidence interval [CI], 0.38-0.98) vs the 30% FIO_2 group. After adjustment for important covariates, the RR of infection in patients administered supplemental oxygen was 0.46 (95% CI, 0.22-0.95; $P = .04$). None of the secondary outcomes varied significantly between the 2 treatment groups.

Conclusions.—Patients receiving supplemental inspired oxygen had a significant reduction in the risk of wound infection. Supplemental oxygen appears to be an effective intervention to reduce SSI in patients undergoing colon or rectal surgery.

► There seems to be no unequivocal way to prevent infections at the site of surgery in all cases, but studies done over several decades have shown that proper antibiotic selection and timing, clipping rather than shaving of hair, maintenance of normothermia and normal blood sugar levels, and an appropriate surgical technique are critical in reducing this risk. In addition, surgeons have been arguing for some years with their anesthesia colleagues about the benefits of higher levels of inspired oxygen applied to patients during surgery. The article by Belda et al shows us the results of clinical trials using different inspired oxygen concentrations intraoperatively for 6 hours after surgery in patients undergoing planned operations. The overall infection rate was 20% (these were colorectal operations in adults) and was significantly reduced in the group of patients receiving 80% inspired oxygen compared with the group receiving 30% oxygen. The absolute risk reduction was 9%, and the relative risk reduction was 39%. If one were to generalize these results, then one would see a 39% reduction in the United States if the estimated number of surgical wound infections was approximately 600,000 each year, and the cost savings would be the better part of a billion dollars.

So, why might oxygen in higher concentrations help in the operating room? One of the primary mechanisms of early bacterial eradication involves oxidative processes in polymorphonuclear leukocytes that depend on oxygen tension. The concept of influencing the risk of surgical site infection by increasing oxygen concentration is attractive, based on the principle that infection risk is dependent on the number of bacteria that reach the surgical wound during an operation and on the host's ability to kill those bacteria during the early wound healing events that follow in the first few hours after surgery. Thus, there is a strong theoretical rationale to support the findings from the study of Belda et al.

The findings from this article, however, are not the end-all, be-all; because other studies looking at the same problem have given somewhat conflicting results, the issue that faces surgeons and anesthesiologists is what to do with all the data. One with myopic vision would say, anyone, adult or child, being operated on for a colorectal procedure should receive added oxygen in the operating room. However, it defies logic that colorectal operations should have a biologically different response to oxygen concentrations compared with other abdominal procedures. Clearly, whether oxygen is the magic bullet or whether other intervention activities are the key, singly or in combination, to preventing wound infection remains to be seen. Who is up to doing a high-quality, quality improvement study to address these issues?

I have one final comment having to do with one other gas that is commonly used in the operating room: nitrous oxide. Folks have been concerned for a while about the possibility that nitrous oxide might increase the risk of surgical wound infections. In vitro evidence indicates that exposure to nitrous oxide inactivates vitamin B12 and, thus, methionine synthetase. The latter enzyme is important, ultimately, for DNA turnover. Even after brief periods of nitrous oxide administration, DNA synthesis remains abnormal until about the fourth postoperative day and does not entirely return to normal until the sixth day. Theoretically, this phenomenon could restrict the formation of new bone marrow cells, including polymorphonuclear white blood cells. Another concern with nitrous oxide is that it inhibits protein formation, which is, again, clearly documented in the laboratory. A third disconcerting property of nitrous oxide is that the gas depresses chemotactic migration by monocytes to areas of inflammation. Recently, investigators in Austria have looked at hundreds of patients given nitrous oxide in the operating room and have compared these patients with others who received other types of anesthetics.[1] The punch line from the study was that nitrous oxide does not increase the incidence of surgical wound infection. Enough said.

J. A. Stockman III, MD

Reference

1. Fleischmann E, Lenhardt R, Kurz A, et al: Nitrous oxide and the risk of surgical wound infection: A randomized study. *Lancet* 365:1101-1107, 2005.

Complete Genome Sequence of USA300, an Epidemic Clone of Community-Acquired Meticillin-Resistant *Staphylococcus aureus*

Diep BA, Gill SR, Chang RF, et al (Univ of California, San Francisco; Univ of California, Berkeley; State Univ of New York at Buffalo; et al)
Lancet 367:731-739, 2006
10–10

Background.—USA300, a clone of meticillin-resistant *Staphylococcus aureus*, is a major source of community-acquired infections in the USA, Canada, and Europe. Our aim was to sequence its genome and compare it with those of other strains of *S aureus* to try to identify genes responsible for its distinctive epidemiological and virulence properties.

Methods.—We ascertained the genome sequence of FPR3757, a multi-drug resistant USA300 strain, by random shotgun sequencing, then compared it with the sequences of ten other staphylococcal strains.

Findings.—Compared with closely related *S aureus*, we noted that almost all of the unique genes in USA300 clustered in novel allotypes of mobile genetic elements. Some of the unique genes are involved in pathogenesis, including Panton-Valentine leucocidin and molecular variants of enterotoxin Q and K. The most striking feature of the USA300 genome is the horizontal acquisition of a novel mobile genetic element that encodes an arginine deiminase pathway and an oligopeptide permease system that could contribute to growth and survival of USA300. We did not detect this element, termed arginine catabolic mobile element (ACME), in other *S aureus* strains. We noted a high prevalence of ACME in *S epidermidis*, suggesting not only that ACME transfers into USA300 from *S epidermidis*, but also that this element confers a selective advantage to this ubiquitous commensal of the human skin.

Interpretation.—USA300 has acquired mobile genetic elements that encode resistance and virulence determinants that could enhance fitness and pathogenicity.

▶ Penicillin resistance on the part of *S aureus* has been with us essentially forever. The semisynthetic methicillin and its derivatives were first introduced in 1959 to counter penicillin-resistant isolates of *S aureus*. We now call these methicillin-resistant *S aureus* or MRSA. Most now in practice were not around at the time, but the first isolation of an MRSA was back in 1961. By the 1990s, most *S aureus* strains were MRSA. This is not new news. What is new news is the emergence of community-acquired (CA) MRSA. CA-MRSA first gained widespread attention with the publication of a case report of 4 deaths in North Dakota and Minnesota in the late 1990s in healthy children. CA-MRSA is different from hospital-acquired MRSA. It is generally not multidrug resistant because its small methicillin resistance element contains none of the accessory resistance genes typically found in hospital MRSA. CA-MRSA is genetically distinct from hospital MRSA, and most strains express a toxin called Panton-Valentine leukocidin, rarely found in hospital isolates. This is a pore-forming toxin that causes necrosis of blood cells and other host tissues, and it is associated with necrotizing pneumonia in children and young adults.

Even more recently has been the emergence of CA-MRSA strains that are causing community-acquired epidemics. It is one of the latter strains that forms the basis of the report of Diep et al, who have described the entire genome sequence of the CA-MRSA strain USA300. This strain is widespread in the United States and is beginning to emerge in Canada and Europe. It seems to be more aggressive than other strains of CA-MRSA because it is frequently found in invasive infections and recent cases of necrotizing fasciitis. A certain gene cluster of this strain apparently enables the bacterium to evade host responses and survive and spread in host tissues. It accomplishes this by inhibiting human peripheral blood mononuclear cells through the action of arginine deiminase.

It seems that members of the genus *Staphylococcus* are getting their act together to share genetic information. As yet, there is no antibiotic to bring the curtain down on this act. We have now begun to see species of MRSA that are resistant to all antibiotics, including the mainstay of MRSA chemotherapy, vancomycin.

One of the best ways to prevent infection spread is good handwashing, preferably with alcohol-based solutions. Sometimes you will run into situations where staff may frown on using such products. See what you would do with the following situation. You are head of your local hospital's infection control program. It is clear that evidence suggests that topical alcohol-based solutions are better than detergent-based cleansers for improving compliance and effectiveness of hand hygiene within hospital settings. Nonetheless, several employees have approached you voicing objections to the use of alcohol-based solutions for this purpose. All of the employees are Muslim and are expressing religious concerns. What is going on here?

In Islam, consumption of alcohol is expressly forbidden and is designated as *haram* in the Qur'an. Alcohol is considered *haram* in Islam because it is a substance leading to *Sukr* (intoxication). For Muslims, any agent or process leading to a disconnection from a state of awareness or consciousness (a state in which he or she may forget the Creator) is called *Sukr*, which is *haram*. Consequently, an enormous taboo has become attached to consumption of alcohol for all Muslims. While it is understood that abstinence from alcohol can have substantial benefits on health, many overlook that alcohol as a medicinal agent is permitted within Islam. Indeed, any substance that man can manufacture or develop in order to alleviate illness or aid health is permitted. In this capacity, the substance is not used as an agent of *Sukr*. For example, cocaine is permitted as a local anesthetic (*halal*, allowed), but inadmissible as a recreational drug (*haram*). This distinction enables the Muslim health care worker to engage in evolving technology and emerging science including acceptance of new applications of substances previously deemed *haram*. The preclusion of alcohol use by the Qur'an has led to a fair amount of confusion on the part of Muslim health care workers in this country and in other parts of the world. It is not a stretch of the interpretation of the Qur'an, however, to say that alcohol can in fact be used for medicinal purposes, and health care workers should be aware of that. Note that at the Saudi Arabian National Guard Health Affairs Hospitals, use of alcohol-based hand rubs has been permitted since 2003, and, in fact, is now mandatory for all staff.

To read more about this topic, see the overview by Ahmed et al.[1]

J. A. Stockman III, MD

Reference

1. Ahmed QA, Memish ZA, Allegranzi B, et al: Muslim healthcare workers and alcohol-based hand rubs. *Lancet* 367:1025-1027, 2006.

Epidemiology of Cat-Scratch Disease Hospitalizations Among Children in the United States
Reynolds MG, Holman RC, Curns AT, et al (Ctrs for Disease Control and Prevention, Atlanta, Ga; Ministry of Public Health, Nonthaburi, Thailand; US Dept of Health and Human Service, Rockville, Md)
Pediatr Infect Dis J 24:700-704, 2005   10–11

Background.—Cat-scratch disease (CSD), caused by infection with *Bartonella henselae*, affects both children and adults but is principally a pediatric disease. Typical CSD is generally benign and self-limited and is characterized by regional lymphadenopathy with fever. Infections can, however, be accompanied by focal or diffuse inflammatory responses (atypical CSD) involving neurologic, organ (liver/spleen), lymphatic or skeletal systems.

Methods.—Pediatric hospitalizations with CSD listed as a diagnosis were examined using the Kids' Inpatient Database for the year 2000. National estimates of CSD-associated hospitalizations, hospitalization rates and various hospitalization statistics were examined for patients younger than 18 years of age.

Results.—During 2000, an estimated 437 (SE 43) pediatric hospitalizations associated with CSD occurred among children younger than 18 years of age in the United States. The national CSD-associated hospitalization rate was 0.60/100,000 children younger than 18 years of age (95% confidence interval, 0.49–0.72) and 0.86/100,000 children younger than 5 years of age (95% CI 0.64–1.07). Accompanying diagnoses included neurologic complications (12%), organ (liver/spleen) involvement (7%) and "other" (5%). Atypical CSD accounted for ~24% of the CSD-associated hospitalizations. The median charge for a CSD-associated hospitalization was $6140 with total annual hospital charges of ~$3.5 million among children in the United States.

Conclusions.—The CSD-associated hospitalization rate among children during 2000 appeared similar to those estimated for the 1980s in the United States, despite significant increases in cat ownership in the intervening time. Early serologic and molecular testing for CSD in children is suggested to minimize unnecessary interventions and promote optimally effective care when supportive measures are required.

▶ CSD is hardly a diagnosis that requires hospitalization, except in a few cases. Nonetheless, way too many kids wind up in the hospital because they have not received a prompt diagnosis and are frequently admitted with a fever of undetermined origin or some complication of CSD for which the causative agent had not previously been identified. It is true that severe CSD can present in either a life-threatening manner or can be associated with severe morbidity. The disease can cause encephalitis, neuroretinitis, osteomyelitis, and hepatitis. Far too often, other infectious agents, malignancies, and autoimmune disorders are mistaken for CSD.

This article tells us a great deal about the assessment and occurrence of CSD in hospitalized patients in the United States. We learn that such hospitalizations tend to be much longer than one should expect and are quite costly, largely because of the spectrum of diagnostic studies that are undertaken, many of which are not necessary. Many of these hospitalizations result from atypical CSD. There really is nothing atypical about encephalitis, hepatitis, and neuroretinitis. All are well-described presentations of CSD, as is osteomyelitis.

It is true that CSD can have protean manifestations. Maybe if, in an era of the electronic medical record, the words *cat-scratch disease* popped up in red with every hospitalization, we would not be missing so much of this disease as part of the differential diagnosis of obscure signs and symptoms.

J. A. Stockman III, MD

Multifocal Bone Marrow Involvement in Cat-Scratch Disease

Hipp SJ, O'Shields A, Fordham LA, et al (Univ of North Carolina, Chapel Hill)
Pediatr Infect Dis J 24:472-474, 2005   10–12

Background.—Several atypical presentations of cat-scratch disease (CSD) have been recognized, including Parinaud oculoglandular disease, encephalopathy, hepatic and splenic abscesses, osteomyelitis with lytic bone lesions, neuroretinitis, and prolonged fevers without a source. It is well recognized that bone involvement in CSD is often reflected by osteolytic lesions, but bone disease without osteolytic lesions has not been well described. Osteolytic lesions were not present in the 2 children with CSD described in this report, but both children had inflammatory bone marrow involvement on MRI studies.

Case 1.—Boy, 10 years, was seen with a fever and left leg and hip pain for 1 month. He was unable to bear weight when febrile; when afebrile he had significantly reduced pain and was more active. The patient had history of exposure to multiple cats and kittens and recalled a scratch across his abdomen 2 months before presentation. The physical examination revealed nonfocal results, and the patient was afebrile at the time. Prior studies for antinuclear antibodies and Epstein-Barr virus, a urinalysis, and blood and urine cultures all yielded negative results. Results of liver function tests, coagulation studies, and electrolyte determinations were normal. Laboratory studies also yielded no clues as to the origin of the fever and leg and hip pain. Blood, urine, and throat cultures were sterile, and a delayed hypersensitivity skin test had negative results. Radiographic examinations included normal plain films of the chest, pelvis, hips, knees, and femurs. A bone scan and CT of the pelvis showed no abnormalities. MRI of the abdomen and pelvis showed multiple foci of increased signal intensity on T2-weighted scans within bone marrow of the sacrum, iliums, and femurs and multiple peripherally enhancing lesions within the liver parenchyma. Ultrasound-guided fine-needle aspiration of 1 of these lesions recovered necrotic debris with a mixed inflammatory infiltrate of neutrophils and activated histiocytes. A bone marrow aspirate and biopsy from the left posterior ilium revealed marked neutrophilic hyperplasia and eosinophilia. On the basis of these findings, the patient was diagnosed with CSD and treated with azithromycin. CSD titers were found to be positive for *Bartonella henselae* and *B quintana*.

Case 2.—Girl, 3 years, was seen with a 3-month history of intermittent fever and associated pain in her arms and legs. She had experienced daily temperature spikes to 40°C in the 15 days before admission. The extremity pain was exacerbated during those spikes to the point that the patient refused to bear weight. She was playful and appeared well during afebrile periods. As with the patient in case 1, laboratory and radiologic examinations were normal and findings on the physical examination were unremarkable, except for a 1- × 1-cm firm, mobile, nontender, right posterior cervical node. Several weeks into the diagnostic evaluation, *Bartonella* titers were found to be positive for *B henselae* and *B quintana*. The patient was treated with azithromycin for 9 days. She continued to complain intermittently of pain in her extremities, and a full-body MRI demonstrated a lesion in the bone marrow in the lateral aspect of the right tibia. This was determined to be a focal infection of the bone marrow caused by *Bartonella*. Azithromycin was administered for 3 weeks, and all symptoms resolved.

Conclusions.—CSD should be an important diagnostic consideration in the evaluation of pediatric patients with prolonged fevers. In both of these cases, the patients were hospitalized for more than 1 week and underwent extensive diagnostic investigations before a diagnosis of CSD was made. The significance of skeletal pain in their clinical presentations was not immediately associated with CSD, and the inability to obtain prompt, accurate serologic results contributed to a significant delay in diagnosis.

▶ This article describes 2 youngsters with CSD who had significant bone involvement. The first was a 10-year-old boy who presented with a fever and left leg and hip pain lasting about a month before he was seen. He had a history of multiple exposures to cats. The physical examination and subsequent hospitalization showed daily temperature spikes to 39° associated with left leg and hip pain. MRI revealed multiple foci of increased signal intensity in the sacrum, iliums, and femurs and multiple enhancing lesions in the liver. CSD titers came back positive for *B henselae* as well as for *B quintana* after being sent to the Center for Disease Control and Prevention. The second youngster, a 3-year-old girl, had a 3-month history of intermittent fevers and pain in her arms. This pain worsened with her fevers. A physical examination showed a firm, nontender right posterior cervical node that was enlarged. A full-body MRI showed a lesion in the bone marrow in the left lateral aspect of the right tibia, which is a finding that was interpreted as a focal infection of the bone marrow, likely linked to CSD because of a rise in *Bartonella* titers.

In both youngsters, the bone findings were most readily confirmed with MRI, not CT scans or plain films. This is true of all bone marrow infections that may not involve the bone itself. In both of these cases, no specific findings were seen on the CT scans, and the radionuclide bone scans themselves had negative findings.

We all know that CSD is an important diagnostic consideration for any child who has a prolonged fever of undetermined origin. In both cases reported, a delayed diagnosis occurred because an MRI was not performed until many other studies had been performed and had yielded negative results. Think about an MRI in a fever of undetermined origin. It and appropriate titers may lead you to a diagnosis of CSD presenting with what appears to be musculoskeletal symptoms.

While on the topic of entities causing febrile illnesses, does the old adage "starve a fever" and "feed a cold" have any basis in fact? Data now do suggest that anorexia could be a prehistoric behavioral adaptation to maintain T helper 2 cells. Starvation apparently increases such cells, which are critical in fighting bacterial infections. Eating, however, stimulates a vagal and neurohormonal output from the gut that promotes T helper 1 cells, which are absolutely critical in fighting many different types of viruses, including, presumably, the virus that causes the common cold.[1] Investigators who have studied this phenomenon are now actively on the trail of whether an apple a day does indeed keep the doctor away.

J. A. Stockman III, MD

Reference

1. Bazar KA, Yun AJ, Lee PY: "Starve a fever and feed a cold": Feeding and anorexia may be adaptive behavioral modulators of autonomic and T helper balance. *Med Hypotheses* 64:1080-1084, 2005.

Human Botulism Immune Globulin for the Treatment of Infant Botulism

Arnon SS, Schechter R, Maslanka SE, et al (California Dept of Health Services, Richmond; Ctrs for Disease Control and Prevention, Atlanta, Ga; Univ of California, Berkeley)
N Engl J Med 354:462-471, 2006

10–13

Background.—We created the orphan drug Human Botulism Immune Globulin Intravenous (Human) (BIG-IV), which neutralizes botulinum toxin, and evaluated its safety and efficacy in treating infant botulism, the intestinal-toxemia form of human botulism.

Methods.—We performed a five-year, randomized, double-blind, placebo-controlled trial statewide, in California, of BIG-IV in 122 infants with suspected (and subsequently laboratory-confirmed) infant botulism (75 caused by type A *Clostridium botulinum* toxin, and 47 by type B toxin); treatment was given within three days after hospital admission. We subsequently performed a 6-year nationwide, open-label study of 382 laboratory-confirmed cases of infant botulism treated within 18 days after hospital admission.

Results.—As compared with the control group in the randomized trial, infants treated with BIG-IV had a reduction in the mean length of the hospital stay, the primary efficacy outcome measure, from 5.7 weeks to 2.6 weeks (P<0.001). BIG-IV treatment also reduced the mean duration of intensive care by 3.2 weeks (P<0.001), the mean duration of mechanical ventilation by 2.6 weeks (P=0.01), the mean duration of tube or intravenous feeding by 6.4 weeks (P<0.001), and the mean hospital charges per patient by $88,600 (in 2004 U.S. dollars; P<0.001). There were no serious adverse events attributable to BIG-IV. In the open-label study, infants treated with BIG-IV within seven days of admission had a mean length of hospital stay of 2.2 weeks, and early treatment with BIG-IV shortened the mean length of stay significantly more than did later treatment.

Conclusions.—Prompt treatment of infant botulism type A or type B with BIG-IV was safe and effective in shortening the length and cost of the hospital stay and the severity of illness.

▶ Many physicians outside of pediatrics are not familiar with the fact that infantile botulism is the most common form of human botulism here in the United States. The clinical entity results from an unusual infectious condition termed intestinal toxemia, in which swallowed spores of *C botulinum*, or rarely certain other forms of clostridia, germinate and temporarily colonize the large intestine, where as vegetative cells they produce botulinum neurotoxin. This toxin is absorbed into the blood and carried to the neuromuscular junction where it binds irreversibly. In the United States, about 100 cases are reported annually, and few are missed since virtually all cases wind up being admitted to the hospital.

Equine botulinum antitoxin has been around for a long time and is used to treat adult patients. It has rarely been used to treat patients with infantile botulism because of its serious side effects, including serum sickness and anaphylaxis, and its short half-life, just 5 to 7 days. Thank goodness for the approval in 2003 of BIG-IV, a human-derived botulism antitoxin that neutralizes botulinum toxin. In the report abstracted, we see exactly how effective BIG-IV is.

To treat babies with infantile botulism, a single IV dose of BIG-IV (50 mg/kg) is all that is needed. While it does not produce an instantaneous cure, it does reduce hospitalization time from an average of 5.7 weeks to just 2.6 weeks, associated with a decrease in hospital charges per patient admission, from $163,400 to $74,800. For the patients described in this report, the total hospital charges avoided were in excess of $34 million. This is no small piece of change.

It is clear that BIG-IV, licensed by the Food and Drug Administration, is a safe and effective treatment for infantile botulism, both type A and type B. Needless to say, treatment should be given as soon as possible. Since the therapy is benign, all suspected cases should be treated before confirmatory testing of feces or enema secretions. It is considered an orphan therapy. Information on it, if you ever need to use it, can be obtained at www.infantbotulism.org or from the Centers for Disease Control and Prevention.

J. A. Stockman III, MD

Effect of BCG Vaccination on Childhood Tuberculous Meningitis and Miliary Tuberculosis Worldwide: A Meta-analysis and Assessment of Cost-effectiveness

Trunz BB, Fine PEM, Dye C (World Health Organization, Geneva; London School of Hygiene and Tropical Medicine)
Lancet 367:1173-1180, 2006　　　　　　　　　　　　　　　　　　　10–14

Background.—BCG vaccine has shown consistently high efficacy against childhood tuberculous meningitis and miliary tuberculosis, but variable efficacy against adult pulmonary tuberculosis and other mycobacterial diseases. We assess and compare the costs and effects of BCG as an intervention against severe childhood tuberculosis in different regions of the world.

Methods.—We calculated the number of tuberculous meningitis and miliary tuberculosis cases that have been and will be prevented in all children born in 2002, by combining estimates of the annual risk of tuberculosis infection, the proportion of infections that lead to either of these diseases in unvaccinated children, the number of children vaccinated, and BCG efficacy.

Findings.—We estimated that the 100.5 million BCG vaccinations given to infants in 2002 will have prevented 29,729 cases of tuberculous meningitis (5th-95th centiles, 24,063-36,192) in children during their first 5 years of life, or one case for every 3435 vaccinations (2771-4177), and 11,486 cases of miliary tuberculosis (7304-16,280), or one case for every 9314 vaccinations (6172-13,729). The numbers of cases prevented would be highest in South East Asia (46%), sub-Saharan Africa (27%), the western Pacific region (15%), and where the risk of tuberculosis infection and vaccine coverage are also highest. At US$2-3 per dose, BCG vaccination costs US$206 dollars (150-272) per year of healthy life gained.

Interpretation.—BCG vaccination is a highly cost-effective intervention against severe childhood tuberculosis; it should be retained in high-incidence countries as a strategy to supplement the chemotherapy of active tuberculosis.

▶ Most of us in the United States do not realize that the bacille Calmette-Guérin (BCG) vaccine is the most widely used immunization throughout the world, with several billion doses having been given over the last few decades. BCG is a live attenuated vaccine derived from a strain of mycobacteria, *Mycobacterium bovis*, and is given to newborns and young infants throughout much of the world. The efficacy of BCG vaccine has been a source of controversy over the years, and it may not prevent infection or adult pulmonary disease, but it is now generally accepted that BCG vaccine is highly effective in preventing severe childhood tuberculosis, including tuberculous meningitis and miliary tuberculosis.

In this article, Trunz et al, from the World Health Organization and the London School of Hygiene and Tropical Medicine, report on the cost-effectiveness of BCG in different regions of the world as part of the prevention of severe childhood tuberculosis. It can be concluded that BCG vaccination is a highly cost-effective intervention and should be retained in those countries with high rates of tuberculosis. The authors calculate that every year, about 1 million doses of BCG vaccination are given to children worldwide, which results in the prevention of about 30,000 cases of tuberculous meningitis and 11,000 cases of miliary tuberculosis before these children reached their fifth birthday. This estimation translates into 1 case of severe childhood tuberculosis prevented for every 2500 inoculations. Without question, BCG vaccination seems to be nearly as cost-effective as short-course chemotherapy for active tubercular disease and, therefore, is considered good value for the money.

Any pediatrician that has seen the devastating effects of tuberculous meningitis should be heartened by the data of Trunz et al. Even in resource-rich countries where there is access to pediatric subspecialty care, infants with tuberculous meningitis continue to have high mortality and morbidity, with 15% of patients dying and up to 50% of infants having serious neurologic sequelae. This report gives a huge boost to believers in the BCG vaccine.

It is unlikely that we will ever see BCG vaccine used here in the United States, but some of our bordering countries might well think about its routine administration. Cost-effectiveness of the vaccine certainly does decrease in those richer countries where tuberculosis infection is low. The authors of this report pose the question whether BCG vaccination should be used in countries that do have adequate resources, being reserved then for high-risk individuals. In countries such as the United Kingdom where routine BCG vaccination of schoolchildren has been stopped, the emphasis is on targeting its administration to high-risk infants and children. We do not take this approach here in the United States.

Even though BCG is not used very much on our shores, we should congratulate the authors of this report for an excellent study, since it provides valuable information underpinning health policies about BCG vaccination worldwide.

J. A. Stockman III, MD

Tuberculosis and Homelessness in the United States, 1994-2003
Haddad MB, Wilson TW, Ijaz K, et al (Centers for Disease Control and Prevention, Atlanta, Ga)
JAMA 293:2762-2766, 2005   10–15

Context.—Tuberculosis (TB) rates among US homeless persons cannot be calculated because they are not included in the US Census. However, homelessness is often associated with TB.

Objectives.—To describe homeless persons with TB and to compare risk factors and disease characteristics between homeless and nonhomeless persons with TB.

Design and Setting.—Cross-sectional analysis of all verified TB cases reported into the National TB Surveillance System from the 50 states and the District of Columbia from 1994 through 2003.

Main Outcome Measures.—Number and proportion of TB cases associated with homelessness, demographic characteristics, risk factors, disease characteristics, treatment, and outcomes.

Results.—Of 185 870 cases of TB disease reported between 1994 and 2003, 11 369 were among persons classified as homeless during the 12 months before diagnosis. The annual proportion of cases associated with homelessness was stable (6.1%-6.7%). Regional differences occurred with a higher proportion of TB cases associated with homelessness in western and some southern states. Most homeless persons with TB were male (87%) and aged 30 to 59 years. Black individuals represented the highest proportion of TB cases among the homeless and nonhomeless. The proportion of homeless persons with TB who were born outside the United States (18%) was lower than that for nonhomeless persons with TB (44%). At the time of TB diagnosis, 9% of homeless persons were incarcerated, usually in a local jail; 3% of nonhomeless persons with TB were incarcerated. Compared with nonhomeless persons, homeless persons with TB had a higher prevalence of substance use (54% alcohol abuse, 29.5% noninjected drug use, and 14% injected drug use), and 34% of those tested had coinfection with human immunodeficiency virus. Compared with nonhomeless persons, TB disease in homeless persons was more likely to be infectious but not more likely to be drug resistant. Health departments managed 81% of TB cases in homeless persons. Directly observed therapy, used for 86% of homeless patients, was associated with timely completion of therapy. A similar proportion in both groups (9%) died from any cause during therapy.

Conclusions.—Individual TB risk factors often overlap with risk factors for homelessness, and the social contexts in which TB occurs are often complex and important to consider in planning TB treatment. Nevertheless, given good case management, homeless persons with TB can achieve excellent treatment outcomes.

▶ One might wonder why a report on TB and homeless people would make it into the YEAR BOOK OF PEDIATRICS. Kids get TB, by and large, from adults with TB, and it is critical for us as pediatric care providers to know about those who are at highest risk for having either active TB or latent TB. It turns out that the homeless are indeed a large reservoir of individuals with TB who may intermingle into and out of families with children. This report shows us that homelessness has persistently cultivated a "pocket of endemicity" for TB, one that continues to be associated with poverty. Countrywide, the number of TB cases associated with homelessness has declined somewhat over the past decade, but certain states have remarkably higher proportions of TB cases associated with homelessness, and the annual number of black homeless patients with TB in southern states has remained unchanged.

Here in the United States, screening for latent TB infection in high-risk populations is a key feature of TB control in both adults and children. Four strategies are currently used to control TB. Passive case finding and treatment serve as the backbone of TB control in all countries throughout the world, including ours. Bacille Calmette-Guérin (BCG) vaccination is used to prevent disseminated complications of TB in children elsewhere but has variable efficacy in preventing pulmonary TB. Environmental controls such as negative-pressure rooms, particulate filters and masks, and UV lights serve to reduce the spread of *Mycobacterium tuberculosis* in health care or occupational settings. Finally, treatment of latent TB infection reduces an individual's risk for developing TB and imparts public health benefits by reducing the pool of latently infected individuals who could develop active TB in the future.

Until recently, however, the only way to make the diagnosis of latent TB was through the use of the tuberculin skin test (TST). However, new diagnostic tests are now available that may improve the ability to make an accurate diagnosis. We all know the limitations of the purified protein derivative (PPD) (mentioned earlier in this chapter). The size of the TST reaction to PPD is used to classify individuals according to their likelihood of infection. Unfortunately, the test does not have the inherent value of indicating the presence or absence of infection with *M tuberculosis*. With the use of current criteria for a positive test result, the TST lacks sensitivity in immunocompromised patients, recently infected persons, very young children, and others. It lacks specificity because many antigens in PPD cross-react with antigens found in environmentally sourced mycobacteria and *Mycobacterium bovis* BCG. In a setting such as the United States where the prevalence of latent infection is low, the predictive value of a positive TST result is necessarily low because most positive results are false positives. To circumvent this problem of low specificity, current recommendations for screening for latent TB suggest that it should be performed in populations where the risk of latent disease is high, effectively increasing the positive predictive value of the TST.

As mentioned elsewhere in this chapter, a new generation of diagnostic tests is currently available that aspire to improve the sensitivity and specificity of TB screening. Two new commercial tests are currently licensed to quantify interferon-γ (IFN-γ) production in response to *M tuberculosis* antigens. There has been a fair amount of controversy about these IFN-γ tests. Nonetheless, some tentative statements can be made at this time about the IFN-γ test compared with the TST. The sensitivity of the IFN-γ test appears adequate to detect latent TB and compares favorably with that of the TST. The specificity of the new test appears to be better than that of the TST, especially in populations vaccinated with BCG. If these findings bear out in different populations, such as children, immunocompromised hosts, and high-risk populations, the IFN-γ test may be a better test for screening than the TST because of the higher specificity. Moreover, there is the theoretic advantage of improving the test characteristics even further as new antigens for *M tuberculosis* are discovered.

Someday, we in pediatric practice may see a blood test replacing the TST-PPD skin test for the detection of TB infection. For the moment, however, the TST remains an imperfect but familiar standard for assessing infection with *M tuberculosis*. IFN-γ assays hold great potential as screening tests for latent tuberculosis because of their promise of improved specificity and convenience. As future studies define the performance of the IFN-γ test in diverse study populations throughout the world, the role of these tests will emerge as either a stand-alone screening test or a companion test to the TST.

To read more on newer ways to make a diagnosis of latent TB infection, see the superb review by Whalen.[1]

J. A. Stockman III, MD

Reference

1. Whalen CC: Diagnosis of latent tuberculosis infection. Measure for measure. *JAMA* 293:2785-2787, 2005.

Discrepancy Between the Tuberculin Skin Test and the Whole-Blood Interferon γ Assay for the Diagnosis of Latent Tuberculosis Infection in an Intermediate Tuberculosis-Burden Country
Kang YA, Lee HW, Yoon HI, et al (Seoul Natl Univ, Republic of Korea)
JAMA 293:2756-2761, 2005   10–16

Context.—A recently developed whole-blood interferon γ (IFN-γ) assay based on stimulation with the *Mycobacterium tuberculosis*–specific antigens early secreted antigenic target 6 and culture filtrate protein 10 shows promise for the diagnosis of latent tuberculosis (TB) infection.

Objective.—To compare the tuberculin skin test (TST) and the whole-blood IFN-γ assay in the diagnosis of latent TB infection according to the intensity of exposure.

Design and Setting.—A prospective comparison between the whole-blood IFN-γ assay and the TST using a 2-TU dose of purified protein derivative RT23 in a population with intermediate TB burden was conducted sequentially between February 1, 2004, and February 28, 2005, in a Korean tertiary referral hospital.

Participants.—Of 273 participants, 220 (95.7%) had received BCG vaccine. Participants were grouped according to their risk of infection: group 1, no identifiable risk of M *tuberculosis* infection (n = 99); group 2, recent casual contacts (n = 72); group 3, recent close contacts (n = 48); group 4, bacteriologically or pathologically confirmed TB patients (n = 54).

Main Outcome Measures.—Levels of agreement between the TST and the IFN-γ assay and the likelihood of infection in the various groups.

Results.—For the TST with a 10-mm induration cutoff, the positive response rate in group 1 was 51%; group 2, 60%; group 3, 71%, and group 4, 78%. For the IFN-γ assay, the positive response rate in group 1 was 4%; group 2, 10%; group 3, 44%; and group 4, 81%. The overall agreement between the TST and the IFN-γ assay in healthy volunteers was κ = 0.16. The odds of a positive test result per unit increase in exposure across the 4 groups increased by a factor of 5.31 (95% confidence interval [CI], 3.62-7.79) for the IFN-γ assay and by a factor of 1.52 (95% CI, 1.20-1.91) for the TST ($P<.001$). Using a 15-mm induration cutoff for the TST did not make a substantial difference to the test results.

Conclusion.—The IFN-γ assay is a better indicator of the risk of M *tuberculosis* infection than TST in a BCG-vaccinated population.

▶ The TST has been used for years for the diagnosis of latent TB infection. Unfortunately, the TST has many limitations, including false-positive test results in individuals who have been vaccinated with bacille Calmette-Guérin (BCG) and in individuals who have infections not related to M *tuberculosis*. The TST measures hypersensitivity response to purified protein derivative (PPD), a relatively crude mixture of antigens, many of which are shared among M *tuberculosis*, *Mycobacterium bovis*, BCG, and several nontuberculous mycobacteria. Cross-reactivities, as well as other factors, significantly influence sensitivity, specificity, positive predictive value, and negative predictive value of the TST. Recently, a whole-blood IFN-γ assay based on the M *tuberculosis*–specific antigens early secreted antigenic target 6 (ESAT-6) and culture filtrate protein 10 (CFP-10) has been introduced for the diagnosis of latent TB infection. This assay is based on the elaboration of inflammatory cytokines by T cells previously sensitized to mycobacterial antigens when they encounter ESAT-6 and CFP-10. In the report abstracted, and the one that follows (Abstract 10–17), it was concluded that the IFN-γ assay based on the ESAT-6 and CFP-10 M *tuberculosis*–specific antigens is indeed a useful method for detecting latent TB infection and very well may ultimately eliminate the limitations of the TST.

Stay tuned to more that will appear in the literature regarding the whole-blood IFN-γ assay for the diagnosis of latent TB infection. It is unlikely that this blood test will replace the PPD here in the United States, but it seems to be the best test to use if you are, for whatever reason, seeing a patient who may previously have been immunized with BCG vaccine. Given the high rates of immigration to the United States, we are seeing more and more such cases. When the PPD gives a positive or equivocally positive result in such individuals, one might need to rely on the IFN-γ assay. The report that follows (Abstract 10–17) tells us a little bit more about this assay in another part of the world, India, where there is a high prevalence of TB.

J. A. Stockman III, MD

***Mycobacterium tuberculosis* Infection in Health Care Workers in Rural India: Comparison of a Whole-Blood Interferon γ Assay With Tuberculin Skin Testing**
Pai M, Gokhale K, Joshi R, et al (Mahatma Gandhi Inst of Med Sciences, Sevagram, India; Univ of California, Berkeley; Univ of California, San Francisco; et al)
JAMA 293:2746-2755, 2005   10–17

Context.—*Mycobacterium tuberculosis* infection in health care workers has not been adequately studied in developing countries using newer diagnostic tests.

Objectives.—To estimate latent tuberculosis infection prevalence in health care workers using the tuberculin skin test (TST) and a whole-blood interferon γ (IFN-γ) assay; to determine agreement between the tests; and to compare their correlation with risk factors.

Design, Setting, and Participants.—A cross-sectional comparison study of 726 health care workers aged 18 to 61 years (median age, 22 years) with no history of active tuberculosis conducted from January to May 2004, at a rural medical school in India. A total of 493 (68%) of the health care workers had direct contact with patients with tuberculosis and 514 (71%) had BCG vaccine scars.

Interventions.—Tuberculin skin testing was performed using 1-TU dose of purified protein derivative RT23, and the IFN-γ assay was performed by measuring IFN-γ response to early secreted antigenic target 6, culture filtrate protein 10, and a portion of tuberculosis antigen TB7.7.

Main Outcome Measures.—Agreement between TST and the IFN-γ assay, and comparison of the tests with respect to their association with risk factors.

Results.—A large proportion of the health care workers were latently infected; 360 (50%) were positive by either TST or IFN-γ assay, and 226 (31%) were positive by both tests. The prevalence estimates of TST and IFN-γ assay positivity were comparable (41%; 95% confidence interval [CI], 38%-45% and 40%; 95% CI, 37%-43%, respectively). Agreement between the tests was high (81.4%; κ = 0.61; 95% CI, 0.56-0.67). Increasing age and years in the health profession were significant risk factors for both IFN-γ assay and TST positivity. BCG vaccination had little impact on TST and IFN-γ assay results.

Conclusions.—Our study showed high latent tuberculosis infection prevalence in Indian health care workers, high agreement between TST and IFN-γ assay, and similar association between positive test results and risk factors. Although TST and IFN-γ assay appear comparable in this population, they have different performance and operational characteristics; therefore, the decision to select one test over the other will depend on the population, purpose of testing, and resource availability.

Epidemiology of Pediatric Tuberculosis Using Traditional and Molecular Techniques: Houston, Texas

Wootton SH, Gonzalez BE, Pawlak R, et al (Baylor College of Medicine, Houston; Univ of Texas, Houston; NIH, Hamilton, Montana)
Pediatrics 116:1141-1147, 2005   10–18

Objective.—To investigate the transmission dynamics of pediatric tuberculosis (TB) by analyzing the clinical characteristics with the molecular profiles of *Mycobacterium tuberculosis* isolates during a 5-year period.

Methods.—A retrospective review of a prospective population-based active surveillance and molecular epidemiology project was conducted in private and public pediatric clinics within Houston and Harris County, Texas. The study population consisted of patients who had pediatric TB diagnosed from October 1, 1995, through September 30, 2000. Cases and potential source cases (PSC) were interviewed using a standardized questionnaire. Available *Mycobacterium tuberculosis* isolates from cases and PSCs were characterized and compared by IS6110 restriction fragment length polymorphism, spoligotyping, and genetic group assignment. Clinical characteristics were described, and molecular characterizations were compared. Data were analyzed by using EpiInfo 6.02b and SAS 8.2.

Results.—A total of 220 (92%) of 238 pediatric TB cases were included. Epidemiologic and clinical findings were consistent with previous studies. Molecular profiles from 3 cases did not match the profile of PSC. Four previously unknown PSCs were identified using molecular techniques. Fifty-one (71.8%) of 71 isolates matched at least 1 other Houston Tuberculosis Initiative TB database isolate and were grouped into 33 molecular clusters. Cases were more likely to be clustered when the patients were younger than 5 years, identified a source case, or were US born.

Conclusions.—Traditional contact tracing may not always be accurate, and molecular characterization can lead to identification of previously unrecognized source cases. Recent transmission plays a significant role in the transmission of TB to children as evident by the high degree of clustering found in our study population.

▶ This study is the first to evaluate the population-based epidemiology of pediatric TB using molecular techniques. The report is significant since TB continues to be a significant health problem here in the United States. As importantly, more than 15% of reported cases here are in the childhood or young adult population (≤24 years of age). These statistics also apply to Houston, the origin of the report, which ranks fourth among large US cities in total number of TB cases reported in children and young adults. Monitoring of TB transmission is usually done by conventional contact tracing, but more recently, molecular analysis has entered the epidemiologist's armamentarium. Characterizing and comparing TB isolates through molecular analysis can identify contacts who are missed by traditional techniques and can estimate the proportion of TB that is attributable to recent transmission, otherwise known as clustering. The data from the Houston study clearly show that traditional contact tracing is hardly always accurate, and molecular characterization is significantly more capable of identifying previously unrecognized source cases.

Molecular epidemiology is the wave of the future. Molecular epidemiology studies of TB allow a fingerprinting of *M tuberculosis*, which is capable of assisting the epidemiologist in defining whether an individual has primary TB versus reactivation TB in many instances. Such techniques, for example, have rid us of an old medical myth that one could tell primary TB from reactivation TB by the findings on the chest x-ray. Old literature suggested that reactivation of infection acquired long ago manifests itself as upper lobe infiltrates and cavitary lesions, and recently acquired disease produces lymphadenopathy, effusions, and lower and middle lung zone infiltrates. Not necessarily so, as we learned in a recent report.[1] With the use of molecular techniques, it has been documented that the time from acquisition of infection to the development of clinical disease does not reliably predict the radiographic appearance of TB. "Classic" reactivation TB on x-ray as we learned it 20 years ago and acute infection with lymphadenopathy are not separable entities. One can look like the other and vice versa.

J. A. Stockman III, MD

Reference

1. Geng E, Kreiswirth B, Burzynski J, et al: Clinical and radiographic correlates of primary and reactivation tuberculosis. A molecular epidemiology study. *JAMA* 293:2740-2745, 2005.

Management of Severe Malaria in Children: Proposed Guidelines for the United Kingdom

Maitland K, Nadel S, Pollard AJ, et al (Kenya Med Research Inst, Kilifi; St Mary's Hosp, London; Univ of Oxford, England; et al)
BMJ 331:337-343, 2005   10–19

Background.—Malaria is the most important vector-borne disease in the world and the most important mosquito-borne infection in the United Kingdom (UK). Malaria is a rare cause of hospital admission in the UK, but it poses a significant health threat for persons traveling in endemic areas. The global increase in long-distance travel has been accompanied by an increase in the incidence of imported malaria in the developed world. Other factors contributing to the increased incidence of imported malaria are immigration and the resurgence of malaria in many tropical countries. *Plasmodium vivax*, once the most common form of imported malaria, has recently been superceded by *P falciparum*, the only form of malaria that can be lethal. The clinical features of malaria are similar in children and adults in the setting of uncomplicated disease; however, in severe disease the clinical spectrum, complications, and management differ between adults and children. Guidelines for the assessment and emergency management of children with imported malaria were outlined.

Overview.—Preventive measures are never 100% effective, so the diagnosis of malaria should be suspected whenever a patient presents with flu-like symptoms and has traveled in a malarious area within the past year. The development of one or more features of severe or complicated malaria in a child is a medical emergency. In most cases of severe malaria, the severity of disease results from a delay in diagnosis and initiation of appropriate treatment in patients with suspected malaria. Oral quinine and chloroquine or pyrimethamine with sulfadoxine should never be prescribed for the treatment of *P falciparum* malaria in children. The emergency assessment of a child with severe malaria should be performed according to Advanced Paediatric Life Support (UK) guidelines. In most cases, frequent reassessment and close monitoring of critically ill children will identify most complications of malaria. Among the most common complications are hypoglycemia, hyperpyrexia, and seizures and posturing. Other common complications include electrolyte derangements, including hyperkalemia or hypokalemia, hypophosphatemia, and hypomagnesemia; metabolic acidosis; and severe malaria anemia.

Conclusions.—The guidelines for management of severe malaria in children proposed in this review should not be viewed as a consensus statement but as recommendations for the initial assessment and identification of children at risk for complications and who require close monitoring or parenteral medication.

▶ This report reminds us that no preventive measure is ever 100% effective and that malaria should be suspected in any patient with flu-like symptoms who has traveled to a malarious area within the preceding year. Actually, here in the United States, since half of malaria cases are homespun, one should think of malaria in any unexplained febrile illness in which the associated symptoms could be compatible with malaria. Chances are you will be overdoing the number of thick prep blood smears, but you cannot make the diagnosis without thinking of it and ordering the right test.

Consider the following scenario.[1] A traveler has recently returned from Africa and now has fever, chills, and a raging headache. He goes to the emergency department. A complete blood cell count and thick prep of the blood smear show anemia, thrombocytopenia, and multiple intraerythrocytic rings of *P falciparum*. Moreover, the patient has labored breathing, acidosis, and altered mental status—dangerous signs warranting immediate parenteral treatment. You are the attending physician. Neither IV quinine nor oral, rectal, or IV artemisinins have been approved by the Food and Drug Administration or are available in the United States. How quickly can you lay your hands on IV quinidine gluconate, the single parenteral antimalarial that is available in this country? The answer is not very quickly since most cardiologists here in the United States have stopped using this IV agent as an antiarrhythmic agent. Most hospitals do not stock it even though the drug's manufacturer, Eli Lilly, has continued to maintain supplies despite the lack of a commercial market, and ships the drug rapidly wherever a patient at a US health care facility needs it. There are reports describing adverse patient outcomes attributable to its limited availability on hospital formularies. It is important to note that the side effects of IV quinidine—QT-segment prolongation, hypotension, and hypoglycemia—also restrict its use to hospitalized patients in cardiac-monitored beds. Although it is potentially lifesaving in a critically ill patient with malaria, the drug can also complicate an already precarious situation unless the patient is closely monitored. We desperately need an antimalarial drug that does not require cardiac monitoring for safe use, especially for US military forces deployed overseas.

Worldwide, malaria causes up to 500 million febrile illnesses and approximately 1 million deaths each year. Drug resistance is increasing rapidly. The number of cases diagnosed here in the United States is likely to escalate as our economy interfaces more closely with parts of the world in which malaria is endogenous. On June 27, 2005, the Bill and Melinda Gates Foundation, which had already donated $150 million toward the development of a malaria vaccine, announced a new round of global health grants totaling $437 million, roughly 20% of which were earmarked to innovative malaria research. On June 30, 2005, President Bush pledged more than $1.2 billion over 5 years to fight malaria in Africa by expanding access to mosquito nets treated with long-lasting insecticides and to indoor spraying, as well as distributing new, effective drug regimens—primarily artemisinin-based combination therapies—through public and private sector outlets in target countries. This initiative was launched in 2006 with an initial $30 million outlay for programs in Tanzania, Uganda, and Angola, and the US government investment could eventually reach more than 175 million people in 15 or more African nations. The cost of treating malaria in Africa as well as the economic downside as a consequence of the illness runs about $12 billion annually, so a relatively modest investment in prevention and treatment could have, theoretically, an extremely cost-effective benefit.

Last, be aware that new data suggest that some individuals are in fact more susceptible than others to malaria, with just 20% of a given population accounting for 80% of all infections.[2] It would seem that some individuals are more attractive to mosquitoes due to factors such as components in their breath and sweat that are not well-understood. Some people just get bitten more often than others. It also turns out that such people not only tend to attract mosquitoes, but the mosquitoes around them are more likely to bite those in the immediate surroundings than elsewhere. If you could just find those individuals who tend to be bitten the most, you might want to stay away from them, at least in malarial areas.

J. A. Stockman III, MD

References

1. McGill A, Panosian C: Making antimalarial agents available in the United States. *N Engl J Med* 353:335-337, 2005.
2. Hampton T: Malarial susceptibility heightened for some. *JAMA* 295:150, 2006.

Paralytic Rabies After a Two Week Holiday in India

Solomon T, Marston D, Mallewa M, et al (Univ of Liverpool, England; Veterinary Laboratories Agency (Weybridge), Surrey, England; Walton Centre for Neurology and Neurosurgery NHS Trust, Liverpool, England; et al)
BMJ 331:501-503, 2005   10–20

Background.—Rabies is an acute infection of the CNS caused by rabies virus or related species in the *Lyssavirus* genus. Rabies virus is usually transmitted through a dog bite. It produces one of the most important viral encephalitides in the world, and at least 40,000 deaths are reported each year. However, rabies has been rare in the United Kingdom: just 12 cases have been reported since 1977. Of those cases, 11 were imported. Most patients with rabies in the United Kingdom were seen with furious rabies, which is characterized by hydrophobia and spasms. A case of paralytic rabies in a tourist who returned from a 2-week vacation in India is reported.

Case Report.—Woman, late 30s, was admitted to a local hospital with lower back pain radiating to the left leg, which had grown progressively worse for 4 days. At admission, she was unable to walk. She also had a headache and had vomited once. On a 2-week holiday in India 3 and a half months earlier, the patient had been nipped on the left leg by a puppy. The wound was slight, and she did not seek medical attention. On examination, the left leg was areflexic, weak, and extremely painful (the patient required morphine), and sensory loss was noted in the L4-S1 dermatomes. The patient had leukocytosis. A CT scan for a prolapsed disk showed normal results. Over the next few days after hospitalization, the patient developed a sore throat and had difficulty swallowing. She also had a swollen left eyelid, a goose pimple rash on her skin, and marked bilateral loss of hearing. A provisional diagnosis of Guillain-Barré syndrome was made, and she was treated with IV immunoglobulin. Her condition continued to deteriorate, and on the 13th day of admission, she had absent oculocephalic reflexes and unreactive pupils. A diagnosis of Bickerstaff's encephalitis was considered. A CT scan of the brain showed normal results. On the 15th day of admission, the infectious diseases unit and neurologists were consulted. On the basis of a history of ascending paralysis after a dog bite in India, investigation for rabies was initiated. Rabies was confirmed by reverse transciptase-polymerase chain reaction analysis. The patient died on the 18th day of admission. Brain tissue was obtained after death through the foramen magnum and supraorbital routes; the diagnosis of rabies was confirmed by both fluorescent antibody testing and polymerase chain reaction analysis.

Conclusions.—Rabies is a risk for any traveler to countries such as India, in which rabies is endemic. Most patients will be seen with the furious form of rabies, which is characterized by hydrophobia, aerophobia, or both; however, up to one third of patients may be seen with the paralytic, or "dumb," form of the disease, which is often more difficult to diagnose. Severe pain in the bitten limb, itching, goose pimples, headache, and fever at presentation, asymmetry of limb weakness, and cells in the CSF are clues of rabies infection.

▶ This article reminds us that when we travel outside the United States, we should be wary of diseases such as rabies. That a British woman died of rabies after being bitten by a dog in Goa, India, highlights the issue of rabies prophylaxis for people who travel to and live in endemic areas. Rabies is an acute, largely incurable, viral encephalomyelitis caused by the bullet-shaped RNA rhabdovirus. It is, indeed, a zoonosis, an animal disease that is transmissible to human beings. Worldwide, most of the 30,000 to 70,000 human deaths annually result from bites from dogs, cats, and wild animals such as foxes, jackals, wolves, mongooses, and raccoons. Skunks and bats are the other culprits. About 90% of deaths from rabies occur in the developing world, and more than half occur in the Indian subcontinent, where dogs that roam freely are largely responsible. The virus is usually transmitted through a transdermal bite or scratch or by contamination of oral mucosa or skin wounds with animal saliva. The incubation period is variable but is typically from 1 to 3 months, after which clinical symptoms appear and a fatal outcome is almost inevitable. Because rabies infection itself cannot be treated, prevention and prophylaxis are paramount. Most of us are not aware that vaccination before exposure does not eliminate the need for treatment after rabies exposure, but it does simplify treatment and may provide protection after unrecognized exposure. Currently, available rabies vaccines containing inactivated virus derived though tissue culture are safe and effective. If you are traveling to a country where rabies is endemic, prophylaxis before exposure involves 3 doses of vaccine given in the deltoid muscle on days 0, 3, and 28, and boosters can be given between 6 and 24 months. Prophylaxis after exposure aims to neutralize the virus before it can enter the CNS and entails wound cleaning, passive immunization with immunoglobulin, and active immunization with vaccine. Individuals who have completed a course of pre-exposure vaccination do not require immunoglobulin and need fewer doses of vaccine in their prophylaxis regimen after exposure. Such treatment is effective in preventing the development of rabies if the recommended regimen is followed precisely.

Wound care is absolutely essential to prevent rabies infection. The wound needs to be thoroughly scrubbed with soap and water or, if available, iodine solution, 40% to 70% alcohol, 0.1% cetrimide or a similar compound, or the virucidal agent povidone, all under local anesthesia, if possible. The rabies virus is killed by sunlight, drying, soap, and the other agents mentioned. In animal experiments, early effective wound cleaning has been shown to prevent rabies.

If one has been in contact with a rabid animal, immunization, although not a medical emergency, should be administered within 24 hours of exposure. Rabies immunoglobulin provides rapid, passive, instantaneous immunity for a relatively short period of time in a previously unvaccinated patient. The intent of immunoglobulin is to allow the active vaccine time to produce an immune response. The dose of immunoglobulin should be given as a single administration and, if possible, infiltrated around the original wound. Individuals who have not been vaccinated before exposure should have postexposure vaccination of 4 to 5 doses over 4 weeks. Those previously vaccinated can have booster doses of active vaccine just on days 0 and 3.

What is the indication for pre-exposure vaccination? For travelers to regions in which rabies is endemic, particularly to remote rural areas where postvaccination techniques might be difficult to obtain, making a decision about pre-exposure rabies vaccination requires an assessment of the risk of being bitten and needing treatment and an assessment of local access to safe and effective rabies immunoglobulin and vaccines. Although we do not think about it very much, in many countries of Africa, Asia, Latin America, and the Middle East, dog rabies is extremely common. To give an example, if you decide to go hiking in a rural area of the Indian subcontinent where dogs commonly roam free, this activity would carry a sufficient risk of exposure, combined with potential difficulties in obtaining early, safe, and effective postexposure prophylaxis, to warrant vaccination before traveling.[1] A good rule of thumb is that wildlife (including dogs and cats) should be appreciated at a distance.

I have one final comment about rabies. In October 2004, in Wisconsin, a 15-year-old girl was given a diagnosis of rabies after having been bitten by a bat a month before. Surprisingly and fortunately, she survived (see Abstract 10–21). She is the second reported survivor of rabies after a bat bite. The first patient was a 9-year-old boy in Ohio who received prompt treatment with rabies vaccine after having been bitten on the thumb by a rabid big-brown bat. The Wisconsin case is unique because the patient received no rabies prophylaxis. This exceptional survival addresses the questions of the pathogenicity of bat rabies and whether bat rabies is the Achilles heel of one of the very few human infections with a near 100% mortality rate. The gene composition of bat rabies is somewhat different than other forms of rabies, which suggests that it might just be a weaker virus.[2]

J. A. Stockman III, MD

References

1. Hankins DG, Rosekrans JA: Overview, prevention and treatment of rabies. *Mayo Clin Proc* 79:671-676, 2004.
2. Lafon M: Bat rabies: The Achilles heel of a viral killer? *Lancet* 366:876-877, 2005.

Survival After Treatment of Rabies With Induction of Coma
Willoughby RE Jr, Tieves KS, Hoffman GM, et al (Med College of Wisconsin, Milwaukee; Ctrs for Disease Control and Prevention, Atlanta, Ga)
N Engl J Med 352:2508-2514, 2005   10–21

Background.—Rabies is a fatal illness in humans. It is characterized by severe encephalopathy and generalized paresis, with death usually occurring within 5 to 7 days after the onset of symptoms if left untreated. Medical management may prolong survival up to 133 days. There is little evidence that any treatment can alter median survival, but 5 persons have survived after receiving immunoprophylaxis before the onset of symptoms. The survival of a patient with rabies who was treated with an intense antiexcitotoxic strategy while the native immune response matured was reported. The patient received no immune prophylaxis.

> *Case Report.*—Girl, 15 years, rescued and released a bat that struck an interior window. During the rescue the girl was bitten by the bat. The wound was washed with peroxide, and no medical attention was sought; thus, the patient did not receive any postexposure prophylaxis. The patient continued to do well until 1 month after the bite, at which time she experienced generalized fatigue and paresthesia of the left hand. Two days later she developed diplopia and unsteadiness. On the third day she developed nausea and vomiting without fever, and a neurologist noted the presence of partial bilateral sixth-nerve palsy and ataxia. Over the next two days she developed blurred vision, left leg weakness, gait abnormality, slurred speech, nystagmus, and tremor of the left arm and was admitted to hospital. The patient was febrile and semiobtunded on admission. Over 2 days she began salivating, with uncoordinated swallowing, and was intubated for airway protection. Treatment included induction of coma while the patient's native immune response matured. A rabies vaccine was not administered. The patient was treated with ketamine, midazolam, ribavarin, and amantadine. A lumbar puncture performed at 8 days after initiation of therapy showed an increased level of rabies antibody; sedation was then tapered. The patient was removed from isolation at day 31 and discharged at day 76. She was alert and communicative at nearly 5 months after hospitalization, but continued to have choreoathetosis, dysarthria, and an unsteady gait.

Conclusions.—This improvised approach to the treatment of rabies—including induction of coma—was a logical extension of previous attempts to prevent complications through aggressive critical care. The uneventful course that followed the induction of coma may suggest that much of the dysautonomia that is characteristic of rabies can be avoided with therapeutic sedation anesthesia. However, the experience with this case must be repeated in other patients and in proof-of-concept experiments in animal models.

▶ This single case report is as important as they come. This 15-year-old girl in whom clinical rabies developed is the only patient known to have ever survived rabies who did not, in some way before the onset of symptoms, receive rabies vaccine or immunoglobulin. She had rescued and released a bat that struck an interior window in her home and sustained a small (5 mm) laceration to her left finger from the bat. The wound was washed with peroxide, and the family sought no medical attention; thus, the patient received no rabies postexposure prophylaxis. Within a month of the bat exposure, she experienced generalized fatigue and paresthesias of the left hand. Two days later, double vision developed followed by nausea and vomiting. She saw a neurologist who noted partial bilateral sixth nerve palsy and ataxia. An MRI was performed, and the findings were unremarkable. Within a day, weakness of the left leg and a gait abnormality were present, followed by fever on the fifth day of illness. Tremors of the left arm developed, and a presumed diagnosis of rabies was made when the history of a bat bite was finally elicited. The patient's clinical course then rapidly deteriorated, and symptoms and signs included salivation, uncoordinated swallowing, dysarthria, myoclonus, and intense tremors of the left arm. Given that no prior patient had ever survived the clinical onset of rabies, her parents were counseled and offered hospice care. Alternatively, the parents were told that the critical care physicians were willing to test a previously untested strategy that combined antiexcitatory and antiviral drugs along with supportive intensive care.

The theory that this young lady's care providers operated under was that the pathology of the human brain in cases of rabies reflected secondary complications rather than any clear primary process, and that a normal immune system might ultimately clear the virus if the patient lived long enough. Prior clinical reports suggested that death from rabies actually resulted from neurotransmitter imbalances and autonomic failure, and that, theoretically, it was possible to survive with excellent supportive care. That is exactly what this young lady was given. She underwent the induction of therapeutic coma using γ-aminobutyric acid–receptor agonism with benzodiazepines and barbiturates, along with N-methyl-D-aspartate (NMDA)-receptor antagonism with ketamine and amantadine as an antiviral agent. These were used to reduce excitotoxicity, brain metabolism, and autonomic reactivity. Basically, the patient was put to sleep and paralyzed. Her clinical course at that point became largely benign, except when the care providers attempted to wake her up and some degree of autonomic hyperreflexia emerged.

This patient, although surviving, was left with some neurologic impairment. She was in the hospital for 76 days. Four months after her initial hospitalization she had dysarthric speech, but she was able to dress herself. She had a normal appetite, ate well, and attended high school part time. She had some mild choreoathetosis and ballismus, which resulted in a lurching gait and fine motor difficulties. She could write legibly, but did so slowly and preferred to type with her index fingers. It was clear at the time she was last seen that her neurologic condition had continued to gradually improve.

Congratulations are to be offered not only to this young lady who survived her rabies, but also to the care providers who gave her such an excellent chance to survive. Recognize, however, that one survivor of rabies does not a series make and in no way changes the overwhelming statistics on clinical rabies. There is no other infectious disease that has such a high case-fatality ratio. This statement remains true. Nonetheless, you can bet that the next patient who is diagnosed with clinical rabies will undergo a management approach very similar to what was described here in *The New England Journal of Medicine* for the very first time.

J. A. Stockman III, MD

Passive Immunization During Pregnancy for Congenital Cytomegalovirus Infection

Nigro G, for the Congenital Cytomegalovirus Collaborating Group (La Sapienza Univ, Rome; et al)
N Engl J Med 353:1350-1362, 2005   10–22

Background.—Currently, there is no effective intervention for a primary cytomegalovirus (CMV) infection during pregnancy.

Methods.—We studied pregnant women with a primary CMV infection. The therapy group comprised women whose amniotic fluid contained either CMV or CMV DNA and who were offered intravenous CMV hyperimmune globulin at a dose of 200 U per kilogram of maternal weight. A prevention group, consisting of women with a recent primary infection before 21 weeks' gestation or who declined amniocentesis, was offered monthly hyperimmune globulin (100 U per kilogram intravenously).

Results.—In the therapy group, 31 women received hyperimmune globulin, only 1 (3 percent) of whom gave birth to an infant with CMV disease (symptomatic at birth and handicapped at two or more years of age), as compared with 7 of 14 women who did not receive hyperimmune globulin (50 percent). Thus, hyperimmune globulin therapy was associated with a significantly lower risk of congenital CMV disease (adjusted odds ratio, 0.02; 95 percent confidence interval, $-\infty$ to 0.15; P<0.001). In the prevention group, 37 women received hyperimmune globulin, 6 (16 percent) of whom had infants with congenital CMV infection, as compared with 19 of 47 women (40 percent) who did not receive hyperimmune globulin. Thus, hyperimmune globulin therapy was associated with a significantly lower risk of congenital CMV infection (adjusted odds ratio, 0.32; 95 percent confidence interval, 0.10 to 0.94; P=0.04). Hyperimmune globulin therapy significantly (P<0.001) increased CMV-specific IgG concentrations and avidity and decreased natural killer cells and HLA-DR+ cells and had no adverse effects.

Conclusions.—Treatment of pregnant women with CMV-specific hyperimmune globulin is safe, and the findings of this nonrandomized study suggest that it may be effective in the treatment and prevention of congenital CMV infection. A controlled trial of this agent may now be appropriate.

▶ Some 15 years ago, an editorial appeared entitled "Congenital Cytomegalovirus Disease: 20 Years Is Long Enough" by Yow and Demmler,[1] who lamented the lack of progress in preventing congenital CMV disease. Since then, progress has been very slow with respect to the development of CMV vaccines. Lacking a CMV vaccine, efforts have focused on developing interventions that would justify universal screening of newborns and pregnant women for CMV infections. The problem is not minor. Some 40,000 infants are born congenitally infected in the United States each year. Of these, about 8000 are at extremely high risk for hearing deficit. It is estimated that 25% of all prelingual hearing deficits are attributable to congenital CMV infection. The report of Nigro et al shows us what is capable of being done to help attenuate the problem of congenital CMV infection.

Although sexual transmission of CMV can occur, most pregnant women acquire CMV infection through exposure to children in their own home or from occupational exposure to children in daycare or elementary school. Exposure typically occurs as the result of contact with contaminated saliva, urine, or fomites such as toys. Approximately 40% of pregnant women with a primary infection will transmit CMV to their fetuses. Rates of transmission are highest when maternal infection occurs in the third trimester. However, the risk of serious fetal injury is greatest when maternal infection occurs in the first trimester or early in the second trimester. It is estimated that somewhere between 10% and 20% of congenitally infected infants will have symptoms identifiable at birth, and up to 20% of this group will die, with the remainder typically having moderate to severe complications. These include growth restriction, microcephaly, enlargement of the ventricles, chorioretinitis, hepatosplenomegaly, hepatitis, thrombocytopenia, and purpuric skin eruption ("blueberry muffin" baby).

Until now, very little could be done for pregnancies affected by CMV infection. Obstetricians have focused their attention on screening selected women considered at high risk for CMV infection and performing amniocentesis to identify infected fetuses. Targeted ultrasonography is then used to identify the severely injured fetus, and pregnancy termination is offered as a management option.[2] The report by Nigro et al changes the whole set of options available to women since it offers the promise of a means to treat and prevent CMV infection. In their study, a large group of pregnant women were identified by routine serologic screening to have primary CMV infection. The vast majority of these women were asymptomatic. A subset of these women had a primary infection more than 6 weeks before enrollment in the study. These women underwent amniocentesis and had CMV detected in amniotic fluid by polymerase chain reaction or culture. The majority of these women elected to receive IV treatment with CMV-specific hyperimmune globulin (200 U/kg of the mother's body weight). The control group was a group of women who declined such therapy. Fifty percent of women who declined therapy had infants who were symptomatic at delivery. In contrast, only 3% of treated women had an infant with clinical CMV disease at birth.

The Nigro study also looked at women who were very recently infected (<6 weeks before enrollment in the immune globulin study). More than 80% of treated pregnancies resulted in infants who were totally free of CMV compared with untreated women who had about a 50% probability of having a CMV-infected infant. These results are impressive.

As impressive as the results of this study are, they are not sufficiently conclusive to warrant jumping on the bandwagon of routine screening of all pregnancies for CMV infection and treating with hyperimmune globulin those pregnancies in which there is a high risk of transmission of CMV to a fetus. The reasons have to do with certain weaknesses in the study (it was not a randomized and controlled trial). As important as the results are, there is some reason to believe that providing antibody to already infected women might not have as dramatic an effect as that observed. By comparison, women with antibodies against herpes simplex are not fully protected from recurrent symptomatic infection. The presence of antibody against varicella-zoster virus does not fully protect a person from future outbreaks of herpes zoster infection. Administration of hyperimmune globulin against HIV has been studied during pregnancy and does not appear to protect the fetus. Moreover, the presence of antibody against CMV does not fully protect the mother or her fetus against reactivation, nor is it protective against subsequent perinatal transmission.

Despite the caveats mentioned, the report of Nigro et al is both provocative and deserving of follow-up with better-designed clinical trials. Such trials should look at the financial and logistical burden associated with screening large obstetric populations for CMV infection, triaging patients with the inevitable false-positive test results, offering amniocentesis and targeted ultrasonography examination of fetuses of women who seroconvert, and treating at-risk women and fetuses with hyperimmune globulin. All of this is a lot of work. About 4 million women become pregnant each year with an intention of carrying their pregnancy. Given a seroconversion rate of approximately 1% during pregnancy, this means that approximately 40,000 women would need intensive follow-up, a daunting task. ...what we really need is an effective CMV vaccine.

J. A. Stockman III, MD

References

1. Yow MD, Demmler LA: Congenital cytomegalovirus disease: 20 years is long enough (editorial). *N Engl J Med* 326:702-703, 1992.
2. Azam AZ, Vial Y, Fawer CL, et al: Prenatal diagnosis of congenital cytomegalovirus infection. *Obstet Gynecol* 97:443-448, 2001.

Vaccine Effectiveness During a Varicella Outbreak Among Schoolchildren: Utah, 2002–2003
Haddad MB, Hill MB, Pavia AT, et al (Ctrs for Disease Control and Prevention, Atlanta, Ga; Utah Dept of Health, Salt Lake City; Salt Lake City Health Dept, Utah; et al)
Pediatrics 115:1488-1493, 2005   10–23

Objectives.—In the context of a chickenpox outbreak involving 2 Utah elementary schools, we conducted an investigation to assess vaccine effectiveness, describe illness severity, and examine risk factors for breakthrough varicella (ie, varicella in those who have been vaccinated).

Methods.—All parents were asked to complete a questionnaire about their child's medical history. Parents of children with recent varicella were interviewed, and vaccination records were verified. Lesions were submitted for polymerase chain reaction testing.

Results.—Questionnaires were returned for 558 (93%) of 597 students in school A and 924 (97%) of 952 students in school B. A total of 83 schoolchildren (57 unvaccinated and 26 vaccinated) had varicella during the October 2002 through February 2003 outbreak period. An additional 17 cases occurred among household contacts, including infants and adults. Polymerase chain reaction analysis recovered wild-type varicella. Vaccine effectiveness was 87%. With 1 notable exception, vaccinated children tended to have milder illness. Risk factors for breakthrough varicella included eczema, vaccination ≥5 years before the outbreak, and vaccination at ≤18 months of age. Restricting analysis to children vaccinated ≥5 years before the outbreak, those vaccinated at ≤18 months of age were more likely to develop breakthrough varicella (relative risk: 9.3; 95% confidence interval: 1.3–68.9).

Conclusions.—The vaccine, administered by >100 health care providers to 571 children during a 7-year time period, was effective. Risk factors for breakthrough varicella suggest some degree of biological interaction between age at vaccination and time since vaccination.

▶ There should be no question that the varicella vaccine is effective, assuming it is administered. Before the licensure of the vaccine in 1995, varicella caused about 11,000 hospitalizations each year in our country and 100 deaths. Since then there have been marked declines not only in the occurrence of varicella but also in hospital admissions for varicella. Despite these declines, chicken pox outbreaks continue to occur, including some outbreaks in vaccinated populations. Outbreaks, in fact, do generate concern that varicella effectiveness is lower under real-life conditions than reported in the literature. In fact, there is some evidence to suggest that this is correct, because varicella effectiveness was only 44% during a 2000-2001 outbreak in a New Hampshire day care and 56% effective during a 2002 outbreak in a Minnesota elementary school.[1,2]

This report by Haddad et al gives us concrete information about hospitalization rates in the post-varicella era compared with the pre-varicella era. The data from the Centers for Disease Control and Prevention (CDC) are clear. Varicella vaccine has resulted in an 88% decrease in varicella-caused hospitalization rates. Ambulatory visits for varicella have decreased by almost 60%.

The varicella vaccine is not a perfect vaccine. Breakthrough varicella does occur, and a recent report confirms that less than 100% protection is associated with the time since vaccination and early age at vaccination. We need to learn more about the epidemiology of varicella here in the United States. As our understanding of the epidemiology of varicella continues to evolve, we will likely develop improved thinking about the long-term benefits and limitations of universal varicella vaccine and, perhaps, the need to give boosters for the vaccine. Elsewhere in this chapter is mention of a combination measles, mumps, rubella and varicella vaccine (Abstract 10–25), which could be used for primary immunization and as a booster. We have to make an imperfect vaccine more perfect, if possible.

In Utah, the vaccine effectiveness was 87% during an outbreak among elementary school-age children.

J. A. Stockman III, MD

References

1. Galil K, Lee D, Strine T, et al: Outbreak of varicella at a day-care center despite vaccinations. *N Engl J Med* 347:1909-1915, 2002.

2. Lee BR, Feaver SL, Miller CA, et al: An elementary school outbreak of varicella attributed to vaccine failure: Policy implications. *J Infect Dis* 190:477-483, 2004.

Impact of Varicella Vaccination on Health Care Utilization

Zhou F, Harpaz R, Jumaan AO, et al (Ctrs for Disease Control and Prevention, Atlanta, Ga)
JAMA 294:797-802, 2005

10–24

Context.—Since varicella vaccine was first recommended for routine immunization in the United States in 1995, the incidence of disease has dropped substantially. However, national surveillance data are incomplete, and comprehensive data regarding outpatient as well as hospital utilization have not been reported.

Objective.—To examine the impact of the varicella vaccination program on medical visits and associated expenditures.

Design, Setting, and Patients.—Retrospective population-based study examining the trends in varicella health care utilization, based on data from the MarketScan databases, which include enrollees (children and adults) of more than 100 health insurance plans of approximately 40 large US employers, from 1994 to 2002.

Main Outcome Measures.—Trends in rates of varicella-related hospitalizations and ambulatory visits and direct medical expenditures for hospitalizations and ambulatory visits, analyzed using 1994 and 1995 as the prevaccination baseline.

Results.—From the prevaccination period to 2002, hospitalizations due to varicella declined by 88% (from 2.3 to 0.3 per 100,000 population) and ambulatory visits declined by 59% (from 215 to 89 per 100,000 population). Hospitalizations and ambulatory visits declined in all age groups, with the greatest declines among infants younger than 1 year. Total estimated direct medical expenditures for varicella hospitalizations and ambulatory visits declined by 74%, from an average of 84.9 million dollars in 1994 and 1995 to 22.1 million dollars in 2002.

Conclusion.—Since the introduction of the varicella vaccination program, varicella hospitalizations, ambulatory visits, and their associated expenditures have declined dramatically among all age groups in the United States.

▶ It has taken a bit of time, but now we finally have solid evidence about the cost effectiveness of the varicella vaccine. Way back in 1994, Lieu and colleagues[1] estimated the cost-effectiveness of a universal childhood varicella vaccination program. Projecting a national vaccination rate of 97% by the sixth year of the program, they estimated a 94% reduction in the incidence of varicella accompanied by an 89% reduction in direct medical costs. It was projected that a varicella vaccination program would save more than $5.00 for every $1.00 spent.

So what has happened in the last decade with the varicella vaccine? The projection of a vaccination rate of 97% was overly optimistic, but data from a variety of sources do indicate reductions of nearly 90% in hospitalization rates for varicella, a 60% reduction in ambulatory visits, and a 74% reduction in cost borne by health care payers. These figures are based on an 80% observed vaccination rate among toddlers.

Just how far off were the original projections about the cost-effectiveness of the varicella vaccine? Off was the cost of the vaccine. The cost of the vaccine has increased more than $10.00 per dose in inflation-adjusted terms since 1995 (when the article abstracted was written, the sector price of each dose of the vaccine was $52.25). Also, there are no solid data about the indirect savings of the varicella vaccine. Indirect savings relate to nondirect savings related to lost time from work on the part of parents. It is possible that the increasing value of work over the past decade may have increased indirect savings beyond what the literature is telling us about the cost-effectiveness of the varicella vaccine.

See the editorial by Davis.[2] You will see confirmation that the varicella vaccine has proven its merit. Also, see the article by Oxman et al (Abstract 2–6) that adds a new understanding about the complete spectrum of the use of the varicella vaccine, that is, to prevent herpes zoster and postherpetic neuralgia in older adults.

J. A. Stockman III, MD

References

1. Lieu TA, Cohci SL, Black SB, et al: Cost effectiveness of a routine varicella vaccination program for US children. *JAMA* 271:375-381, 1984.
2. Davis MM: Varicella vaccine, cost-effectiveness analyses and the vaccination policy. *JAMA* 294:845-846, 2005.

Evaluation of a Quadrivalent Measles, Mumps, Rubella and Varicella Vaccine in Healthy Children
Shinefield H, Black S, Digilio L, et al (Univ of California San Francisco; Kaiser Permanente Vaccine Study Ctr, Oakland, Calif; Primary Physicians Research, Pittsburgh, Pa; et al)
Pediatr Infect Dis J 24:665-669, 2005   10–25

Background.—A quadrivalent measles, mumps, rubella and varicella vaccine would facilitate universal immunization against all 4 diseases, improve compliance and immunization rates and decrease the number of injections given to children and visits to physicians' offices.

Objectives.—To evaluate 1- and 2-dose regimens of a combined measles, mumps, rubella and varicella vaccine (ProQuad, referred to as MMRV) manufactured with a varicella component of increased potency.

Methods.—In this partially blind, multicenter study, 480 healthy 12- to 23-month-old children were randomized to receive either MMRV and placebo or M-M-R®II and VARIVAX. Injections were given concomitantly at separate sites. Subjects randomized to receive MMRV and placebo received a second dose of MMRV 90 days later. Subjects were followed for 42 days after each vaccination for adverse experiences. Immunogenicity was evaluated 6 weeks after each vaccination.

Results.—Measles-like rash and fever during days 5-12 were more common after the first dose of MMRV (rash, 5.9%; fever, 27.7%) than after M-M-R®II and VARIVAX (rash, 1.9%; fever, 18.7%). The incidence of other adverse events were similar between groups. Response rates were >90% to all vaccine components in both groups. Geometric mean titers to measles and mumps were significantly higher after 1 dose of MMRV than after administration of M-M-R®II and VARIVAX. The second dose of MMRV elicited slight to moderate increases in measles, mumps and rubella antibody titers and a substantial increase in varicella antibody titer (from 13.0 to 588.1 glycoprotein antigen-based enzyme-linked immunosorbent assay units/mL).

Conclusion.—A 1- or 2-dose regimen of MMRV is generally well-tolerated when administered to 12- to 23-month-old children and has a safety and immunogenicity profile similar to that of M-M-R®II and VARIVAX administered concomitantly.

Dose-Response Study of a Quadrivalent Measles, Mumps, Rubella and Varicella Vaccine in Healthy Children

Shinefield H, for the Dose Selection Study Group for Proquad (Univ of California San Francisco; et al)
Pediatr Infect Dis J 24:670-675, 2005   10–26

Background.—A combined measles, mumps, rubella and varicella (MMRV) vaccine would facilitate universal immunization against 4 diseases by decreasing the number of injections and thus enhancing compliance and coverage rates. If a second dose of varicella vaccine were to be recommended, MMRV could be used to administer a routine second dose of M-M-R®II with the added advantage of boosting varicella-zoster virus (VZV) antibody titers.

Methods.—Subjects 12–23 months of age received a single injection of 1 of 3 lots of an MMRV vaccine (ProQuad) containing high, middle or low VZV potency, or VARIVAX given concomitantly with M-M-R®II. Recipients of MMRV received a second injection of MMRV ~90 days later.

Results.—We enrolled 1559 subjects in the study. Antibody response rates to VZV 6 weeks after 1 injection of high potency MMRV (88.6%) or 2 injections of MMRV of any varicella potency (99.7–100%) were similar to the response rates after concomitant administration of M-M-R®II and VARIVAX (93.1%). The second injection of MMRV boosted VZV antibody titers. Antibody responses to measles, mumps and rubella were ≥98%, similar to the control, after 1 or 2 injections of MMRV. MMRV was generally well-tolerated during the 42 days after vaccination.

Conclusions.—One injection of high potency MMRV resulted in antibody responses to the 4 vaccine components equivalent to those found after concomitant administration of M-M-R®II and VARIVAX. A second injection of MMRV resulted in a significant boost in VZV antibody. This boost may translate into enhanced immunogenicity against varicella, which is known to correlate with increased protection.

▶ The preceding 2 reports (Abstracts 10–25 and 10–26) provide us with important information about the potential for using a combination vaccine that includes protection against MMRV. There have been earlier studies that have suggested that such a combination does not provide adequate protection against varicella, an issue addressed in the first report, which studies a combination vaccine that uses a higher varicella vaccine dose in combination with MMR than had been previously used. The results of this study are unequivocal: the combination vaccine with the higher varicella component produces exactly the same antibody titers against varicella as when the varicella vaccine is given separately.

The findings from these studies are very important. Currently, here in the United States, almost all children are vaccinated against MMR by 4 to 6 years old with a standard 2-dose regimen. The data are not as good with respect to varicella where in 2003, just 84% of children here were vaccinated against varicella before 36 months old, recognizing also that state-to-state coverage with this vaccine varied from a low of 60% to a high of 93%. This failure to completely immunize would be largely eliminated if there were a combination MMRV vaccine. An additional advantage would be the fact that the varicella vaccine component in an MMRV vaccine could also be given as a booster, as is currently true of MMR. Currently, a second dose of varicella vaccine is not recommended for children younger than 13 years despite the fact that 1% to 2% of vaccinated children per year will in fact have breakthrough varicella. Low VZV antibody titers 6 weeks postvaccination correlate with a higher probability of developing breakthrough varicella, and a second dose of varicella vaccine clearly has been documented to increase varicella titers.

Without question, the availability of a safe and effective combination MMRV vaccine would offer significant advantages. The combined quadrivalent vaccine would decrease the number of injections administered to children and potentially increase immunization rates. In addition, a quadrivalent vaccine would offer a convenient method to administer a second dose of varicella vaccine, a recommendation that many believe is long past due.

One final comment about vaccine studies. Our hats should be off to the Kaiser Permanente Vaccine Study Center in California. Shinefield et al, using the resources of Kaiser Permanente, have on many occasions assisted those in primary care by clarifying for us best practices with respect to vaccine use. Three cheers and many kudos should be tossed these investigators' way.

J. A. Stockman III, MD

Screening for HIV: A Review of the Evidence for the US Preventive Services Task Force

Chou R, Huffman LH, Fu R, et al (Oregon Health & Science Univ, Portland)
Ann Intern Med 143:55-73, 2005   10–27

Background.—HIV infection affects 850,000 to 950,000 persons in the United States. The management and outcomes of HIV infection have changed substantially since the U.S. Preventive Services Task Force issued recommendations in 1996.

Purpose.—To synthesize the evidence on risks and benefits of screening for HIV infection.

Data Sources.—MEDLINE, the Cochrane Library, reference lists, and experts.

Study Selection.—Studies of screening, risk factor assessment, accuracy of testing, follow-up testing, and efficacy of interventions.

Data Extraction.—Data on settings, patients, interventions, and outcomes were abstracted for included studies; quality was graded according to criteria developed by the Task Force.

Data Synthesis.—No trials directly link screening for HIV with clinical outcomes. Many HIV-infected persons in the United States currently receive diagnosis at advanced stages of disease, and almost all will progress to AIDS if untreated. Screening based on risk factors could identify persons at substantially higher risk but would miss a substantial proportion of those infected. Screening tests for HIV are extremely (>99%) accurate. Acceptance rates for screening and use of recommended interventions vary widely. Highly active antiretroviral therapy (HAART) substantially reduces the risk for clinical progression or death in patients with immunologically advanced disease. Along with other adverse events, HAART is associated with an increased risk for cardiovascular complications, although absolute rates are low after 3 to 4 years.

Limitations.—Data are insufficient to estimate the effects of screening and interventions on transmission rates or in patients with less immunologically advanced disease. Long-term data on adverse events associated with HAART are not yet available.

Conclusions.—Benefits of HIV screening appear to outweigh harms. The yield from screening higher-prevalence populations would be substantially higher than that from screening the general population.

▶ This is the first of 2 reports that were contracted for by the Agency for Healthcare Research in Quality (AHRQ) to help all of us better understand the evidence underlying the need for screening for HIV infection. There are likely to be just about 1 million persons here in the United States infected with HIV, 25% of whom are unaware of their diagnosis. The latter group, if untreated, will eventually have AIDS, which remains the seventh leading cause of death in persons 15 to 24 years old and is the fifth leading cause of death in persons 25 to 44 years old here in the United States. In addition, the annual incidence of AIDS has remained steady at about 40,000 per year in the United States. This figure includes infection through mother-to-child (vertical) transmission, with approximately 300 infants infected each year. Women are the fastest growing group of persons with new HIV diagnoses, and an estimated 6000 to 7000 HIV-positive women give birth each year in the United States. Some 40% of infected babies are born to mothers who were not prenatally detected with HIV infection before delivery.

So what are the current recommendations about HIV screening (as of 2006)? The United States Preventative Services Task Force (USPSTF) makes these recommendations. USPSTF strongly recommends that clinicians screen all adolescents and adults at increased risk for HIV infection. Individual risk for HIV infection is assessed through a careful patient history. Those at increased risk (as determined by prevalence rates) include boys and men who have had sex with males; those having unprotected sex with multiple partners; past or present injection drug users; those who exchange money for sex or drugs or who have sex partners who do; individuals whose past or present sex partners were HIV infected, bisexual, or injection drug users; persons being treated for sexually transmitted diseases; and persons with a history of blood transfusion between 1978 and 1985. Also considered at increased risk are persons who request an HIV test despite reporting no individual risk factors, because this approach is likely to include individuals (including many teens) not willing to disclose high-risk behaviors. This "at-risk" recommendation of the USPSTF is listed as a grade A recommendation, indicating that there is good evidence that the provision of such screening services provides important health outcomes and that benefits substantially outweigh harms. It should be noted that the USPSTF makes no recommendations for or against routinely screening adolescents and adults who are not at increased risk of HIV infection. In fact, this is a grade C recommendation, meaning that the evidence is only fair at best that such universal screening can improve large-group health outcomes and that the balance of benefits and harms is too close to justify a recommendation. The yield of screening such teens and adults without risk factors would be expectedly low and potential harm associated with screening has been found in some studies. The conclusion has been that the benefit of screening adolescents and adults without risk factors for HIV is too small (relative to potential harms) to justify such a recommendation.

This commentary closes with a question about immunosuppression. An 8-year-old patient in your practice has AIDS, acquired perinatally. He is immunocompromised. His family wishes to take him from New York City to Disneyland. They ask you whether or not it would be important for him to bring bottled water with him for his flight. You scratch your head a bit trying to figure out whether there might be a problem for immunosuppressed patients who drink aircraft water. If you were to research this topic, what would you find?

Recently, the Environmental Protection Agency (EPA) conducted a round of water quality sampling of 169 randomly selected domestic and international aircraft at 12 major airports here in the United States. Samples were obtained from galley water taps and lavatory faucets for each aircraft. About one-sixth (or 17.2%) of the aircraft tested carried water contaminated with total coliform bacteria at unacceptable levels. These findings have prompted the EPA to advise that passengers with compromised immune systems or other health concerns request canned or bottled beverages and avoid drinking tea or coffee that is not made with bottled water. The EPA informed airlines about this problem and 6 months later repeated their study, finding that almost 13% of 158 aircraft still carried water positive for coliform bacteria in unacceptable amounts.

These latest results warrant continued scrutiny, according to the EPA, which continues to review existing regulations and guidance regulations and is working with other federal agencies to develop a final rule that would ensure safe drinking water on all aircraft. If you want to read more about this, go to the EPA web site and see the actual data (http://www.epa.gov/airlinewater/).

J. A. Stockman III, MD

Prenatal Screening for HIV: A Review of the Evidence for the US Preventive Services Task Force
Chou R, Smits AK, Huffman AH, et al (Oregon Health & Science Univ, Portland)
Ann Intern Med 143:38-54, 2005   10–28

Background.—Each year in the United States, 6000 to 7000 women with HIV give birth. The management and outcomes of prenatal HIV infection have changed substantially since the U.S. Preventive Services Task Force issued recommendations in 1996.

Purpose.—To synthesize current evidence on risks and benefits of prenatal screening for HIV infection.

Data Sources.—MEDLINE, the Cochrane Library, reference lists, and experts.

Study Selection.—Studies of screening, risk factor assessment, accuracy of testing, follow-up testing, and efficacy of interventions.

Data Extraction.—Data on settings, patients, interventions, and outcomes were abstracted for included studies; quality was graded according to criteria developed by the Task Force.

Data Synthesis.—No published studies directly link prenatal screening for HIV with clinical outcomes. In developed countries, the rate of mother-to-child transmission from untreated HIV-infected women is 14% to 25%. Targeted screening based on risk factors would miss a substantial proportion of infected women. "Opt-out" testing policies appear to increase uptake rates. Standard HIV testing is highly (>99%) sensitive and specific, and initial studies of rapid HIV tests found that both types of testing had similar accuracy. Rapid testing can facilitate timely interventions in persons testing positive. Recommended interventions (combination antiretroviral regimens, elective cesarean section in selected patients, and avoidance of breastfeeding) are associated with transmission rates of 1% to 2% and appear acceptable to pregnant women.

Limitations.—Long-term safety data for antiretroviral agents are not yet available. Data are insufficient to accurately estimate the benefits of screening on long-term maternal disease progression or other clinical outcomes, such as horizontal transmission.

Conclusions.—Identification and treatment of asymptomatic HIV infection in pregnant women can greatly decrease mother-to-child transmission rates.

▶ In the years 1999 to 2001, some 280 to 370 HIV-infected infants were born yearly in the United States. As noted in the previous commentary, a large percentage of these babies were born to mothers not known to have HIV infection prior to delivery. As of 3 years ago, about 5000 cumulative deaths from perinatally acquired AIDS had occurred here on our shores, highlighting the magnitude of the problem of vertical transmission of HIV infection.[1]

We now know when HIV infection is likely to be transmitted vertically, that is, mother to child. This can occur during pregnancy (antepartum), during labor and delivery (intrapartum), and after delivery (postnatal). In the absence of breast feeding, antepartum transmission is thought to account for 25% to 40% of cases of mother-to-child transmission with the remaining cases occurring during labor and delivery. This risk can be lessened by labor management techniques that minimize contact between infected maternal blood and the fetus. Breast feeding is thought to be the only important means of postnatal transmission between mothers and children and accounts for 44% of infant cases in settings with high breast-feeding rates. It is also known that higher maternal viral loads and lower CD4 cell counts are associated with an increased risk for transmission from mother to baby.

This study of the evidence for screening for HIV in pregnant women as a method of reducing mother to child transmission of HIV infection shows us exactly how effective screening is. Antiretroviral therapy markedly reduced vertical transmission. Screening is of value for all women because seropositive prevalence rates for HIV are now running between 0.15% and 5% here in the United States, varying with region, at-risk populations, and so forth. Depending on the study one reads, just 8% to 57% of HIV-infected women have an identifiable risk factor, indicating that all women should be screened during pregnancy.

The results of this study show the benefits of universal HIV screening during pregnancy. This does not mean that no harms are associated with such screening. A very small number of women will have false-positive rapid tests for HIV and may briefly receive antiretroviral prophylaxis unnecessarily. Positive tests should always be repeated. No one wants to see a woman undergo elective pregnancy termination on the basis of inaccurate test results, should that be a woman's consideration if she were to think she was HIV-positive.

In the absence of antiretroviral prophylaxis, the risk of mother-to-child transmission of HIV runs 14% to 25% in developed countries and 13% to 42% in countries with high rates of breast feeding. The landmark pediatric AIDS clinical trials group study found that 3-phase mother and infant zidovudine regimen in non–breast-feeding women starting at 14 to 34 weeks gestation (median, 26 weeks gestation) through 6 weeks postpartum decreased the risk for transmission from about 25% to 8% when compared with that of placebo. Now we are seeing multidrug regimens that are producing even better results. Elective cesarean section also decreases vertical transmission.

The data regarding universal screening of all pregnant women for HIV are so strong that the USPSTF recommends that clinicians screen all pregnant women. They consider this also a grade A recommendation. The USPSTF has found good evidence that both standard and FDA-approved rapid screening tests accurately detect HIV infection in pregnant women and that the approaches used are found to be acceptable by women. Early detection of maternal HIV infection allows for discussion of elected cesarean section, avoidance of breast feeding, and the introduction of antiviral therapies. The recommendation by the USPSTF also notes that there is no evidence of an increase in fetal anomalies or other fetal harm associated with currently recommended antiviral regimens with the exception of efavirenz. The latter drug has been recently classified as a class D in pregnancy showing positive evidence of human fetal risk.

If you want to read more about screening for HIV and statements of the US Preventative Services Task Force, see the excellent summary of this in a recent *Annals of Internal Medicine* article.[2]

J. A. Stockman III, MD

References

1. Centers for Disease Control and Prevention: HIV/AIDS surveillance report, 2003 (vol 15) [on-line], http://www.cdc.gov/hiv/stats/2003SurveillanceReport.htm. (accessed December 6, 2005).
2. United States Preventative Services Task Force, Agency for healthcare research and quality. Screening for HIV: Recommendation statement. *Ann Intern Med* 143:32-37, 2005.

Role of Sexual Behavior in the Acquisition of Asymptomatic Epstein-Barr Virus Infection: A Longitudinal Study
Woodman CBJ, Collins SI, Vavrusova N, et al (Univ of Birmingham, England; Univ of Palacky, Olomouc, Czech Republic; VU Med Ctr, Amsterdam; et al)
Pediatr Infect Dis J 24:498-502, 2005   10–29

Background.—The natural history of Epstein-Barr virus (EBV) infection is poorly defined. We report the prevalence and subsequent incidence of EBV infection in a cohort of sexually active young women and explore the social and sexual determinants of incident infections.

Methods.—The study population was drawn from a cohort of young women, who were recruited for a longitudinal study of risk factors for early cervical neoplasia. A case-control analysis, nested within the cohort of 45 women for whom the first EBV sample tested was EBV-negative and who had further follow-up, was undertaken. EBV serostatus was determined in serum with a synthetic peptide-based enzyme-linked immunosorbent assay; EBV DNA was measured in cervical smears with the use of quantitative polymerase chain reaction.

Results.—Of 1023 women 15–19 years of age included in this analysis, 978 (95.6%) tested positive for antibodies to EBV in their first serum sample. Of 45 women who tested negative, 22 subsequently acquired an asymptomatic EBV infection; the median time to seroconversion was 25 months (range, 1–60 months), and the median age at seroconversion was 18 years (range, 16–21 years). The risk of seroconversion increased with increasing number of sexual partners [compared with 1 partner, odds ratio (OR) was 1.28 for 2 partners and 2.23 for 3 or more; χ^2_{TREND} 5.02; df 1; $P <$ 0.05] and was greatest when a new sexual partner had been acquired in the 2 years before seroconversion (OR 4.78; χ^2 4.62; df 1; $P < 0.05$). EBV DNA was detected in 9 of 14 women who seroconverted and who also provided cervical samples.

Conclusions.—In susceptible young women, the acquisition of EBV infection is associated with their sexual behavior.

▶ It has been known for some time that in the pediatric population, the greatest rate of seroconversion to EBV occurs in the preschool-age child, presumably as the result of exposure to 1 or more other children who have this common infection. If one makes it past this period without infection, one can grow up to be a teen or young adult who is seronegative, in which case, as this report shows, the risk of acquiring EBV is directly related to interactions with the opposite sex, including interactions involving sexual activity. It has been strongly hypothesized that infectious mononucleosis in teens and young adults is usually acquired from transfer of saliva and that, in young adults, this is more likely after the onset of sexual activity. Although this hypothesis has been widely accepted, only limited evidence can be adduced to support an actual association between the acquisitions of EBV infection in teens and young adults and their sexual behavior. An association with the number of sexual partners and early age of first intercourse has been reported for patients with infectious mononucleosis but not for those with asymptomatic infection.[1] In this report by Woodman et al, there does seem to be a clear link between sexual behavior and the acquisition of EBV infection, including asymptomatic infection.

No study to date has clearly indicated, or even remotely indicated, the possibility of transmission of EBV by actual intercourse. Yes, infectious virus has been detected in the female genital tract, but this is most likely the consequence of infection in lymphocytes in an actively infected individual and does not necessarily indicate viral replication in the genital tract. Thus, EBV remains a "kissing" infection with some kisses being sweeter than wine by being a setup for disease transmission.

J. A. Stockman III, MD

Reference

1. Crawford DH, Swerdlow AC, Higgins C, et al: Sexual history and Epstein-Barr virus infection. *J Infect Dis* 186:731-736, 2002.

Effect of Hepatitis B Immunisation in Newborn Infants of Mothers Positive for Hepatitis B Surface Antigen: Systematic Review and Meta-analysis

Lee C, Gong Y, Brok J, et al (Copenhagen Univ Hosp; Tri-Service Gen Hosp, Taipei, Taiwan; Heart of England NHS Trust, Birmingham)

BMJ 332:328-331, 2006   10–30

Objective.—To evaluate the effects of hepatitis B vaccine and immunoglobulin in newborn infants of mothers positive for hepatitis B surface antigen.

Design.—Systematic review and meta-analysis of randomised clinical trials.

Data Sources.—Electronic databases and hand searches.

Review Methods.—Randomised clinical trials were assessed for methodological quality. Meta-analysis was undertaken on three outcomes: the relative risks of hepatitis B occurrence, antibody levels to hepatitis B surface antigen, and adverse events.

Results.—29 randomised clinical trials were identified, five of which were considered high quality. Only three trials reported inclusion of mothers negative for hepatitis B e antigen. Compared with placebo or no intervention, vaccination reduced the occurrence of hepatitis B (relative risk 0.28, 95% confidence interval 0.20 to 0.40; four trials). No significant difference in hepatitis B occurrence was found between recombinant vaccine and plasma derived vaccine (1.00, 0.71 to 1.42; four trials) and between high dose versus low dose vaccine (plasma derived vaccine 0.97, 0.55 to 1.68, three trials; recombinant vaccine 0.78, 0.31 to 1.94, one trial). Compared with placebo or no intervention, hepatitis B immunoglobulin or the combination of plasma derived vaccine and hepatitis B immunoglobulin reduced hepatitis B occurrence (immunoglobulin 0.50, 0.41 to 0.60, one trial; vaccine and immunoglobulin 0.08, 0.03 to 0.17, three trials). Compared with vaccine alone, vaccine plus hepatitis B immunoglobulin reduced hepatitis B occurrence (0.54, 0.41 to 0.73; 10 trials). Hepatitis B vaccine and hepatitis B immunoglobulin seem safe, but few trials reported adverse events.

Conclusion.—Hepatitis B vaccine, hepatitis B immunoglobulin, and vaccine plus immunoglobulin prevent hepatitis B occurrence in newborn infants of mothers positive for hepatitis B surface antigen.

▶ Hepatitis B vaccine and immunoglobulin, solely or in combination, do reduce hepatitis B occurrence in newborn infants of mothers who are seropositive for hepatitis B surface antigen. In this meta-analysis of 29 randomized controlled trials of newborns given vaccination or immunoglobulin in their first month, Lee et al have conclusively shown that immunization against hepatitis B will reduce the occurrence of infection. There was no significant difference between low-dose and high-dose vaccine nor between recombinant and plasma-derived vaccine, but vaccine plus immunoglobulin was superior to vaccine alone.

The data from this report are important since we already know that the risk of perinatal transmission is associated with the hepatitis B e antigen status of the mother. If a mother is positive for both hepatitis B surface antigen and e antigen, 70% to 90% of her children will become chronically infected. If a mother is positive for the surface antigen only, the risk of transmission is significantly lower. In either situation, it is worth administering the hepatitis B vaccine and hepatitis B immunoglobulin. The data from this study show that hepatitis B vaccination prevents the occurrence of hepatitis B in the newborn infants of mothers positive for hepatitis B surface antigen.

The recommended schedules for immune prophylaxis against hepatitis B vary among countries. The meta-analysis was unable to show any significant difference among different doses, schedules, and forms of plasma-derived vaccine and recombinant vaccine on hepatitis B occurrence. It should be noted that the findings of this report are mainly based on immune prophylaxis for infants of mothers positive for hepatitis B surface antigen and hepatitis B e antigen. The applicability of these findings to mothers negative for hepatitis B e antigen, therefore, is somewhat limited. Most, as noted above, would give the vaccine as well as immunoprophylaxis in both situations.

See the report that follows (Abstract 10–31), which tells us how using molecular biological tools can identify hepatitis B outbreaks more precisely.

J. A. Stockman III, MD

Identifying a Hepatitis B Outbreak by Molecular Surveillance: A Case Study

Fisker N, Carlsen NLT, Kolmos HJ, et al (Odense Univ Hosp, Denmark)
BMJ 332:343-345, 2006   10–31

Background.—An outbreak of infection is usually recognized when an unexpectedly high number of cases of a clinical illness are observed. In the case of hepatitis B infection, the incubation period is long, and a significant number of infected people, particularly children and the immunocompromised host, may remain asymptomatic. These factors may increase the risk of prolonged and unrecognized outbreaks. In Denmark, universal childhood hepatitis B immunization has not been implemented, and vaccination is not required for health workers performing invasive procedures. Phylogenetic analysis of hepatitis B virus have been used to investigate recognized outbreaks, to identify suspected chains of transmission, and to prove unusual reservoirs or routes of infection. The unraveling of an outbreak of asymptomatic hepatitis B on a pediatric ward after the incidental identification of a single case of hepatitis B was presented.

Case Report.—A child was diagnosed with an acute asymptomatic hepatitis B infection during preparation for bone marrow transplantation at a Danish hospital. Screening for hepatitis B had been negative 2 years earlier, and testing of repository blood donation samples and follow-up samples from all involved blood donors were negative for the virus. The patient had no contact with known hepatitis B cases during the suspected incubation period. As part of a research program, strains of the hepatitis B virus consecutively detected in the area had been partially sequenced. The patient's sequence (the hepatitis B epi strain) was identical to that of a known hepatitis B carrier who had been admitted to the ward 14 months earlier. It was suggested that more cases might therefore be involved in the transmission. An investigation was conducted, including hepatitis B testing for all patients admitted in the period from the source patient's initial admission until procedures were corrected, inspection of the ward by the hospital's infection control team, and a review of hospital records of infected patients. Hepatitis B infection was found to correlate significantly with the insertion of a central venous catheter. Disease category, time of initial admission, age, and sex were unrelated to hepatitis B transmission. The only identifiable breaches in hygiene were found in the ward's preparation rooms, and these were corrected. It was concluded that unintentional contamination of multidose vials and other IV preparations may have occurred because both sterile and non-sterile procedures were performed in the preparation room.

Conclusions.—The recognition and control of the spread of the hepatitis B virus outbreak described in this report was possible because of the availability of a DNA sequences library compiled from patients with hepatitis B in the local area. Surveillance may be a valuable tool in reducing hospital-based transmission.

▶ It should be noted that this is the first hepatitis B outbreak report that identifies all victims of a hepatitis B outbreak following recognition of only one asymptomatic case. If the outbreak had not been tracked down using molecular tools, chances are that many patients would have ultimately become infected to the point of clinical disease.

Data from this report and the previous one add critical information to our knowledge of hepatitis B. Chronic infection with hepatitis B virus (HBV) accounts for an enormous burden of disease worldwide, including up to half of all cases of cirrhosis, endstage liver disease, and hepatocellular carcinoma. With the development of a safe and effective vaccine in the early 1980s, hepatitis B became a preventable disease. Routine hepatitis B vaccination of newborns in Taiwan and China, areas of the world with high rates of hepatitis B, was followed by significant declines in the rates of chronic hepatitis B and hepatocellular carcinoma. In the United States where the disease is uncommon, the incidence of new cases is currently 75% lower than before the introduction of the vaccine.

As importantly as prophylaxis has been, hepatitis B has also become a treatable disease. Several agents are now approved for therapy of chronic hepatitis B here in the United States with several more in the pipeline. Current choices include interferon alfa (standard and pegylated) and 3 oral antiviral agents (lamivudine, adefovir dipivoxil, and entecavir). Entecavir, the newest of the antiviral agents approved for chronic hepatitis B, is a guanosine analog with marked activity against HBV DNA polymerase both in vitro and in vivo. These have unequivocally been shown to be helpful in diminishing the rates of cirrhosis and hepatocellular carcinoma.

All licensed agents are effective in suppressing HBV DNA levels and improving liver enzymes and hepatic histology, but it is still unclear exactly who should be treated, with which agent or combination of agents, and for how long. What monitoring as well as what end points to measure the success or failure of treatment remain unknown. Only time and a number of new studies will answer these questions.

J. A. Stockman III, MD

Entecavir Versus Lamivudine for Patients With HBeAg-Negative Chronic Hepatitis B
Lai C-L, for the BEHoLD AI463027 Study Group (Queen Mary Hosp, Hong Kong; et al)
N Engl J Med 354:1011-1020, 2006   10–32

Background.—Entecavir is a potent and selective antiviral agent that has demonstrated efficacy in phase 2 studies in patients with hepatitis B e antigen (HBeAg)–negative chronic hepatitis B.

Methods.—In this phase 3, double-blind trial, we randomly assigned 648 patients with HBeAg-negative chronic hepatitis B who had not previously been treated with a nucleoside analogue to receive 0.5 mg of entecavir or 100 mg of lamivudine once daily for a minimum of 52 weeks. The primary efficacy end point was histologic improvement (a decrease by at least two points in the Knodell necroinflammatory score, without worsening of fibrosis).

Results.—Histologic improvement after 48 weeks of treatment occurred in 208 of 296 patients in the entecavir group who had adequate baseline liver-biopsy specimens that could be evaluated (70 percent), as compared with 174 of 287 such patients in the lamivudine group (61 percent, P=0.01). More patients in the entecavir group than in the lamivudine group had undetectable serum hepatitis B virus (HBV) DNA levels according to a polymerase-chain-reaction assay (90 percent vs. 72 percent, P<0.001) and normalization of alanine aminotransferase levels (78 percent vs. 71 percent, P=0.045). The mean reduction in serum HBV DNA levels from baseline to week 48 was greater with entecavir than with lamivudine (5.0 vs. 4.5 log [on a base-10 scale] copies per milliliter, P<0.001). There was no evidence of resistance to entecavir. Safety and adverse-event profiles were similar in the two groups.

Conclusions.—Among patients with HBeAg-negative chronic hepatitis B who had not previously been treated with a nucleoside analogue, the rates of histologic improvement, virologic response, and normalization of alanine aminotransferase levels were significantly higher at 48 weeks with entecavir than with lamivudine. The safety profile of the two agents was similar, and there was no evidence of viral resistance to entecavir.

A Comparison of Entecavir and Lamivudine for HBeAg-Positive Chronic Hepatitis B

Chang T-T, for the BEHoLD AI463022 Study Group (Natl Cheng Kung Univ, Tainan, Taiwan; et al)

N Engl J Med 354:1001-1010, 2006   10–33

Background.—Entecavir is a potent and selective guanosine analogue with significant activity against hepatitis B virus (HBV).

Methods.—In this phase 3, double-blind trial, we randomly assigned 715 patients with hepatitis B e antigen (HBeAg)–positive chronic hepatitis B who had not previously received a nucleoside analogue to receive either 0.5 mg of entecavir or 100 mg of lamivudine once daily for a minimum of 52 weeks. The primary efficacy end point was histologic improvement (a decrease by at least two points in the Knodell necroinflammatory score, without worsening of fibrosis) at week 48. Secondary end points included a reduction in the serum HBV DNA level, HBeAg loss and seroconversion, and normalization of the alanine aminotransferase level.

Results.—Histologic improvement after 48 weeks occurred in 226 of 314 patients in the entecavir group (72 percent) and 195 of 314 patients in the lamivudine group (62 percent, P=0.009). More patients in the entecavir group than in the lamivudine group had undetectable serum HBV DNA levels according to a polymerase-chain-reaction assay (67 percent vs. 36 percent, P<0.001) and normalization of alanine aminotransferase levels (68 percent vs. 60 percent, P=0.02). The mean reduction in serum HBV DNA from baseline to week 48 was greater with entecavir than with lamivudine (6.9 vs. 5.4 log [on a base-10 scale] copies per milliliter, P<0.001). HBeAg seroconversion occurred in 21 percent of entecavir-treated patients and 18 percent of those treated with lamivudine (P=0.33). No viral resistance to entecavir was detected. Safety was similar in the two groups.

Conclusions.—Among patients with HBeAg-positive chronic hepatitis B, the rates of histologic, virologic, and biochemical improvement are significantly higher with entecavir than with lamivudine. The safety profile of the two agents is similar, and there is no evidence of viral resistance to entecavir.

▶ Hepatitis B vaccine has been around for a while now. Here in the United States where the disease is somewhat more uncommon than in other parts of the world, the incidence of new cases has dropped remarkably. It is still with us, however, and therefore it is worthwhile to see reports such as these (Abstracts 10–32 and 10–33) that show how effective newer antiviral agents are. There are several therapeutic modalities approved for treatment of chronic hepatitis B in the United States. Current choices include interferon alfa (both standard and pegylated) and 3 oral antiviral agents (lamivudine, adefovir dipivoxil, and most recently, entecavir). The reason for the need for these agents is the enormous burden of disease resulting from HBV, namely, end-stage liver disease with cirrhosis and hepatocellular carcinoma. Effective agents would be expected to minimize or eliminate these long-term complications of hepatitis B infection.

Among the antiviral agents, entecavir is the newest one approved for chronic hepatitis B. It is a guanosine analogue with marked activity against HBV DNA polymerase in vitro and in vivo. As we see in the reports by Lai et al (Abstract 10–32) and Chang et al (Abstract 10–33) in this year's YEAR BOOK OF PEDIATRICS, human trials show that entecavir has few side effects and very potent activity against HBV. In many patients, serum HBV DNA levels become undetectable with antiviral treatment, and just as impressive is that entecavir is associated with little or no antiviral resistance.

Clearly, antiviral agents are not the magic bullet for hepatitis B infection. The central problem is that all current therapies do not truly eradicate HBV, nor do they cure the infection. For all we know, they have to be used indefinitely. For now, they do offer the greatest hope for treatment of chronic hepatitis B by controlling HBV replication and arresting or halting the progression of liver disease. The data do seem to indicate that entecavir should be considered as the primary therapy for certain forms of hepatitis B infection such as HBeAg-negative chronic hepatitis B, certainly in patients not previously treated with other nucleoside analogues.

J. A. Stockman III, MD

Safety and Efficacy of an Attenuated Vaccine Against Severe Rotavirus Gastroenteritis

O'Ryan M, for the Human Rotavirus Vaccine Study Group (Univ of Chile, Santiago; et al)

N Engl J Med 354:11-22, 2006   10–34

Background.—The safety and efficacy of an attenuated G1P[8] human rotavirus (HRV) vaccine were tested in a randomized, double-blind, phase 3 trial.

Methods.—We studied 63,225 healthy infants from 11 Latin American countries and Finland who received two oral doses of either the HRV vaccine (31,673 infants) or placebo (31,552 infants) at approximately two months and four months of age. Severe gastroenteritis episodes were identified by active surveillance. The severity of disease was graded with the use of the 20-point Vesikari scale. Vaccine efficacy was evaluated in a subgroup of 20,169 infants (10,159 vaccinees and 10,010 placebo recipients).

Results.—The efficacy of the vaccine against severe rotavirus gastroenteritis and against rotavirus-associated hospitalization was 85 percent (P<0.001 for the comparison with placebo) and reached 100 percent against more severe rotavirus gastroenteritis. Hospitalization for diarrhea of any cause was reduced by 42 percent (95 percent confidence interval, 29 to 53 percent; P<0.001). During the 31-day window after each dose, six vaccine recipients and seven placebo recipients had definite intussusception (difference in risk, -0.32 per 10,000 infants; 95 percent confidence interval, -2.91 to 2.18; $P=0.78$).

Conclusions.—Two oral doses of the live attenuated G1P[8] HRV vaccine were highly efficacious in protecting infants against severe rotavirus gastro-enteritis, significantly reduced the rate of severe gastroenteritis from any cause, and were not associated with an increased risk of intussusception.

▶ It has been some years since the first licensed rotavirus vaccine (RotaShield) was withdrawn from the US market. This was less than a year after its introduction because it became apparent that the vaccine was associated with an uncommon but potentially life-threatening adverse event— intussusception—at an estimated rate of 1 incident per 10,000 vaccine recipients. For a short while, elsewhere in the world, this vaccine continued to be used largely because of the profound problem rotavirus causes, particularly in the undeveloped world. It soon became apparent, however, that it was untenable to continue the use of this vaccine in developing countries when the "better-off" countries, such as the United States, had stopped its use. The manufacture of the first rotavirus vaccine was halted, and hope was lost for a vaccine that could have prevented much severe diarrhea, and death, around the world. As it turns out, 2 vaccine manufacturers accepted the challenge of producing a safe vaccine, and 2 reports have appeared in *The New England Journal of Medicine* showing promising results of large clinical trials of these 2 new rotavirus vaccines.

The 2 new vaccine products are Rotateq from Merck and Rotarix from GlaxoSmithKline. Both vaccines are orally administered and intended to be given to infants at the same time as their immunizations for diphtheria, pertussis, and tetanus. The vaccines differ in their approaches, strains, and formulations. Rotarix is a monovalent vaccine derived from the most common human rotavirus strain, G1P[8], that has been attenuated by serial passage, and is administered in 2 oral doses 1 to 2 months apart. This vaccine strain replicates in the gut, is shed by more than 50% of patients receiving the vaccine after the first dose, and (like natural rotavirus infections) provides cross-protection against most other serotypes. By contrast, Rotateq is a pentavalent vaccine based on a bovine strain, WC3, that contains 5 human-bovine reassortant viruses. WC3 is naturally attenuated for humans but is not broadly cross-protective. Each reassortant virus contains a single gene encoding a major outer capsid protein from the most common human serotypes. The bovine virus grows less well in the human intestine, so the aggregate titer required to immunize a child is greater. In addition, the vaccine strains are infrequently shed in the stool, and 3 oral doses are required, with at least a month between doses.

Despite the differences between the vaccines, both vaccines demonstrate a very high efficacy profile. The differences in observed efficacy against severe rotavirus disease (85% for Rotarix and 98% for Rotateq) may very well be explained by differences in the classification of disease severity and the populations studied. GlaxoSmithKline conducted its trials primarily among infants of poor and middle-income families in Latin America, whereas Merck tested its vaccine in the United States and Finland. In Latin America, Rotarix vaccination

Absent the rotavirus vaccine, about 20% of physician visits for diarrhea and about 30% of hospitalizations for diarrhea have been attributable to rotavirus infections here in the United States. This translates into an estimated 400,000 physician visits and 50,000 hospitalizations annually, with an economic impact exceeding $1 billion per year. The majority of these costs relate to direct medical care including hospitalizations. Nonetheless, the aggregate estimated non-medical cost runs in the $22 million range annually.

Rotavirus = not chump change.

J. A. Stockman III, MD

Reference

1. Lee BP, Azimi PH, Staat MA, et al: Nonmedical costs associated with rotavirus disease requiring hospitalization. *Pediatr Infect Dis J* 24:984-988, 2005.

West Nile Virus Infection Among Pregnant Women in a Northern Colorado Community, 2003 to 2004
Paisley JE, Hinckley AF, O'Leary DR, et al (Univ of Colorado, Denver; Poudre Valley Hosp, Fort Collins, Colo; Ctrs for Disease Control and Prevention, Fort Collins, Colo)
Pediatrics 117:814-820, 2006   10–36

Objective.—Since West Nile virus (WNV) was first detected in New York in 1999, it has spread across North America and become a major public health concern. In 2002, the first documented case of intrauterine WNV infection was reported, involving an infant with severe brain abnormalities. To determine the frequencies of WNV infections during pregnancy and of intrauterine WNV infections, we measured WNV-specific antibodies in cord blood from infant deliveries after a community-wide epidemic of WNV disease.

Methods.—Five hundred sixty-six pregnant women who presented to Poudre Valley Hospital (Fort Collins, CO) for delivery between September 2003 and May 2004 provided demographic and health history data through self-administered questionnaires and hospital admission records. Umbilical cord blood was collected from 549 infants and screened for WNV-specific IgM and IgG antibodies with enzyme-linked immunosorbent assays, with confirmation by plaque-reduction neutralization tests. Newborn growth parameters, Apgar scores, and hearing test results were recorded.

Results.—Four percent (95% confidence interval: 2.4–5.7%) of cord blood samples tested positive for WNV-specific IgG antibodies. No cord blood samples were positive for WNV-specific IgM antibodies. There were no significant differences between infants of seropositive and seronegative mothers with respect to any of the growth parameters or outcomes measured.

Conclusions.—Intrauterine WNV infections seemed to be infrequent. In our study, WNV infection during pregnancy did not seem to affect adversely infant health at birth. Larger prospective studies are necessary to measure more completely the effects of maternal WNV infection on pregnancy and infant health outcomes.

▶ The WNV saga is now exactly 8 years old. The virus is a flavivirus transmitted to humans primarily through the bite of infected mosquitoes. Just 5 years ago, the first documented case of intrauterine WNV infection was reported. This involved an infant who appeared grossly normal at birth but had bilateral chorioretinitis and severe cystic destruction of temporal and occipital cerebral tissue. Shortly after this case report, 4 additional cases of infection during pregnancy were reported. Of the 4, 3 infections apparently resulted in no fetal infection or adverse outcome for the infants. In one instance, an otherwise normal premature infant was not tested for WNV infection, so we do not know the outcome of that case. It was also in 2002 that probable transmission via breast milk was reported, but without apparent health consequences for the infant.

This report from Colorado is important because it gives us a better understanding of exactly how common WNV infection is during pregnancy and also provides us with precise information about fetal outcomes. WNV was first detected in Colorado, the site of this report, in 2002 when WNV-positive birds and 14 human cases were reported. The following year, almost 3000 human disease cases were reported in Colorado. Many of these were near Fort Collins, a community of 125,000 people located 65 miles north of Denver on the Front Range of the Rocky Mountains. A single hospital, Poudre Valley Hospital, serves Fort Collins and surrounding communities and is the only birthing hospital for the area, thus allowing for the ability to carefully document the prevalence in pregnant women of WNV infection.

What we learn from the Colorado experience is critical to the understanding of how much of a role this virus plays in pregnancy. The Colorado report is the first study to evaluate the seroprevalence of WNV antibodies among pregnant women and their offspring. This seroprevalence was 4%. Importantly, none of the newborn infants of infected mothers had detectable WNV-specific IgM antibodies. We do not know enough about an infant's ability to produce antibody to be sure that no infants were infected. It is possible that some congenitally infected infants (such as perhaps those infected during the first trimester) do not produce detectable concentrations of WNV-specific IgM antibodies in response to infection. What we do know from this report, however, is that women with WNV infection do not seem to have any greater risk of delivering preterm, of having infants with low birth weight, or of having infants with intrauterine growth problems.

The data from this report should provide some degree of reassurance that infection with the WNV during pregnancy will not commonly result in congenital WNV infection or serious problems in the neonatal period. This is not to say that it will not in some infants cause problems, however.

See the Oncology chapter (Abstract 16–5) for a report of WNV infection in a teenage boy with acute lymphocytic leukemia in remission.

J. A. Stockman III, MD

Bone Marrow Transplantation for Severe Combined Immune Deficiency

Grunebaum E, Mazzolari E, Porta F, et al (Univ of Toronto; Univ of Brescia, Italy)
JAMA 295:508-518, 2006   10–37

Context.—Bone marrow transplantation (BMT) using stem cells obtained from a family-related, HLA-identical donor (RID) is the optimal treatment for patients with severe combined immune deficiency (SCID). In the absence of an RID, HLA-mismatched related donors (MMRDs) are often used. However, compared with RIDs, use of MMRDs for BMT is associated with reduced survival and inferior long-term immune reconstitution. Use of HLA-matched unrelated donors (MUDs) represents another potential alternative for BMT.

Objective.—To compare outcomes and immune reconstitution in a large cohort of patients with SCID who received RID, MUD, or MMRD BMT.

Design, Setting, and Patients.—Retrospective study of medical records from 94 infants diagnosed as having SCID who received BMT between 1990 and 2004 at 1 Canadian and 1 Italian pediatric referral center. Thirteen, 41, and 40 patients received RID, MUD, and MMRD BMT, respectively.

Main Outcome Measures.—Survival and graft failure, along with incidence of graft-vs-host disease, infections, and other complications; immune reconstitution was assessed in children who survived for more than 2 years after BMT.

Results.—Survival after RID BMT was highest. Twelve (92.3%) of 13 patients who received RID BMT, 33 (80.5%) of 41 who received MUD BMT, and 21 (52.5%) of 40 patients who received MMRD BMT survived. Compared with MMRD BMT, survival was significantly higher with RID ($P = .008$) or with MUD ($P = .03$). Graft failures and need for repeat BMT were more common in patients receiving MMRD BMT than in those who underwent MUD BMT. Long-term reconstitution of a full T-cell repertoire was achieved more frequently following MUD BMT (94.7%) than after MMRD BMT (61.1%) ($P = .02$). Acute graft-vs-host disease was documented in 73.1% of patients following MUD BMT but in only 45% after MMRD BMT ($P = .009$). Conversely, interstitial pneumonitis was observed more frequently after MMRD BMT (14 [35.0%] of 40) than after MUD BMT (3 [7.3%] of 41; $P = .002$).

Conclusion.—Our study suggests that in the absence of a relative with identical HLA, MUD BMT may provide better engraftment, immune reconstitution, and survival for patients with SCID than MMRD BMT.

▶ Most pediatricians will not be involved with the care of a patient with SCID. The disease is just too rare (1 in 50,000 to 1 in 100,000 live births). Death in this disease is universal unless treated by hematopoietic stem cell transplantation. The treatment of choice is from an RID, which unfortunately is available only for a minority of patients with SCID. If this modality of therapy is available, the long-term survival is well over 90%. This survival falls to about 50% in patients undergoing MMRD BMT. Better than this is the use of MUD bone marrow, as we see in this report. Not only does MUD bone marrow result in a significant increase in survival of patients with SCID, but it also results in excellent long-term immune reconstitution. In this series, more than 80% of patients receiving such a transplant had robust immune reconstitution. An 80% cure rate for an otherwise lethal disease is not bad. Yes, there is a chance of graft-vs-host disease, but this can usually be managed.

This is the last entry in this chapter, so we will close with a query. Some have suggested that marriage leads to illness. Speculation aside, what is the largest epidemic of illness related to marriages that occurred on one weekend in one city? It turns out that a single bakery is accountable for causing a gastroenteritis outbreak at 46 weddings that took place over one weekend back in 2002. The norovirus involved affected 39% of the wedding guests who partook of the contaminated wedding cakes. Some 2,700 people developed barfing and loose stools. Two bakery workers had experienced a norovirus-type illness during the week before the wedding weekend, but they could not take off work since they had to complete the order for the 46 wedding cakes. Every single cake was handled directly by these 2 people who applied the finishing touches to each cake. Yes indeed, getting married can be injurious to your health.[1]

J. A. Stockman III, MD

Reference

1. Friedman DS, Heisey-Grove D, Argyros F, et al: An outbreak of norovirus gastroenteritis associated with wedding cakes. *Epidemiol Infect* 133:1057-1063, 2005.

11 Miscellaneous

Can We Abolish Skull X Rays for Head Injury?
Reed MJ, Browning JG, Wilkinson AG, et al (Royal Hosp for Sick Children, Edinburgh, Scotland)
Arch Dis Child 90:859-864, 2005

11–1

Objectives.—To assess the effect of a change in skull x ray policy on the rate of admission, use of computed tomography (CT), radiation dose per head injury, and detection of intracranial injuries; and to compare the characteristics of patients with normal and abnormal head CT.

Design.—Retrospective cohort study.

Setting.—UK paediatric teaching hospital emergency department.

Patients.—1535 patients aged between 1 and 14 years with a head injury presenting to the emergency department between 1 August 1998 and 31 July 1999 (control period), and 1867 presenting between 1 August 2002 and 31 July 2003 (first year of new skull x ray policy).

Intervention.—Hospital notes and computer systems were analysed and data were collected on all patients presenting with a head injury.

Results.—The abolition of skull x rays in children aged over 1 year prevented about 400 normal skull x rays being undertaken in period 2. The percentage of children undergoing CT rose from 1.0% to 2.1% with no change in the positive CT pick up rate (25.6% v 25.0%). There was no significant change in admission rate (10.9% v 10.1%), and a slight decrease in the radiation dose per head injury (0.042 mSv compared to 0.045 mSv).

Conclusions.—Skull x rays can be abandoned in children aged 1 to 14 without a significant increase in admission rate, radiation dose per head injury, or missed intracranial injury. The mechanism and history of the injury and a reduced Glasgow coma scale are probably the most important indicators of significant head injury in children.

▶ This article is from Great Britain. There, the National Institute for Clinical Effectiveness (NICE) sets guidelines for a number of different clinical entities in terms of practice management. NICE guidelines suggest that skull radiographs have a role combined with high-quality inpatient observation but only where CT is not available. In Scotland, the Intercollegiate Guideline Network guidelines place more emphasis on skull radiographs in situations in which risk factors for fractures or intracranial injuries exist, although it is generally acknowledged that skull fractures in children are less commonly associated with intracranial injuries; therefore, their detection is less helpful than in the adult population. Here in the United States, virtually all management guidelines omit the need for skull radiographs, and CT is the predominant scanning mode. In the United States, up to 60% of head-injured patients will go on to have a CT, and resultant low positivity rates run between 5% and 10%. Even when results are positive, fewer than 30% of those with intracranial abnormalities on CT scanning go on to require neurosurgical intervention. It does seem appropriate to go right to CT; however, one must recognize the problem with the positive predictive value of such an expensive test. Also, one must recognize that, even if a routine skull series is performed, plain radiographs of the skull are frequently misread in a false-positive or false-negative way. Most pediatricians also recognize that severe intracranial injuries can occur in the absence of a skull fracture.

If one puts all these facts into a bag and shakes them up, what comes out is the conclusion of this article from Great Britain, that is, that skull radiographs can be abandoned in children between the ages of 1 and 14 years without a significant increase in misdiagnosis, which, however, is obviously dependent on where you practice and how good your history and physical examination skills are.

While on the topic of things having to do with radiology, recognize that the typical primary care physician here in the US receives some 800 chemistry reports, 40 radiology reports, and 12 pathology reports each week.[1] Some 83% of primary care physicians surveyed report delays in receipt of such tests and only 41% of primary care physicians indicate they are satisfied with how test results are managed. US Courts have placed a clear onus on the radiologist to communicate abnormal radiology findings with many cases in which the radiologist has been found personally negligent for not making such efforts.[2] Furthermore, where efforts were in fact made to contact clinicians, the radiologist was still found to be negligent because communication was inadequately documented. Part of the reason for the problem has to do with the national shortage of radiologists. Pediatric radiologists seem to do a better job at communication than their adult counterparts (personal observation), but unfortunately pediatric radiology, workforce wise, is in trouble. Approximately 3% of all radiologists, some 800 to 900 physicians, are pediatric radiologists. Depending on how pediatric radiology is defined, two thirds to three quarters of pediatric radiologists spend 70% or more of their clinical work time doing pediatric radiology. While the number of pediatric radiologists has been growing, that growth is fairly slow and evidence currently exists that there is a likely shortage here in the United States. This situation is likely to become worse based on several factors. The workload of the radiology profession is increasing rapidly, fueled largely by scientific advances (new imaging techniques and advances in existing techniques) that allow radiology to do more for patients. Findings of a recent report suggest that the number of pediatric radiologists is not likely to expand to meet this growing need.[3]

With respect to the average age of a pediatric radiologist, it is unexpectedly older than one might anticipate. The average age is 55 years, which exceeds the average age of any of the medical subspecialties of pediatrics (the next oldest subspecialty average age is 54 in the field of pediatric nephrology, with the youngest average age of pediatric medical subspecialist being the emergency medicine physician at age 44). Among the pediatric subspecialties boarded by the American Board of Pediatrics, if pediatric radiology were to fit in in comparison to these specialties, it would be the 10th down the line in terms of size, with nephrology having almost the same number of subspecialists, and pediatric hematology-oncology and cardiology having more than twice as many subspecialists as there are pediatric radiologists.

One final comment about pediatric radiology, unlike general radiology and the other specialties of radiology, pediatric radiology has a disproportionate number of women practicing in the field. Specifically, one third or more of pediatric radiologists are women versus just 19% for the other subspecialties of radiology in hospital-based academic practices. Pediatric radiologists who spend more than 70% of their clinical work time in pediatrics indicate that they would like to have a significant reduction in their workload even if it meant a corresponding reduction in income.

J. A. Stockman III, MD

References

1. Poon EG, Gandhi TK, Sequist TD, et al: I wish I had seen this test result earlier! *Arch Intern Med* 164:2223-2228, 2004.
2. Garvey CJ, Connolly S: Radiology reporting—where does the radiologist's duty end? *Lancet* 367:443-445, 2006.
3. Marewitz L, Sunshine JH: A portrait of pediatric radiologists in the United States. *AJR* 186:12-22, 2006.

Simulation of Pediatric Trauma Stabilization in 35 North Carolina Emergency Departments: Identification of Targets for Performance Improvement

Hunt EA, Hohenhaus SM, Luo X, et al (Johns Hopkins Univ, Baltimore, Md; Duke Univ, Durham, NC)
Pediatrics 117:641-648, 2006
11–2

Objective.—Trauma is the leading cause of death in children. Most children present to community hospital emergency departments (EDs) for initial stabilization. Thus, all EDs must be prepared to care for injured children. The objectives of this study were to (1) characterize the quality of trauma stabilization efforts in EDs and (2) identify targets for educational interventions.

Methods.—This was a prospective observational study of simulated trauma stabilizations, that is, "mock codes," at 35 North Carolina EDs. An evaluation tool was created to score each mock code on 44 stabilization tasks. Primary outcomes were (1) interrater reliability of tool, (2) overall performance by each ED, and (3) performance per stabilization task.

Results.—Evaluation-tool interrater reliability was excellent. The median number of stabilization tasks that needed improvement by the EDs was 25 (57%) of 44 tasks. Although problems were numerous and varied, many

EDs need improvement in tasks uniquely important and/or complicated in pediatric resuscitations, including (1) estimating a child's weight (17 of 35 EDs [49%]), (2) preparing for intraosseous needle placement (24 of 35 [69%]), (3) ordering intravenous fluid boluses (31 of 35 [89%]), (4) applying warming measures (34 of 35 [97%]), and (5) ordering dextrose for hypoglycemia (34 of 35 [97%]).

Conclusions.—This study used simulation to identify deficiencies in stabilization of children presenting to EDs, revealing that mistakes are ubiquitous. ED personnel were universally receptive to feedback. Future research should investigate whether interventions aimed at improving identified deficiencies can improve trauma stabilization performance and, ultimately, the outcomes of children who present to EDs.

▶ Three cheers for Hunt et al. They have created a model simulation that allows EDs delivering care to children to assess how "ready" and complete they are to receive and to care for a pediatric emergency. The EDs involved agreed to the study, which included a "surprise" presentation to the ED triage area of a child-sized mannequin. One clinical vignette consisted of a 3-year-old child brought in by his mother. The triage nurse was told that the child had fallen off a tall slide, did not move for a while, and had been very sleepy since the fall. He was described as lying quietly in his mother's arms and breathing spontaneously, with dried blood on his face. The triage nurse was instructed to proceed as if this were a true emergency requiring a code. This particular study was quite expansive, involving a visit to one third of all the EDs in North Carolina. The findings, however, are probably not unique to North Carolina and showed many mistakes requiring the need for additional training to manage children in EDs.

You should be aware that there is a strong push, and some urgency, to move to an all-or-none measurement of quality reporting. Currently, there are at least 3 different options for calculating performance on multiple, discreet measures for the same condition. One is the item-by-item measurement, which takes each item being measured and scores the measurement separately even though multiple measurements of different items may have been performed. Another approach is known as the composite measurement, in which performance on the provision of several elements of care is reported by computing a percentage across all patients and criterion indicators. Let us say that there are 4 recommended measurement objectives and a patient receives 3 of these 4. A hospital or physician whose performance is assessed with a composite measurement would get credit for delivering 3 elements. The third option is known as the all-or-none measurement. A percentage is determined by applying an all-or-none rule at the patient level. For example, in pneumonia care, the denominator would be the number of patients eligible to receive the discreet measurement elements of care, and the numerator would be the number of patients who actually received all the care for which the specific patient was eligible. No partial credit is given.

In measurement terms, the all-or-none approach of process quality was recently described by Nolan and Berwick.[1] The all-or-none approach of process quality yields a picture quite different from either the item-by-item approach or the composite approach. According to the 2004 National Healthcare Quality Report, for example, the item-by-item measurement shows the following performance standards in diabetes care: hemoglobin A_{1c} testing, 90.0%; lipid profiling, 93.8%; retinal examinations, 69.7%; foot examinations, 66.3%; and influenza vaccination, 56.5%.[2] However, all 5 of these interventions reached only 32.1% of all eligible patients. HealthPartners, an integrated care system based in Minneapolis and the first major health care organization that has reported all-or-none measurements, found typical performance ranging from 37.4% to 92.4% for each of the 7 process measures of diabetes care, but only 7.6% of patients received all 7 interventions.[3]

Pay attention to the all-or-none measurement of quality performance. It does raise the bar in the journey to high-quality health care. Patients seem to recognize this as a better methodology for assessing whether they get total care. It also fosters a systems perspective to quality improvement, and it clearly offers a more sensitive scale for assessing improvements. According to item-level process measures, many hospitals are achieving more than 90% compliance with individual elements of care, and this leaves little room on the scale for setting goals and measuring progress. High scores seem to dampen enthusiasm for further improvement, even if overall reliability for complete processes remains low. If 5 items in a measurement set are statistically independent and each allows 90% reliability, only 59% of patients will actually receive all the care they need, an example of why all-or-none measurement raises the bar.

One final comment on quality care in the emergency room. The most powerful predictor of waiting times in emergency departments is the time of arrival. Analysis of data from more than 75,000 patients to see who waits the longest and who leaves without being seen found that patient characteristics were far less important than the time they presented themselves to an emergency room. Arriving at night, on a Monday or Sunday, and during the autumn were linked to significantly longer waits. When analyzing what patient was most likely to bolt from an emergency room because of a lack of patience with respect to waiting, it was a young male who self-referred to the emergency room. These individuals tended to be those who would leave without being seen.[4]

Some would say that quality with respect to patient care is not an all-or-none phenomenon. Then again, why can it not be?

J. A. Stockman III, MD

References

1. Nolan T, Berwick DM: All-or-none measurement raises the bar on performance. *JAMA* 295:1168-1170, 2006.
2. Agency for Healthcare Research in Quality: *2004 National Healthcare Quality Report.* Washington, DC, US Department of Health and Human Services, AHRQ Publication 05-0013, 2004.
3. Amundsen G, Wehrle D: HealthPartners: 2004 clinical indicators report, http://www.healthpartners.com/files/24880.pdf, accessed March 21, 2006.
4. Goodacre S, Webster A: Who waits longest in the emergency department and who leaves without being seen? *Emerg Med J* 22:93-96, 2005.

Pediatric Emergencies on a US-Based Commercial Airline

Moore BR, Ping JM, Claypool DW (Mayo Clinic and College of Medicine, Rochester, Minn)
Pediatr Emerg Care 21:725-729, 2005   11–3

Objectives.—The purpose of this investigation was to determine the incidence and character of pediatric emergencies on a US-based commercial airline and to evaluate current in-flight medical kits.

Methods.—In-flight consultations to a major US airline by a member of our staff are recorded in an institutional database. In this observational retrospective review, the database was queried for consultations for all passengers up to 18 years old between January 1, 1995, and December 31, 2002. Consultations were reviewed for type of emergency, use of the medical kit, and unscheduled landings.

Results.—Two hundred twenty-two pediatric consultations were identified, representing 1 pediatric call per 20,775 flights. The mean age of patients was 6.8 years. Fifty-three emergencies were preflight calls, and 169 were in-flight pediatric consultations. The most common in-flight consultations concerned infectious disease (45 calls, 27%), neurological (25 calls, 15%), and respiratory tract (22 calls, 13%) emergencies. The emergency medical kit was used for 60 emergencies. Nineteen consultations (11%) resulted in flight diversions (1/240,000 flights), most commonly because of in-flight neurological (9) and respiratory tract (5) emergencies. International flights had a higher incidence than domestic flights of consultations and diversions for pediatric emergencies.

Conclusions.—The most common in-flight pediatric emergencies involved infectious diseases and neurological and respiratory tract problems. Emergency medical kits should be expanded to include pediatric medications.

▶ There is no more chilling series of words to be heard than, "Is there a doctor on board the plane?" The chill comes from the expectation that a physician is a physician is a physician; in other words, that any physician can take care of any problem. This article from Rochester, Minnesota, gives us some information about what an in-flight emergency involving a pediatric patient might entail. We learn that in 2001, US commercial airliners flew 547 million passengers, accounting for 613 billion passenger miles. Estimates of in-flight medical emergencies occurring on flights vary between 0.003% (1/333 flights per year) and 0.0005% (1/1900 flights per year). The usual emergencies occurring at any age include trauma, syncope, and gastrointestinal tract, cardiac, respiratory tract, psychiatric, and neurological illnesses. Somewhere between 21 and 72 in-flight deaths occur per year on commercial carriers in the United States. Most of these deaths are natural deaths in elderly patients, commonly attributable to cardiac and pulmonary disease. Unfortunately, no central registry exists for these emergencies; therefore, true incidence figures are undetermined. In-flight emergency reporting to the US Department of Transportation is not mandatory unless death occurs or a flight is diverted.

If you are called to assist in an emergency, please be aware that you may not be totally on your own. Some airlines, for example, contract for services to assist in a medical emergency; these contract services are on the ground and available by phone. For example, the Mayo Clinic Departments of Emergency Medicine and Medical Transportation Service and the Division of Aerospace Medicine provide in-flight consultation to a large major US airline. This airline provides service to approximately 10% of all US passengers. All data related to the consultations provided are collected in the Mayo In-Flight Advisory Reports database. It is this database that was the source of the information provided in the article, and it gives us excellent insights regarding in-flight emergencies involving children.

The Mayo In-Flight Advisory Registry recorded some 222 pediatric emergency consultations between 1995 and 2002, which represented about 9.2% of consultations for all passengers. The math is fairly clear. There was 1 pediatric emergency consultation for every 20,775 flights. The average age of the pediatric patient needing emergency attention was 6.8 years. Of all the pediatric emergencies, 60 required opening the onboard emergency medical kit, mostly for neurologic, allergic, gastrointestinal, and infectious disease emergencies. Just 11% of emergencies caused the flights to make an unscheduled landing (which is a rate of about 1 in one quarter million flights). The most common causes of diversion were neurologic and respiratory tract emergencies. The average cost of a diversion was about $50,000. All the neurologic emergencies resulting in diversion were on account of seizures, most of which were grand mal, lasting for an extended period of time. Asthma was the basis for diversion for respiratory tract problems.

You should be aware that the mean cabin pressure during air flight is equivalent to an altitude of approximately 6900 feet (slightly lower than the atmospheric pressure found in Aspen, Colorado). This will correspond to a decrease in alveolar partial pressure of oxygen from 109 mm Hg at sea level to 70 mm Hg at 7000 feet. This can have some cardiovascular and pulmonary effects in children who have pre-existing conditions such as anemia or cardiopulmonary disease.

One final comment: when a pediatric emergency occurs on a flight of a US-based airline, the onboard emergency kit is usually ill-equipped to manage it. The Federal Aviation Administration requires large aircraft to contain emergency medical kits, and this requirement was first implemented in 1986. The cost is fairly minimal ($94 per year per aircraft). The original design of the kits was modified in 1994 to include protective gloves and was modified again in 2001 to include automatic external defibrillators. Medications in these kits are fairly limited and mostly consist of glucose, epinephrine, diphenhydramine, and nitroglycerin. Although not required to, most airlines carry a supplemental medical kit that includes some medications appropriate for children. There is no standardization of this supplemental medical kit across airlines. Of course, all airlines carry oxygen for emergency purposes. The limited supply of medications means that children with seizures or asthma are unable to be treated in flight because aircraft do not carry antiepileptics or inhaled β_2-agonist inhalers. Children with in-flight fevers usually cannot be treated because the emergency kits do not include liquid forms of antipyretics. The easiest way to obtain some of these medications is to ask the passengers on the flight what they might have on their persons. Most times, however, these are not in an appropriate dose form for children's use.

One concluding comment about in-flight illnesses. Some are caused by the airlines themselves. Most of us have undoubtedly noticed that airlines no longer serve meals on many flights here in the US. Passengers are encouraged instead to purchase their snacks from airport fast-food restaurants and carry them onboard. Not at all bad because you have a choice of what you eat and you can avoid food-borne illness occasionally associated with airline meals. For example, in August 2004 and reported recently on cnn.com, 45 passengers in 22 states and Japan, Australia, and American Samoa experienced illness caused by *Shigella sonnei*. The likely source of this was contaminated carrots in a salad prepared by Gate Gourmet, Inc, that has facilities in 30 countries and provides meals to many airlines. Chances are the plane "facilities" were quite occupied as a result of Gate Gourmet. Bon appetite![1]

Now you have the skinny on in-flight emergencies involving children. Fly the friendly skies, knowing that you will have to keep your wits about you because you will have limited options to manage problems as they occur.

J. A. Stockman III, MD

Reference

1. Airline food (editorial). *Pediatr Infect Dis* 24:1, 2005.

Pediatric Intravenous Insertion in the Emergency Department: Bevel Up or Bevel Down?

Black KJL, Pusic MV, Harmidy D, et al (Dalhousie Univ, Halifax, Nova Scotia, Canada; Univ of British Columbia, Vancouver, Canada; Montreal Children's Hosp; et al)
Pediatr Emerg Care 21:707-711, 2005   11–4

Objective.—Intravenous catheters are usually inserted with the bevel facing up. Bevel down may be superior in small and/or dehydrated children. We seek to determine whether there is a difference in the success rate of intravenous insertion using these 2 methods.

Methods.—We recruited children requiring an intravenous catheter in the emergency department where there was time to obtain consent. Patients were randomized to have the first attempt bevel up or bevel down. If the first attempt was unsuccessful, the alternate technique was used on second attempt. Attempts beyond 2 were not tracked.

Results.—We recruited 428 patients. Data are available from 396 (201 bevel-up and 195 bevel-down techniques). At least 63 different nurses participated. The nurses participated in the study a median number of 2 times (maximum, 36). Four nurses used the bevel-down technique more than 10 times. The success rate on first attempt was 75.6% (95% confidence interval [CI], 69.8–81.4) for bevel up and 60% (95% CI, 53.2–66.8) for bevel down.

The success rate on second attempt was 56.8% (95% CI, 45.30–68.2) for bevel up and 42.9% (95% CI, 30.3–55.5) for bevel down. In the subgroup of infants weighing less than 5 kg, there was no difference between the 2 techniques on the first attempt, with bevel up having a success of 33% (95% CI, 8.4–57.6) and bevel down 30% (95% CI, 4.1–55.9).

Conclusions.—The bevel-up technique performed superior to bevel-down technique in this study. The bevel-down technique might be useful in small infants.

▶ It is interesting to see how local custom dictates how needles are placed. This article looks at whether bevel up or bevel down is best. Most in North America insert the needle with the bevel facing upward; in some places (for example, in Belgium), the bevel down technique is more prevalent. Some textbooks suggest that the bevel-down technique may be superior in the small or dehydrated child. This goes way back to a study done by Filston and Johnson more than 30 years ago.[1] The theory behind this recommendation is that, with the bevel down, the tip of the needle is less likely to pierce the opposite side of a small blood vessel.

The folks from Canada who now have actually studied whether bevel up or bevel down is best tell us that the success rates in an emergency department setting on first attempt to put a needle in is 75.6% for bevel up and 60% for bevel down. The success rate on second attempt is 56.8% for bevel up and 42.9% for bevel down. For infants weighing less than 15 kg, essentially no difference was found between the 2 techniques on the first attempt: the bevel up approach had a success rate of 33%, and the bevel down approach had a success rate of 30%.

The findings of this article will not change anyone's current attitudes toward what technique for needle insertion they personally prefer. New safety catheters are now being introduced across North America. These new IV catheters are designed to be inserted only with the bevel up. Perhaps these new needles will take the preferences out of our hands.

J. A. Stockman III, MD

Reference

1. Filston HC, Johnson DG: Percutaneous venous cannulation in newborns and infants: A method for catheter insertion without "cut down." *Pediatrics* 48:896-901, 1971.

Clinical and Laboratory Manifestations of Kikuchi's Disease in Children and Differences Between Patients With and Without Prolonged Fever

Chuang C-H, Yan D-C, Chiu C-H, et al (Chang Gung Children's Hosp, Kweishan, Taoyuan, Taiwan; Chang Gung Mem Hosp, Kewishan, Taoyuan, Taiwan)
Pediatr Infect Dis J 24:551-554, 2005   11–5

Background.—Kikuchi's disease (KD) is characterized by cervical lymphadenopathy with or without fever. It has been recognized worldwide but seldom reported in pediatric patients.

Methods.—From January 1985 through December 2001, 64 patients younger than 18 years of age with pathologic proof of KD were enrolled in this study. The clinical manifestations, laboratory data and outcomes were reviewed.

Results.—There were 35 male patients and 29 female patients with age ranging from 2 to 18 years and a median age of 16. All patients had cervical lymphadenopathy except 1 who had generalized lymphadenopathy. Lymph nodes of 32 patients (50%) were painful or tender or both. Lymphadenopathy was unilateral in 52 patients (82.5%). Lymphadenopathy associated with fever was observed in 21 patients (32.8%). Other signs such as skin rash, hepatomegaly or body weight loss were less common. Twenty-six patients (40.6%) had leukopenia and 2 patients had leukocytosis. Nearly one-fourth of the patients had mild liver dysfunction. Virologic or immunologic studies were normal in most patients. Patients with prolonged fever were more likely to have leukopenia ($P < 0.05$). All patients recovered, but 1 developed systemic lupus erythematosus 5 years later, and the other had vasculitis syndrome 2 years later.

Conclusions.—The clinical presentation of KD in pediatric patients is similar to that of adults. KD is a benign, self-limiting disease; prolonged fever occurred only in 32.8% of pediatric patients in our cohort. Leukopenia was the only feature significantly associated with prolonged fever.

Kikuchi-Fujimoto Disease Is a Rare Cause of Lymphadenopathy and Fever of Unknown Origin in Children: Report of Two Cases and Review of the Literature

Scagni P, Peisino MG, Bianchi M, et al (Children's Hosp Regina Margherita, Torino, Italy; Univ of Torino, Italy)
J Pediatr Hematol Oncol 27:337-340, 2005   11–6

Background.—Kikuchi-Fujimoto disease (KFD) is an unusual histiocytic necrotizing lymphadenitis with a higher prevalence among young Asian adults, mainly women. KFG is benign and self-limiting and has rarely been reported in children; thus, it is frequently confused with malignant melanoma. Two cases of KFD in Italian children of Caucasian origin were described and implications for management were discussed.

Case 1.—Boy, 11, was seen with a 6-week history of high-grade fever, fatigue, weight loss, and swelling on both sides of the neck. The parents described recent onset of sweats and a transient generalized erythematous skin rash 2 weeks after the initial fever. The patient had been treated with antibiotics for presumed infection with no improvement. He appeared ill and anorexic on admission, with a weight loss of 2 kg and an axillary daily spiking fever of up to 40°C.

The only finding on physical examination was a bilateral cervical chain of lymph nodes approximately 0.8 to 1 cm in diameter. Laboratory findings were significant only for a mild normochromic, normocytic anemia, leukopenia, and elevated lactate dehydrogenase. The erythrocyte sedimentation rate was also elevated. The clinical picture of fever, general malaise, and night sweats persisted during the investigation, and a presumptive diagnosis of a neoplastic condition prompted aggressive investigation with CT, US, and ^{99}Tc scintigraphy, all of which were unrevealing.

Findings on excisional biopsy of one of the enlarged cervical nodes revealed an architecture completely distorted by diffuse necrosis. Flow cytometry showed the residual lymphoid cells to be T cells, and human leukocyte antigen–DR was highly expressed. The histologic findings and clinical data were consistent with KFD.

Case 2.—Boy, 13, was referred for 2 months of persistent fever, weakness, and fatigue associated with left cervical and supraclavicular lymphadenopathy and increased volume of the left parotid gland. He had been treated 2 weeks earlier with a 7-day course of amoxicillin for presumed bacterial lymphadenitis, with only minimal reduction in parotid gland volume. The family and personal histories were negative for lymphoproliferative disorder. On admission, the boy was febrile (38°C), and physical examination showed a tender, nonfluctuant mass in the left side of the neck. No other lymphadenopathies were observed, nor was hepatosplenomegaly observed.

Laboratory studies revealed mild leukopenia, neutropenia, and thrombocytopenia. Neck and parotid US revealed localized cervical lymphadenopathy, with multiple nodes measuring 0.7 to 2.4 cm, and left parotidomegaly with several hypo-anechoic areas inside. Abdominal US and chest radiograph results were normal, as was ^{99}Tc scintigraphy. CT scans of the neck, chest, and abdomen confirmed previous findings. Bone marrow was normal.

Discussion.—Histiocytic necrotizing lymphadenitis, or KFD, is an unusual self-limiting cause of cervical lymphadenitis. In both cases, the patients recovered spontaneously after 2 to 3 months with symptomatic care in the first case and no specific therapy in the second case. Although KFD is rare in children, it should be considered in the differential diagnosis of many systemic disorders.

There is no specific diagnostic tool for KFD, and the histologic features can be misleading. Therefore, a clinical suspicion in directing the workup and detailed collaboration between clinicians and pathologists are critical to ensuring an accurate diagnosis and minimizing unnecessary investigations and inappropriate or aggressive treatments.

▶ If you have not seen a case of Kikuchi disease, you should read this report in detail since sooner or later you will run into one, even in a general pediatric practice. Kikuchi disease is also known as histiocytic necrotizing lymphadenitis. It was first reported back in 1972 in Japan. Children and young adults presenting with this disorder show cervical lymphadenopathy. This is usually painful and tender.

The disease is usually associated with fever and may have other signs and symptoms including skin rash, hepatomegaly, and weight loss. The most consistent laboratory finding historically in this disease is leukopenia. There are no diagnostic laboratory tests to unequivocally confirm the disease, which is largely based on the clinical presentation and on lymph node biopsy evidence of paracortical necrosis surrounded by a prominent collar of histiocytes with crescentic nuclei, immunoblasts, and plasmacytoid monocytes. Neutrophils are absent from the lymph node pathology. No one as yet knows what the cause of Kikuchi disease is.

This series reported out of Taiwan is important because it provides us with information on a total of 64 pediatric patients with the disorder. This series makes it the largest single series reported out of a single children's hospital. The series informs us of exactly how patients with Kikuchi disease present, both clinically and in the laboratory. As can be seen in the abstract, a variety of findings are present, but the single most common abnormality is cervical lymphadenopathy. Other findings are variable.

Fever was present in only one third of cases. Just 40% of cases had leukopenia. Prolonged fever occurred in 32.8% of patients in this report, which allows one to add Kikuchi disease to the causes of prolonged fever and fever of undetermined origin.

The previous report (Abstract 11–5) gives us additional insights on Kikuchi disease. You will note that the title of this article refers to Kikuchi-Fujimoto disease. It was in 1972 that, in separate articles, this disease was first described. One article was by Kikuchi and the other by Fujimoto et al.[1,2] You can be the one who argues over whether one should call this disease Kikuchi disease or Kikuchi-Fujimoto disease. In all fairness, the 2 reports that appeared in 1972 had a total of 4 authors: Kikuchi, Fujimoto, Kojima, and Yamaguchi, so why not call it by all 4 authors' names?

J. A. Stockman III, MD

References

1. Kikuchi M: Lymphadenitis following focal reticulum cell hyperplasia with nuclear debris and phagocytes. *Acta Haematol Jpn* 35:379-380, 1972.
2. Fujimoto Y, Kojima Y, Yamaguchi K: Cervical subacute necrotizing lymphadenitis. *Naika* 30:920-927, 1972.

Early Experience With Pay-for-Performance: From Concept to Practice
Rosenthal MB, Frank RG, Li Z, et al (Harvard School of Public Health, Boston; Brigham and Women's Hosp, Boston; Harvard Med School, Boston)
JAMA 294:1788-1793, 2005   11–7

Context.—The adoption of pay-for-performance mechanisms for quality improvement is growing rapidly. Although there is intense interest in and optimism about pay-for-performance programs, there is little published research on pay-for-performance in health care.

Objective.—To evaluate the impact of a prototypical physician pay-for-performance program on quality of care.

Design, Setting, and Participants.—We evaluated a natural experiment with pay-for-performance using administrative reports of physician group quality from a large health plan for an intervention group (California physician groups) and a contemporaneous comparison group (Pacific Northwest physician groups). Quality improvement reports were included from October 2001 through April 2004 issued to approximately 300 large physician organizations.

Main Outcome Measures.—Three process measures of clinical quality: cervical cancer screening, mammography, and hemoglobin A_{1c} testing.

Results.—Improvements in clinical quality scores were as follows: for cervical cancer screening, 5.3% for California vs 1.7% for Pacific Northwest; for mammography, 1.9% vs 0.2%; and for hemoglobin A_{1c}, 2.1% vs 2.1%. Compared with physician groups in the Pacific Northwest, the California network demonstrated greater quality improvement after the pay-for-performance intervention only in cervical cancer screening (a 3.6% difference in improvement [$P = .02$]). In total, the plan awarded $3.4 million (27% of the amount set aside) in bonus payments between July 2003 and April 2004, the first year of the program. For all 3 measures, physician groups with baseline performance at or above the performance threshold for receipt of a bonus improved the least but garnered the largest share of the bonus payments.

Conclusion.—Paying clinicians to reach a common, fixed performance target may produce little gain in quality for the money spent and will largely reward those with higher performance at baseline.

▶ Pay-for-performance (P4P) has not been on the radar screen of most pediatricians, at least until recently. We have been late on the tsunami that has affected our adult counterparts. The reason why has to do with the fact that pediatric measures have been tardy in their development in comparison with measures applicable to adult care. Also, the agencies responsible for Medicare and Medicaid have been able to put into place the equivalent of P4P measures for Medicare, but not so easily for Medicaid, which is administered largely by states that have not yet gotten their acts together. Federal control over Medicare allows implementation of P4P in a wholesale, seamless manner. Since there is very little Medicare reimbursement in pediatrics (essentially only for chronic renal disease requiring dialysis), there has been little in the way of P4P initiatives related to the care of children.

This is not to say that a variety of health care plans, employer coalitions, etc, are not using P4P to improve the quality of care provided, including pediatric care. The rationale for P4P comes almost entirely from experience with incentives in other industries. Only 90 randomized controlled trials of P4P have been reported in the literature as of 2005, and even these are not clearly applicable to current P4P because they all have focused on performance for a single indicator or a single aspect of disease (eg, preventive care), whereas most current P4P initiatives use multiple indicators for multiple conditions and types of care.[1] The report of Rosenthal et al offers an excellent example of how current and future research should proceed. These investigators evaluated what would be considered to be a natural experiment using administrative reports from 2 groups, one of which received P4P incentives for cervical cancer screening, mammography, and hemoglobin A_{1c} testing in diabetic patients. They found that paying to reach a common, fixed performance target produced little gain and largely rewarded those with a high performance at baseline. This does not mean that P4P does not work, simply that in the design of this particular approach, it did not work.

To read more about P4P research, see the excellent editorial that appeared in *JAMA*.[2]

J. A. Stockman III, MD

References

1. Baker G, Carter B: *Provider Pay-for-Performance Incentive Programs: 2004 National Study Results.* San Francisco, Med-Vantage, 2005.
2. Dudley RA: Pay-for-performance research: How to learn what clinicians and policy makers need to know (editorial). *JAMA* 294:821-823, 2005.

Use of Personal Child Health Records in the UK: Findings From the Millenium Cohort Study

Walton S, and the Millenium Cohort Study Child Health Group (Inst of Child Health, London)
BMJ 332:269-270, 2006

11–8

Objectives.—The personal child health record (PCHR) is a record of a child's growth, development, and uptake of preventive health services, designed to enhance communication between parents and health professionals. We examined its use throughout the United Kingdom with respect to recording children's weight and measures of social disadvantage and infant health.

Design.—Cross sectional survey within a cohort study.

Setting.—UK.

Participants.—Mothers of 18 503 children born between 2000 and 2002, living in the UK at 9 months of age.

Main Outcome Measures.—Proportion of mothers able to produce their child's PCHR; proportion of PCHRs consulted containing record of child's last weight; effective use of the PCHR (defined as production, consultation, and child's last weight recorded).

Results.—In all, 16 917 (93%) mothers produced their child's PCHR and 15 138 (85%) mothers showed effective use of their child's PCHR. Last weight was recorded in 97% of PCHRs consulted. Effective use was less in children previously admitted to hospital, and, in association with factors reflecting social disadvantage, including residence in disadvantaged communities, young maternal age, large family size (four or more children; incidence rate ratio 0.87; 95% confidence interval 0.83 to 0.91), and lone parent status (0.88; 0.86 to 0.91).

Conclusions.—Use of the PCHR is lower by women living in disadvantaged circumstances, but overall the record is retained and used by a high proportion of all mothers throughout the UK in their child's first year of life. PCHR use is endorsed in the National Service Framework for Children and has potential benefits which extend beyond the direct care of individual children.

▶ In Great Britain, all parents are given a personal health record booklet on their children. This booklet is used as the main record of a child's growth, development, and documentation of preventive health services. The report abstracted shows us how many mothers, in fact, keep this record intact and how accurate the information is. Just 7% of mothers could not produce their child's personal health record, and it was up to date in 97% of cases...outstanding!

Although the use of the personal health record booklet is lower among mothers living in disadvantaged circumstances, overall, the booklet is retained and used by a huge proportion of mothers across the United Kingdom, at least during a child's first year of life. Walton et al have documented in their study of more than 18,000 mothers and children in the Millennium Cohort Study, performed between 2000 and 2002, that even in disadvantaged areas, 90% of mothers keep these records and keep them up to date.

Great Britain seems to be way ahead of the United States not only in the use of PCHRs, retained by parents, but also with respect to the implementation of the electronic medical record. Here in the United States, we pediatricians lag behind family physicians in the percentage of us who have electronic medical record capability. Interestingly, many more pediatricians practice in multi-member practices than family physicians, and one would think that implementation of an electronic medical record would be more cost-effective in such circumstances. We need to become believers. If other countries, and other disciplines within our own country, can do a better job than us, what's holding us back?

J. A. Stockman III, MD

Paper Versus Computer: Feasibility of an Electronic Medical Record in General Pediatrics

Roukema J, Los RK, Bleeker SE, et al (Sophia Children's Hosp, Rotterdam, The Netherlands)

Pediatrics 117:15-21, 2006

11–9

Background.—Implementation of electronic medical record systems promises significant advances in patient care, because such systems enhance readability, availability, and data quality. Structured data entry (SDE) applications can prompt for completeness, provide greater accuracy and better ordering for searching and retrieval, and permit validity checks for data quality monitoring, research, and especially decision support. A generic SDE application (OpenSDE) to support documentation of patient history and physical examination findings was developed and tailored for the domain of general pediatrics.

Objective.—To evaluate OpenSDE for its completeness, uniformity of reporting, and usability in general pediatrics.

Methods.—Four (trainee) pediatricians documented data for 8 first-visit patients in the traditional, paper-based, medical record and immediately thereafter in OpenSDE (electronic record). The 32 paper records obtained served as the common data source for data entry in OpenSDE by the other 3 physicians (transcribed record). Data entered by 2 experienced users, with all patient information present in the paper record, served as the control record. Data entry times were recorded, and a questionnaire was used to assess users' experiences with OpenSDE.

Results.—Clinicians documented 44% of all available patient information identically in the paper and electronic records. Twenty-five percent of all patient information was documented only in the paper record, and 31% was present only in the electronic record. Differences were found in patient history and physical examination documentation in the electronic record; more information was missing for patient history (38%) than for physical examination (15%). Furthermore, physical examination contained more additional information (39%) than did patient history (21%). The interobserver agreement of documentation of patient information from the same data source was fair to moderate, with κ values of 0.39 for patient history and 0.40 for physical examination. Data entry times in OpenSDE decreased from 25 minutes to <15 minutes, indicating a learning effect. The questionnaire revealed a positive attitude toward the use of OpenSDE in daily practice.

Conclusion.—OpenSDE seems to be a promising application for the support of physician data entry in general pediatrics.

▶ Please do not conclude that having this particular article in the YEAR BOOK OF PEDIATRICS in any way is an endorsement for the software used in the study. OpenSDE was developed in the Department of Medical Informatics, Erasmus Medical Center, to support the structured recording of patient data in any clinical domain. OpenSDE, as a medical record, uses a tree of medical concepts that represents the available descriptive options physicians would normally use in their office. The use of the electronic medical record did seem to capture more clinical information. Approximately 31% additional information was observed to be entered in the electronic medical record versus a handwritten medical record. This extra information was found almost entirely on the physical examination component of the medical record, with the medical history actually being a bit leaner in the electronic version.

One of the many purposes of using an electronic medical record is to reduce medical errors. Recall that the report from the Institute of Medicine back in 1999 estimated that somewhere between 44,000 and 98,000 people die each year because of a medical error.[1] The Physicians Insurance Association of America indicates that medication errors are the second most frequent and second most expensive procedure causing medical liability claims. Only a few studies, however, have investigated this problem in any detail, and even fewer have looked at outpatient prescriptions written for children. One study shows an error rate of 14% to 21% in prescriptions written by family medicine residents, and another has found that 6% of all prescriptions contain an error of some sort.[2,3] The report that follows (Abstract 11–10) looks at error rates in prescriptions written by residents in a pediatric emergency department and tells us that one or more errors on a prescription written by a pediatric resident may be found in more than 50% of prescriptions written. Most of the time, these errors relate to incomplete directions, but more serious problems were also frequently found. Curiously, third-year residents had error rates in prescription writing that were just as bad as those of first-year residents. Read this report in more detail.

J. A. Stockman III, MD

References

1. Kohn LT, Corrigan JM, Donaldson MS (eds): *To Err Is Human: Building a Safer Health System. Report of the Institute of Medicine.* Washington, DC, National Academy Press, 1999.
2. Howell RR, Jones KW: Prescription-writing errors and markers: The value of knowing the diagnosis. *Fam Med* 25:104-106, 1993.
3. Johnson KB, Butta JK, Donohue PK, et al: Discharging patients with prescriptions instead of medications: Sequelae in a teaching hospital. *Pediatrics* 97:41-45, 1997.

Prescription Writing Errors in the Pediatric Emergency Department
Taylor BL, Selbst SM, Shah AEC (Alfred I duPont Hosp for Children, Wilmington, Del; Jefferson Med College, Philadelphia)
Pediatr Emerg Care 21:822-827, 2005   11–10

Objectives.—To determine the frequency, type, and severity of written prescription (RX) errors in a pediatric emergency department with attention to specialty and level of training of the residents who wrote the RXs.

Methods.—Copies of RXs written by residents in a pediatric emergency department during a 6-month period were matched with pediatric emergency department records. Investigators evaluated individual RXs. Errors were noted and grouped into categories. Severity of errors was scaled, based on predetermined criteria (from previously published articles). The prescribing physician's specialty and level of training were documented. Discharge instructions were reviewed to determine if RX errors were later clarified.

Results.—There were 358 RXs eligible for overall descriptive analysis. A total of 212 RXs (59%) contained 311 errors. Discharge instructions ameliorated 16% of the RXs containing an error. Minor omissions were the most common error (62%), followed by incomplete directions (23%), dose/directions errors (6%), and unclear quantity to dispense (5%). In analysis of resident specialty and level of training, 339 RXs, written by 47 residents, were included. RXs written by pediatric residents were less likely to have an error (48%) than those by emergency medicine (81%), family medicine (76%), or combined internal medicine/pediatrics residents (100%). First year residents' RXs were errant 59%, second year residents 42%, and third year residents 69% of the time. The majority of RXs with errors (77%) were categorized as insignificant. Nineteen percent of RXs were defined as a problem and were unlikely to be filled. Less than 5% of errors were significant, and none were serious or severe.

Conclusions.—RX errors are very common in the pediatric emergency department. Pediatric-specific experience was more influential than level of training on reducing the likelihood of error.

▶ The data from this report speak for themselves, so we will ask a question about accidents that can land in the emergency room. Most data suggest that there is an increase in accident rate probability during times that individuals are using their cell phones. You are trying to educate a teen population about this problem. One of the teens asks a very logical question: "Is there any lower risk of an accident if a driver uses a hands-free cell phone?"

One study that was sponsored by the Insurance Institute for Highway Safety[1] has shown that there is no reduction in accident risk rate with the use of a hands-free cell phone as opposed to one that an individual must hold. The design of this study was quite interesting. It looked at individuals who were on mobile phones shortly before or during an accident. With permission of the individuals who were driving, the cell phone records of these individuals were examined for the 24-hour period during which the crash occurred as well as a period 72 hours after. A driver's use of a mobile phone up to 10 minutes before a crash was associated with a 4-fold increased likelihood of crashing. This risk was elevated irrespective of whether or not a hands-free device was used. Gender did not affect the risk either.

Two of the automobiles in this editor's stable are equipped with Bluetooth® technology, including voice activation. This means that his cell phone can be anywhere on his person and the calls are picked up through the internal system of the automobile allowing a totally hands-free phone use. This was not a free option and one that was paid for thinking that this would permit talking and driving at the same time. The research provided by the Insurance Institute for

Highway Safety, however, suggests that this was wishful thinking and money perhaps wasted.

J. A. Stockman III, MD

Reference

1. McEvoy SP, Stevenson MR, McCartt AT et al: Role of mobile phones in motor vehicle crashes resulting in hospital attendance: A case-crossover study. *BMJ* 331:428-430, 2005.

The Costs of a National Health Information Network

Kaushal R, and the Cost of National Health Information Network Working Group (Brigham and Women's Hosp, Boston; Harvard Med School, Boston; Cornell Med School, New York; et al)
Ann Intern Med 143:165-173, 2005   11–11

Background.—The use of information technology may result in a safer and more efficient health care system. However, consensus does not exist about the structure or costs of a national health information network (NHIN).

Objectives.—To describe the potential structure and estimate the costs of an NHIN.

Design.—Cost estimates of an NHIN model developed by an expert panel.

Setting.—U.S. health care system.

Measurements.—An expert panel estimated the existing and the expected prevalence in 5 years of critical information technology functionalities. They then developed a model of an achievable NHIN by defining key providers, functionalities, and interoperability functions. By using these data and published cost estimates, the authors determined the cost of achieving this model NHIN in 5 years given the current state of information technology infrastructure.

Results.—To achieve an NHIN would cost $156 billion in capital investment over 5 years and $48 billion in annual operating costs. Approximately two thirds of the capital costs would be required for acquiring functionalities and one third for interoperability. Ongoing costs would be more evenly divided between functionality and interoperability. If the current trajectory continues, the health care system will spend 24 billion dollars on functionalities over the next 5 years or about one quarter of the cost for functionalities of a model NHIN.

Limitations.—Because of a lack of primary data, the authors relied on expert estimates.

Conclusions.—While an NHIN will be expensive, $156 billion is equivalent to 2% of annual health care spending for 5 years. Assessments such as this one may assist policymakers in determining the level of investment that the United States should make in an NHIN.

▶ No one will argue with the fact that health care here in the United States lags behind other industries in investment and in the use of information technology in its front-line processes. The Institute of Medicine in the United States has clearly said that it is critical for us to advance information technology to achieve health care goals. In the 2004 State of the Union Address, President George W. Bush noted that "by computerizing health records, we can avoid dangerous medical mistakes, reduce cost and improve care." In late April 2004, he created a new position of national health information technology coordinator at the US Department of Health and Human Services and named Dr David Brailer to this role. By July 2004, a NHIN conference was convened, which began to make recommendations regarding the needs here in the United States for full implementation of a NHIN. Senators Bill Frist and Hillary Clinton co-authored an editorial in the Washington Post calling for more information technology in health care, but we in the United States still lag behind other countries. The United Kingdom and Canada, for example, have made major investments in the health care information infrastructure. The United Kingdom's government has allocated more than $8 billion and the Canadian government has invested some $1.5 billion (Canadian), recognizing that much more will actually be needed. In Great Britain, the government has committed to providing all the requisite support, which, of course, is necessary there because the government funds the National Health Service.

This article is an analysis of just what it may take to get the United States on the map when it comes to the creation of an NHIN. The estimate is that it will cost in excess of $150 billion, which is the equivalent of about 2% of annual health care expenditures over a 5-year period. Is it worth the investment? You betcha. The rub here in the United States is the lack of any centralized process for the development of such a network. Such a system obviously will be developed in a joint manner between government and the private sector, and standards must be set to allow interoperability as systems are developed. These systems must also be compliant with the Health Insurance Portability and Accountability Act (HIPAA). Whatever the final cost of such a system and the time necessary to implement this system, the effect in terms of benefits to this society will be obvious.

J. A. Stockman III, MD

Challenges to Implementing the National Programme for Information Technology (NPfIT): A Qualitative Study

Hendy J, Reeves BC, Fulop N, et al (London School of Hygiene and Tropical Medicine)

BMJ 331:331-334, 2005   11–12

Objectives.—To describe the context for implementing the national programme for information technology (NPfIT) in England, actual and perceived barriers, and opportunities to facilitate implementation.

Design.—Case studies and in depth interviews, with themes identified using a framework developed from grounded theory.

Setting.—Four acute NHS trusts in England.

Participants.—Senior trust managers and clinicians, including chief executives, directors of information technology, medical directors, and directors of nursing.

Results.—The trusts varied in their circumstances, which may affect their ability to implement the NPfIT. The process of implementation has been suboptimal, leading to reports of low morale by the NHS staff responsible for implementation. The overall timetable is unrealistic, and trusts are uncertain about their implementation schedules. Short term benefits alone are unlikely to persuade NHS staff to adopt the national programme enthusiastically, and some may experience a loss of electronic functionality in the short term.

Conclusions.—The sociocultural challenges to implementing the NPfIT are as daunting as the technical and logistical ones. Senior NHS staff feel these have been neglected. We recommend that national programme managers prioritise strategies to improve communication with, and to gain the cooperation of, front line staff.

▶ This article from Great Britain shows us some of the challenges in implementing a national program for health information technology, which is a problem that we are also wrestling with in the United States. The difference in Great Britain is that the Brits began to seriously deal with facilitated information exchange much earlier than we did here in the United States. In 1998, the British NHS executive set a target for all NHS Trusts to have electronic patient records in place by no later than the year 2005. The process has been going a bit more slowly than anticipated. By the spring of 2003, just 3% of Trusts were meeting the target. When it was recognized that things were lagging behind schedule, the British government began to throw huge amounts of money at the problem, and the current aim is for electronic patient records to be implemented across all of England by the end of 2007. It is just possible that that target will be met, and this would be years ahead of anything that is likely to occur in the United States.

This article tells us what some of the problems have been in Great Britain in implementing a common electronic health record system at a national level. The key to success there has been the appointment of what there is called a technology supremo in the Department of Health. We, in the United States, during the first Bush administration, saw the appointment of Dr David Brailer into a similar role in Washington. As the "czar" for health information technology development, Dr Brailer had been going gung-ho in the development of common standards for electronic health records before his untimely resignation in early 2006.

In Great Britain, the individual who has the corresponding role to our information "czar," the man with the technology plan is Richard Granger. Unlike Brailer, an internist by background, Mr Granger is not a physician. His first job, in 1987 after a degree in geology from Bristol University, was in the oil industry. It involved collecting data from sensors around and beneath oil rigs. This experience in information technology and data collection was enough to convince him that it was going to be a powerful and general influence in society. Two years later, he left to join Andersen Consulting, working on the computerization of the United Kingdom's social security benefit system. In 1998, he became a partner in Deloitte Consulting, where he organized London's congestion charging scheme. The success of this scheme launched him into his current role as Information Technology Supremo in the Department of Health in Great Britain. He appears to be doing a bang-up job and is really getting things done there.

By the way, if you are not familiar with London's congestion charging scheme, it was a colossal project. It is currently in effect. Basically, the system scans license numbers on plates of cars being driven into London Center City. These readings are computerized, and drivers are seamlessly charged £8.00 as a fee for the privilege of driving within the inner city part of London. Needless to say, Richard Granger made few friends when he was managing the streets of London but is doing much better in his present job.

See the article by Kaushal and colleagues (Abstract 11–11) for some estimates of the cost of a national health information network here in the United States.

J. A. Stockman III, MD

Disciplinary Action by Medical Boards and Prior Behavior in Medical School

Papadakis MA, Teherani A, Banach MA, et al (Univ of California, San Francisco; Federation of State Med Boards, Dallas; Thomas Jefferson Univ, Philadelphia; et al)
N Engl J Med 353:2673-2682, 2005

11–13

Background.—Evidence supporting professionalism as a critical measure of competence in medical education is limited. In this case–control study, we investigated the association of disciplinary action against practicing physicians with prior unprofessional behavior in medical school. We also examined the specific types of behavior that are most predictive of disciplinary action against practicing physicians with unprofessional behavior in medical school.

Methods.—The study included 235 graduates of three medical schools who were disciplined by one of 40 state medical boards between 1990 and

TABLE 1.—Description of the 740 Violations Among 235 Physicians That Led to Disciplinary Action on the Part of 40 State Medical Boards

Type of Violation	No. (%)
Unprofessional behavior	
Use of drugs or alcohol*	108 (15)
Unprofessional conduct	82 (11)
Conviction for a crime	46 (6)
Negligence	42 (6)
Inappropriate prescribing or acquisition of controlled substances	39 (5)
Violation of a law or order of the board, of a consent or rehabilitation order, or of probation	32 (4)
Failure to conform to minimal standards of acceptable medical practice	31 (4)
Sexual misconduct	29 (4)
Failure to meet requirements for continuing medical education or other requirements	26 (4)
Fraud or inappropriate billing practices (e.g., Medicare billing irregularities)	20 (3)
Failure to maintain adequate medical records	19 (3)
Failure to report adverse actions against oneself in accordance with rules of the board	10 (1)
Conduct that might defraud or harm the public	10 (1)
Other (less than 1% of any single category)	57 (8)
Total	551 (74)
Incompetence	
Health-related problems, incompetence, or impairment	44 (6)
Unknown†	
Violation imposed by another board or agency	87 (12)
License revocation or suspension	28 (4)
Inappropriate treatment or diagnosis of patients or malpractice	7 (1)
Other or not available (less than 1% of any single category)	23 (3)
Total	145 (20)

*The decision to categorize the use of drugs or alcohol as unprofessional behavior was based on the customary practice of medical boards to discipline physicians for such use if they commit acts that endanger patients. Physicians who have used drugs or alcohol but have not endangered patients may be referred to the diversion programs of medical boards and generally do not face disciplinary action.

†The category of unknown violations includes those that could not be ascribed to unprofessional behavior or to incompetence.

(Reprinted by permission of *The New England Journal of Medicine from Papadakis MA, Teherani A, Banach MA, et al: Disciplinary action by medical boards and prior behavior in medical school. N Engl J Med* 353:2673-2682, 2005. Copyright 2005, Massachusetts Medical Society. All rights reserved.)

2003 (case physicians) (Table 1). The 469 control physicians were matched with the case physicians according to medical school and graduation year. Predictor variables from medical school included the presence or absence of narratives describing unprofessional behavior, grades, standardized-test scores, and demographic characteristics. Narratives were assigned an overall rating for unprofessional behavior. Those that met the threshold for unprofessional behavior were further classified among eight types of behavior and assigned a severity rating (moderate to severe).

Results.—Disciplinary action by a medical board was strongly associated with prior unprofessional behavior in medical school (odds ratio, 3.0; 95 percent confidence interval, 1.9 to 4.8), for a population attributable risk of disciplinary action of 26 percent. The types of unprofessional behavior most strongly linked with disciplinary action were severe irresponsibility (odds ratio, 8.5; 95 percent confidence interval, 1.8 to 40.1) and severely diminished capacity for self-improvement (odds ratio, 3.1; 95 percent confidence interval, 1.2 to 8.2). Disciplinary action by a medical board was also associated with low scores on the Medical College Admission Test and poor grades in the first two years of medical school (1 percent and 7 percent population attributable risk, respectively), but the association with these variables was less strong than that with unprofessional behavior.

Conclusions.—In this case-control study, disciplinary action among practicing physicians by medical boards was strongly associated with unprofessional behavior in medical school. Students with the strongest association were those who were described as irresponsible or as having diminished ability to improve their behavior. Professionalism should have a central role in medical academics and throughout one's medical career.

▶ It should probably come as no surprise that the apple does not fall far from its tree. In the instance of disciplinary action by medical boards and prior behavior in medical school, the apple is the individual who is being sanctioned by his state medical-licensing board, and the tree is that same individual some years previously when that individual was in medical school. How surprising is it that this study found that physicians who were disciplined by state medical-licensing boards were 3 times as likely to have displayed unprofessional behavior in medical school when compared with their peers. The report of Papadakis et al provides evidence from 3 medical schools of the association between disciplinary action by state medical boards against practicing physicians and a documented lack of professional behavior (particularly irresponsibility, diminished capacity for self-improvement, and poor initiative) when those physicians were medical students.

Currently, the organizations engaged with assessing competency across the continuum of medical education have defined the domains of behavior that are essential for physicians to meet these competencies. The Liaison Committee on Medical Education, the Accreditation Council for Graduate Medical Education, and the American Board of Medical Specialties and its member boards, including the American Board of Pediatrics, have defined these domains of behavior. Central to these is professionalism, the domain of competence that remains the most difficult to measure. What the work of Papadakis et al does is to add more understanding to what elements of professionalism truly correlate. Lack of professionalism seems to be typified by the presence of irresponsibility and resistance to improvement, which are the most significance predictors of unprofessional behavior as defined by sanctions imposed by state medical-licensing boards.

It is no longer possible for us to claim we cannot measure professionalism at any stage of one's career. Papadakis et al have documented the types of behavior that serve as metrics for identifying students and physicians at greatest risk for unprofessional behavior and in need of remediation. If we are expected to be a self-regulating profession, we must accept the responsibility for dealing with those elements within our profession who are "ill" and in need of therapy. The American Board of Pediatrics receives notification from the Federation of State Medical Boards of actions that have been taken against those within our niche of the medical profession. It seems fairly clear that a large percentage of individuals who get into trouble with their medical license are individuals who showed the seeds of this problem way back when, even during their pediatric residency. All too often we think that misbehavior is a one-time affair. It may be, but then again it may be symptomatic of a lifelong problem that needs to be tackled head on. Let's not shy away from our responsibility as teachers, professional peers, and colleagues to those in need of help or remediation.

Last, one of the worst behaviors we see from time to time is cheating on high-stakes examinations. Fortunately, we now have ways to detect such cheating using readily available software. One such software is Acinonyx, which is written in C++, and recently was shown how to be effective when used in a study of the 11 examinations held by the Royal College of Pediatrics and Child Health in Great Britain. Some 11,518 candidates took the examinations and the software compared more than 6 million possible pairs of answers of candidates. There appeared to be abnormalities in 8 of the examinations showing 13 anomalies compatible with cheating. In all instances, the pair of examinees that were linked together were found to have been examined in the exact same testing center and for most of these when seating plans were looked at, the problem examinations showed that the 2 candidates were sitting side by side. This suggests that, at least in Great Britain, one anomalous pair of results is found for every 1000 examinations studied using cheating software.[1]

Many testing organizations use such software. In some instances, the software can detect anomalies that are of benefit to the candidate when they are picked up. For example, if a candidate has a "sequence error" in filling out their answer sheet if it is done with a paper and pencil examination, the computer will detect that. In other words, if a candidate, let's say, is on average answering questions 88% of the time correctly to a certain point in the examination and then begins to perform poorly, chances are very good that the candidate began to transpose answers incorrectly somewhere at the point in which he began to do poorly. Many testing organizations will recognize such a problem and allow a candidate to be retested in such circumstances without any penalty.

J. A. Stockman III, MD

Reference

1. McManus IC, Lissauer T, Williams SE: Detecting cheating in written medical examinations by statistical analysis of similarity of answers: Pilot study. *BMJ* 330:1064-1066, 2005.

Medical Students' Exposure to and Attitudes About Drug Company Interactions: A National Survey

Sierles FS, Brodkey AC, Cleary LM, et al (Rosalind Franklin Univ of Medicine and Surgery, North Chicago; Univ of Pennsylvania, Philadelphia; State Univ of New York, Syracuse; et al)

JAMA 294:1034-1042, 2005

11–14

Context.—While exposure to and attitudes about drug company interactions among residents have been studied extensively, relatively little is known about relationships between drug companies and medical students.

Objective.—To measure third-year medical students' exposure to and attitudes about drug company interactions.

Design, Setting, and Participants.—In 2003, we distributed a 64-item anonymous survey to 1143 third-year students at 8 US medical schools, exploring their exposure and response to drug company interactions. The schools' characteristics included a wide spectrum of ownership types, National Institutes of Health funding, and geographic locations. In 2005, we conducted a national survey of student affairs deans to measure the prevalence of school-wide policies on drug company–medical student interactions.

Main Outcome Measures.—Monthly frequency of students' exposure to various activities and gifts during clerkships, and attitudes about receiving gifts.

Results.—Overall response rate was 826/1143 (72.3%), with range among schools of 30.9%-90.7%. Mean exposure for each student was 1 gift or sponsored activity per week. Of respondents, 762/818 (93.2%) were asked or required by a physician to attend at least 1 sponsored lunch. Regarding attitudes, 556/808 (68.8%) believed gifts would not influence their practices and 464/804 (57.7%) believed gifts would not affect colleagues' practices. Of the students, 553/604 (80.3%) believed that they were entitled to gifts. Of 183 students who thought a gift valued at less than $50 was inappropriate, 158 (86.3%) had accepted one. The number of students who simultaneously believed that sponsored grand rounds are educationally helpful and are likely to be biased was 452/758 (59.6%). Students at 1 school who had attended a seminar about drug company–physician relationships were no more likely than the nonattending classmates to show skepticism. Of the respondents, 704/822 (85.6%) did not know if their school had a policy on these relationships. In a national survey of student affairs deans, among the 99 who knew their policy status, only 10 (10.1%) reported having school-wide policies about these interactions.

Conclusions.—Student experiences and attitudes suggest that as a group they are at risk for unrecognized influence by marketing efforts. Research should focus on evaluating methods to limit these experiences and affect the development of students' attitudes to ensure that physicians' decisions are based solely on helping each patient achieve the greatest possible benefit.

▶ Nationally, very few medical schools have policies regarding drug company–student interactions, and as noted in the study, very few students are even aware of the presence or absence of such policies at their own schools. The article, representing a survey of more than 1000 medical students from across the United States, clearly shows that students are a soft target for drug companies. Respondents from 8 medical schools received an average of 1 gift or sponsored event each week. Almost all the students had eaten sponsored lunches and accepted pens or coffee mugs from drug representatives. More than four fifths had also attended sponsored grand rounds, and about half had accepted gifts of textbooks. Eighty percent of third-year students believe that they were entitled to such gifts from drug companies, and two thirds said that gifts and other direct marketing would not influence their practice. One wonders why medical students think that drug companies offer such perks if they did not think they would influence those receiving the perks?

It is clear that medical students in the United States are not as skeptical as they should be about marketing tactics of drug companies. Drug companies surely do a lot of good, but at the same time, they can produce undue influence on those who market their products. Seventy percent of those who participated in the survey believed that drug company materials were, in fact, a good way to learn about new drugs, and 90% described sponsored grand rounds as helpful and educational. While these benefits may, in fact, be good, they come at a price that has to do with a potential compromise of one's professionalism.

Those who have control of the oversight of medical students and residents somehow believe they can walk the fine line of taking money from drug companies to sponsor lunches, grand rounds, and other "educational" events. Others believe that there is no fine line to walk and that it comes with strings attached any time you accept support.

The problem described for medical students does not stop there. Pharmaceutical companies here in the US spend more than $20 billion a year on marketing. It has been estimated that approximately 90% of this marketing is specifically directed at physicians. This is an amount that is far in excess of the amount of money spent on research or direct consumer advertising. It is currently estimated that pharmaceutical companies spend approximately $13,000 a year per physician here in the United States on marketing activities.[1]

J. A. Stockman III, MD

Reference

1. Charatan F: Doctors told to shun rewards from industry as size of payments become clear. *BMJ* 332:255, 2006.

Neurobehavioral Performance of Residents After Heavy Night Call vs After Alcohol Ingestion

Arnedt JT, Owens J, Crouch M, et al (Brown Med School, Providence, RI; Rhode Island Hosp, Providence; E P Bradley Hosp, Providence, RI)
JAMA 294:1025-1033, 2005

11–15

Context.—Concern exists about the effect of extended resident work hours; however, no study has evaluated training-related performance impairments against an accepted standard of functional impairment.

Objectives.—To compare post-call performance during a heavy call rotation (every fourth or fifth night) to performance with a blood alcohol concentration of 0.04 to 0.05 g% (per 100 mL of blood) during a light call rotation, and to evaluate the association between self-assessed and actual performance.

Design, Setting, and Participants.—A prospective 2-session within-subject study of 34 pediatric residents (18 women and 16 men; mean age, 28.7 years) in an academic medical center conducted between October 2001 and August 2003, who were tested under 4 conditions: light call, light call with alcohol, heavy call, and heavy call with placebo.

Interventions.—Residents attended a test session during the final week of a light call rotation (non–post-call) and during the final week of a heavy call rotation (post-call). At each session, they underwent a 60-minute test battery (light and heavy call conditions), ingested either alcohol (light call with alcohol condition) or placebo (heavy call with placebo condition), and repeated the test battery. Performance self-evaluations followed each test.

Main Outcome Measures.—Sustained attention, vigilance, and simulated driving performance measures; and self-report sleepiness, performance, and effort measures.

Results.—Participants achieved the target blood alcohol concentration. Compared with light call, heavy call reaction times were 7% slower (242.5 vs 225.9 milliseconds, $P < .001$); commission errors were 40% higher (38.2% vs 27.2%, $P < .001$); and lane variability (7.0 vs 5.5 ft, $P < .001$) and speed variability (4.1 vs 2.4 mph, $P < .001$) on the driving simulator were 27% and 71% greater, respectively. Speed variability was 29% greater in heavy call with placebo than light call with alcohol (4.2 vs 3.2 mph, $P = .01$), and reaction time, lapses, omission errors, and off-roads were not different. Correlation between self-assessed and actual performance under heavy call was significant for commission errors ($r = -0.45$, $P = .01$), lane variability ($r = -0.76$, $P < .001$), and speed variability ($r = -0.71$, $P < .001$), but not for reaction time.

Conclusions.—Post-call performance impairment during a heavy call rotation is comparable with impairment associated with a 0.04 to 0.05 g% blood alcohol concentration during a light call rotation, as measured by sustained attention, vigilance, and simulated driving tasks. Residents' ability to judge this impairment may be limited and task-specific.

▶ After 3 or 4 alcoholic drinks, most of us are somewhat uninhibited and overconfident, if not three sheets to the wind. Apparently, being on call has a similar effect. In this article, researchers paid 34 young pediatric residents some $400 each to complete a series of performance tests after 4 weeks of light on-call duty and after 4 weeks of heavy duty. The residents also did the same test after enough vodka and tonic (with lime, of course) to bring their blood alcohol concentrations to 0.04 to 0.05 mg/mL. Compared with light duties, the heavy call rotation (90 h/wk and 1 in 4 or 5 nights on-call) significantly reduced the residents' ability to drive a simulator and impaired their performance on tests of vigilance and sustained attention. The residents' performance after a month of heavy duties was largely indistinguishable from their performance after several vodka and tonics. Reaction times and attention were similarly impaired, and drinking or heavy call duty made the residents equally likely to swerve off the road or to crash in a driving simulator. Keeping to a steady speed seemed particularly difficult for tired but sober residents. In fact, speed variability in the driving simulator was 30% better when well rested but drunk in comparison with testing when tired.

Thus, it is that too many work hours may, in fact, be detrimental. This is not new news. In fact, it is hard to believe that these residents were actually working 90 hours a week because that is in violation of current guidelines from the Accreditation Council for Graduate Medical Education. In the United Kingdom, resident work hours will soon decline to fewer than 50 hours a week. If we ever get to that point in the United States, we have to seriously ask ourselves the question of whether we can continue to adequately train residents in the period of time that we now do so. Are we up to the challenge of extending our residency in general pediatrics to 4 years?

This commentary closes with a totally unrelated subject, religion. What exactly is the religious affiliation breakdown of physicians in the United States? The following table, created with data taken from Curlin et al, provides the answer.[1]

Affiliation	Physicians	Population
Protestant	38.8%	54.7%
Catholic	21.7%	26.7%
Jewish	14.1%	1.9%
None	10.6%	13.3%
Hindu	5.3%	0.2%
Muslim	2.7%	0.5%
Orthodox	2.2%	0.5%
Mormon	1.7%	0.4%
Buddhist	1.2%	0.2%
Other	1.8%	1.6%

NOTE: Percentages do not add up to 100 due to rounding.

J. A. Stockman III, MD

Reference

1. Curlin F, Lantos JD, Roach CJ, et al: Religious characteristics of US physicians: A national survey. *J Gen Intern Med* 20:629-634, 2005.

The Changing Composition of the Pediatric Medical Subspecialty Workforce

Mayer ML, Preisser JS (Univ of North Carolina, Chapel Hill)
Pediatrics 116:833-840, 2005

11–16

Objectives.—To characterize the composition of the pediatric subspecialty workforce in terms of the distribution of women and international medical graduates (IMGs) across pediatric medical subspecialties and to determine whether the proportions of board-certified pediatric subspecialists who are women or IMGs differ between graduation cohorts.

Study Design.—We used board certification data from the American Board of Pediatrics. Within each pediatric subspecialty, we classified physicians into 2 groups, ie, recent graduates, defined as those who completed medical school after January 1, 1987, and nonrecent graduates, who completed medical school before that date. We calculated the percentage of female physicians for each subspecialty and computed 95% confidence intervals around those estimates to identify male-dominated subspecialties. Using Pearson χ^2 tests, we compared the percentages of women between the 2 graduation cohorts for each subspecialty. Similar calculations were performed for the percentage of IMGs in each subspecialty. Sensitivity analyses were performed with data from the 2002 American Medical Association Physician Masterfile.

Results.—For 9 of 16 pediatric medical subspecialties studied, the percentages of board-certified women were significantly greater in the recent cohort than in the nonrecent cohort. Subspecialties that remain predomi-

TABLE 5.—Percentages of Trainees Who Were Women, According to Fellowship Type and Year, Among Third-Year Fellows (ABP Data, 2003)

Pediatric Subspecialty	Female, %					
	1998	1999	2000	2001	2002	2003
Allergy/immunology	NA	NA	NA	NA	NA	NA
Adolescent medicine	70.6	55.6	65.0	63.6	60.9	81.8
Cardiology	28.8	39.7	35.1	38.2	50.0	35.3
Critical care	40.0	42.0	42.7	46.4	47.0	35.3
Emergency medicine	52.8	51.5	57.9	52.4	49.2	44.3
Endocrinology	70.4	58.1	60.5	72.7	46.0	64.6
Gastroenterology	41.9	36.4	35.5	28.9	47.4	44.9
Hematology/oncology	47.3	50.6	47.9	57.1	51.1	53.3
Infectious diseases	46.3	58.3	47.9	57.4	51.9	62.2
Neurodevelopment	NA	NA	NA	NA	NA	NA
Neonatology	50.7	45.9	48.4	55.1	47.3	49.4
Nephrology	35.7	52.2	57.9	35.3	40.9	58.8
Pulmonology	51.7	38.2	45.5	44.8	48.6	35.0
Rheumatology	50.0	33.3	85.7	90.0	53.8	80.0
Sports medicine	NA	NA	NA	NA	NA	NA

Data source: ABP 2003-2004 workforce data (available at: www.abp.org/stats/wrkfrc/menu1.htm). Developmental and behavioral medicine was excluded because of inconsistencies in the number of years of training across programs. NA indicates data not available.

(Courtesy of Mayer ML, Preisser JS: The changing composition of the pediatric medical subspecialty workforce. *Pediatrics* 116:833-840, 2005. Reproduced by permission of *Pediatrics*.)

nantly male in the recent graduation cohort include cardiology, critical care medicine, gastroenterology, pulmonology, and sports medicine (Table 5). In contrast, the percentages of board-certified IMGs were significantly lower for 6 of the 16 specialties studied; endocrinology and gastroenterology remain relatively reliant on IMGs.

Conclusions.—For the majority of pediatric medical subspecialties, concerns that the predominance of women in pediatric training may negatively affect the supply of subspecialists are likely unfounded; however, a small number of procedure-based specialties, as well as sports medicine, continue to rely disproportionately on men. There do not seem to be consistent differences in the role of IMGs across the pediatric medical subspecialties between recent and nonrecent graduates, which may reflect differing tendencies to become certified.

▶ This report attempts to define whether the increasing number of women in the pediatric workforce in any way influences the numbers of individuals going into subspecialty training in pediatrics. The report also attempts to tell us whether changing numbers of IMGs affect subspecialty workforce numbers. Traditionally, more women than men have gone into general pediatrics, and more men than women into subspecialty training. Tradition does not always repeat itself, and what we are seeing is an increasing number of women who have become interested in subspecialty training. This partially accounts for the significant rise in the number of subspecialty trainees in recent years. It is true that there has been a falloff in the number of IMGs entering general pediatric residency training and that because of this, there has been some decline in their numbers going into subspecialty training. However, this decline has been offset by the numbers of American medical school graduates, so subspecialty training numbers have held their own in recent years.

In February 2006, the American Board of Pediatrics began to publish, in serial form, all aspects of its workforce database. The first of these reports appeared in the *Journal of Pediatrics*.[1] In 1991, approximately 60% of residents completing general pediatric residency training indicated a desire to go into general pediatric practice. This percentage reached its peak in 1998 at 73%. It was around this time that we began to appreciate a serious shortage of pediatric subspecialists. Fortunately since then, interest in pediatric subspecialties has significantly increased.

Residency matching data from 2006 showed that interest in general pediatric residency training continues to be very strong despite periodic concerns that we may be training too many pediatric generalists. It is apparent that the need for pediatricians continues. Thus far, there is no end in sight for the number of generalists or subspecialists that we need in our discipline.

The trends we are seeing in pediatrics provide an interesting contrast to trends occurring at the medical school level here in the United States. The 2005-2006 entering class of American medical schools was the largest ever. As of mid-October 2005, a total of 17,004 first-time medical students had enrolled during that academic year. This figure amounts to a 2.1% gain over 2004 and represents the largest expansion in percentage terms since 1978. The class was selected from amongst 37,364 applicants. These applicants themselves represent a 4.6% increase from the previous year. Applicant numbers previously had declined for 6 consecutive years from 1997 to 2002 before ultimately rebounding by 3.4% in 2003. Among all US medical schools, about half had increased their class size with 22 schools showing gains of 5% or more, and 7 schools registering increases of more than 11%. These increases have come on the heels of the Association of American Medical Colleges' call in February 2005 for a 15% increase in medical school enrollments by 2015 based on concerns about a physician shortage here in the United States. Growth in the US population, especially in those over age 65, seems to be fueling the demand for physicians.

Men, rather than women, constitute a greater percentage of growth in the first year of medical school entering class this year. Data show a 5.8% increase in the number of male applicants, bringing the totals for male and female applicants to just about even. Men accounted for 50.2% of the total applicant pool this year after 2 consecutive years in which women have been in the minority. Women still hold a thin majority of 50.7% among first-time applicants to medical school this year. Men seem to be a bit more tenacious in reapplying.

Among ethnic and racial groups, the 2005-2006 entering class saw a 6.4% increase among Hispanic applicants to medical school. Among Hispanics, Mexican-American students had the largest percentage increase—7.9%. Applications from prospective Asian students rose 8.1%. Asian students made up a full 20% of all applicants to medical school. Black applicant numbers were holding steady with 2809 applicants. Native American applicants decreased while Native Hawaiian and Pacific Islander applicants rose slightly.

If you are wondering what institutions are increasing their class size the most, they are Florida State University College of Medicine (up 38%), Brown Medical School (up 20%) and Joan C. Edwards School of Medicine at Marshall University (up 15%). Others showing substantial gains include the University of Miami School of Medicine (14%), Northeastern Ohio Universities School of Medicine (13%), University of Missouri-Kansas City School of Medicine (12%), and Jefferson Medical College of Thomas Jefferson University (11%).[2]

J. A. Stockman III, MD

References

1. Althouse LA, Stockman JA: Pediatric workforce: A look at general pediatrics data from the American Board of Pediatrics. *J Pediatr* 148:166-169, 2006.
2. Harris S: Size of entering class top 17,000 for biggest percentage gained since 1978. *Reporter* 15(no. 2):1-4, 2005.

The Physician-Scientist Career Pipeline in 2005: Build It, and They Will Come
Ley TJ, Rosenberg LE (Washington Univ, St Louis; Princeton Univ, NJ)
JAMA 294:1343-1351, 2005   11–17

Context.—Physician-scientists play a unique and critical role in medical research. Nonetheless, a number of trends followed during the 1980s and

1990s revealed that this career pathway was in serious jeopardy. Physician-scientists were declining in number and were getting older. A variety of factors were thought to contribute to this problem, including increasing indebtedness of medical school graduates caused by rapidly rising medical school tuition costs.

Objective.—To evaluate the impact of recently initiated programs from the National Institutes of Health (NIH) and several not-for-profit institutions designed to revitalize the physician-scientist career pipeline.

Design.—We assessed recent trends in the physician-scientist career pipeline using data obtained from the NIH, the American Medical Association, the Association of American Medical Colleges, and other sources.

Main Outcome Measures.—Total numbers of physicians performing research, grant application numbers and success rates for MDs, MD-PhDs, and PhDs at various stages in their careers, interest in research among medical students, medical school tuitions and postgraduate salaries, numbers and composition of applicants for NIH loan repayment programs, and gender distribution of young physician-scientists.

Results.—The number of physician-scientists in the United States has been in a steady state for the past decade, but funded physician-scientists are significantly older than they were 2 decades ago. However, the study of early career markers over the past 7 to 10 years has demonstrated increasing interest in research careers by medical students, steady growth of the MD-PhD pool, and a new burst of activity in the "late bloomer" pool of MDs (individuals who choose research careers in medical school or in residency training), fueled by loan repayment programs that were created by the NIH in 2002. Several recent trends for more established physician-scientists have also suggested improvement.

Conclusions.—Although it is too early to assess the impact of these indicators on the long-term career pathway, the recent growth in activity in the physician-scientist career pipeline is an encouraging development. Continued funding of these new programs, coupled with sustained support for physician-scientists committed to the pathway, will be required to maintain these positive trends.

▶ Gosh knows that we in pediatrics need more physician–scientists. This article suggests that the macrolevel problem related to all disciplines of medicine is not very different than what we see here in pediatrics. While the number of physician–scientists in our country is at a relatively steady state, the age of these scientists is increasing fairly rapidly. As the article shows, there has been a burst in activity to entice individuals into science careers in medicine, and it does appear that we are beginning to see some payoffs in this regard, including in pediatrics, although as a primary care discipline, we have a tougher job creating the image of a need for physician–scientists.

So what is the overall status of the physician workforce in the United States? Without question, the health care workforce has expanded rapidly in recent years: nonphysician providers, graduates of international medical schools, and osteopaths augment a stable supply of about 16,000 graduates per year from US medical schools. Some experts believe that we need to increase the output of our medical schools on the basis of the growing US economy, the growing population (particularly the growing number of elderly people), and the possibility of enhancing the position of allopathic medicine in American health care. Many others, however, say that we do not need more physicians or, at least, not many more. There seems to be no debate that we need at least a small increase to meet the country's growing population needs and to offset the decreased number of graduates of international medical schools who now come to the United States. The naysayers believe that educating and training many more physicians would be unnecessary and expensive, especially when it should be possible to distribute the current supply of physicians more effectively to enhance efficiency. Such naysayers have also commented that research has shown that having more physicians does not necessarily equal improved health. To substantially increase the number of US-trained physicians will be expensive and will take many years, and few expect that it would actually improve the health of the US population. Perhaps the most basic difference between researchers who call for a large increase in the number of American medical school graduates and those who do not is in the answer to whether we should base physician supply on patient demand and traditional physician practices or on a more idealized vision of health care delivery that includes greater physician efficiency and alternative care providers.

How is the debate shaking out? The Association of American Medical Colleges recently recommended increasing medical school production by 15%, which works out to 2800 new graduates each year by 2015 and a total of about 30,000 new physicians by 2020. The Association of American Medical Colleges suggests that this is not a lot of new physicians for a nation that will have a population of more than 330 million and 54 million people older than 65 years by 2020. Indeed, we have more than 200,000 physicians who are currently practicing who are also older than 55 years and will likely be retiring in the next decade or two. At the same time, doctors are working fewer hours. This debate, as you might suspect, will rage on and on well beyond most of our lifespans.

I have one final comment about physician supply, having to do with geography. Currently, the physician supply concentrates in areas where doctors want to live: in cities and nearby suburban locations. The physician supply in rural locations is typically smaller. The National Health Services Corporation, which reduces medical school loans in return for a few years of service in underserved areas, already promotes practice in underserved areas. The concept of service to an underserved region as a payback for public support of medical education could be expanded to other incentive programs. Right now, all medical school graduates have, in fact, received a substantial taxpayer subsidy for their medical education, and one could require public service of virtually everyone; however, this would obviously be an unpopular solution to the problem. Active manipulation of physician distribution and specialization practices (controlling what specialties physicians can choose) is a common practice in many countries but would be a radical departure from US political and economic traditions. To read more on this fascinating topic that all of us should pay a great deal of attention to, see the excellent summary by Wilson.[1]

Most readers of the YEAR BOOK OF PEDIATRICS know that Dr Frank Oski and I co-edited the YEAR BOOK for many years. Frank died a bit more than 10 years ago, but his wisdom lingers on in many of his now famous quotations, one of which relates to the topic of the report abstracted, physician scientists.

Frank once commented: "As a medical student, I aspired to lasting fame, I craved factual certainty, and I thirsted for a meaningful vision of human life—so I became a physician scientist. This is like becoming an archbishop so you can meet girls."

J. A. Stockman III, MD

Reference

1. Wilson GF: US needs more physicians soon, but how many more is debatable. *Ann Intern Med* 143:469-472, 2005.

The Metrics of the Physician Brain Drain
Mullan F (George Washington Univ, Washington, DC)
N Engl J Med 353:1810-1818, 2005   11–18

Background.—There has been substantial immigration of physicians to developed countries, much of it coming from lower-income countries. Although the recipient nations and the immigrating physicians benefit from this migration, less developed countries lose important health capabilities as a result of the loss of physicians.

Methods.—Data on the countries of origin, based on countries of medical education, of international medical graduates practicing in the United States, the United Kingdom, Canada, and Australia were obtained from sources in the respective countries and analyzed separately and in aggregate. With the use of World Health Organization data, I computed an emigration factor for the countries of origin of the immigrant physicians to provide a relative measure of the number of physicians lost by emigration.

Results.—International medical graduates constitute between 23 and 28 percent of physicians in the United States, the United Kingdom, Canada, and Australia, and lower-income countries supply between 40 and 75 percent of

TABLE 1.—Characteristics of International Medical Graduates (IMGs) in Physician Workforces of the United States, the United Kingdom, Canada, and Australia

Country	No. of Physicians Per 100,000 Population	Total No. of IMGs	% of IMGs in Workforce	% of IMGs from Lower-Income Countries	% of IMGs from the Three Other Developed Countries
United States	293	208,733	25.0	60.2	6.5
United Kingdom	231	39,266	28.3	75.2	2.5
Canada	220	15,701	23.1	43.4	22.3
Australia	271	14,346	26.5	40.0	33.5

these international medical graduates. India, the Philippines, and Pakistan are the leading sources of international medical graduates. The United Kingdom, Canada, and Australia draw a substantial number of physicians from South Africa, and the United States draws very heavily from the Philippines. Nine of the 20 countries with the highest emigration factors are in sub-Saharan Africa or the Caribbean.

Conclusions.—Reliance on international medical graduates in the United States, the United Kingdom, Canada, and Australia is reducing the supply of physicians in many lower-income countries (Table 1).

▶ This article speaks to a topic that has been buried below the surface of active debate here in the United States. Although the United States, United Kingdom, Canada, and Australia have never formally adopted policies of meeting medical service needs with international medical school graduates (IMGs), the heavy reliance by these countries on physicians trained elsewhere suggests that they would have substantial physician shortages without IMGs staying in these countries. Pressures are mounting on all 4 countries that receive IMGs to increase the supply of physicians in practice. In the United Kingdom, for example, a commitment has been made to achieve a rapid increase of 9500 qualified physicians by accommodation of new medical schools and increased recruitment from abroad. Canada is adding residency positions to accommodate more IMGs and is streamlining immigration and training requirements to facilitate the direct entry of IMGs into practice. In the United States, a number of professional organizations and academic leaders as well as the Institute of Medicine's Committee on Graduate Medical Education have called for measures to augment the numbers of physicians in practices. These developments suggest that the demand for IMGs in the United States, United Kingdom, Canada, and Australia is likely to continue into the near future, exacerbating current trends.

The point here is fairly obvious. The equivalent of a brain drain of physicians is occurring from parts of the world where health services might possibly be improved if this brain drain did not occur. Between 23% and 28% of medical professionals practicing in the United Kingdom, United States, Canada, and Australia were trained abroad. In the United States and United Kingdom, most of these IMGs (60% and 75%, respectively) come from developing countries that can ill afford to lose them. Caribbean countries and those in subSaharan Africa lose the greatest proportion of their homegrown doctors to this brain drain. More than 40% of students graduating in Jamaica eventually emigrate to the United Kingdom, United States, Canada, or Australia. More than 30% of graduates from Haiti do the same. Ghana loses about 30% of its graduates, and South Africa loses about 20%. The Indian subcontinent is also a big donor, especially Sri Lanka, where more than a quarter of medical graduates immigrate to higher income countries.

Although the benefits to the recipient countries are obvious—without foreign doctors, a serious shortage of health professionals would occur in the United States—it is equally clear that a hemorrhage of talented ambitious graduates on the huge scale that occurs every year must damage the already impoverished health care systems that paid for their training. It is true that all 4 developed countries that are the subject of this article in the *New England Journal of Medicine* do, in fact, need more physicians. Given the fact that even some highly intelligent applicants to medical school never make it in because of the limited capacity we have in our medical schools, why can't we train more of our own? We cannot solve our own workforce problem on the backs of impoverished countries.

J. A. Stockman III, MD

Comparison of the Instructional Efficacy of Internet-Based CME With Live Interactive CME Workshops: A Randomized Controlled Trial

Fordis M, King JE, Ballantyne CM, et al (Baylor College of Medicine; Kelsey Research Found and Kelsey-Seybold Clinic, Houston)
JAMA 294:1043-1051, 2005   11–19

Context.—Despite evidence that a variety of continuing medical education (CME) techniques can foster physician behavioral change, there have been no randomized trials comparing performance outcomes for physicians participating in Internet-based CME with physicians participating in a live CME intervention using approaches documented to be effective.

Objective.—To determine if Internet-based CME can produce changes comparable to those produced via live, small-group, interactive CME with respect to physician knowledge and behaviors that have an impact on patient care.

Design, Setting, and Participants.—Randomized controlled trial conducted from August 2001 to July 2002. Participants were 97 primary care physicians drawn from 21 practice sites in Houston, Tex, including 7 community health centers and 14 private group practices. A control group of 18 physicians from these same sites received no intervention.

Interventions.—Physicians were randomly assigned to an Internet-based CME intervention that could be completed in multiple sessions over 2 weeks, or to a single live, small-group, interactive CME workshop. Both incorporated similar multifaceted instructional approaches demonstrated to be effective in live settings. Content was based on the National Institutes of Health National Cholesterol Education Program—Adult Treatment Panel III guidelines.

Main Outcome Measures.—Knowledge was assessed immediately before the intervention, immediately after the intervention, and 12 weeks later. The percentage of high-risk patients who had appropriate lipid panel screening and pharmacotherapeutic treatment according to guidelines was documented with chart audits conducted over a 5-month period before intervention and a 5-month period after intervention.

Results.—Both interventions produced similar and significant immediate and 12-week knowledge gains, representing large increases in percentage of items correct (pretest to posttest: 31.0% [95% confidence interval {CI}, 27.0%-35.0%]; pretest to 12 weeks: 36.4% [95% CI, 32.2%-40.6%]; $P <$ .001 for all comparisons). Chart audits revealed high baseline screening rates in all study groups (≥93%) with no significant postintervention change. However, the Internet-based intervention was associated with a significant increase in the percentage of high-risk patients treated with pharmacotherapeutics according to guidelines (preintervention, 85.3%; postintervention, 90.3%; $P = .04$).

Conclusions.—Appropriately designed, evidence-based online CME can produce objectively measured changes in behavior as well as sustained gains in knowledge that are comparable or superior to those realized from effective live activities.

▶ This study speaks for itself. If there is anything worthwhile, we can learn from CME course work, it is to respect the wishes of those to whom we provide care. A Canadian study[1] that sought the opinion of more than 1,000 people seeking health care found that, overwhelmingly, folks like, and prefer, the old-fashioned term "patient". Alternatives such as consumer, client, customer, partner, and survivor all evoked moderate to strong dislike, in some to the point of emesis.

J. A. Stockman III, MD

Reference

1. Deber RB, Kraetschmer N, Urowitz S, et al: Patient, consumer, client, or customer: What do people want to be called? *Health Expectations* 8:345-351, 2005.

Major Epidemiological Changes in Sudden Infant Death Syndrome: A 20-Year Population-based Study in the UK

Blair PS, Sidebotham P, Berry PJ, et al (Univ of Bristol, England; St Michaels Hosp, Bristol, England)
Lancet 367:314-319, 2006   11–20

Background.—Results of case-control studies in the past 5 years suggest that the epidemiology of sudden infant death syndrome (SIDS) has changed since the 1991 UK Back to Sleep campaign. The campaign's advice that parents put babies on their back to sleep led to a fall in death rates. We used a longitudinal dataset to assess these potential changes.

Methods.—Population-based data from home visits have been collected for 369 consecutive unexpected infant deaths (300 SIDS and 69 explained deaths) in Avon over 20 years (1984–2003). Data obtained between 1993 and 1996 from 1300 controls with a chosen "reference" sleep before interview have been used for comparison.

Findings.—Over the past 20 years, the proportion of children who died from SIDS while co-sleeping with their parents, has risen from 12% to 50% (p<0.0001), but the actual number of SIDS deaths in the parental bed has halved (p=0.01). The proportion seems to have increased partly because the Back to Sleep campaign led to fewer deaths in infants sleeping alone—rather than because of a rise in deaths of infants who bed-shared, and partly because of an increase in the number of deaths in infants sleeping with their parents on a sofa. The proportion of deaths in families from deprived socio-economic backgrounds has risen from 47% to 74% (p=0.003), the prevalence of maternal smoking during pregnancy from 57% to 86% (p=0.0004), and the proportion of pre-term infants from 12% to 34% (p=0.0001). Although many SIDS infants come from large families, first-born infants are now the largest group. The age of infants who bed-share is significantly smaller than that before the campaign, and fewer are breastfed.

Interpretation.—Factors that contribute to SIDS have changed in their importance over the past 20 years. Although the reasons for the rise in deaths when a parent sleeps with their infant on a sofa are still unclear, we strongly recommend that parents avoid this sleeping environment. Most SIDS deaths now occur in deprived families. To better understand contributory factors and plan preventive measures we need control data from similarly deprived families, and particularly, infant sleep environments.

▶ It has taken some time, but the US experience with the back-to-sleep program in the prevention of sudden infant death has been replicated elsewhere; this study took place in Europe. In the developed world, SIDS is responsible for more infant deaths beyond the neonatal period than any other cause. Unfortunately, SIDS has only gradually been recognized as a serious health risk. Since the back-to-sleep campaign showed its initial successes, we have recognized other risk factors for SIDS including the use of soft pillows, smoking during pregnancy, and secondhand smoke. We in the United States should not be patting ourselves on the back any too quickly about the timeliness with which the back-to-sleep program was put into place since the prone sleeping position was identified as a risk factor as early as 1944 in New York.[1] Actually, Great Britain began its back-to-sleep campaign 3 years before the start of our campaign back in 1994.

We are now at the point that we need to fine-tune our directions in order to further prevent SIDS. Beyond the back-to-sleep program, we need to deal with issues related to unemployed single mothers younger than 20 years, preterm delivery, active maternal smoking during pregnancy and secondary smoking during infancy, cosleeping, and the need for breast-feeding.

J. A. Stockman III, MD

Reference

1. Abramson H: Accidental mechanical suffocation in infants. *Pediatrics* 25:404-413, 1944.

Predicting the Risk for Sudden Infant Death Syndrome From Obstetric Characteristics: A Retrospective Cohort Study of 505 011 Live Births

Smith GCS, White IR (Cambridge Univ, England; Inst of Public Health, Cambridge, England)

Pediatrics 117:60-66, 2006   11–21

Objective.—We sought to develop a simple robust method for assessing the risk for sudden infant death syndrome (SIDS) on the basis of obstetric characteristics.

Methods.—A population-based retrospective cohort study was conducted of data from the linked Scottish Morbidity Record, Stillbirth and Infant Death Enquiry and General Registrar's Office database of births and deaths, encompassing births in Scotland between 1992 and 2001. All women who had a singleton live birth between 24 and 43 weeks' gestation and for whom data were available ($n = 505\,011$), divided into model development and validation samples, were studied. The main outcome measure was death of the infant in the first year of life as a result of SIDS.

Results.—The risk for SIDS was modeled in the development sample using logistic regression with the following predictors: maternal age, parity, marital status, smoking, and the birth weight and the gender of the infant. When the model was evaluated in the validation sample, the area under the receiver operating characteristic curve was 0.84 and the incidence of SIDS was 0.7 per 10 000 (95% confidence interval: 0.3–1.4) among 126 253 women in the lower 50% of predicted risk and 29.7 per 10 000 (95% confidence interval: 23.4–37.2) among the 25 250 women in the top 10% of predicted risk. A logistic-regression model then was developed for the whole population, and the output was converted into adjusted likelihood ratios. These are tabulated and provide a simple method for assessing the risk for SIDS associated with any combination of obstetric characteristics.

Conclusions.—A model that uses maternal characteristics and outcome at birth is predictive of the risk for SIDS. This model is presented in a simple form that allows calculation of the individual risk for SIDS.

▶ Many studies have noted a relationship between pregnancy outcome and the risk of SIDS, such as inverse associations between birth weight percentile and gestational age. Women who have complications in a pregnancy, such as intrauterine growth restriction and preterm birth, are known to be at increased risk of the same outcomes in future pregnancies, an association that implies that women who have a baby who ultimately dies of SIDS would be expected to be at increased risk of intrauterine growth restriction and preterm birth in other pregnancies. Recently, a report verified that women whose infants die of SIDS are indeed more likely to have complications in other pregnancies.[1] The recurrence of pregnancy complications predisposing to SIDS could, in fact, partially explain why women have pregnancies resulting in more than one baby who ultimately dies of SIDS.

The report of Smith and White takes us one step further in refining our understanding about pregnancy characteristics as a set of risk factors for the birth of a child who might die of SIDS. These investigators have done us a service by showing us what the range is for the risk of SIDS (0.7 to 29.7 per 10,000), depending on what problems a woman has during her pregnancy or what risk factors she otherwise experiences during her pregnancy. To do this calculation, all one needs is age at pregnancy, parity (per birth), marital status of the mother, smoking status of the mother, sex of the infant, and infant birth weight. Toss all these factors into an equation and you can predict the probability of SIDS far better than has ever been done in the past.

This commentary closes with a query, are you aware of the historical origins of the word "autopsy?" The word autopsy is derived from the Latin *autopsia*, meaning "seeing for one's self." The word autopsy has been in use since the 17th century to refer to postmortem examination of the human body to reveal evidence of organic disease or to discover medical causes of death. Before the 18th century, anatomical dissections were fairly commonplace, but it was rare for autopsies to be done purely to investigate disease processes or to ascertain cause of death. Not until the 20th century did postmortem examinations become the preserve of hospital and forensic pathologists, by which time the word autopsy had displaced the hitherto preferred term "necropsy."[2]

J. A. Stockman III, MD

References

1. Smith GCS, Wood AM, Pell JP, et al: Sudden infant death syndrome and complications in other pregnancies. *Lancet* 366:2107-2111, 2005.
2. Clark MJ: Autopsy. *Lancet* 366:1767, 2005.

Abdominal Injury Due to Child Abuse

Barnes PM, Norton CM, Dunstan FD, et al (Cardiff Univ, Penarth, England; Hope Hosp, Salford, England)
Lancet 366:234-235, 2005   11–22

Abstract.—Diagnosis of abuse in children with internal abdominal injury is difficult because of limited published work. We aimed to ascertain the incidence of abdominal injury due to abuse in children age 0-14 years. 20 children (identified via the British Paediatric Surveillance Unit) had abdominal injuries due to abuse and 164 (identified via the Trauma Audit and Research Network) had injuries to the abdomen due to accident (112 by road-traffic accidents, 52 by falls). 16 abused children were younger than 5 years. Incidence of abdominal injury due to abuse was 2.33 cases per million children per year (95% CI 1.43–3.78) in children younger than 5 years. Six abused children died. 11 abused children had an injury to the gut (ten small bowel) compared with five (all age >5 years) who were injured by a fall (relative risk 5.72 [95% CI 2.27–14.4]; p=0.0002). We have shown that small-bowel injuries can arise accidentally as a result of falls and road-traffic accidents but they are significantly more common in abused children. Therefore, injuries to the small bowel in young children need special consideration, particularly if a minor fall is the explanation (Table 2).

karyotyping only if the fetal NT thickness is increased would reduce the economic costs, provide rapid delivery of results, and identify 99% of the clinically significant chromosomal abnormalities.

▶ Without question, combining US (to detect NT) with maternal serum screening improves the ability to prenatally diagnose Down syndrome. NT measurement is now well established, but it is difficult to implement as a population-based screening program because of a shortage of adequately trained sonographers, with consequent problems with quality assurance. Various approaches to screening for Down syndrome in utero have been developed. Most of these use a combination of tests. Combined strategies include "integrated screening," with calculation of risk delayed until after the second stage of screening, and "contingent screening," in which women whose first-trimester screening results show them to be at high risk are offered chorionic villus sampling as a definitive test. Those with very low risk results are reassured, and those in the middle progress to the second stage of second-trimester screening. Clearly, uncertainty remains about the optimal combination of different screening tests. Whichever package of tests proves most effective, diagnosing, or as is much more common, excluding Down syndrome, still relies on invasive techniques. Midpregnancy amniocentesis and earlier transabdominal chorionic villus sampling have miscarriage rates of about 1%.

Chitty et al describe a series of almost 17,500 women whose infants had increased fetal NT and who had chorionic villus sampling with 2 different kinds of chromosome analysis. The study that these researchers undertook was to determine what the most cost-effective method is in the judicial use of karyotyping. The investigators found that those at high risk should have full karyotyping on chorionic villus samples. Analysis by qf-PCR is cheaper and faster, but will not detect all significant abnormalities. They suggest that qf-PCR be used to screen all cases, reserving full karyotyping only for the 10% of cases with fetal NT of 4 mm or more, an approach that would identify 99% of significant chromosomal abnormalities. This would result in a 60% reduction in cost compared with full karyotyping for all.

J. A. Stockman III, MD

First-Trimester or Second-Trimester Screening, or Both, for Down's Syndrome
Malone FD, for the First- and Second-Trimester Evaluation of Risk (FASTER) Research Consortium (Royal College of Surgeons in Ireland, Dublin; et al)
N Engl J Med 353:2001-2011, 2005   11–24

Background.—It is uncertain how best to screen pregnant women for the presence of fetal Down's syndrome: to perform first-trimester screening, to perform second-trimester screening, or to use strategies incorporating measurements in both trimesters.

Methods.—Women with singleton pregnancies underwent first-trimester combined screening (measurement of nuchal translucency, pregnancy-associated plasma protein A [PAPP-A], and the free beta subunit of human chorionic gonadotropin at 10 weeks 3 days through 13 weeks 6 days of gestation) and second-trimester quadruple screening (measurement of alpha-fetoprotein, total human chorionic gonadotropin, unconjugated estriol, and inhibin A at 15 through 18 weeks of gestation). We compared the results of stepwise sequential screening (risk results provided after each test), fully integrated screening (single risk result provided), and serum integrated screening (identical to fully integrated screening, but without nuchal translucency).

Results.—First-trimester screening was performed in 38,167 patients; 117 had a fetus with Down's syndrome. At a 5 percent false positive rate, the rates of detection of Down's syndrome were as follows: with first-trimester combined screening, 87 percent, 85 percent, and 82 percent for measurements performed at 11, 12, and 13 weeks, respectively; with second-trimester quadruple screening, 81 percent; with stepwise sequential screening, 95 percent; with serum integrated screening, 88 percent; and with fully integrated screening with first-trimester measurements performed at 11 weeks, 96 percent. Paired comparisons found significant differences between the tests, except for the comparison between serum integrated screening and combined screening.

Conclusions.—First-trimester combined screening at 11 weeks of gestation is better than second-trimester quadruple screening but at 13 weeks has results similar to second-trimester quadruple screening. Both stepwise sequential screening and fully integrated screening have high rates of detection of Down's syndrome, with low false positive rates.

▶ This report reminds us how controversial the prenatal screening for Down syndrome remains. The current standard of care is second-trimester screening, but the report abstracted compares first-trimester screening for Down syndrome with second-trimester screening and with screening in both trimesters. The results demonstrate that first-trimester screening for Down syndrome is highly effective, but combinations of measurements of markers from both the first and second trimesters yield higher detection rates and fewer false-positives. The report also shows that using both nuchal translucency and serum markers in the first trimester is more effective in screening for Down syndrome than using either alone. At 11 weeks' gestation, adding serologic markers to the determination of nuchal translucency increases the detection rate of Down syndrome from 70% to almost 90%, with a false-positive rate of 5%. A 5% false-positive rate is still quite high.

This report concludes that when there is appropriate quality control for the measurement of nuchal translucency, first-trimester combined screening is a powerful tool for the detection of Down syndrome. See the preceding report (Abstract 11–23), which tells us more about screening for Down syndrome that involves the detection of nuchal translucency.

J. A. Stockman III, MD

Risk of Death for Children With Down Syndrome and Sepsis

Garrison MM, Jeffries H, Christakis DA (Univ of Washington, Seattle; Children's Hosp and Regional Med Ctr, Seattle, Wash)
J Pediatr 147:748-752, 2005   11–25

Objective.—To determine differences in case fatality rates between children with and without Down syndrome.

Study Design.—We used the Pediatric Health Information System (PHIS) database, which includes demographic and diagnostic data from freestanding children's hospitals. Using Poisson regression, we determined the risk of mortality from sepsis for children with Down syndrome, after controlling for potential confounding factors.

Results.—A total of 35,645 patients met our inclusion criteria, of which 3936 (11%) died during hospitalization. Altogether, 620 of the included patients also had a diagnosis of Down syndrome; 106 (17%) of these died during hospitalization. Children with Down syndrome had significantly elevated risk of mortality (mortality rate ratio = 1.30; 95% confidence interval = 1.06 to 1.59) after adjusting for potential confounding factors including demographics, pathogens, and concomitant conditions.

Conclusions.—Children with Down syndrome and sepsis have elevated risk of mortality. These findings have implications for treatment decisions, communications about prognosis, and future research.

▶ These investigators have used the PHIS database to determine the risk of death from sepsis in children with Down syndrome. They looked at an overall child population of more than 35,000 youngsters, including 620 who had a diagnosis of Down syndrome. Children with Down syndrome had a significantly elevated risk of death from sepsis with a mortality ratio of 1.3 after adjustment was made for confounding factors such as demographics, pathogens, and concomitant conditions. Youngsters with Down syndrome tended to be younger on average than other patients with sepsis and, of course, had a higher probability of having congenital heart disease. The most common organism causing sepsis was one or another species of *Staphylococcus*.

As seen in the article by de Hingh et al (Abstract 11–26), children with Down syndrome have a variety of immune peculiarities that may be among the reasons why they have a higher risk of infection. de Hingh et al have performed immunophenotyping on peripheral blood lymphocytes from almost 100 children with Down syndrome ranging in age from 1 to 20 years with an average age of 7 years. They found a diminished expansion of T and B lymphocytes with age, which strongly suggests that the immune system of patients with Down syndrome is not the same as that in children without the disorder.

Those affected with Down syndrome do have a much higher prevalence of immune-related disorders. These include a higher probability of developing celiac disease, hypothyroidism, thyrotoxicosis, chronic hepatitis, and diabetes mellitus. It may well be that an alteration in peripheral blood lymphocytes in children with Down syndrome is the key factor in this increased probability of developing immune-related disorders as well as an increase in the risk of death from sepsis.

J. A. Stockman III, MD

Intrinsic Abnormalities of Lymphocyte Counts in Children With Down Syndrome

de Hingh YCM, van der Vossen PW, Gemen EFA, et al (Je-roen Bosch Hosp, 's-Hertogenbosch, The Netherlands; Erasmus Med Centre, Rotterdam, The Netherlands; Rijnstate Hosp, Arnhem, The Netherlands)
J Pediatr 147:744-747, 2005   11–26

Objective.—Down syndrome (DS) is associated with an increased frequency of infections, hematologic malignancies, and autoimmune diseases, suggesting that immunodeficiency is an integral part of DS that contributes significantly to the observed increased morbidity and mortality. We determined the absolute counts of the main lymphocyte populations in a large group of DS children to gain further insight into this immunodeficiency.

Study Design.—In a large group of children with DS (n = 96), the absolute numbers of the main lymphocyte subpopulations were determined with 3-color immunophenotyping using the lysed whole-blood method. The results were compared with previously published data in healthy children without DS.

Results.—In healthy children with DS, the primary expansion of T and B lymphocytes seen in healthy children without DS in the first years of life was severely abrogated. The T-lymphocyte subpopulation counts gradually reached more normal levels with time, whereas the B-lymphocyte population remained severely decreased, with 88% of values falling below the 10th percentile and 61% below the 5th percentile of normal.

Conclusions.—The diminished expansion of T and B lymphocytes strongly suggests that a disturbance in the adaptive immune system is intrinsically present in DS and is not a reflection of precocious aging. Thymic alterations have been described in DS that could explain the decreased numbers of T lymphocytes, but not the striking B lymphocytopenia, seen in these children.

▶ Since the preceding several commentaries related all the new information about Down syndrome this editor knows, and since this chapter opened on the subject of emergency care, we close with a question related to this field. You are a pediatric emergency medicine physician who has just finished fellowship training. You see an ad in a professional journal for a temporary position as a pediatric emergency medicine specialist in a new hospital in Qatar. You apply and are accepted for this position, but before going, decide to read up a little bit about trauma in Qatar. Lo and behold you find one specific entity accounts for 2.6% of all childhood injuries in the United Arab Emirates. The entity is one that has no reported incidence here in the United States. What is that entity?

Camel-related injuries in the pediatric age group account for some 2.6% of all injuries in children and adolescents in the Middle East. Almost all of these injuries are seen in camel jockeys. Camel racing is extremely common in the Middle East, and most camel-related injuries in the pediatric age group result from injuries to older children and adolescents who frequently are the camel jockeys, even in sanctioned races. There is no lower limit of age for camel jockeys. As far as camel jockey injuries are concerned, head injury is the most devastating problem with more than half of injured children having sustained such injuries from camel jockeying. Although the majority of these injuries are mild, they can be severe, including skull fractures.[1] Needless to say, these youngsters also sustain many fractured bones, liver lacerations, splenic injuries, and injuries to the bowel.

There is one type of fracture that is considered to be absolutely unique to camel jockeys. This fracture has a name: "camel jockeys' tibial fracture," a fracture caused by compression rotation of the part of the leg below the knee between the trunks of adjacent racing camels. This injury is so common that some sanctioned camel races create separate tracks for each camel to obviate contact between 2 racing animals.

Thank goodness we do not see "camel"-related injuries here in the US, other than those caused by the tobacco industry.

J. A. Stockman III, MD

Reference

1. Nawaz A, Matta H, Hamchou M, et al: Camel-related injuries in the pediatric age group. *J Pediatr Surg* 40:1248-1251, 2005.

12 Musculoskeletal

A Multi-Disciplinary Study of the Ocular, Orthopedic, and Neurologic Causes of Abnormal Head Postures in Children
Nucci P, Kushner BJ, Serafino M, et al (Univ of Milan, Italy; Univ of Wisconsin, Madison)
Am J Ophthalmol 140:65-68, 2005   12–1

Purpose.—To determine the relative frequency that abnormal head postures in children are caused by orthopedic, ophthalmologic, or neurologic disorders, respectively.

Design.—A prospective, consecutive case series.

Methods.—Children found to have an abnormal head posture on routine pediatric examination underwent an evaluation by a pediatric ophthalmologist, pediatric orthopedist, and pediatric neurologist. The study was conducted in northwestern Italy.

Results.—In the 63 children evaluated, the cause of the abnormal head posture was orthopedic in 35, ocular in 25, and neurologic in 5. In 8 patients, no specific cause could be found. The most common orthopedic cause was

TABLE 1.—Etiology of Abnormal Head Posture as a Function of Age

Etiology	1/2 to 2 Years of Age, N	2-5 Years of Age, N	5-8 Years of Age, N	Total - All Ages, N
Ocular				
Duane's syndrome	2	4	0	6
Nystagmus	2	1	1	4
SOP	0	2	10	12
Brown's syndrome	0	1	2	3
Total ocular	4	8	13	25
Orthopedic				
CMT	17	8	6	31
Klippel-Feil	2	1	1	4
Total orthopedic	19	9	7	35
Neurologic				
Psychomotor delay	0	3	1	4
Brain tumor	0	1	0	1
Total neurologic	0	4	1	5
Unknown	6	1	1	8

Abbreviations: SOP, Superior oblique muscle palsy; *CMT,* congenital muscular torticollis.
(Reprinted by permission of the publisher from Nucci P, Kushner BJ, Serafino M, et al: A multidisciplinary study of the ocular, orthopedic, and neurologic causes of abnormal head postures in children. *Am J Ophthalmol* 140:65-68, 2005. Copyright 2005 by Elsevier Science Inc.)

congenital muscular torticollis, which accounted for 31 patients. The most common ocular cause was superior oblique muscle palsy, which accounted for 12 patients. In 2 patients neck muscle contracture suggested an orthopedic cause, however, the tight neck muscles were secondary to a head tilt caused by superior oblique muscle palsy.

Conclusions.—When the cause of an abnormal head posture is not obvious, a multi-disciplinary approach including ophthalmologic, neurologic, and orthopedic specialists may be helpful (Table 1).

▶ There is not a pediatrician who has been around for a while who has not seen a number of cases of abnormal head posture. This is a relatively common problem in children, and its estimated incidence is 1% to 1.5%. Common causes of abnormal head posture include congenital muscular torticollis, caused by tightness of the sternocleidomastoid muscle, ocular problems, and disorders of the CNS. Interestingly, as common as the problem of head tilting is, this article is the first study to look at a large number of children to determine the causes of the disorder. We learn, as anyone would suspect, that congenital muscular torticollis accounts for about half of all cases of abnormal head postures in children. Superior oblique muscular weakness is the next most common cause. Other causes of head tilting occur much less frequently. Neurologic causes of abnormal head posture include space-occupying lesions within the brain, postinflammatory conditions, and focal dystonia.

In addition to the neuromuscular causes of abnormal head posture, numerous ocular causes other than superior oblique muscle palsy also exist. Lateral rectus muscle palsy, nystagmus, strabismus, Brown's syndrome, and Duane's syndrome all can result in a head tilt, a face turn, or a chin-up or a chin-down position.

All too quickly, we jump to tightness of the sternocleidomastoid muscle as the cause of head tilting. We need to think beyond congenital muscular torticollis so that we do not miss other equally significant causes of the problem. The article by Dudkiewicz et al (see Abstract 12–2) brings us up-to-date about the US diagnosis of congenital muscular torticollis in infants.

J. A. Stockman III, MD

Congenital Muscular Torticollis in Infants: Ultrasound-Assisted Diagnosis and Evaluation

Dudkiewicz I, Ganel A, Blankstein A (Chaim Sheba Med Ctr, Tel Hashomer, Israel)
J Pediatr Orthop 25:812-814, 2005   12–2

Abstract.—Ultrasonography is considered the modality of choice for differentiating congenital muscular torticollis from other pathologies in the neck. The authors present their experience with ultrasound examination for the evaluation and management of congenital muscular torticollis. Twenty-six infants, 14 boys and 12 girls, age ranging from 1 to 16 weeks, with torticollis and a palpable mass were examined. Ultrasound showed a well-defined mass in the sternocleidomastoid muscle. The lesions ranged in size from 8 to 15.8 mm on maximal transverse diameter, with length ranging from 13.7 to 45.8 mm. Clinically the torticollis disappeared between 1 to 6 weeks, with complete clinical reduction of the palpated mass between 2 and 8.5 weeks. The ultrasonographic disappearance of the mass was delayed by an average of 2 weeks in comparison to the clinical disappearance of the mass. Ultrasound is advocated for the diagnosis and follow-up of congenital muscular torticollis because it noninvasively provides reliable and dynamic information without sedation.

▶ Congenital muscular torticollis (CMT) is a common problem that is usually seen at birth or shortly thereafter. It is not at all uncommon to have a history of birth trauma, difficult delivery, or a breech delivery in affected youngsters. The condition causes a unilateral contraction of the sternocleidomastoid muscle fibers forcing the infant to hold the head tilted toward the affected side. On physical examination, the head is tilted toward the involved muscle, the chin is rotated toward the contralateral shoulder, and neck range of motion is significantly limited. A mass in the sternocleidomastoid muscle region is palpable. Most children with CMT recover totally with time, but the abnormal position and limitation of head motion may result in asymmetric pressure in the growing cranium and may affect craniofacial growth and development of the spine, which may cause progressive deformity of the skull (plagiocephaly) and facial hemihypoplasia. Thus, it is critical to make a diagnosis early to begin physical therapy.

Physical examination can detect torticollis with a mass in the sternocleidomastoid muscle, but it cannot always differentiate these findings from tumors, cysts, or other pathologic conditions. Ultrasound (US) has been increasingly used to demonstrate the fibrotic lesion within the sternocleidomastoid muscle and has been proposed as the modality of choice for differentiating CMT from other pathologic conditions in the head and neck. The current article adds to our knowledge of just how good US is in the diagnosis and evaluation of youngsters with CMT. The article shows that babies with CMT do have hyperechoic areas in affected muscles relative to normal muscle in many babies. In virtually all babies, the masses are surrounded by a hyperechoic rim, and there is excellent demonstration of the mass margins.

When you see infants who appear to have torticollis, refer them for a US study. If the problem is caused by CMT, you should be able to readily make the diagnosis. If CMT is excluded, as the previous article indicates (see Abstract 12–1), look for ocular and neurologic causes of the head tilt.

J. A. Stockman III, MD

Treatment of Lateral Epicondylitis With Botulinum Toxin: A Randomized, Double-Blind, Placebo-Controlled Trial

Wong SM, Hui ACF, Tong P-Y, et al (North District Hosp, Hong Kong; Chinese Univ of Hong Kong; Prince of Wales Hosp, Hong Kong)
Ann Intern Med 143:793-797, 2005   12–3

Background.—Lateral epicondylitis, or tennis elbow, is a common cause of chronic elbow pain and wrist extensor dysfunction in adults, affecting 1% to 3% of the general population annually. Tennis elbow is characterized by localized tenderness around the lateral epicondyle, and pain can be reproduced by resisted extension of the wrist or middle finger with the elbow in a straight position. No consensus exists on the optimal treatment, but many opinions are available. Whether an injection of botulinum toxin is more effective than placebo for pain reduction in adults with lateral epicondylitis was determined.

Methods.—A randomized, double-blind, placebo-controlled trial was conducted in outpatient clinics at a university hospital and a district hospital in Hong Kong. Sixty patients with lateral epicondylitis were given a single injection of 60 units of botulinum toxin type A or normal saline placebo. The primary outcome measure was a change in subjective pain as measured by a 100-mm visual analog scale (VAS) ranging from 0 to 10 at 4 weeks and again at 12 weeks. All patients completed posttreatment follow-up.

Results.—The mean VAS scores in the botulinum group at baseline and at 4 weeks were 65.5 mm and 25.3 mm, respectively. Respective scores for the placebo group at baseline and 4 weeks were 66.2 mm and 50.5 mm. At week 12, the mean VAS scores were 23.5 mm for the botulinum group and 43.5 mm for the placebo group. Grip strength was not statistically significantly different between groups at any time. In 1 patient, symptoms persisted until week 12, whereas none of the patients in the placebo group had the same experience. At 4 weeks, 10 patients in the botulinum group and 6 patients in the placebo group experienced weak finger extension on the same side as the injection site.

Conclusions.—Botulinum toxin injections may provide improvement in pain over 3 months in patients with lateral epicondylitis. However, these injections may be associated with digital paralysis and weakness of finger extension.

▶ Who would have thought that the 127th use of botulinum toxin would be described after its introduction as part of the management of strabismus more than 30 years ago? So what is the 127th use of botulinum toxin? It is to treat tennis elbow, otherwise known as lateral epicondylitis.

This use of botulinum toxin to treat pain is quite intriguing. The authors of this article randomly assigned 60 patients with long-standing pain who received 60 units of botulinum toxin or placebo. All patients received injections at the same location relative to the lateral epicondyle. At 4 weeks and again at 12 weeks, pain scores were distinctly lower in the botulinum toxin treatment group than in the placebo group. Exactly how botulinum toxin may work is unsettled in the case of epicondylitis. The obvious mechanism of actions would either be direct pain reduction or relief of muscle tension. The authors did measure muscle weakness by grip strength and did not find any serious decrease in muscle strength, which implies that pain reduction may have been attributable to other sources, such as a direct analgesic effect of botulinum toxin. Anyone with tennis elbow will find the results of this article quite heartening because botulinum toxin injections are less noxious than other therapies for lateral epicondylitis, such as corticosteroids or surgery. Botulinum toxin can also provide long-lasting results.

It will be interesting to see whether additional uses of botulinum toxin to control pain evolve. Animal investigations suggest that botulinum toxin may alter the physiologic processes of pain through modulation of substance P, glutamate, and calcitonin gene-related peptide. These substances are present at cholinergic nerve endings and are believed to play important roles in pain sensation. Anecdotal reports exist about the possible analgesic effects of botulinum toxin on conditions in which pain is the predominant issue, including conditions such as migraine headaches and nonneurologic musculoskeletal conditions. Pain syndromes such as lateral epicondylitis, intractable daily headaches, and visceral pain may soon become potentially new indications for botulinum therapy.

As we await more data on the use of botulinum toxin for control of pain syndromes, its use for conditions for which its clinical indications are now well understood expands. These include relief of excessive muscle contractions in dystonia, hemifacial spasms, and other hyperkinetic disorders, spasticity from a stroke, cerebral palsy, brain trauma and multiple sclerosis, and hyperhidrosis in autonomic disorders. It has also been used to help control weight gain. When injected into the gastric antrum, it delays gastric emptying, which increases one's sensation of satiety. Other uses include control of headaches and pain disorders, as well as its many cosmetic uses.

While on the topic of sports-related injuries, have you ever wondered whether baseball catchers might be at unusual risk for certain types of hand injury as the result of repetitive ball catching? In fact, there are no studies of this phenomenon in the pediatric population, but recently, a report appeared about young professional baseball catchers that might be of some relevance to all of us.[1] Professional catchers receive more than 100 pitches per game with baseballs that are thrown at more than 90 miles per hour. Researchers at Wake Forest University, Baptist Medical Center in Winston-Salem, North Carolina, asked 36 minor-league ballplayers of the various fielding positions whether they experience pain in either their catching or throwing hands during or between games. Using ultrasound and blood pressure tests, the researchers also assessed whether each hand's blood vessels had been damaged. Indeed problems were found. The majority of problems were in catchers rather than other types of field position players. Almost all of the problems were in the glove hand. All the catchers evaluated described hand pain during games and several said they had chronic pain in the hand that was frequently pounded by fastballs. Few of the other players had any similar symptoms. Five catchers definitively showed altered blood flow in their gloved hand, a significantly higher proportion than among the other players.

Stay tuned for more and more uses for botulinum toxin. My favorite is its injection into the tongues of mothers-in-law who talk too much.

J. A. Stockman III, MD

Reference

1. A problem at hand for catchers (editorial). *Science News* 168:41-42, 2005.

Simple Wrist Ganglia in Children: A Follow-up Study

Calif E, Stahl S, Stahl S (Rambam Med Ctr, Haifa, Israel)
J Pediatr Orthop B 14:448-450, 2005   12–4

Background.—Ganglions are the most common soft tissue tumors of the wrist and hand. The pattern of wrist ganglia in children has been largely inferred from studies based in the general population; few studies have been done in children. The incidence of ganglions in children is reported to be lower than that in adults. However, the precise incidence in children is uncertain, and the reported rates are probably underestimated because most children do not complain of pain, have little if any functional impairment, and do not ask for medical attention. Treatment methods in adults are associated with high recurrence rates. These rates are reported to be even higher in children. Surgical intervention is associated with an inherent risk of complications. The natural history of pediatric ganglia was characterized, and the indications for surgical intervention were defined.

Methods.—A retrospective review was conducted of the medical charts of all children younger than 17 years with simple wrist ganglia who were treated and followed up for at least 2 years at one unit between the 1993 and 2003.

Results.—Over 10 years, 34 children younger than 17 years (22 girls and 12 boys) were consecutively treated at one unit. The average age at presentation was 10 years, 2 months (range, 4 months-16 years and 8 months). The average follow-up was 34 months (range, 30-56 months). Dorsal ganglions were present in 16 patients (47%), volar ganglions were present in 11 patients (32.4%), and retinacular ganglions were present in 7 patients (20.6%). Most of the children (29) were treated conservatively, and spontaneous resolution occurred in 27 of these patients within an average of 9 months. Four patients were treated by aspiration; among these patients, a recurrence was observed in 1 patient, and 1 underwent surgical excision without a recurrence.

Conclusions.—Conservative management is recommended in conjunction with reassurance of the child and parents. Surgery should be considered for ganglions with an atypical appearance or for those that elicit complaints and for larger cysts that do not show signs of resolution within 1 year.

▶ One sees a lot more wrist ganglia in adults than in children, but they do also occur in the younger population. Technically, ganglia are soft tissue tumors usually seen on the wrist and hand. In most instances, these are cysts, are asymptomatic, and are rarely of any great clinical significance. They can enlarge, however, and can be in locations that are annoying or present aesthetic problems. In most instances, given their benign nature, their recurrence rate, and the inherent risk associated with surgical intervention, a conservative approach to their management seems wise. Surgical resection of ganglia is a well-established modality of treatment in adults. Reported recurrence rates are only about 5%. However, the outcome of surgical resection in children is much less favorable, and recurrence rates are 2 to 3 times higher than in adults. The inherent risks of surgery in a child are also significantly greater.

We learn from this article that if you leave ganglia alone, you are leaving well enough alone. The behavior of pediatric wrist ganglia differs from the behavior of those in adults in that they tend to follow a much more benign course that generally ends in spontaneous remission. Surgery may be indicated if a ganglion is associated with pain, weakness, or an atypical appearance and for cases that do not seem to go away over a long period of time (in excess of a year).

When I was growing up, a common treatment of a ganglion on one's hand or wrist was to smash the thing with a heavy object. It was usually done with a large book of literature or a family bible, the latter presumably adding some greater effectiveness over a work of Steinbeck. This manner of therapy frequently did the trick.

On a very peripherally-related topic, are you aware of the oldest description of writer's cramp? This description of writer's cramp may be found in the 1713 revised edition *De Morbis Artificum*. This work is generally held to be the foundation for the field of occupational medicine since it included discussions of the dangers of toxic inhalation by workers in various occupations and many other occupational disorders. It was written by Ramazzini. Ramazzini noted the occupational hazards of being a scribe and a notary. He observed 3 classes of maladies associated with these occupations: those from constant sitting, constant writing, and mental strain from frequent tedious calculations. In terms of the dangers of constant writing, Ramazzini wrote: "An acquaintance of mine, a notary by profession, still living, used to spend his whole life continually engaged in writing, and he made a good deal of money from it; first he began to complain of intense fatigue in the whole arm, but no remedy would relieve this, and finally the whole right arm became completely paralyzed. In order to offset this infirmity, he began to train himself to write with his left, but it too before very long was attacked with the same malady." What Ramazzini was describing we now call writer's cramp, a form of focal dystonia of the hand in which an individual, usually someone whose occupation requires a significant amount of writing, has paresis or even paralysis when attempting to write despite having no weakness in the hand on standard clinical testing, no musculoskeletal problems in the arm that could account for the inability to write, and no lesions of the central nervous system or peripheral nerves demonstrable by standard imaging and electrophysiology techniques such as a CT, MRI, nerve conduction studies, or electromyography.

As far as treatment was concerned, Ramazzini offered only one: rubbing salves. Shame he didn't know about Botox, now the most commonly employed therapy for writer's cramp![1]

J. A. Stockman III, MD

Reference

1. Altschuler EL: Ramazzini and writer's cramp. *Lancet* 365:938, 2005.

Fetal Breech Presentation Predisposes to Subsequent Development of Septic Arthritis of the Hip
Cieslak TJ, Rajnik M (San Antonio Military Pediatric Ctr, Tex)
Pediatr Infect Dis J 24:650-652, 2005   12–5

Background.—Fetal breech presentation is associated with neonatal hip instability and congenital hip dislocation. Experience with a neonate with concomitant breech deformation sequence and group B streptococcal septic arthritis of the hip prompted the authors to question whether breech positioning in utero is a predisposing factor for development of septic arthritis postnatally. The possibility of a link between breech presentation and septic arthritis of the hip in neonates was investigated.

Methods.—Both septic arthritis of the hip and breech presentation are relatively rare occurrences, so a very large patient population was needed. The Patient Administration Systems and Biostatistics Activity (PASBA) is an element of the US Army's Medical Command in San Antonio, TX. Use of the PASBA database offered the potential for very large numbers of patients available through retrospective query. Records of mothers with a diagnosis of breech presentation were cross-matched with those of children with a diagnosis of septic arthritis of the pelvis and thigh.

Results.—From January 1989 through September 2002 there were 949,483 live births at US Army, Navy, and Air Force hospitals throughout the world. Of these, 31,986 (3.4%) were complicated by fetal breech presentation. In the first year of life, 4 cases (0.012%) of septic arthritis subsequently occurred among the breech group, compared with 28 cases (0.003%) among the 917,497 nonbreech infants.

When children old enough to have an appropriate length of follow-up were studied to age 6 years, 197 cases of septic arthritis were documented in the nonbreech group and 8 cases occurred in the breech group. The relative risk of septic arthritis of the hip among breech children was 4.1 in the first year of life. Relative risk was not increased beyond the first year of life.

Conclusion.—Fetal breech presentation is a predisposing factor for the development of septic hip in the first year of life.

▶ We have known for some time that breech delivery is associated with certain problems including congenital hip dislocation. This report extends our knowledge. Given the relative rarity of breech presentation (3% to 4% of potential deliveries) and of septic arthritis of the hip (1.2 to 2.6 cases per 100,000 children), one might question how one would ever document a potential relationship between the two. What the authors here have done is to look at the huge inpatient and ambulatory database provided by the US Army Medical Command which keeps biostatistical information on literally hundreds and hundreds of thousands of individuals, including all pregnancies that are in the military database.

Using the PASBA database, it was possible to electronically query for the following diagnosis group codes: live birth, breech conversion, fetal breech presentation, breech extraction, and septic arthritis of the pelvis and thigh. Over a 13-year period, almost 1 million live births occurred at US Army, Navy, and Air Force hospitals worldwide. Of the deliveries, 3.37% were breech. Four cases of septic arthritis occurred among the breech group compared with 28 cases in the remainder of the better part of a million deliveries. These data, therefore, showed a relative risk of septic arthritis of the hip among children whose gestation involved breech presentation as being 4.1 during the first year of life. No increased relative risk was seen beyond the first year of life.

Thus, it seems that there is a smoking gun when it comes to a potential relationship between breech presentation and septic arthritis of the hip. Obviously, breech presentation is a relatively small component of all septic arthritis, but, nonetheless, the latter is something we should be concerned about in any baby who is born by breech delivery who presents with fever and hip signs.

As important as these data are, the other important aspect of this report is the "power" of large databases. There are not many places one can go to find 1 million deliveries with all of the medical codes that go with these deliveries. Those receiving care through the military are, indeed, a captive audience whose experiences we can all learn from.

J. A. Stockman III, MD

Growth-Reductive Therapy in Children With Marfan Syndrome
Rozendaal L, and the Dutch Marfan Working Group (Leiden Univ, The Netherlands; et al)
J Pediatr 147:674-679, 2005   12–6

Objectives.—To determine the accuracy and precision of 2 height-prediction methods in Marfan syndrome and to assess the growth-reductive effect and side effects of sex hormone treatment.

Study Design.—In a retrospective study in 31 untreated (17 boys) and 43 treated patients (21 boys) with Marfan syndrome, we assessed bone age and predicted adult height by 2 methods. The accuracy of the methods was assessed in the untreated group. The effect of therapy was corrected for outcome in the untreated group and other confounding variables with multivariate analysis.

Results.—Accuracy strongly varied with sex, chronological age, and prediction method. Overall precision was low. Treatment was started at a mean age of 12.8 ± 1.4 years (boys) and 11.4 ± 1.2 years (girls). With multiple regression analysis, a statistically significant effect was observed only in boys using a pharmacologic dosage (5.5 cm, 95% CI 0.96-10.1 cm; $P = .02$). Side effects were worsening of acne and weight and muscle gain.

Conclusions.—In adolescents with Marfan syndrome, the accuracy and precision of 2 height-prediction methods were limited. The apparent growth-reductive effect of sex hormone treatment appears similar to earlier reports on adolescents with constitutional tall stature. There were no clinically important short-term side effects.

▶ In case you forgot, Marfan syndrome, a systemic disorder of connective tissue, was first described more than 100 years ago by a Parisian professor of pediatrics, Antoine-Bernard Marfan, who reported the association of long slender digits and other skeletal abnormalities in a 5-year-old girl named Gabrielle. Two to three individuals are affected per 10,000 in the US population. Many with the diagnosis are missed because similar manifestations are common in otherwise unaffected individuals. While the disorder is an autosomal dominant, about 25 percent of cases are sporadic due to de novo mutations. Thus, a family history of Marfan syndrome is not always present as an obvious risk factor. Both boys and girls are affected.

If you are going to be looking for cases of Marfan syndrome in the pediatric population at large, check out basketball and volleyball players. Tall stature with dolichostenomelia (long-bone overgrowth) leads to an increased prevalence in certain athletes, particularly basketball and volleyball players. In fact, some have recommended screening of such athletes with echocardiography. Kinoshita and coworkers[1] screened 455 basketball and volleyball players in high school, college, and professional sports. Of these, 1% had aortic enlargement with a diameter greater than 4.6 cm at the aortic root, and 2 were diagnosed with Marfan syndrome.

It is tall stature that is the subject of the report abstracted by Rozendaal et al. Excessive growth and tall stature are common features of Marfan syndrome and have a substantial impact on the physical and psychologic well-being of affected adolescents and adults. This report shows how accurately one can predict adult height in a youngster with Marfan syndrome. Prediction methods are, in fact, quite imprecise, showing the variability in final height of many of these patients. If, however, it is obvious that a child will be "excessively" tall before growth is completed, the standard therapies for reducing bone growth do, in fact, work in subjects with Marfan syndrome. Treatment with sex hormones can dramatically reduce final height, an especially important aspect of management in girls with the disorder.

If you are concerned about a diagnosis of Marfan syndrome but are unsure of it, think about genetic testing, but also realize the limitations in such testing. The role of genetic testing in establishing a diagnosis remains limited, since more than 500 mutations resulting in the disorder have been cataloged in an international registry. Over 90% of these mutations are known as "private" mutations unique to an individual or to an individual's family. All of these mutations seem to occur within the *FBN1* gene, which encodes the matrix protein fibrillin 1. If you do make the diagnosis, attention to detail in terms of prevention of long-term complications is critical. β-Blockers are used in virtually everyone to delay or prevent aortic aneurysm and dissection. Lifestyle modifications to decrease the risk of aortic dissection are important. Patients should be counseled not to engage in contact sports, competitive athletics, or isometric exercises. Also, if you are caring for a teenage girl, you should begin to talk about counseling related to pregnancy. There is a high risk of aortic dissection during pregnancy, directly related to the size of the aortic root before pregnancy.

The above are just a few insights into what is thought to be modern thinking about the diagnosis and management of Marfan syndrome. To read much more in the way of the details, see the superb review by Judge and Dietz.[2]

J. A. Stockman III, MD

References

1. Kinoshita N, Nimura J, Obayashi C, et al: Aortic root dilatation among young competitive athletes: Echocardiographic screening of 1929 athletes between 15 and 34 years of age. *Am Heart J* 139:723-728, 2000.
2. Judge DP, Dietz HC: Marfan's syndrome. *Lancet* 366:1965-1976, 2005.

Recombinant Osteoprotegerin for Juvenile Paget's Disease
Cundy T, Davidson J, Rutland MD, et al (Univ of Auckland, New Zealand; LabPlus, Auckland, New Zealand; Auckland City Hosp, New Zealand; et al)
N Engl J Med 353:918-923, 2005   12–7

Background.—In the autosomal recessive bone disease juvenile Paget's disease, bone turnover is greatly accelerated. The result is progressive deformity, growth retardation, and deafness when the cochlea is involved. Mutations in the gene encoding for osteoprotegerin have been identified as the culprit causing most cases of juvenile Paget's disease. Osteoprotegerin inhibits the activity of bone-resorbing cells (osteoclasts). The disease in effect develops because of osteoprotegerin deficiency. Treatment of two adult siblings with the disease using recombinant osteoprotegerin was reported.

Methods.—The brother and sister both had juvenile Paget's disease and were 24 and 31 years old, respectively. Both had first developed bony deformity about age 5 years and were restricted to wheelchairs by age 15 years. After evaluating their physical condition and obtaining biochemical profiles, bone densitometry, radiographs, and quantitative scintigraphy, treatment with recombinant osteoprotegerin was begun. To find the correct dose, injections were given at 3-week intervals using escalating doses. Measures of serum calcium and phosphate levels as well as urine markers were done each day for 5 days after the injection, then two to three times a week for 15 days. When a dose was found to inhibit bone turnover effectively, it was continued at 3-week intervals. Bone resorption was monitored throughout the process to ensure the dose remained effective. Plasma samples were also obtained to detect any antibodies to the recombinant osteoprotegerin.

Results.—Nadir values of the urine markers were obtained 3 to 8 days after a single dose of 0.1 mg/kg of recombinant osteoprotegerin. Increasing the dose to 0.3 mg/kg reduced the urine markers further and dropped plasma calcium and phosphate levels. Because hypocalcemia developed, the dose was held at 0.3 mg/kg. The dose interval was shortened to once weekly because the longer interval accomplished only transient suppression of N-telopeptide excretion. After 25 weeks of treatment for the man and 31 weeks for the woman, the dose was increased to 0.4 mg/kg, which suppressed N-telopeptide excretion for 8 months. Transient mild symptoms of hypocalcemia developed in both patients, along with transient mild elevations of plasma parathyroid hormone levels. Bone pain was decreased according to both patients. Some increase in bone density occurred in each patient. Significant improvement in bone turnover was detected radiographically, with healing of lytic lesions and improved radiographic density. The most serious complication was an exacerbation of the woman's asthma requiring hospitalization for one night 3 days after her second injection. Treatment was discontinued after 15 months. Bone turnover returned to the previous accelerated pattern.

Conclusions.—Recombinant osteoprotegerin given as a subcutaneous injection once a week was able to completely suppress the accelerated bone turnover of juvenile Paget's disease. Bone formation was also reduced secondarily. Continued treatment reduced the rate of bone turnover, as shown by decreased skeletal clearance of technetium-99m–labeled methylene diphosphonate, increased cortical bone mass, and improved radiographic findings. The anticipated side effects of hypophosphatemia and hypocalcemia with secondary hyperparathyroidism developed, but were managed. When therapy was withdrawn, accelerated bone turnover resumed.

▶ The culprit in Paget's disease is the osteoclast. Osteoclasts have the unique molecular machinery needed to tear bone apart. Mature osteoclasts attach to bone matrix by way of an integrin seal. In Paget's disease, osteoclasts veraciously dissolve skeletal minerals with acid and dissolve bone matrix with enzymes and then release the resorption products into the circulation. Once they are done feeding, they detach and migrate to other bone sites. The mechanism of action in Paget's disease is similar to the bone problem seen in a number of other skeletal disorders, including bone metastases, the hypercalcemia of malignant disease, osteoporosis, and renal osteodystrophy. Thus, whatever is found to be perhaps good for the management of Paget's disease may also turn out to be helpful for this wider spectrum of more common disorders.

There are two new drugs now for the treatment of Paget's disease. One is zoledronic acid and the other is osteoprotegerin. Both act by inhibiting osteoclast function, but in different ways. Zoledronic acid acts primarily by impairing key metabolic pathways of the mature osteoclast and, perhaps, by stabilizing bone against resorption. Osteoprotegerin acts primarily by inhibiting osteoclastogenesis. Osteoprotegerin is a recombinant protein.

Osteoprotegerin was discovered through the basic studies that led to the elucidation of the long-sought pathway that coupled bone formation to bone resorption—a pathway regulated by bone marrow mesenchymal cells and osteoblasts. The recombinant protein attaches to a receptor that blocks the action of osteoclasts. In one sense, juvenile Paget's disease could be thought of as osteoprotegerin deficiency. As we see in this report, it works extremely well and this portends good news for the application of this recombinant product to other bone resorption diseases. As one also sees, treatment intervals vary from months to years with these new agents so that they seem to be long-lasting in their effects. Although we do not know about any long-term side effects, one might be a bit concerned about oversuppression of resorption of bones since bone remodeling is a healthy process in and of itself. The fear is that inhibition of skeletal metabolic activity might lead to a phenomenon known as "frozen bone" syndrome, involving bones that no longer are metabolically active in a healthy way.

Juvenile Paget's disease is an inherited disorder. It is an autosomal recessive disease. Little did Dr Paget know when he first described the disorder (back in 1887) that the juvenile variety would ultimately be described to arise from inactivating mutations in the gene that encodes osteoprotegerin. In the last 50 years we have gone through a litany of relatively ineffective therapies (anti-inflammatory agents, mithramycin, bisphosphonates, etc) before we have come upon zoledronic acid and recombinant osteoprotegerin. The journey of over 120 years from the descriptions by Sir James Paget to the present time began with small steps, ultimately culminating in huge leaps in the last few years.

J. A. Stockman III, MD

Cheerleading-related Injuries to Children 5 to 18 Years of Age: United States, 1990–2002
Shields BJ, Smith GA (Children's Hosp, Columbus, Ohio; Ohio State Univ, Columbus)
Pediatrics 117:122-129, 2006   12–8

Objective.—To describe the epidemiology of cheerleading-related injuries among children in the United States.

Design.—A retrospective analysis of data for children 5 to 18 years old from the National Electronic Injury Surveillance System (NEISS) of the US Consumer Product Safety Commission, 1990–2002.

Methods.—Sample weights provided by the NEISS were used to make national estimates of cheerleading-related injuries. Injury rates were calculated for the most frequently occurring types of injury using cheerleading participation data.

Results.—An estimated 208 800 children (95% confidence interval [CI]: 166 620–250 980) 5 to 18 years of age were treated in US hospital emergency departments for cheerleading-related injuries during the 13-year period of 1990–2002. The number of injuries increased by 110% from 10 900 in 1990 to 22 900 in 2002, with an average of 16 100 (95% CI: 12 848–19 352) injuries per year ($P < .01$). The average age of injured children was 14.4 years (median: 15.0 years); 97% were female; and 85% of injuries occurred to children 12 to 17 years old. The number of injuries per 1000 participants per year was greater for 12- to 17-year-olds (8.1) than for 6- to 11-year-olds

(1.2) for all cheerleading-related injuries combined (P < .01; relative risk [RR]: 6.49; 95% CI: 6.40–6.58), as well as for injuries grouped by body part injured and type of injury. The body parts injured were lower extremity (37.2%), upper extremity (26.4%), head/neck (18.8%), trunk (16.8%), and other (0.8%). Injury diagnoses were strains/sprains (52.4%), soft tissue injuries (18.4%), fractures/dislocations (16.4%), lacerations/avulsions (3.8%), concussions/closed head injuries (3.5%), and other (5.5%). Children in the 12- to 18-year age group were more likely to sustain strains or sprains to the lower extremity than 5- to 11-year-olds (P < .01; RR: 1.62; 95% CI: 1.50-1.88). The majority of patients with cheerleading-related injuries was treated and released from the emergency department (98.7%). Patients sustaining fractures or dislocations were more likely to be admitted to the hospital than those sustaining other types of injury (P < .01; RR: 5.30; 95% CI: 3.29-6.43).

Conclusions.—To our knowledge, this study is the first to report numbers, rates, and trends of cheerleading-related injuries to children using a nationally representative sample. Cheerleading is an important source of injury to girls. The number of cheerleading-related injuries more than doubled during the 13-year study period. A set of uniform rules and regulations directed at increasing the safety of cheerleading, that are universally enforced, should be implemented. Mandatory completion of a safety training and certification program should be required of all cheerleading coaches. Establishment of a national database for cheerleading-related injuries would facilitate the development and evaluation of injury-prevention strategies based on epidemiologic evidence.

▶ In March 2006, the national television news highlighted a student who fell from the top of a pyramid while cheerleading, falling straight down on her head. Briefly unconscious, she awoke after being placed on a stretcher with her head taped so as to prevent any worsening of a potential spinal injury. The youngster did perfectly fine, and the amusing part of the scenario was that as she was being rushed off the court on the stretcher, she continued her cheerleading maneuvers with her arms and hands in an almost seizure-like activity, a testimony to the bravado and dedication, if not the smarts, of teens who engage in certain cheerleading activities. The report by Shields and Smith from Ohio gives us a sense of just how common cheerleading injuries are. The report is an important one because it is the first study to tell us national estimates, rates, and trends of cheerleading-related injuries to children.

Cheerleading injuries run the gamut from strains and sprains to injuries of the lower back and head and neck. The most serious injuries are associated with maneuvers such as pyramid formations and basket tosses.

While we do not hear much about serious cheerleading injuries, the National Center for Catastrophic Sport Injury Research has reported that cheerleading accounts for more than 50% of catastrophic injuries to female sports participants.[1] Some high schools and colleges are more enlightened than others in dealing with the problem. For example, on March 11, 2002, the University of Nebraska (Lincoln) Athletic Department issued a press release stating that cheerleading stunts and tumbling would be banned in an effort to protect their student athletes from unnecessary injury. The decision was based on the observation that cheerleading was responsible for the majority of catastrophic injuries to female college and high school athletes. One University of Nebraska cheerleader had already been seriously injured, having fractured her neck while doing a handspring at practice. It would seem that history does not have much university memory since a year later, a new athletic director at the university reversed the ruling of the previous athletic director and again allowed the cheerleading squad to resume stunts and tumbling in their routines.

There is nothing routine about a cheerleading activity that routinely causes injury. Three cheers for Shields and Smith who have enlightened us about this problem in a meaningful way. It is up to the rest of us to cheer on investigators such as these.

In closing this chapter of the YEAR BOOK, we end with a question. Have you ever heard of a disorder known as "cyclist palsy?" Long-distance cyclists are prone to "cyclist palsy" due to prolonged gripping of the handlebars of a bicycle. Nerve conduction studies performed on 28 adults after a 420-mile cycle event confirmed that motor latencies of the deep branch of the ulnar nerve were commonly significantly prolonged. Three individuals also developed carpal tunnel syndrome as a result of cyclist palsy. Fortunately, nerves to the little finger are not significantly affected, allowing that finger to be used for whatever important activities that are not able to be accomplished by other fingers.[2]

J. A. Stockman III, MD

References

1. Mueller FO: Catastrophic head injuries and high school and collegiate sports. *J Athl Train* 36:312-315, 2001.
2. Handberry J: Cyclist palsy. *Am J Sports Med* 33:1224-1230, 2005.

13 Neurology and Psychiatry

Tick Paralysis: Atypical Presentation, Unusual Location
Daugherty RJ, Posner JC, Henretig FM, et al (Univ of Pennsylvania, Philadelphia; Poison Control Ctr Philadelphia; New Jersey Dept of Health and Senior Services, Trenton)
Pediatr Emerg Care 21:677-680, 2005   13–1

Background.—Tick paralysis is an uncommon disease in the United States. It affects primarily young children in the Southeastern, Rocky Mountain, and Pacific Northwest regions of the country. The typical presentation is that of asymmetric ascending paralysis with intact sensation and mental status. Although cranial nerve involvement has been observed, it has been a late finding in patients with progressive weakness of the lower extremities, followed by upper extremity weakness. Two patients who were seen over 2 months with tick paralysis are described. Both cases occurred in the Philadelphia area, a region in which tick paralysis rarely occurs.

   Case 1.—In May 2003, a previously healthy female child, 5 years, presented with diplopia and progressive weakness. On the evening before presentation, the child complained of double vision. She awoke early in the morning crying that she was unable to see, secondary to severe diplopia. Her mother reported that her speech was slurred and that she was unable to sit up or walk. The patient had no history of a fever, headache, photophobia, neck stiffness, abdominal pain, or diarrhea. She had vomited once. The family lived in southern New Jersey and had 2 pet dogs. There were no known toxic exposures, recent travel, or contact with ill individuals.
   Case 2.—In July 2003, female child, 7 years, was seen with a 2-day history of a rapidly ascending paralysis and ataxia. The child had first complained of severe pain in both lower extremities and then clumsiness had developed. Over the next day, she became unable to walk and had difficulties feeding herself because of weakness in her upper extremities. The patient denied headaches, photophobia, fever, vomiting, diarrhea, or other constitutional symptoms. Her family also lived in southern New Jersey and owned a pet dog.

Discussion.—In both cases, an engorged tick was found on the scalp area and removed. Both patients recovered quickly after removal of the tick. The index of suspicion for tick paralysis was low in these cases because of the geographic location; tick paralysis is a rare occurrence in the greater Philadelphia region. It was determined that, in both cases, the most likely area of tick exposure was near their homes. The disease is generally a disease of school-age children and seems to predominate in young girls with long hair, presumably because of difficulty in detecting the tick. The atypical presentation of the first patient and the further occurrence of a second patient in an area in which the diagnosis is rarely made suggest the need to maintain a high index of suspicion for the disease in patients seen with acute onset of cranial nerve dysfunction or muscle weakness. Tick paralysis can be diagnosed simply by performing a careful history and physical examination. The tick can usually be found attached to the scalp, but the axilla and pubic regions should also be checked.

▶ This article should remind us that tick paralysis can present in very unusual ways. The first child in this case report was a 5-year-old in whom the preliminary diagnosis was Guillain-Barré syndrome, Miller-Fisher variant. She had ptosis of the right eyelid with bilateral cranial nerve VI weakness, bilateral facial nerve diplegia, right greater than left, and dysarthria. Before being admitted to the ICU for management of Guillain-Barré syndrome, the patient's mother found an engorged tick attached to the child's left parietal scalp area. The tick was a typical female *Dermacentor variabilis*. By the next day, the youngster, who had some generalized weakness, was able to get out of bed and walk around with minimal assistance.

The second patient reported was a 7-year-old with a history of rapidly ascending paralysis and ataxia. A neurologic examination showed moderate weakness of the muscles of the lower extremity. The distal muscles were affected more severely than were the proximal muscles. In the upper extremities, mild weakness of the biceps and triceps muscles was noted. Mild ptosis of the right eyelid was present, but an examination of the remainder of the cranial nerves showed that they were intact. An engorged tick was palpated on the posterior scalp and removed. Within 24 hours, with only observation, all symptoms had resolved. These 2 cases are similar to 1 reported not long ago of a child who was seen with a Bell's palsy in whom a tick was found attached to a tympanic membrane.

Tick paralysis is a relatively rare condition, and the most common offending tick is *D variabilis*. The toxin produced is an ixobotoxin. This toxin affects sodium flux across axonal membranes and results in a presynaptic junction that fails to release acetylcholine. This mechanism of action differs slightly from that of botulinum toxin, in which presynaptic acetylcholine release is inhibited by interference with the somatosome–cell membrane docking–fusing complex. Nevertheless, the clinical effects are very similar, although botulinum toxin typically produces a descending paralysis with profound early bulbar involvement. Tick paralysis traditionally follows a very distinct course of ascending weakness. The children may be ataxic or clumsy. This finding is usually due to CNS side effects of the toxin on the cerebellum or is due to neuromuscular weakness of the lower extremities. All this progresses fairly rapidly, often in a matter of just a few hours, and quickly spreads to involve the trunk and upper extremities. Cranial nerve paralysis follows.

The lesson to be learned from the report of these 2 youngsters is that a careful physical examination should be made of anyone presenting with weakness. Ticks in the scalp are frequently overlooked. Ticks in the ear canal are even more frequently overlooked unless a complete physical examination is performed. Removal of the tick almost always results in rapid and often dramatic resolution of symptoms, usually within just a few hours.

Ticks are miserable creatures that none of us like. They not only cause tick paralysis but also are potential carriers of Rocky Mountain spotted fever, babesiosis, ehrlichiosis, tularemia, tick-borne relapsing fever, Colorado tick fever, and Lyme disease. Combinations of these tick-borne diseases have been reported in single individuals.

J. A. Stockman III, MD

Long-term Stimulant Medication Treatment of Attention-Deficit/Hyperactivity Disorder: Results From a Population-Based Study

Barbaresi WJ, Katusic SK, Colligan RC, et al (Mayo Clinic, Rochester, Minn)
J Dev Behav Pediatr 27:1-10, 2006   13–2

Abstract.—The purpose of this study was to offer detailed information about stimulant medication treatment provided throughout childhood to 379 children with research-identified attention-deficit hyperactivity disorder (ADHD) in the 1976-1982 Rochester, MN, birth cohort. Subjects were retrospectively followed from birth until a mean of 17.2 years of age. The complete medical record of each subject was reviewed. The history and results of each episode of stimulant treatment were compared by gender, DSM-IV subtype of ADHD, and type of stimulant medication. Overall, 77.8% of subjects were treated with stimulants. Boys were 1.8 times more likely than girls to be treated. The median age at initiation (9.8 years), median duration of treatment (33.8 months), and likelihood of developing at least one side effect (22.3%) were not significantly different by gender. Overall, 73.1% of episodes of stimulant treatment were associated with a favorable response. The likelihood of a favorable response was comparable for boys and girls. Treatment was initiated earlier for children with either ADHD combined type or ADHD hyperactive-impulsive type than for children with ADHD predominantly inattentive type and duration of treatment was longer for ADHD combined type. There was no association between DSM-IV subtype and likelihood of a favorable response or of side effects. Dextroamphetamine and methylphenidate were equally likely to be associated with a favorable response, but dextroamphetamine was more likely to be associated with side effects. These results demonstrate that the *effectiveness* of stimulant medication treatment of ADHD provided throughout childhood is comparable to the *efficacy* of stimulant treatment demonstrated in clinical trials.

► For more on the topic of ADHD, tune in to the American Academy of Pediatrics educational tool on this topic as part of eQIPP (www.aap.org). On a different neurologic topic, what is "gelastic syncope"?

Gelastic syncope refers to laughter-related syncope, an autonomic nervous system disorder. For some patients, laughter is no laughing matter. During periods of laughter, the average individual actually is performing a Valsalva maneuver. In those who are prone to vasovagal syncope, performing a Valsalva maneuver may trigger a whole host of autonomic instability problems resulting in a fall in blood pressure uncompensated for by an increase in heart rate. Recently, an adult male was referred for episodes of syncope preceded by intense laughter. He had had at least 10 episodes of these in the preceding 20 years before he was fully evaluated with a tilt table test, where during a Valsalva maneuver done in the sitting position a drop in blood pressure was recorded. About 14 seconds into the Valsalva maneuver, the patient lost consciousness (systolic blood pressure 20 mmHg; heart rate 57 beats per minute) and jerking movements appeared. After a few seconds in the recumbent position, he recovered completely and told the doctors: "See, I've been telling you all along this is what happens."[1]

Remember the phenomenon of gelastic syncope. There is a similar phenomenon called gelastic seizures that may or may not be related to autonomic instability. If you are curious about the word gelastic, it comes from the Greek word gelos, meaning laughter.

J. A. Stockman III, MD

Reference

1. Braga SS, Manni R, Pedretti RFE: Laughter-induced syncope. *Lancet* 366:426, 2005.

Progressive Multifocal Leukoencephalopathy in a Patient Treated With Natalizumab

Langer-Gould A, Atlas SW, Green AJ, et al (Stanford Univ, Calif; Univ of California, San Francisco)
N Engl J Med 353:375-381, 2005   13–3

Background.—Progressive multifocal leukoencephalopathy (PML) is a rare oligodendroglial infection caused by the polyomavirus JC virus. PML is most often found in persons infected with HIV, but it has also been reported in immunocompromised patients receiving prolonged treatment with methotrexate, cyclophosphamide, and azathioprine. PML has not been reported in persons with multiple sclerosis, even though these medications are frequently used in the treatment of this disease. The clinical course of a patient with multiple sclerosis in whom PML developed during treatment with interferon beta-1a and natalizumab was described.

Case Report.—Man, 23, in 1983, had a 1-month episode of right hemianesthesia, his first symptoms of what would prove to be relapse-remitting multiple sclerosis. In 1998, a malignant melanoma was excised from his back with negative margins. His history was also notable for Ramsay Hunt syndrome with auricular zoster in 1998 and a cleft lip and palate. A sister also had relapsing-remitting multiple sclerosis. The patient started receiving weekly IM injections of interferon beta-1a in 1998. In 2002, he was enrolled in a clinical trial of natalizumab. In November 2004, the patient's physician observed uncharacteristic, inappropriate behavior in the patient in a routine study visit. The patient subsequently reported difficulty with concentration and attentiveness. He also developed progressive left hemiparesis, dysarthria, and cognitive impairment. MRI of the brain showed new and extensive abnormalities. Despite treatment with corticosteroids, cidofovir, and IV immune globulin, the patient's condition deteriorated rapidly and he became quadriparetic, globally aphasic, and minimally responsive. Natalizumab therapy was discontinued; however, changes consistent with an immune-reconstitution inflammatory syndrome developed. The patient was treated with systemic cytarabine, and within 2 months his condition had improved. By May 2005, he was starting to walk and to have meaningful conversations regarding his clinical deterioration. However, the patient still had disabling ataxia, cognitive impairment, mild neglect, and mild left hemiparesis.

Conclusions.—Cidofovir, an antiviral agent, has been used successfully in the treatment of HIV-associated PML. However, cidofovir does not kill glial cells infected with the JC virus. Cytarabine kills JC virus in vitro. This case suggests that the the potential exists for some degree of recovery from natalizumab-associated PML.

▶ This report, along with the one that follows (Abstract 13–4), reminds us of the risks inherent in using drugs that interfere with the normal trafficking of lymphocytes. As noted in the Gastroenterology chapter (Abstract 7–12), natalizumab is being increasingly used as part of the management of both Crohn disease and multiple sclerosis. Natalizumab is a humanized monoclonal antibody to the T-cell adhesion molecule known as α_4 integrin. This antibody would be expected to suppress T-cell function. The agent was approved by the Food and Drug Administration for the treatment of multiple sclerosis in November 2004, but the manufacturer, Biogen Idec, has been conducting continuing clinical trials with the agent to clarify its role in the treatment of a number of medical conditions. It was as a result of the 2 reports appearing in this chapter of the YEAR BOOK OF PEDIATRICS that Biogen Idec put a halt to the sales and testing of this drug. As of this writing, just 3 of 3000 patients have developed the neurologic complications reported. Close surveillance has continued to detect further active or subclinical cases of PML.

As with all new therapies that have had complications, a dilemma arises. On one hand, integrin blockers seem to have great promise. On the other hand, a complication such as PML can be fatal. Cases demonstrating serious consequences of innovative therapy pose sobering issues to investigators and the manufacturers of therapeutic agents. From everything we know, Biogen Idec did act responsibly in the design of its clinical trials and was more than responsible in quickly withdrawing its therapeutic agent when there appeared to have been a problem. What happened to the several patients has taught us all a great lesson, namely that fatal viruses lurking within many of us are just waiting to be unleashed if we tinker with our immune system. Natalizumab is a potent tinkerer.

J. A. Stockman III, MD

Progressive Multifocal Leukoencephalopathy Complicating Treatment With Natalizumab and Interferon Beta-1a for Multiple Sclerosis

Kleinschmidt-DeMasters BK, Tyler KL (Univ of Colorado, Denver; Denver Veterans Affairs Med Ctr)
N Engl J Med 353:369-374, 2005   13-4

Background.—Progressive multifocal leukoencephalopathy (PML) is associated with high rates of morbidity and mortality and occurs nearly exclusively in immunocompromised patients. A patient with multiple sclerosis who died of PML after receiving natalizumab as part of a clinical trial was described.

Case Report.—Woman, 41, who was right-handed, began to experience numbness and burning pain in her right foot and leg and tingling numbness and clumsiness in her right hand in June 1999, and eventually received a diagnosis of relapsing-remitting multiple sclerosis. The patient had a history of migraine and transient numbness of the left hand. In April 2002, the patient was enrolled in a randomized, placebo-controlled, parallel-group, multicenter study to determine the efficacy and safety of natalizumab combined with interferon beta-1a in patients with relapsing-remitting multiple sclerosis. The patient received a total of 30 doses of natalizumab by IV infusion at 4-week intervals. In November 2004, the patient reported new problems with hand-eye coordination. A mental status examination showed a decreased fund of information, minor errors on 3-dimensional drawing tests and tests of mathematics ability, and reduced immediate recall on a word-learning test. By December 2004, she had right-sided numbness and found it difficult to carry on a conversation. MRI evaluation showed a large area of abnormal signal in the left frontal lobe posteriorly. Right-sided hemiparesis with an extensor plantar response was also noted. The patient's condition continued to deteriorate, and she was hospitalized in February 2005. She was unresponsive and had a right-sided gaze preference. She died 2 weeks after admission. PML was diagnosed at autopsy based on the presence of JC viral DNA in the CSF. Nearly all the tissue sections from both cerebral hemispheres showed either macroscopic or microscopic PML lesions. There was extensive tissue destruction and cavitation in the left frontoparietal area, large numbers of bizarre astrocytes, and inclusion-bearing oligodendrocytes, which were positive for JC virus DNA.

Conclusions.—This patient with multiple sclerosis developed PML after receiving natalizumab as part of a clinical trial. The possibility of a contributory role of interferon beta-1a in this patient's PML cannot be excluded, as she received interferon beta-1a therapy for more than 2 years. However, there have been no reports of PML in patients receiving interferon beta-1a monotherapy.

Neurotropic Viruses and Cerebral Palsy: Population Based Case-Control Study

Gibson CS, MacLennan AH, Goldwater PN, et al (Univ of Adelaide, Australia; Dept of Health, Adelaide, Australia)
BMJ 332:76-79, 2006   13–5

Objective.—To investigate the association between cerebral palsy and direct evidence for perinatal exposure to neurotropic viruses.

Design.—Population based case-control study.

Setting.—Adelaide Women's and Children's Hospital Research Laboratory.

Participants and Main Outcome Measures.—Newborn screening cards of 443 white case patients with cerebral palsy and 883 white controls were tested for viral nucleic acids from enteroviruses and herpes viruses by using polymerase chain reaction. Herpes group A viruses included herpes simplex viruses 1 and 2 (HSV-1 and HSV-2), Epstein-Barr virus (EBV), cytomegalovirus (CMV), and human herpes virus 8 (HHV-8), and herpes group B viruses included varicella zoster virus (VZV) and human herpes viruses 6 and 7 (HHV-6 and HHV-7).

Results.—The prevalence of viral nucleic acids in the control population was high: 39.8% of controls tested positive, and the prevalence was highest in preterm babies. The detection of herpes group B viral nucleic acids increased the risk of developing cerebral palsy (odds ratio 1.68, 95% confidence interval 1.09 to 2.59).

Conclusions.—Perinatal exposure to neurotropic viruses is associated with preterm delivery and cerebral palsy.

▶ The role of postnatal infection, such as catastrophic meningitis or encephalitis in infancy or early childhood, as a cause of cerebral palsy is clear-cut. What is not so clear-cut is the part played by infection in congenital or neonatal cerebral palsy. The study by Gibson et al represents a case-controlled investigation into this issue and reports the prevalence of neurotropic viral nucleic acid in blood spots from routine neonatal screening. The blood spots were looked at retrospectively in infants who ultimately were determined to have cerebral palsy. Herpes group A (including CMV) nucleic acids were found more often in neonatal blood spots of preterm infants than in control infants born at term, and these were found more often in infants who subsequently received a diagnosis of cerebral palsy in comparison with control infants. These findings lead to the suggestion that there is a linkage.

It is important to read the findings of this report in some detail. Using the infants' dried blood spots, investigators retrospectively looked for HSV-1 and HSV-2, EBV, CMV, HHV-6, HHV-7, and HHV-8, and VZV. Some 40% of all infants had dried blood spots that tested positive for one or more of these viruses. Some 26.7% of infants tested positive for CMV. Much higher prevalences were found in infants who were ultimately shown to have developed cerebral palsy.

Prior estimates based on prospective studies of mothers who have had a primary CMV infection in pregnancy suggest that 5% to 10% of cases of cerebral palsy might be attributable to this virus. Also, evidence of the role of perinatal maternal infection in preterm pregnancy, itself a cause of cerebral palsy, is increasing. A large number of studies have found an excess of surrogate markers of perinatal infections in preterm and term infants who were later found to have cerebral palsy, although the extent to which these associations reflect a direct causal relationship is unclear.

Needless to say, the finding of evidence of a virus in a dry blood spot specimen does not equate with causality when it comes to cerebral palsy. The presence of such viruses may be a marker for something else, but where there is smoke there is definitely fire, and we should pay careful attention to the conclusions of this report.

It was in the early 1960s that President Kennedy invoked a war against mental retardation, a condition his family had experienced. All too often, cerebral palsy and mental retardation coexist, although clearly not in all cases. In the 50 years or so since the war was "declared," we have seen a decrease in the prevalence of mental retardation here in the United States, but only those forms of mental retardation for which there are identifiable etiologies. Brosco et al show that in 1950, some 16.5% of all mental retardation was caused by a small constellation of disorders including congenital syphilis, Rh hemolytic disease of the newborn, measles, Haemophilus influenzae, type B meningitis, congenital hypothyroidism, phenylketonuria, and congenital rubella syndrome.[1] These disorders now constitute just 0.005% of all newly diagnosed cases of mental retardation here in the United States. The rub is that what constituted the etiology of the remainder of the 83.5% of mental retardation cases back in the 1950s is still with us. Once again, mental retardation and cerebral palsy are not one in the same, but all too often the etiologies overlap.

J. A. Stockman III, MD

Reference

1. Brosco JP, Mattingly M, Sanders LM: Impact of specific medical interventions on reducing the prevalence of mental retardation. *Arch Pediatr Adolesc Med* 160:302-309, 2006.

The Relevance of Fecal Soiling as an Indicator of Child Sexual Abuse: A Preliminary Analysis

Mellon MW, Whiteside SP, Friedrich WN (Mayo Clinic, Rochester, Minn)
J Dev Behav Pediatr 27:25-32, 2006   13–6

Abstract.—Encopresis is typically characterized as resulting from chronic constipation with overflow soiling but has been portrayed as an indicator of sexual abuse. The predictive utility of fecal soiling as an indicator of sexual abuse status was examined. In a retrospective analysis of three comparison groups of 4–12 year olds, we studied 466 children documented and treated for sexual abuse; 429 psychiatrically referred children with externalizing problems and 641 normative children recruited from the community, with the latter two samples having abuse ruled out. Standardized parent report measures identified soiling status and sexual acting out behaviors. Multiple regression analysis was used to predict abuse status in each group. Reported soiling rates were 10.3% (abuse), 10.5% (psychiatric), and 2% (normative), respectively. The soiling rate in the abused group differed significantly from that of the normative group, but not from the psychiatric group. Similar rates of soiling were reported among abused children, with and without penetration, and the psychiatric sample. Rates of sexualized behavior were reported significantly more often by the abused group versus both the psychiatric and normative groups and were a better predictor of abuse status. The positive predictive value of soiling as an indicator of abuse was 45% versus 63% for sexual acting out. The psychiatric sample displayed significantly more dysregulated behavior than the sexually abused sample. The predictive utility of fecal soiling as an indicator of sexual abuse in children is not supported. Soiling seems to represent one of many stress-induced dysregulated behaviors. Clinicians should assume the symptom of soiling is most likely related to the typical pathology and treat accordingly.

▶ Some have suspected that there is a subset of children with encopresis who have this problem as a result of sexual abuse. For example, Krugman[1] advised in a clinical report that physicians consider the possibility of sodomy in children with a long-standing history of encopresis. Indeed, the published literature contains several studies pertaining to the association between sexual abuse and soiling in children. Morrow et al[2] studied 23 boys in a psychiatric treatment program and found that 36% were soiling. Two thirds of those who were soiling had likely been sodomized. Boon[3] reviewed 30 inpatients in a child psychiatry hospital with encopresis and found that sexual abuse appeared to be the precipitating factor in 16% of those children. On the other hand, Foreman and Thambirajah[4] found no examples of sexual abuse in a sample of 63 encopretic children referred to a psychiatric clinic.

What we see in the report from the Mayo Clinic is a very large study of 466 children with documented sexual abuse who are compared with 429 psychiatrically referred children and 641 normal children recruited from the same community. The study examined the potential relationship between fecal soiling and child abuse. The results of this study do demonstrate significantly higher rates of occasional fecal soiling in a group of children with known sexual victimization compared with a normal sample of children. There was, however, no difference in the rate of occasional fecal soiling between a group of children with known sexual abuse compared with children who were referred for psychiatric problems. Moreover, classifying a child as abused based on the presence of "occasional" soiling is as likely to be incorrect as correct. The authors concluded that the single behavioral symptom of occasional fecal soiling is not useful in identifying sexual abuse in children.

The data from this report do not mean that we should not think of sexual abuse when we are seeing children with encopresis. Recognize, however, that encopresis alone cannot be used as a marker of sexual abuse of a child. The number of children who have encopresis, for the multitude of reasons children have this problem, far outweighs the occasional child who has encopresis as a result of sexual abuse.

J. A. Stockman III, MD

References

1. Krugman R: Recognition of sexual abuse in children. *Pediatr Rev* 8:25-30, 1986.
2. Morrow J, Yeager C, Otnow-Lewis D: Encopresis and sexual abuse in a sample of boys in residential treatment. *Child Abuse Negl* 21:11-18, 1997.
3. Boon F: Encopresis and sexual assault. *J Am Acad Child Adolesc Psychiatr* 30:509-510, 1991.
4. Foreman D, Thambirajah M: Letter to the editor. *Child Abuse Negl* 22:337, 1996.

Rates of Adult Schizophrenia Following Prenatal Exposure to the Chinese Famine of 1959-1961

St Clair D, Xu M, Wang P, et al (Shanghai Jiao Tong Univ, People's Republic of China; Chinese Academy of Sciences, Wuhu, People's Republic of China; Peking Univ, Shanghai, People's Republic of China; et al)
JAMA 294:557-562, 2005   13–7

Context.—Schizophrenia is a common major mental disorder. Intrauterine nutritional deficiency may increase the risk of schizophrenia. The main evidence comes from studies of the 1944-1945 Dutch Hunger Winter when a sharp and time-limited decline in food intake occurred. The most exposed cohort conceived during the famine showed a 2-fold increased risk of schizophrenia.

Objective.—To determine whether those who endured a massive 1959-1961 famine in China experienced similar results.

Design, Setting, and Participants.—The risk of schizophrenia was examined in the Wuhu region of Anhui, one of the most affected provinces. Rates were compared among those born before, during, and after the famine years. Wuhu and its surrounding 6 counties are served by a single psychiatric hospital. All psychiatric case records for the years 1971 through 2001 were examined, and clinical and sociodemographic information on patients with schizophrenia was extracted by researchers who were blinded to the nature of exposure. Data on number of births and deaths in the famine years were available, and cumulative mortality was estimated from later demographic surveys.

Main Outcome Measures.—Evidence of famine was verified, and unadjusted and mortality-adjusted relative risks of schizophrenia were calculated.

Results.—The birth rates (per 1000) in Anhui decreased approximately 80% during the famine years from 28.28 in 1958 and 20.97 in 1959 to 8.61 in 1960 and 11.06 in 1961. Among births that occurred during the famine years, the adjusted risk of developing schizophrenia in later life increased significantly, from 0.84% in 1959 to 2.15% in 1960 and 1.81% in 1961. The mortality-adjusted relative risk was 2.30 (95% confidence interval, 1.99-2.65) for those born in 1960 and 1.93 (95% confidence interval, 1.68-2.23) for those born in 1961.

Conclusion.—Our findings replicate the Dutch data for a separate racial group and show that prenatal exposure to famine increases risk of schizophrenia in later life.

▶ This study of St Clair et al reports an association between prenatal exposure to severe maternal nutritional deficiency and a risk for the development of schizophrenia in adulthood. From 1959 through 1961, there was a profound famine in China that afforded the opportunity to undertake this study years later. The findings are similar to the linkage between nutrition during pregnancy and the development of schizophrenia as a result of the Dutch Hunger Winter of 1944-1945. It was at that time that the German army blockaded foodstuffs to the western Netherlands as punishment for Dutch involvement in the planned allied invasion of Europe. Before the blockade, the food supply had been adequate; in May 1945, after the German retreat, food again became quite plentiful. During the intervening months, however, the Dutch population, particularly in larger cities, received increasingly meager rations of food, a circumstance rendered especially difficult by an unusually harsh winter. Dutch women who were pregnant in October 1944 experienced a famine and malnutrition unlike anything ever recorded before in civilized populations. Children born of such pregnancies showed a 2-fold increased risk of schizophrenia in later life, a statistic equally applicable to men and women. Indeed, the schizophrenia findings from the Dutch and the Chinese famine studies are in remarkable agreement. St Clair et al reported a 2-fold increased risk of schizophrenia among individuals prenatally exposed to famine both overall and for each sex separately.

Why there is a link between maternal starvation before delivery and the subsequent development of schizophrenia remains speculative. Most suspect that this has something to do with folate deficiency and its consequences on DNA methylation in the developing brain.

Needless to say, a phenomenon similar to what occurred in the Netherlands more than 6 decades ago is now taking place in certain parts of Africa where "state-sponsored" starvation is endemic. In a few decades, we may very well see mental disorders developing in survivors of the Darfur famine.

A couple of additional comments about schizophrenia: there are some who believe that evidence exists that schizophrenia has been present for only approximately the last 200 years of our history. As potential proof of this are casebooks from asylums. Casebooks from asylums for the mentally ill from the end of the 18th century have no descriptions of patients with a disease that at all resembles schizophrenia, while later editions in the early 19th century do contain the beginnings of potential descriptions of this psychiatric entity. Furthermore, the only known description possibly consistent with schizophrenia prior to 1800 is the Edgar ("Poor Mad Tom") character in Shakespeare's King Lear.[1] In fact, there is no clear description of schizophrenia until the middle of the 19th century.[2] Conversely, descriptions of substance abuse, mania, temporal lobe epilepsy and antisocial personality disorder, heavy metal poisoning, and even porphyric madness have been consistently logged for many centuries or even millennia.[3]

So, in evolutionary history, is schizophrenia a truly new diagnostic entity? The answer is not really clear. Absence of evidence is not evidence of absence. Nevertheless, history tends to report unusual phenomenon fairly accurately, and we see no accurate history that catalogs any incidence or occurrence of schizophrenia more than 200 years ago.

Last, recent information suggests there may be a link between schizophrenia and immune disorders. Having a history of autoimmune disease is associated with a 45% increase in the risk of schizophrenia, at least according to data from a Danish study. In a large epidemiological study, 9 autoimmune disorders had higher prevalence among patients with schizophrenia, and 12 autoimmune diseases had higher prevalence among parents of those with schizophrenia. Thyrotoxicosis, celiac disease, acquired hemolytic anemia, interstitial cystitis, and Sjogren's syndrome had higher prevalence among both patients and relatives of patients. Believers of the mind-body theory should read the Danish report in some detail.[4]

J. A. Stockman III, MD

References

1. Bark NM: Did Shakespeare know schizophrenia? The case of Poor Mad Tom in King Lear. *Br J Psychiatr* 146:436-438, 1985.
2. Altschuler EL: One of the oldest cases of schizophrenia in Gogol's diary of a mad man. *BMJ* 323:1475-1477, 2001.
3. Altschuler EL: Schizophrenia and the Chinese famine of 1959-1961. *JAMA* 294:2968, 2005.
4. Eaton WW, Byrne M, Ewald H, et al: Association of schizophrenia and autoimmune diseases: linkage of Danish national registers. *Am J Psychiatr* 163:521-528, 2006.

Randomised Controlled Trial of Animal Facilitated Therapy With Dolphins in the Treatment of Depression

Antonioli C, Reveley MA (Univ of Leicester Med School, England)
BMJ 331:1231-1234, 2005   13–8

Objective.—To evaluate the effectiveness of animal facilitated therapy with dolphins, controlling for the influence of the natural setting, in the treatment of mild to moderate depression and in the context of the biophilia hypothesis.

Setting.—The study was carried out in Honduras, and recruitment took place in the United States and Honduras.

Design.—Single blind, randomised, controlled trial.

Participants.—Outpatients, recruited through announcements on the internet, radio, newspapers, and hospitals.

Results.—Of the 30 patients randomly assigned to the two groups of treatment, two dropped out of the treatment group after the first week and three withdrew their consent in the control group after they had been randomly allocated. For the participants who completed the study, the mean severity of the depressive symptoms was more reduced in the treatment group than in the control group (Hamilton rating scale for depression, $P = 0.002$; Beck depression inventory, $P = 0.006$). For the sample analysed by modified intention to treat and last observation carried forward, the mean differences for the Hamilton and Beck scores between the two groups was highly significant ($P = 0.007$ and $P = 0.012$, respectively).

Conclusions.—The therapy was effective in alleviating symptoms of depression after two weeks of treatment. Animal facilitated therapy with dolphins is an effective treatment for mild to moderate depression, which is based on a holistic approach, through interaction with animals in nature.

► This article appears to be the first randomized, single-blind, controlled trial of animal facilitated therapy with dolphins. Before assigning the study as a suitable entry for "Ripley's Believe It or Not," you might want to think about the implications of the findings of this study first. I had not been in tune with the latest literature on the topic of biophilia, which is the basis for the findings in this study, which used dolphins to treat human disease. In the biophilic vision, the manifestation of emotions and the affiliation with nature are thought to be an innate human tendency. Those devotees of biophilia believe that disrupting the affiliation with nature results in the loss of biophilic equilibrium and alters our psychological health. The findings from this article add some credence, perhaps, to believers in biophilia. The authors of the article suggest that the biophilic method of intervention for depression represents a new emphasis in psychiatry and has the potential to bring alternative clinical strategies to the treatment of emotional disorders.

It is probably worth reading this article in detail to learn more about animal facilitated therapy. Clearly, it is not for everyone. First of all, when it comes to depression and dolphin therapy, you have to know or learn how to snorkel.

Secondly, you have to live in an area where there are trained dolphins or be willing to fly to such a place. Gosh knows what that may cost.

One final comment: in case you are not aware, *Tursiops truncatus* is the proper name for the bottle-nosed dolphin, the type of dolphin indigenous to Sea World.

J. A. Stockman III, MD

Paternal Depression in the Postnatal Period and Child Development: A Prospective Population Study

Ramchandani P, and the ALSPAC Study Team (Univ of Oxford, England; Univ of Bristol, England; Univ of Rochester, NY)

Lancet 365:2201-2205, 2005   13–9

Background.—Depression is common and frequently affects mothers and fathers of young children. Postnatal depression in mothers affects the quality of maternal care, and can lead to disturbances in their children's social, behavioural, cognitive, and physical development. However, the effect of depression in fathers during the early years of a child's life has received little attention.

Methods.—As part of a large, population-based study of childhood, we assessed the presence of depressive symptoms in mothers (n=13 351) and fathers (n=12 884) 8 weeks after the birth of their child with the Edinburgh postnatal depression scale (EPDS). Fathers were reassessed at 21 months. We identified any subsequent development of behavioural and emotional problems in their children (n=10 024) at age 3.5 years with maternal reports on the Rutter revised preschool scales.

Findings.—Information was available for 8431 fathers, 11,833 mothers, and 10,024 children. Depression in fathers during the postnatal period was associated with adverse emotional and behavioural outcomes in children aged 3.5 years (adjusted odds ratio 2.09, 95% CI 1.42-3.08), and an increased risk of conduct problems in boys (2.66, 1.67-4.25). These effects remained even after controlling for maternal postnatal depression and later paternal depression.

Interpretation.—Our findings indicate that paternal depression has a specific and persisting detrimental effect on their children's early behavioural and emotional development.

▶ A tremendous amount of literature deals with postpartum depression in women and the effects thereof on their offspring, but virtually nothing exists in the literature about postpartum depression in fathers and what the impact might be on their offspring. The article abstracted opens a new chapter on child developmental research. The researchers have included fathers in the equation. Fathers have existed as long as there have been children, and it should be expected that the well-being of the father would have some effect on his baby.

Research on maternal postpartum depression would fill a library; it is possibly one of the most researched areas in developmental psychopathology. To see what happens when the father is depressed, the investigators asked a simple question, does paternal depression in the postnatal period in any way affect infant development? The answer is an unequivocal yes. Fathers know that interaction with their babies is important. More and more young fathers and mothers want to take care of their infants together. In many countries other than our own, paternal leave is automatic. In Finland, for example, fathers can take 3 weeks leave with part pay immediately after a baby is born or later in infancy and can also share the paternal leave with the mother. The significant majority of all new fathers in Finland used this opportunity for paternal leave in 2003.[1]

It is no longer acceptable that we say men lack "the maternal instinct." Indeed, mothers seem well adapted to care for their babies, but there is nothing inherently defined that says that mothers are more sensitive to their babies than fathers might be. This article by Ramchandani and colleagues adds to our understanding about the role of fathering by suggesting that infants are, in fact, sensitive to their fathers' presence. You can bet that there will be much more in the way of mainstream research into infant development, psychopathology, and the role of a new father.

One final comment, this having to do with the opposite of depression, happiness. Most of us feel a little bit better on days in which we have some money in our wallet, but it is generally been considered debatable whether wealth makes you happy? Does it? It indeed is debatable whether wealth makes you happy, but it does influence your risk of dying, at least according to one recent study.[2] That study showed that each additional dollar of income results in a slightly smaller risk of death. Using mathematical wizardry to model what happens when you apply this to a national population over three years, New Zealand investigators found that the overall mortality would be reduced by 14% after a 10% to 40% increase in everyone's income.

If you believe these data, Warren Buffet should have Methuselah genes.

J. A. Stockman III, MD

Reference

1. *Statistical Yearbook of the Social Insurance Institution, Finland 2003.* Helsinki, Social Insurance Institution, 2004.
2. Blakely T, Wilson N: Shifting dollars, saving lives: What might happen to mortality rates, and socio-economic inequalities in mortality rates, if income was redistributed? *Soc Sci Med* 62:2024-2034, 2006.

Suicidal Ideation Among Urban Nine and Ten Year Olds

O'Leary CC, Frank DA, Grant-Knight W, et al (Boston Univ; Harvard Med School, Boston)
J Dev Behav Pediatr 27:33-39, 2006
13–10

Abstract.—Little is known about rates and correlates of suicidal ideation among nonclinical samples of preadolescents from low-income urban backgrounds. Using the Children's Depression Inventory, we measured suicidal ideation in 131 preadolescent urban children (49% female, 90% African American/Caribbean) participating in an ongoing prospective longitudinal study of prenatal cocaine exposure and children's outcome. Suicidal ideation was reported by 14.5% of the children in this sample at 9 to 10 years of age. Children's reports of depressive symptoms, exposure to violence, and distress symptoms in response to witnessing violence were associated with suicidal ideation, but prenatal cocaine exposure, parent-rated child behavior, and caregivers' psychological distress symptoms were not. Suicidal ideation may be more prevalent among preadolescents from urban, low-income backgrounds than clinicians suspect, particularly among children exposed to violence.

► This report is a subset study of a long-term sample of inner-city children with prenatal exposure to cocaine. The authors found that 14.5% of 9- and 10-year-old poor, largely minority children have suicidal ideation. Of note, this finding was in all children being followed, and suicidal ideation was not significantly associated with exposure to cocaine, gender, race, or foster or adoptive placement. In most cases, suicidal ideation was significantly associated with self-reported depressive symptoms.

What is important about the study is that most of us have assumed that 9 and 10 year olds have a low rate of depression and cognitively are less likely to frame suicidal thoughts compared with a junior high or high school peer. Clearly, we do not understand what makes a 5-, 7-, 9-, or 11-year-old child commit suicide, but they do. We do not have accurate figures, however, on the rate of suicide. When it comes to adolescents, clinical depression seems to occur at a rate of 5000 to 10,000 per 100,000, with completed suicide occurring at a rate of 11 per 100,000. If the data of O'Leary are correct, the rate of suicidal ideation in prepubertal children is on the order of 14,500 per 100,000. These are staggering numbers. For more on the topic of suicidal ideation, see the commentary of Jellinek.[1]

While on the topic of cocaine, who is likely to be the most famous physician who was a cocaine addict? A little background is in order about cocaine and the medical field to answer this question. In 1884, cocaine, the alkaloid derivative of the coca plant treasured by the Incas, became all the rage among the medical cognoscenti. In July of that year, for example, Sigmund Freud published a detailed monograph on cocaine. Although Freud's series of experiments on himself and others demonstrated many of cocaine's effects, in the monograph he glossed over a critical one that had immediate applications, the drug's properties as a local anesthetic. It was in late October of 1884 that William Halsted, the most famous of all surgeons, began his own experiments with this "wonder drug" as a local anesthetic, showing how infiltrating the sensory nerves and blocking major nerve trunks could be safely facilitated. He published his findings in the *New York Medical Journal* in 1885, but it was soon clear that he had begun to use his own experimental drug. In February and March of 1886, Halsted was sailing on a schooner bound for the Windward islands and very craftily had brought with him a large supply of cocaine with the sincere hope of gradually cutting down his dose and weaning himself off the drug. Despite his careful calculations, he could not satisfy his addictive hunger and actually ran out of cocaine long before the ship was nearing its destination. One night, it is recorded, that thousands of miles out to sea, the cocaine-obsessed Halsted lay awake in his rocking hammock until his bunkmate's telltale snoring indicated slumber. At that point Halsted sneaked out of his cabin, prowled about until he located the captain's medicine chest, and absconded back to his cabin with the entire ship's supply of cocaine.

Halsted's addiction came to light during his time at Johns Hopkins Hospital in Baltimore. His close friend, William Welsh, had become professor of pathology at the newly established Johns Hopkins Hospital and enticed his friend, Halsted, from New York City to join the Baltimore faculty. Very shortly after joining the faculty, where he was named surgeon-in-chief in 1889, he was noted to have difficulty with attentiveness in the operating room, frequently dropping out in the middle of surgeries. Most famously, William Osler recalled in 1890 that he had seen the surgeon having severe chills and suspected that Halsted was addicted to morphine and to cocaine and was going through withdrawal. Osler gained the surgeon's trust and over time Halsted was able to reduce the amount of cocaine that he was addicted to less than "three grains" daily.

Historians believe that William Halsted never really became "clean" and remained an addict to the day of his death. He had a particular pension for having his soiled linens sent to a laundry in Paris, which may or may not have sent him back more than just clean shirts. It should also be noted that in the early days of Johns Hopkins, as was true of virtually every other medical institution, cocaine and morphine were not locked up in operating rooms.[2]

J. A. Stockman III, MD

References

1. Jellinek M: Suicide ideation in prepubertal children: What does it mean? What to do? *J Dev Behav Pediatr* 27:40-41, 2006.
2. Markel H: The accidental addict. *N Engl J Med* 352:966-968, 2005.

Trends in Suicide Ideation, Plans, Gestures, and Attempts in the United States, 1990-1992 to 2001-2003

Kessler RC, Berglund P, Borges G, et al (Harvard Med School, Boston; Univ of Michigan, Ann Arbor; Mexican Inst of Psychiatry, Mexico City; et al)
JAMA 293:2487-2495, 2005   13–11

Context.—Little is known about trends in suicidal ideation, plans, gestures, or attempts or about their treatment. Such data are needed to guide and evaluate policies to reduce suicide-related behaviors.

Objective.—To analyze nationally representative trend data on suicidal ideation, plans, gestures, attempts, and their treatment.

Design, Setting, and Participants.—Data came from the 1990-1992 National Comorbidity Survey and the 2001-2003 National Comorbidity Survey Replication. These surveys asked identical questions to 9708 people aged 18 to 54 years about the past year's occurrence of suicidal ideation, plans, gestures, attempts, and treatment. Trends were evaluated by using pooled logistic regression analysis. Face-to-face interviews were administered in the homes of respondents, who were nationally representative samples of US English-speaking residents.

Main Outcome Measure.—Self-reports about suicide-related behaviors and treatment in the year before interview.

Results.—No significant changes occurred between 1990-1992 and 2001-2003 in suicidal ideation (2.8% vs 3.3%; $P=.43$), plans (0.7% vs 1.0%; $P=.15$), gestures (0.3% vs 0.2%; $P=.24$), or attempts (0.4%-0.6%; $P=.45$), whereas conditional prevalence of plans among ideators increased significantly (from 19.6% to 28.6%; $P=.04$), and conditional prevalence of gestures among planners decreased significantly (from 21.4% to 6.4%; $P=.003$). Treatment increased dramatically among ideators who made a gesture (40.3% vs 92.8%) and among ideators who made an attempt (49.6% vs 79.0%).

Conclusions.—Despite a dramatic increase in treatment, no significant decrease occurred in suicidal thoughts, plans, gestures, or attempts in the United States during the 1990s. Continued efforts are needed to increase outreach to untreated individuals with suicidal ideation before the occurrence of attempts and to improve treatment effectiveness for such cases.

▶ It is unfortunate that, despite our better ability to treat the causes of suicide, suicide thoughts, plans, gestures or attempts at suicide have not significantly decreased here in the United States over the last decade or more. Although a growing body of literature has shed light on the intensity, duration, and follow-up required to treat mental disorders, comparable data on the optimal treatment of suicidal thoughts and behavior are few and far between and are only just beginning to emerge. In light of the controversy about the role of antidepressants and suicidal ideation among adolescents, identifying whether emerging treatments have the potential to ameliorate suicidal ideation in some individuals while potentially worsening it others will be important.

While some take their own lives, in certain parts of the world, physicians are actively assisting in the death of patients. One is referring here to the Groningen protocol, which defines criteria for euthanasia in severely ill newborns.[1] In The Netherlands, active euthanasia of certain newborns is becoming increasingly more common. Infants with severe forms of spina bifida seem to be the target babies. This is a shame because mandatory folic acid fortification would have prevented the development of spina bifida in a large percentage of babies who are being euthanized. The failure of the Dutch government and many other governments to require folic acid fortification remains the tragic policy error.[2] One hopes that physicians always try to do the "right thing." Sometimes the right thing is not to be proactive in hastening death, including the death of tiny babies with complex medical problems.

This is the last entry in the Neurology and Psychiatry chapter, so we will conclude this commentary with a question on a modifier of human behavior, stress. Words and the meaning of words in medicine are a critical part of practice. It is important, at times, to know the derivation of some of the terms we use. What is the derivation of the word "stress?" Hayward gives us the answer to this query.[3] Stress derives from the Latin verb, *stringo [stingere]*, meaning to bind or draw tight, but also to graze, touch, pluck, or prune. The word entered the English language in the 14th century as a modified form of distress or distrain. In early uses, it referred to a physical hardship or trial, but by the 16th century, it also indicated a form of physical injury. In these early uses, stress was seen as an unpleasant condition of the environment rather than of the individual. It was not until the 17th century that the word began to refer to an inner state. This inner state was described throughout the 1800s as one that could lead to physical illness. The idea that the body's response to environmental conditions might have long-term consequences was proposed formally by William Osler (1849-1919). In 1934, Walter B. Cannon (1871-1945) provided experimental evidence of this process when he showed the increased production of adrenaline in animals subject to stressors.

Whatever the historical origins of the word stress may be, the term currently refers to mental or physical states, minor irritants, life crises, verbal emphasis, and problematic forces in engineering and dentistry. Stress can be good or bad, and even when good, too much of a good thing can be bad.

J. A. Stockman III, MD

References

1. Verhagen E, Sauer PJJ: The Groningen protocol: Euthanasia in severely ill newborns. *N Engl J Med* 352:959-962, 2005.
2. Oakley GP: Euthanasia in severely ill newborns (letter). *N Engl J Med* 352:2354, 2005.
3. Hayward R: Stress. *Lancet* 365:2001, 2005.

14 Newborn

Vitamin C and Vitamin E in Pregnant Women at Risk for Pre-eclampsia (VIP Trial): Randomised Placebo-Controlled Trial

Poston L, for the Vitamins in Pre-eclampsia (VIP) Trial Consortium (King's College London)

Lancet 367:1145-1154, 2006   14-1

Background.—Oxidative stress could play a part in pre-eclampsia, and there is some evidence to suggest that vitamin C and vitamin E supplements could reduce the risk of the disorder. Our aim was to investigate the potential benefit of these antioxidants in a cohort of women with a range of clinical risk factors.

Methods.—We did a randomised, placebo-controlled trial to which we enrolled 2410 women identified as at increased risk of pre-eclampsia from 25 hospitals. We assigned the women 1000 mg vitamin C and 400 IU vitamin E (RRR α tocopherol; n=1199) or matched placebo (n=1205) daily from the second trimester of pregnancy until delivery. Our primary endpoint was pre-eclampsia, and our main secondary endpoints were low birthweight (<2.5 kg) and small size for gestational age (<5th customised birthweight centile). Analyses were by intention to treat. This study is registered as an International Standard Randomised Controlled Trial, number ISRCTN 62368611.

Findings.—Of 2404 patients treated, we analysed 2395 (99.6%). The incidence of pre-eclampsia was similar in treatment and placebo groups (15% [n=181] *vs* 16% [n=187], RR 0.97 [95% CI 0.80-1.17]). More low birthweight babies were born to women who took antioxidants than to controls (28% [n=387] *vs* 24% [n=335], 1.15 [1.02-1.30]), but small size for gestational age did not differ between groups (21% [n=294] *vs* 19% [n=259], 1.12 [0.96-1.31]).

Interpretation.—Concomitant supplementation with vitamin C and vitamin E does not prevent pre-eclampsia in women at risk, but does increase the rate of babies born with a low birthweight. As such, use of these high-dose antioxidants is not justified in pregnancy.

► Preeclampsia produces a lot of problems not only for mothers but also their soon-to-be-delivered infants. This report focuses on preeclampsia prevention. The VIP study is a well-conducted trial in which 2410 women with clinical risk factors predisposing them to develop preeclampsia were randomly allocated in blinded fashion to receive antioxidant supplementation (1000 mg vitamin C and 400 IU vitamin E) or placebo before 22 weeks' gestation. This VIP study of vitamin supplementation was based on an interesting but still not established hypothesis (ie, the roles of antioxidant excess and exaggerated systemic inflammatory response in the causation of preeclampsia) that seemed to have considerable supporting data, but was not without its critics. Earlier, smaller studies did suggest that antioxidant vitamin supplementation might be of some help. Unfortunately, it turns out that this intervention not only failed to decrease the incidence of preeclampsia, but might also have been responsible for an increase in adverse outcomes. Preeclampsia appeared 8 days earlier and may have been more severe in the supplemented group, as significantly more of these women required parenteral antihypertensives, magnesium sulfate, or both. Supplementation was also associated with more gestational hypertension and fetal jeopardy. Birth weights were significantly lower, and there were significantly more unexplained deaths after 24 weeks' gestation, higher rates of cord-blood acidosis, and lower 5-minute Apgar scores in supplemented women.

What is a bit strange about the findings of this report is that adverse outcomes were observed with the administration of vitamins in amounts that do not exceed what are considered to be maximum daily tolerable allowances. These findings are consistent vitamins A and D studies during pregnancy. Adverse outcomes were seen when these vitamins were taken at maximal (but acceptable) dosage by women participating in a high-protein supplementation study.[1]

Without question, preventing preeclampsia or decreasing its severity would considerably reduce maternal-fetal morbidity in our country and worldwide. Unfortunately, vitamin C and vitamin E are just 2 more failures in a long lineage of failures that have included aspirin, calcium supplementation, and vitamins A and D. The search goes on for the magic bullet.

This is the first entry in the Newborn chapter, which contains much information on pregnancies, so we will close with a query about pregnancy. A couple comes to see you in anticipation of the completion of a successful pregnancy. During this prenatal visit they offhandedly ask you whether or not you think the child whom you will be caring for as a pediatrician will be a boy or a girl. The only significant history is that this couple did experience some difficulty getting pregnant and had tried for more than 12 months before conception occurred. What is your bet as to the sex of the infant? If you did not know, the time taken to get pregnant is positively related to the chance of having a baby boy in couples conceiving naturally. The proportions of X- and Y-chromosomes bearing sperm in human semen are equal, but more boys than girls are normally born under any circumstance. Male embryos and fetuses have a greater risk of attrition in utero than their female counterparts, and therefore male excess is still likely to be larger at the time of conception. It remains unexplained, however, what is responsible, presumably at some point between insemination and conception, for the greater probability of Y-bearing sperms fusing with the ovum. One hypothesis relates to experiments showing that Y-bearing sperms swim faster than X-bearing sperms in viscous fluids. For natural conception, human sperms have to penetrate cervical mucous, the viscosity of which varies among and within women. Since mucal viscosity also influences the probability of conception, one might expect that natural conceptions that take longer to achieve are more likely to be male than quick conceptions. In fact, this is true. A recent report analyzed 5,283 Dutch women who gave birth to singletons between July 2001 and July 2003. Among women with times to pregnancy longer than 12 months, the probability of male offspring was 57.6%, whereas the proportion of male births among women with shorter times to pregnancy was as expected at about 51.1%. These findings are consistent with the hypothesis that more viscous cervical mucous reduces the chance of conception, but increases the chance of male offspring.

Thus it is that households in which it takes a long time to get pregnant are more likely not to have an offspring that is sugar and spice and all things nice.[2]

J. A. Stockman III, MD

References

1. Rush D, Stein M, Susser M: A randomized controlled trial of prenatal nutritional supplementation in New York City. *Pediatrics* 65:683-697, 1980.
2. Smits LJM, Bie RA, Essed GG, et al: Time to pregnancy and sex of offspring: Cohort study. *BMJ* 331:1437, 2005.

Effect of Treatment of Gestational Diabetes Mellitus on Pregnancy Outcomes

Crowther CA, for the Australian Carbohydrate Intolerance Study in Pregnant Women (ACHOIS) Trial Group (Univ of Adelaide, Australia; et al)
N Engl J Med 352:2477-2486, 2005
14–2

Background.—We conducted a randomized clinical trial to determine whether treatment of women with gestational diabetes mellitus reduced the risk of perinatal complications.

Methods.—We randomly assigned women between 24 and 34 weeks' gestation who had gestational diabetes to receive dietary advice, blood glucose monitoring, and insulin therapy as needed (the intervention group) or routine care. Primary outcomes included serious perinatal complications (defined as death, shoulder dystocia, bone fracture, and nerve palsy), admission to the neonatal nursery, jaundice requiring phototherapy, induction of labor, cesarean birth, and maternal anxiety, depression, and health status.

Results.—The rate of serious perinatal complications was significantly lower among the infants of the 490 women in the intervention group than among the infants of the 510 women in the routine-care group (1 percent vs. 4 percent; relative risk adjusted for maternal age, race or ethnic group, and parity, 0.33; 95 percent confidence interval, 0.14 to 0.75; P=0.01). However, more infants of women in the intervention group were admitted to the neonatal nursery (71 percent vs. 61 percent; adjusted relative risk, 1.13; 95 percent confidence interval, 1.03 to 1.23; P=0.01). Women in the intervention group had a higher rate of induction of labor than the women in the routine-care group (39 percent vs. 29 percent; adjusted relative risk, 1.36; 95

percent confidence interval, 1.15 to 1.62; P<0.001), although the rates of cesarean delivery were similar (31 percent and 32 percent, respectively; adjusted relative risk, 0.97; 95 percent confidence interval, 0.81 to 1.16; P=0.73). At three months post partum, data on the women's mood and quality of life, available for 573 women, revealed lower rates of depression and higher scores, consistent with improved health status, in the intervention group.

Conclusions.—Treatment of gestational diabetes reduces serious perinatal morbidity and may also improve the woman's health-related quality of life.

▶ This article reminds us how common gestational diabetes is. It occurs in 2% to 9% of all pregnancies. The article also reminds us that the risk of perinatal mortality is not increased with gestational diabetes, but the risk of macrosomia is, along with certain other complications that include shoulder dystocia, birth injuries (such as bone fractures and nerve palsies), and postpartum neonatal hypoglycemia. Long-term studies of babies born of mothers with gestational diabetes have also shown an increase in the subsequent risk of impaired glucose tolerance, obesity, and, possibly, impaired intellectual achievement. What has remained unknown is whether screening and treatment to reduce maternal glucose levels in women with gestational diabetes would, in any way, diminish the neonatal problems seen in babies born of these mothers. The Australian Carbohydrate Intolerance Study in Pregnant Women trial tells us the answer to whether screening and treatment make a difference. It does.

In this article, we see that the offspring of women who are tightly managed for their gestational diabetes as compared with the offspring of women in a routine care group had a significantly reduced risk of a composite primary outcome measure that included perinatal death, shoulder dystocia, bone fractures, and nerve palsy (1% vs 4%). There were 5 deaths (3 stillborns and 2 neonatal deaths) among the offspring of mothers in the routine care group as compared with none in the intervention group. Macrosomia (defined as a birth weight of 4 kg or greater) was significantly more common among infants of mothers in the routine care group than among infants of mothers in the intervention group (21% vs 10%). Postpartum assessment of mood and quality of life, performed in a subgroup of the women, indicated improved health status in the intervention group, which suggests that being aware of the diagnosis or the need for frequent monitoring had no negative effect on their quality of life.

The data from this article come none too soon. Recent evidence indicates a worrisome rise in the prevalence of gestational diabetes. This presumably is the result of the recent increase seen in maternal obesity. There seems to be little argument left these days for not screening and treating women at risk. They, as well as their babies, are better off.

For more on the topic of gestational diabetes mellitus, see the superb editorial by Greene and Solomon.[1]

One concluding comment about adverse risk factors during pregnancy. Folks who smoke frequently say the reason they smoke is that it calms them down. The question we ask is whether women who smoke during pregnancy have offspring who are calmer, or less calm than their peers? The answer to this query comes from a comprehensive study examining smoking during pregnancy and the risk for hyperkinetic disorders in the offspring of mothers who smoked while their babies were still in utero.[2] It is clear that women who smoke during pregnancy do not have calm babies. In fact, smoking during pregnancy increases the risk of offspring having hyperkinetic disorders by some 3-fold. This is true even after one corrects for socioeconomic factors, a history of mental disorder in parents/siblings, low birth weight, premature delivery, and abnormal Apgar scores.

She who smokes during pregnancy to stay calm is going to need a lot more cigarettes later on during child-rearing years to stay calm around offspring who are bouncing off walls.

J. A. Stockman III, MD

References

1. Greene MF, Solomon CG: Gestational diabetes mellitus: Time to treat. *N Engl J Med* 352:2544-2546, 2005.
2. Linnet KM, Wisborg K, Obel C, et al: Smoking during pregnancy and the risk for hyperkinetic disorder in offspring. *Pediatrics* 116:462-467, 2005.

Randomized Trial of Liberal Versus Restrictive Guidelines for Red Blood Cell Transfusion in Preterm Infants
Bell EF, Strauss RG, Widness JA, et al (Univ of Iowa, Iowa City)
Pediatrics 115:1685-1691, 2005   14–3

Objective.—Although many centers have introduced more restrictive transfusion policies for preterm infants in recent years, the benefits and adverse consequences of allowing lower hematocrit levels have not been systematically evaluated. The objective of this study was to determine if restrictive guidelines for red blood cell (RBC) transfusions for preterm infants can reduce the number of transfusions without adverse consequences.

Design, Setting, and Patients.—We enrolled 100 hospitalized preterm infants with birth weights of 500 to 1300 g into a randomized clinical trial comparing 2 levels of hematocrit threshold for RBC transfusion.

Intervention.—The infants were assigned randomly to either the liberal- or the restrictive-transfusion group. For each group, transfusions were given only when the hematocrit level fell below the assigned value. In each group, the transfusion threshold levels decreased with improving clinical status.

Main Outcome Measures.—We recorded the number of transfusions, the number of donor exposures, and various clinical and physiologic outcomes.

Results.—Infants in the liberal-transfusion group received more RBC transfusions (5.2 ± 4.5 [mean ± SD] vs 3.3 ± 2.9 in the restrictive-transfusion group). However, the number of donors to whom the infants were exposed was not significantly different (2.8 ± 2.5 vs 2.2 ± 2.0). There was no difference between the groups in the percentage of infants who avoided transfusions altogether (12% in the liberal-transfusion group versus 10% in the less weight loss during the first 10 days of life, the higher the risk of broncho-pulmonary dysplasia. This is an important observation. Compared with the dismal outcome of infants with bronchopulmonary dysplasia in the 1980s, the outcome of infants with this disorder has not improved significantly. Given the increasing numbers of low birth weight infants, the actual number of infants with this disorder is also increasing, meaning that bronchopulmonary dysplasia is becoming an even more serious cause of long-term problems, including neurodevelopmental difficulties. Any intervention that could reduce its incidence would be of great clinical importance. Keeping infants free of fluid overload is one such maneuver to help minimize the problem.

J. A. Stockman III, MD

References

1. Bell EF, Warburton D, Stonstreet BS, et al: Effective fluid administration on the development of symptomatic patent ductus arteriosus and congestive heart failure in premature infants. *N Engl J Med* 302:598-604, 1980.
2. Oh W, Poindexter BB, Perritt R, et al: Association between fluid intake and weight loss during the first ten days of life and risk of bronchopulmonary dysplasia in extremely low birth weight infants. *J Pediatr* 147:786-790, 2005.

A Controlled, Randomized, Double-Blind Trial of Prophylaxis Against Jaundice Among Breastfed Newborns
Gourley GR, Li Z, Kreamer BL, et al (Oregon Health and Science Univ, Portland; Univ of Wisconsin, Madison)
Pediatrics 116:385-391, 2005   14-5

Objectives.—Neonatal jaundice is a greater problem for infants fed breast milk, compared with formula. This study tested the hypotheses that feeding breastfed newborns β-glucuronidase inhibitors during the first week after birth would increase fecal bilirubin excretion and would reduce jaundice without affecting breastfeeding deleteriously.

Methods.—Sixty-four breastfed newborns were randomized to 4 groups, ie, control or receiving 6 doses per day (5 mL per dose) of L-aspartic acid, enzymatically hydrolyzed casein (EHC), or whey/casein (W/C) for the first week. L-aspartic acid and EHC inhibit β-glucuronidase. Transcutaneous bilirubin levels (primary outcome) were measured daily (Jaundice Meter [Minolta/Air Shields, Hatboro, PA] and Bilicheck [Respironics, Pittsburgh, PA]). All stools were collected, and fecal bile pigments, including bilirubin diglucuronide, bilirubin monoglucuronides, and bilirubin, were analyzed with high-performance liquid chromatography. Follow-up assessments included day 7 body weight, day 6/7 prebreastfeeding/postbreastfeeding weights, maternal ratings, and ages at formula introduction and breast-feeding cessation.

Results.—The groups were comparable at entry. Overall, the L-aspartic acid, EHC, and W/C groups had significantly lower transcutaneous bilirubin levels than did the control group (75.8%, 69.6%, and 69.2%, respectively, of the control mean, 8.53 mg/dL, at the bilirubin peak on day 4). The L-aspartic acid, EHC, and W/C groups had significantly lower transcutaneous bilirubin levels on days 3 to 7. Fecal bile pigment excretion was greatest in the L-aspartic acid group, significantly greater than control values. There were no significant differences in dosages, follow-up measurements, and maternal ratings.

Conclusions.—Use of minimal aliquots of L-aspartic acid and EHC for β-glucuronidase inhibition results in increased fecal bilirubin excretion and less jaundice, without disruption of the breastfeeding experience. Decreased jaundice in the W/C group, which lacked a β-glucuronidase inhibitor, suggests a different mechanism.

▶ Many have argued that breast milk–induced hyperbilirubinemia could never be a cause of kernicterus. Nonetheless, if you look at the US Kernicterus Registry, 98% of the infants in the registry were breast-fed.[1] Also, in a large retrospective study, breast-feeding was the second highest independent factor (odds ratio, 5.7) associated with serum bilirubin concentrations of 25 mg/dL or greater.[2] Breast-feeding in and of itself is unlikely to ever cause kernicterus but can compound, in a very adverse way, a bad situation when other risk factors for kernicterus (eg, dehydration or alloimmunization) are present.

Because most do agree that breast-feeding can, on occasion, create a situation that puts an infant at risk of the consequences of a high bilirubin level, it is reasonable to consider ways to prevent jaundice. In the article abstracted, Gourley et al have tested the hypothesis that giving breast-fed newborn infants oral β-glucuronidase inhibitors during the first week of life increases fecal bilirubin excretion and reduces levels of jaundice in breast-fed babies. The hypothesis is based on the known observation that β-glucuronidase potentiates the enterohepatic circulation of bilirubin by deconjugating intestinal bilirubin conjugates, which produces a bilirubin that is better absorbed by the intestine. In utero, such deconjugation facilitates bilirubin clearance via the placenta. After birth, however, the enterohepatic circulation of bilirubin delays bilirubin clearance. Breast milk is rich in β-glucuronidase. Routine infant formulas have negligible amounts of this enzyme. Infants consuming such formulas have significantly less jaundice than breast-fed infants. The major β-glucuronidase inhibitor in casein hydrolysate is L-aspartic acid, and it is the latter that was used in this study to show that it would reduce levels of jaundice and increase bilirubin clearance.

L-aspartic acid is easily administered to babies, and as the authors of this article speculate, wouldn't it be wonderful if breast-fed babies could have the best of both worlds, that is, the advantages of exclusive breast-feeding plus a decreased risk of hyperbilirubinemia associated with exclusive formula feeding. The results of the study do show that significant reductions in bilirubin levels can be achieved with no negative effect on breast-feeding with the administration of small daily amounts of selected key ingredients of currently available infant formulas. Naysayers, including the breast-feeding purists, might not go along with this approach, but it does seem to make sense; nonetheless, we will have to see how theory plays out in practice. It is true that the occurrence of kernicterus is rare, but the costs associated with traditional approaches to "preventing" kernicterus (eg, home phototherapy, switching from breast milk to formula, and other therapies) are substantial.

J. A. Stockman III, MD

References

1. Johnson LH, Bhutani VK, Brown AK: System-based approach to management of neonatal jaundice and prevention of kernicterus. *J Pediatr* 140:396-403, 2002.
2. Newman TB, Xiong B, Gonzales VM, et al: Prediction and prevention of extreme hyperbilirubinemia in a mature health maintenance organization. *Arch Pediatr Adolesc Med* 154:1140-1147, 2000.

Post-phototherapy Neonatal Bilirubin Rebound: A Potential Cause of Significant Hyperbilirubinaemia
Kaplan M, Kaplan E, Hammerman C, et al (Shaare Zedek Med Ctr, Jerusalem)
Arch Dis Child 91:31-34, 2006   14–6

Aim.—To determine the incidence of post-phototherapy neonatal plasma total bilirubin (PTB) rebound.

Methods.—A prospective clinical survey was performed on 226 term and near-term neonates treated with phototherapy in the well baby nursery of the Shaare Zedek Medical Center from January 2001 to September 2002. Neonates were tested for PTB 24 hours (between 12 and 36 hours) after discontinuation of phototherapy, with additional testing as clinically indicated. The main outcome measure, significant bilirubin rebound, was defined as a post-phototherapy PTB $\geq$256 μmol/l. Phototherapy was not reinstituted in all cases of rebound, but rather according to clinical indications.

Results.—A total of 30 (13.3%) neonates developed significant rebound (mean (SD) PTB 287 (27) μmol/l, upper range 351 μmol/l). Twenty two of these (73%) were retreated with phototherapy at mean PTB 296 (29) μmol/l. Multiple logistic regression analysis showed significant risk for aetiological risk factors including positive direct Coombs test (odds ratio 2.44, 95% CI 1.25 to 4.74) and gestational age <37 weeks (odds ratio 3.21, 95% CI 1.29 to 7.96). A greater number of neonates rebounded among those in whom phototherapy was commenced $\leq$72 hours (26/152, 17%) compared with >72 hours (4/74, 5.4%) (odds ratio 3.61, 95% CI 1.21 to 10.77).

Conclusion.—Post-phototherapy neonatal bilirubin rebound to clinically significant levels may occur, especially in cases of prematurity, direct Coombs test positivity, and those treated $\leq$72 hours. These risk factors should be taken into account when planning post-phototherapy follow up.

▶ Everyone is familiar with postphototherapy rebound in bilirubin levels, but this report shows us just how common and significant this rebound can be in some infants. The problem is at its worst in infants who have a positive direct Coombs test and those who are born prematurely. The rebound is greatest in infants who are treated with phototherapy very early on (<3 days of age). The definition of significant rebound in this report was a 25% increase in bilirubin levels over the routine indication for discontinuing phototherapy—the beginning of the range of the 95th centile for bilirubin levels after the first 2 to 3 days of life.

The information provided by this report should not necessarily be equated with dangerous levels of bilirubin, nor should it imply the need for a decision to reinstitute phototherapy in all cases. It does mean, however, that these infants do need to be watched carefully, since a few infants did in fact have their bilirubin creep back to levels that would potentially be considered dangerous, particularly in infants with a positive Coombs test.

If you need to look up the current recommendations of the American Academy of Pediatrics with respect to the guidelines for management of hyperbilirubinemia, see the following website: www.bilitool.org. The prudent early use of phototherapy, a noninvasive, safe, and intrinsically inexpensive treatment, has eliminated most potential cases of bilirubin encephalopathy without the need for additional measures, albeit at the cost of some overtreatment. The effectiveness of phototherapy is such that the need for exchange transfusion even in very busy neonatal units now has become very low. A recent review of the latter topic shows that only 8 of 55,128 infants of all birth weights (1.5 exchanges per 10,000 live births) born between 1988 and 1997 at William Beaumont Hospital required an exchange transfusion, and similarly, from 1992 to 2002, a combined total of fewer than 6 infants per year, on average, received an exchange transfusion at very large referral perinatal centers in Cleveland, Ohio.[1] Be it good or bad, we have a whole cohort of residents, and now fellows in training in neonatal-perinatal medicine, who have never even seen an exchange transfusion performed, much less having performed one themselves.

J. A. Stockman III, MD

Reference

1. McDonagh AF, Maisels MJ: Bilirubin unbound: Deja vu all over again? *Pediatrics* 117:523-525, 2006.

Bronze Baby Syndrome and the Risk of Kernicterus
Bertini G, Dani C, Fonda C, et al (Univ of Florence, Italy; Meyer Pediatric Hosp, Florence, Italy; Gen Hosp of Camposampiero, Padova, Italy)
Acta Paediatr 94:968-979, 2005   14–7

Aim.—The problem of kernicterus in infants with bronze baby syndrome (BBS) has been reviewed on the basis of cases reported in the literature. In addition, a new case concerning an infant with severe Rh haemolytic disease, who presented with BBS and who has developed neurological manifestations of kernicterus with magnetic resonance images showing basal ganglia abnormalities, is presented. In this patient, the total serum bilirubin (TSB) concentration ranged from 18.0 to 22.8 mg/dl (306 to 388 µmol/l) and the bilirubin/albumin (B/A) ratio was 6.0 (mg/g) (6.8 is the value at which an exchange transfusion should be considered). The case presented is important due to the fact that kernicterus appeared after an exchange transfusion

the development of PPHN including male sex, nonvertex presentation, meconium staining of the amniotic fluid, neonatal sepsis, and pneumonia. Maternal risk factors include a lower educational level, fever, urinary tract infection, diabetes, cesarean section, antenatal use of nonsteroidal anti-inflammatory agents, and tobacco use.

To the long list of risk factors for PPHN, we must now add maternal use of SSRIs. Chambers et al have found that infants born to women who took SSRIs during the second half of pregnancy have 5 to 6 times the expected risk of developing PPHN. This suggests that perhaps as many as 1 infant of 100 mothers who are exposed to SSRIs will have PPHN. If you run the math for how many women are taking SSRIs and how many of them are likely to be pregnant, one can calculate that approximately 4000 of the 4 million infants born per year here in the United States would be exposed to the risk of PPHN. If PPHN were to develop in 1 infant per 100 exposed, one can calculate that about 40 SSRI-related cases of PPHN are occurring in the United States each year.[1] You can see why, because of these low numbers, it has taken so long for anybody to set off an alarm about the use of SSRIs during pregnancy.

These new data about SSRIs and their use during pregnancy create a number of complications for clinicians. Depression is not a rare event at any time, much less during pregnancy. Data suggest that 10% or more of pregnant women have clinical depression. While it is preferable to manage depression in pregnant women without the use of antidepressants, it is not always possible to take this approach. SSRIs have been the class of drugs of choice for nonpregnant women who have moderate to severe depression because of their track record of minimal side effects. Given the data from Chambers et al, there is a pressing need to compare SSRIs with other forms of treatment to determine what forms of treatment are the safest and most effective for pregnant women with depression in order to avoid the problem of PPHN. Given the relative rarity of PPHN, one wonders whether the benefit-to-risk ratio continues to favor the use of SSRIs for significantly depressed women who are pregnant. Depression is not good for anyone, much less those who are carrying a baby.

J. A. Stockman III, MD

Reference

1. Mils JL: Depressing observations on the selective use of SSRIs during pregnancy. *N Engl J Med* 354:636-638, 2006.

Underwater Birth and Neonatal Respiratory Distress
Kassim Z, Sellars M, Greenough A (King's College, London)
BMJ 330:1071-1072, 2005   14–9

Background.—In 1992 the United Kingdom's House of Commons Select Health Committee produced a report on maternity services that recommended that all hospitals should provide women with the option, where practical, of giving birth in a birthing pool. A subsequent surveillance study of all National Health Service maternity units between 1994 and 1996 found that 0.6% of all deliveries in England and Wales occurred in water. One report has suggested that water births have become popular among mothers and midwives because the buoyancy and warmth of the water promote natural labor and, at the same time, provide a noninvasive, safe, and effective form of pain management. However, these birthing pools also present potential risks to the newborn. In this case report, a baby developed respiratory distress as a result of aspiration after an underwater birth.

> *Case Report.*—A full-term male infant weighing 3150 g was born in the birthing pool of an National Health Service maternity ward. The mother was a 34-year-old, healthy primagravida who had an uneventful pregnancy. The baby was born underwater and required no resuscitation; however, at a review 1 hour after birth, the baby was grunting. The grunting persisted, and the baby was admitted to the neonatal ICU at 3 hours of age. He had no fever but was tachypneic and had intercostal recession and nasal flaring. The baby needed supplementary oxygen to maintain his oxygen saturation level at ≥92%, and the need for supplemental oxygen persisted for 9 hours. He was screened for infection and began a course of antibiotics. Respiratory distress persisted for 48 hours, and the patient was not allowed anything by mouth. IV fluid was administered until the patient's recovery. Chest radiographs obtained soon after admission to the neonatal ICU showed widespread changes consistent with aspiration of the birthing pool water. Follow-up radiography on day 3 showed resolution of the abnormalities, and the infection screen showed negative results. Follow-up evaluation at 3 months showed that the patient was symptom free.

Conclusions.—It has been suggested by some researchers that babies can drown only when submerged, only if they are already severely compromised, and are literally on their last breath. However, it has been shown that, in lambs, mechanisms that prevent breathing until the lamb is in contact with cold water can be overridden by sustained hypoxia. In a birthing pool, some babies with unrecognized hypoxia may gasp water. The present case report highlights the adverse effects of aspiration of water in birthing pools. Practitioners and parents should be aware of these potential risks so that the mother can make a fully informed decision as to the place of delivery.

▶ This article is from the King's College Hospital in London where, apparently, underwater birthing is not only tolerated but also supported by the presence of a birthing pool on the labor ward. While the common teaching is that babies born under water do not suffer ill consequences, this is hardly true, as this single case report provides testimony and proof of. The full-term baby born at King's College Hospital must have taken a hearty breath underwater because he had chest x-ray findings consistent with partial drowning. Several other cases with similar findings have been reported.[1]

In addition to water aspiration and subsequent pulmonary edema, other adverse neonatal outcomes after water birth have been noted in the literature. These include water intoxication, hyponatremia, hypoxic ischemic encephalopathy, and pneumonia.[2,3]

It is hard to decide whether underwater birthing is a temporary fad or an established alternative to routine methods of delivery. Data do support the fact that immersion during labor is associated with significant reductions in the use of epidural, spinal, or paracervical analgesia; reports of pain are also decreased. Whether these benefits outweigh the risks of the procedure has not been carefully studied. It seems entirely logical to conclude that human beings are not like fishes or whales. Being born under water is like rolling the dice in a lottery in which the odds are ultimately against you.

J. A. Stockman III, MD

References

1. Ruth E, Gilbert P, Tookey A: Prenatal mortality and morbidity among babies delivered in water: Surveillance study and postal survey. *BMJ* 319:483-487, 1999.
2. Pinette MG, Wax J, Wilson E: The risks of underwater birth. *Am J Obstet Gynecol* 190:1211-1215, 2004.
3. Cluett ER, Nikodem BC, McCandilish RE, et al: Immersion in water in pregnancy, labor and birth. *Cochran Database Syst Rev* 1:cd000111, 2005.

Outcome After Neonatal Continuous Negative-Pressure Ventilation: Follow-up Assessment

Telford K, Waters L, Vyas H, et al (Univ of Nottingham, England; Queen's Med Ctr, Nottingham, England; Univ of Leicester, England)
Lancet 367:1080-1085, 2006   14–10

Background.—A previous randomised trial of continuous negative extrathoracic pressure (CNEP) versus standard treatment for newborn infants with respiratory distress syndrome raised public concerns about mortality and neonatal morbidity. We studied the outcome in late childhood of children entered into the trial to establish whether there were long-term sequelae attributable to either mode of ventilation.

Methods.—Outpatient assessment of neurological outcome, cognitive function, and disability was done by a paediatrician and a psychologist using standardised tests. 133 of 205 survivors from the original trial were assessed at 9-15 years of age. Of the original pairs randomly assigned to each ventilation mode, the results from 65 complete pairs were available. The primary outcome was death or severe disability.

Findings.—Primary outcome was equally distributed between groups (odds ratio for the CNEP group 1.0; 95% CI 0.41-2.41). In unpaired analysis there was no significant difference between treatment modalities (1.05; 0.54-2.06). Full IQ did not differ significantly between the groups, but mean performance IQ was 6.8 points higher in the CNEP group than in the conventional-treatment group (95% CI 1.5-12.1). Results of neuropsychological testing were consistent with this finding, with scores on language production and visuospatial skills being significantly higher in the CNEP group.

Interpretation.—We saw no evidence of poorer long-term outcome after neonatal CNEP whether analysis was by original pairing or by unpaired comparisons, despite small differences in adverse neonatal outcomes. The experience of our study indicates that future studies of neonatal interventions with the potential to influence later morbidity should be designed with longer-term outcomes in mind.

▶ This is an important report. Back in the early 1990s, Samuels et al[1] did a randomized controlled trial of CNEP ventilation as an additional modality for treatment of respiratory distress syndrome. Normally, support for infants and young children with respiratory failure is usually achieved by intubation and positive pressure ventilation. However, this approach can damage the immature lung, increases the risk for secondary infection, and requires analgesia for sedation. To avoid these hazards, Samuels et al developed new equipment for improving respiratory support with CNEP. There did appear to be advantages for CNEP in terms of fewer days spent on oxygen in the first 2 months of life, and fewer infants developed chronic lung disease. However, on secondary analysis, there seemed to be a higher mortality, and more infants receiving CNEP had abnormalities on cranial US and pneumothoraces, although the differences did not appear to be significant.

After the publication of the Samuels report, concerns were raised by parents whose children had been included in the trial that CNEP might have led to a greater risk of death or to the occurrence of disability in their children. Concerns were also raised about the conduct of the CNEP trial, concerns that ultimately led to a British inquiry which recommended that the report should have its data carefully audited. Indeed, the study by Telford et al, reported above, was commissioned by the National Health Service in Great Britain to establish whether there were long-term consequences of the treatment with CNEP. The concern was that the tight neck seal needed for CNEP might have compromised cerebral circulation, leading to an excess of disabilities in infants managed with CNEP. What we learn from the Telford study is that not only were deaths not excessive with CNEP in those who had been entered into the earlier clinical trial, but IQ in fact was 6.8 points higher in those treated with CNEP. Results of neuropsychologic testing were consistent with this finding, and scores on language development and visual spacial skills were significantly higher in the CNEP group.

So, will we see a massive shift to CNEP? The answer is almost certainly no. The CNEP study that showed better outcomes in comparison with positive pressure ventilation took place well over a decade ago, and in the interval period, there have been marked improvements in positive pressure ventilation and the greater use of surfactant, nitric oxide, high-frequency oscillation ventilation, and better ventilators. All have reduced the need for long-term ventilation of premature infants.

Samuels and Southall, who first reported the CNEP data, were almost criminalized in Great Britain because of concerns about the way they originally carried out their study. Samuels and Southall were suspended from practice

References

1. Vain NE, Szyld EG, Prudent LM, et al: Oropharyngeal and nasopharyngeal suctioning of meconium-stained neonates before delivery of their shoulders: Multicenter randomized controlled trial. *Lancet* 364:597-602, 2004.
2. Grand RJ, Watkins JB, Torti FM: Development of the human gastrointestinal tract: A review. *Gastroenterology* 70:790-810, 1976.

Neurodevelopmental Outcomes of Premature Infants Treated With Inhaled Nitric Oxide

Mestan KKL, Marks JD, Hecox K, et al (Univ of Chicago)
N Engl J Med 353:23-32, 2005   14–12

Background.—Chronic lung disease and severe intraventricular hemorrhage or periventricular leukomalacia in premature infants are associated with abnormal neurodevelopmental outcomes. In a previous randomized, controlled, single-center trial of premature infants with the respiratory distress syndrome, inhaled nitric oxide decreased the risk of death or chronic lung disease as well as severe intraventricular hemorrhage and periventricular leukomalacia. We hypothesized that infants treated with inhaled nitric oxide would also have improved neurodevelopmental outcomes.

Methods.—We conducted a prospective, longitudinal follow-up study of premature infants who had received inhaled nitric oxide or placebo to investigate neurodevelopmental outcomes at two years of corrected age. Neurologic examination, neurodevelopmental assessment, and anthropometric measurements were made by examiners who were unaware of the children's original treatment assignment.

Results.—A total of 138 children (82 percent of survivors) were evaluated. In the group given inhaled nitric oxide, 17 of 70 children (24 percent) had abnormal neurodevelopmental outcomes, defined as either disability (cerebral palsy, bilateral blindness, or bilateral hearing loss) or delay (no disability, but one score of less than 70 on the Bayley Scales of Infant Development II), as compared with 31 of 68 children (46 percent) in the placebo group (relative risk, 0.53; 95 percent confidence interval, 0.33 to 0.87; $P=0.01$). This effect persisted after adjustment for birth weight and sex, as well as for the presence or absence of chronic lung disease and severe intraventricular hemorrhage or periventricular leukomalacia. The improvement in neurodevelopmental outcome in the group given inhaled nitric oxide was primarily due to a 47 percent decrease in the risk of cognitive impairment (defined by a score of less than 70 on the Bayley Mental Developmental Index) ($P=0.03$).

Conclusions.—Premature infants treated with inhaled nitric oxide have improved neurodevelopmental outcomes at two years of age.

Inhaled Nitric Oxide for Premature Infants With Severe Respiratory Failure

Van Meurs KP, for the Preemie Inhaled Nitric Oxide Study (Stanford Univ, Palo Alto, Calif; et al)
N Engl J Med 353:13-22, 2005   14–13

Background.—Inhaled nitric oxide is a controversial treatment for premature infants with severe respiratory failure. We conducted a multicenter, randomized, blinded, controlled trial to determine whether inhaled nitric oxide reduced the rate of death or bronchopulmonary dysplasia in such infants.

Methods.—We randomly assigned 420 neonates, born at less than 34 weeks of gestation, with a birth weight of 401 to 1500 g, and with respiratory failure more than four hours after treatment with surfactant to receive placebo (simulated flow) or inhaled nitric oxide (5 to 10 ppm). Infants with a response (an increase in the partial pressure of arterial oxygen of more than 10 mm Hg) were weaned according to protocol. Treatment with study gas was discontinued in infants who did not have a response.

Results.—The rate of death or bronchopulmonary dysplasia was 80 percent in the nitric oxide group, as compared with 82 percent in the placebo group (relative risk, 0.97; 95 percent confidence interval, 0.86 to 1.06; $P=0.52$), and the rate of bronchopulmonary dysplasia was 60 percent versus 68 percent (relative risk, 0.90; 95 percent confidence interval, 0.75 to 1.08; $P=0.26$). There were no significant differences in the rates of severe intracranial hemorrhage or periventricular leukomalacia. Post hoc analyses suggest that rates of death and bronchopulmonary dysplasia are reduced for infants with a birth weight greater than 1000 g, whereas infants weighing 1000 g or less who are treated with inhaled nitric oxide have higher mortality and increased rates of severe intracranial hemorrhage.

Conclusions.—The use of inhaled nitric oxide in critically ill premature infants weighing less than 1500 g does not decrease the rates of death or bronchopulmonary dysplasia. Further trials are required to determine whether inhaled nitric oxide benefits infants with a birth weight of 1000 g or more.

▶ By now, most of us have come to appreciate the value of surfactant as part of the management or prevention of the respiratory distress syndrome in premature infants. Unfortunately, however, a subset of babies continue to develop severe respiratory failure, often associated with pulmonary hypertension. In these cases, inhaled nitric oxide is used to selectively dilate pulmonary blood vessels and improve the ventilation–profusion matching. The article abstracted tells us what inhaled nitric oxide will do when administered to critically ill preterm infants weighing less than 1500 g. It also tells us what nitric oxide cannot do. An article by Mestan et al (see Abstract 14–12) adds additional information on the neurologic and developmental outcomes of babies so treated. We learn that nitric oxide can improve cognitive and neurodevelopmental outcomes at 2 years of age. In contrast, the article by Van Meurs et al

(Abstract 14–13) reports that treatment with inhaled nitric oxide results in no overall improvement in the rate of survival to hospital discharge and even suggests that worse outcomes may occur in a subset of infants who have birth weights of less than 1 kg. It takes a careful read of these 2 articles together to understand the discrepant results. In the Mestan et al study, the average birth weight of the premature infants was 992 g. In contrast, the infants in the study by Van Meurs et al were considerably smaller (839 g) and less mature (26 weeks vs 27.4 weeks). Almost half of the babies in the Van Meurs et al study had a birth weight of less than 750 g. The difference in the racial composition is also striking in these 2 studies. Seventy percent of the infants in the trial by Mestan et al and 35% in the trial by Van Meurs et al were black. Race or ethnic group is a very crude marker of potential biological differences in drug responses, known as pharmacogenomics.

So what do we learn from these 2 studies that brings us closer to an understanding of what we should do in clinical practice? An editorial by Martin and Walsh[1] helps us with the interpretation. They suggest that the tiniest and most severely ill babies with birth weights of 1000 g or less may, in fact, not benefit from nitric oxide. The sobering finding of increased rates of mortality and hemorrhagic or ischemic brain injury with inhaled nitric oxide therapy in this subset of babies should not be ignored and may be the result of biologically toxic byproducts such as peroxynitrite from the combination of nitric oxide with the high oxygen concentration to which these very sick babies are exposed. In contrast, however, less ill preterm babies might, in fact, benefit from this therapy, both in the short term and in the long term, as suggested by the data of Mestan et al.

The ultimate conclusion to the nitric oxide saga is that we need more data. Currently, there are several multicenter randomized trials of prolonged inhaled nitric oxide exposure beginning shortly after birth in preterm babies. Pending the results of these trials, one would be wise to be very cautious in the use of nitric oxide, particularly for the very tiny preterm baby.

J. A. Stockman III, MD

Reference

1. Martin RJ, Walsh MC: Inhaled nitric oxide for preterm infants: Who benefits? *N Engl J Med* 353:82-84, 2005.

Transition of Extremely Low-Birth-Weight Infants From Adolescence to Young Adulthood: Comparison With Normal Birth-Weight Controls
Saigal S, Stoskopf B, Streiner D, et al (McMaster Univ, Hamilton, Ont, Canada; Univ of Toronto; Michigan State Univ, East Lansing)
JAMA 295:667-675, 2006
14–14

Context.—Traditionally, educational attainment, getting a job, living independently, getting married, and parenthood have been considered as markers of successful transition to adulthood.

Objective.—To describe and compare the achievement and the age at attainment of the above markers between extremely low-birth-weight (ELBW) and normal birth-weight (NBW) young adults.

Design, Setting, and Participants.—A prospective, longitudinal, population-based study in central-west Ontario, Canada, of 166 ELBW participants who weighed 501 to 1000 g at birth (1977-1982) and 145 sociodemographically comparable NBW participants assessed at young adulthood (22-25 years). Interviewers masked to participant status administered validated questionnaires via face-to-face interviews between January 1, 2002, and April 30, 2004.

Main Outcome Measures.—Markers of successful transition to adulthood, including educational attainment, student and/or worker role, independent living, getting married, and parenthood.

Results.—At young adulthood, 149 (90%) of 166 ELBW participants and 133 (92%) of 145 NBW participants completed the assessments at mean (SD) age of 23.3 (1.2) years and 23.6 (1.1) years, respectively. We included participants with neurosensory impairments (ELBW vs NBW: 40 [27%] vs 3 [2%]) and 7 proxy respondents. The proportion who graduated from high school was similar (82% vs 87%, $P = .21$). Overall, no statistically significant differences were observed in the education achieved to date. A substantial proportion of both groups were still pursuing postsecondary education (47 [32%] vs 44 [33%]). No significant differences were observed in employment/school status; 71 (48%) ELBW vs 76 (57%) NBW young adults were permanently employed ($P = .09$). In a subanalysis, a higher proportion of ELBW young adults were neither employed nor in school (39 [26%] vs 20 [15%], $P = .02$ by Holm's correction); these differences did not persist when participants with disabilities were excluded. No significant differences were found in the proportion living independently (63 [42%] vs 70 [53%], $P = .19$), married/cohabitating (34 [23%] vs 33 [25%], $P = .69$), or who were parents (16 [11%] vs 19 [14%], $P = .36$). The age at attainment of the above markers was similar for both cohorts.

Conclusion.—Our study results indicate that a significant majority of former ELBW infants have overcome their earlier difficulties to become functional young adults.

▶ This report from Canada adds to our information about what happens to ELBW infants as they transition from adolescence to adulthood. We see that in many instances, former ELBW infants do seem to overcome their earlier difficulties as they transition into young adulthood. Among the few articles on ELBW survivors as young adults, the most notable is that of Hack et al,[1] which describes a cohort of 20-year-old inner-city very low birth weight survivors from Cleveland compared with NBW peers. A significantly lower proportion of adults who were very low birth weight infants had graduated from high school (74% vs 83%), and fewer previously very low birth weight infant males, compared with females, were enrolled in postsecondary education (30% vs 53%). A study by Cooke[2] performed a survey of a hospital-based cohort of 19- to 22-year-old very low birth weight survivors attending mainstream schools in Liverpool, England. A higher proportion of very low birth weight young adults compared with NBW young adults had vocational qualifications (54% vs 23%), fewer were at universities or had completed a degree (23% vs 58%), and a higher proportion were in paid employment (44% vs 27%).

The study by Saigal et al seems to suggest that children who survive ELBW circumstances and who did not incur substantial neurologic deficits, but may have had subtle defects, need to be considered from a lifespan perspective, as recovery from these deficits may not be evident until adulthood. The few studies of young adults who were born preterm seem to suggest that recovery of function may occur, in that participants were doing better than predicted in their health, behavior, and social and emotional functioning. In any event, it is good news to see that against our expectations and many odds, a significant majority of ELBW young adults have overcome earlier difficulties to become functional members of society.

See the report by Allin et al (Abstract 14–17). This report suggests that young adults who were born very preterm have somewhat different personality styles than their term-born peers. You will need to read this report, which appeared in *Pediatrics*, to decide whether the findings coincide with your own experiences. The authors suggest that premature children and adolescents may be at risk of developing personality traits that could predispose them to later mental illnesses.

One final comment about newborns: special boxes that allow mothers to abandon their newborn babies with no questions asked have now spread throughout Western Europe from Germany down through Italy. For example, Germany and Hungary introduced such boxes in separate but similar initiatives about 5 years ago to help prevent dozens of deaths of newborn babies abandoned on the streets. Such boxes are high tech, modern equivalents of the old medieval foundling wheels operated by orphanages in Padua from about 1400 until 1888. Such wheels were a circular wooden board, half inside and half outside the orphanages run by nuns. Mothers would place their unwanted newborns on the board and ring a bell. The nuns would spin the board to find the child. The modern day incubators, dubbed "baby boxes" by the European media, are installed in hospital walls and can be opened from the inside or outside, much like a bank deposit box. Mothers place the baby inside the heated box and can leave it safe in the knowledge that heat sensors will alert a trained medical expert to the baby's presence.

If you would like to see a picture of a baby box, see the summary by Chapman.[3]

J. A. Stockman III, MD

References

1. Hack M, Flannery DJ, Schluchter M, et al: Outcomes in young adulthood for very low birth weight infants. *N Engl J Med* 346:149-157, 2002.
2. Cooke RW: Health, lifestyle and quality of life for young adults born very preterm. *Arch Dis Child* 89:201-206, 2004.
3. Chapman C: Italy introduces "baby boxes" to save the lives of abandoned newborn babies. *BMJ* 332:322, 2006.

Chronic Conditions, Functional Limitations, and Special Health Care Needs of School-aged Children Born With Extremely Low-Birth-Weight in the 1990s

Hack M, Taylor HG, Drotar D, et al (Case Western Reserve Univ, Cleveland, Ohio)

JAMA 294:318-325, 2005   14–15

Context.—Information on the school-age functioning and special health care needs of extremely low-birth-weight (ELBW, <1000 g) children is necessary to plan for medical and educational services.

Objective.—To examine neurosensory, developmental, and medical conditions together with the associated functional limitations and special health care needs of ELBW children compared with normal-birth-weight (NBW) term-born children (controls).

Design, Setting, and Participants.—A follow-up study at age 8 years of a cohort of 219 ELBW children born 1992 to 1995 (92% of survivors) and 176 NBW controls of similar sociodemographic status conducted in Cleveland, Ohio.

Main Outcome Measures.—Parent Questionnaire for Identifying Children with Chronic Conditions of 12 months or more and categorization of specific medical diagnoses and developmental disabilities based on examination of the children.

Results.—In logistic regression analyses adjusting for sociodemographic status and sex, ELBW children had significantly more chronic conditions than NBW controls, including functional limitations (64% vs 20%, respectively; odds ratio [OR], 8.1; 95% confidence interval [CI], 5.0-13.1; $P<.001$), compensatory dependency needs (48% vs 23%, respectively; OR, 3.0; 95% CI, 1.9-4.7; $P<.001$), and services above those routinely required by children (65% vs 27%, respectively; OR, 5.4; 95% CI, 3.4-8.5; $P<.001$). These differences remained significant when the 36 ELBW children with neurosensory impairments were excluded. Specific diagnoses and disabilities for ELBW vs NBW children included cerebral palsy (14% vs 0%, respectively; $P<.001$), asthma (21% vs 9%; OR, 3.0; 95% CI, 1.6-5.6; $P = .001$), vision of less than 20/200 (10% vs 3%; OR, 3.1; 95% CI, 1.2-7.8; $P = .02$), low IQ of less than 85 (38% vs 14%; OR, 4.5; 95% CI, 2.7-7.7; $P<.001$), limited academic skills (37% vs 15%; OR, 4.2; 95% CI, 2.5-7.3; $P<.001$), poor motor skills (47% vs 10%; OR, 7.8; 95% CI, 4.5-13.6; $P<.001$), and poor adaptive functioning (69% vs 34%; OR, 6.5; 95% CI, 4.0-10.6; $P<.001$).

Conclusion.—The ELBW survivors in school at age 8 years who were born in the 1990s have considerable long-term health and educational needs.

▶ A recent report out of California, where careful data are kept on all low birthweight and very low birthweight infants, shows that this group of babies accounts for the largest majority of hospitalization costs for the newborn age category admission.[1] This should come as no surprise, but what is surprising is the magnitude of the impact of being born significantly prematurely. The average length of stay for low birthweight infants in California nurseries ranges from 6.2 to 68.1 days, whereas the average hospital stay for infants weighing more than 2500g at birth is just 2.3 days. Overall, very low birthweight infants account for just 0.9% of all cases, but 35.7% of hospital costs, whereas low birthweight infants account for 5.9% of cases, but 56.6% of total hospital cost. In the aggregate, such pregnancies generate more than $1.6 billion in medical cost in this one state alone. Needless to say, anything that increases the ability of a woman to hold on to a pregnancy, even for a little bit longer, will markedly diminish the type of expenditures we currently are seeing.

J. A. Stockman III, MD

Reference

1. Schmitt SK, Sneed L, Phibbs CS: Cost of newborn care in California: A population-based study. *Pediatrics* 117:154-160, 2006.

Changes in Neurodevelopmental Outcomes at 18 to 22 Months' Corrected Age Among Infants of Less Than 25 Weeks' Gestational Age Born in 1993-1999

Hintz SR, for the National Institute of Child Health and Human Development Neonatal Research Network (Stanford Univ, Palo Alto, Calif; et al)
Pediatrics 115:1645-1651, 2005   14–16

Background.—Increased survival rates for extremely preterm, extremely low birth weight infants during the postsurfactant era have been reported, but data on changes in neurosensory and developmental impairments are sparse.

Objective.—To compare neuromotor and neurodevelopmental outcomes at 18 to 22 months' corrected age for infants of <25 weeks' estimated gestational age (EGA) who were born in the 1990s.

Methods.—This was a multicenter, retrospective, comparative analysis of infants of <25 weeks' EGA, with birth weights of 501 to 1000 g, born between January 1993 and June 1996 (epoch I) or between July 1996 and December 1999 (epoch II), in the National Institute of Child Health and Human Development Neonatal Research Network. Neurodevelopmental assessments were performed at 18 to 22 months' corrected age. Logistic-regression models were constructed to evaluate the independent risk of cerebral palsy, Mental Development Index of <70, Psychomotor Development Index of <70, and neurodevelopmental impairment.

Results.—A total of 366 patients in epoch I and 473 patients in epoch II were evaluated. Prenatal steroid use, cesarean section, surfactant treatment, bronchopulmonary dysplasia, and severe retinopathy of prematurity were more likely in epoch II, whereas Apgar scores of <5 at 5 minutes, patent ductus arteriosus, and severe intraventricular hemorrhage were more likely in epoch I. The prevalences of cerebral palsy, Psychomotor Development Index of <70, and neurodevelopmental impairment were similar between epochs.

The prevalences of Mental Development Index of <70 were 40% for epoch I and 47% for epoch II. Regression analysis revealed that epoch II was an independent risk factor for Mental Developmental Index of <70 (epoch I versus II: odds ratio: 0.63; 95% confidence interval: 0.45-0.87) but not for other outcomes.

Conclusions.—Early childhood neurodevelopmental outcomes among infants of <25 weeks' EGA are not improving in the postsurfactant era, despite more aggressive perinatal and neonatal treatment. Later childhood follow-up assessment is needed to delineate trends in severe cognitive impairment in this extremely high-risk group.

▶ These articles by Hack et al (Abstract 14–15) and Hintz et al (Abstract 14–16) are part of the continuing saga of information that is evolving around outcomes for extremely low birth weight infants. The long-term outcome for extremely low birth weight infants weighing less than 1000 g at birth remains of great interest to parents; the public; a broad variety of professional groups including educators, psychologists, and health care planners; and obstetricians, neonatologists, pediatricians, and all other medical specialists involved in the care of these children. Studies performed before 1990 showed that the absolute numbers of low-birth weight infants who survived had significant disabilities. Advances in perinatal care in the last 15 years however, have led to improvements, largely as the result of the widespread use of antenatal steroids and postnatal surfactant, which have dramatically reduced the mortality of high-risk infants. Partly because of these advances, which have diminished the prevalence of intracranial hemorrhaging and have improved pulmonary functioning, there has been hope for a reduction in the proportion of low-birth weight infant survivors who might have long-term disabilities. Studies to document this have been few, at least until these 2 articles.

The study of Hack et al (Abstract 14–15) reports outcomes at 8 years of age for more than 200 low-birth weight infants who survived the newborn period. The results show that the low-birth weight infant group did have substantially worse outcomes than did their normal birth weight peers in every type of assessment, although the difference may be less than that expected by many obstetricians and pediatricians as well as other professionals or lay persons. The most severe problems occurred almost exclusively in very low birth weight infants. Some 60% of these babies grow up to be children with major neurosensory impairments, including cerebral palsy, deafness, and blindness. Some 6% require the use of a wheelchair. One percent require tube feedings, and 6% to 10% have difficulty eating, difficulty using the toilet, or are unable to play or socialize with others.

It is difficult to compare the results of the study by Hack et al with previous studies because of differences in design. There is some suggestion, however, that the proportion of low-birth weight infant survivors with adverse outcomes has not necessarily decreased in those who have been born in the last 10 years or so. Indeed, this proportion may have increased, likely partly because of the liberal use of postnatal pharmacologic doses of steroids to prevent or treat chronic lung disease during the 1990s, which has allowed more at-risk babies to actually survive.

The article by Hintz et al (Abstract 14–16) also shows that advances in perinatal and neonatal medicine in the past 10 to 20 years have resulted in improved survival rates for premature and very low birth weight infants but that early childhood neurodevelopmental outcomes do not seem to be improved, despite more aggressive perinatal and neonatal treatment options.

One final comment about neurodevelopmental outcomes in graduates of our nurseries, this having to do with the cognitive cost of being a twin. Evidence from comparisons within families of twins as opposed to singletons in Great Britain shows that at age 7, the mean IQ score of twins is 5.3 points lower and at age 9, 6.0 points lower than that of singletons in the same family. If adjusted for birthweight and gestational age, the IQ difference between twins and singletons drops to 2.6 points.[1] It would appear that twins have substantially lower IQ in childhood when compared to their peers who are single born within the same family. This observation cannot be explained by confounding due to socioeconomic, maternal, or other family characteristics. The reduced prenatal growth and shorter gestation of twins may explain perhaps two thirds of the difference in IQ in childhood.

J. A. Stockman III, MD

Reference

1. Ronalds GA, Stavola BL, Leon DA: The cognitive cost of being a twin: Evidence from comparisons within families in the Aberdeen children of the 1950s cohort study. *BMJ* 331:1306-1309, 2005.

Personality in Young Adults Who Are Born Preterm
Allin M, Rooney M, Cuddy M, et al (King's College, London; Mercy Univ Hosp, Grenville Place, Cork, Ireland; Royal Free and Univ College Med School, London)
Pediatrics 117:309-316, 2006   14–17

Introduction.—Very preterm birth (VPT; <33 weeks' gestation) is associated with later neuromotor and cognitive impairment, reduced school performance, and psychiatric morbidity. Several follow-up studies have demonstrated increased anxiety and social rejection and reduced self-esteem in preterm children and adolescents, but few studies have examined the effects of preterm birth on adult personality.

Methods.—We assessed 108 VPT individuals and 67 term-born controls at ages 18 to 19 years with the Eysenck Personality Questionnaire-Revised, short form (EPQ-RS). This questionnaire rates 3 dimensions of personality: extraversion (sociability, liveliness, sensation seeking); neuroticism (anxiety, low mood, low self-esteem); and psychoticism (coldness, aggression, predisposition to antisocial behavior). A fourth scale, "lie," which measures dissimulation, is also derived.

Results.—VPT individuals had significantly lower extraversion scores, higher neuroticism scores, and higher lie scores than term-born controls, after controlling for age at assessment and socioeconomic status. *P* scores were not significantly different between the 2 groups. There was a gender difference in that the increased neuroticism and decreased extraversion scores were accounted for mainly by VPT females. Associations between EPQ-RS scores and neonatal status, adolescent behavioral ratings, and body size at 18 to 19 years were assessed by using Kendall partial correlations, correcting for age at assessment and socioeconomic status. Gestational age, indices of neonatal hypoxia, and neonatal ultrasound ratings were not correlated with EPQ-RS scores. Birth weight was weakly associated with increased lie scores. Rutter Parents' Scale score, a measure of adolescent psychopathology, was associated with an increased neuroticism score. Poor social adjustment in adolescence was associated with an increased lie score. Height and weight at 18 to 19 years were not associated with EPQ-RS, but reduced occipitofrontal circumference was associated with both decreased extraversion and increased lie scores.

Conclusions.—Young adults who are born VPT have different personality styles from their term-born peers. This may be associated with an increased risk of psychiatric difficulties.

▶ The information provided by this report pretty much speaks for itself, so rather than commenting further, we will ask a question having to do with pregnancy prevention. For the next year, you will be a medical missionary on a group of remote islands in the South Pacific. As you read up on the populations you are about to serve, you learn that the native population has no access to traditional forms of contraception. In order to better serve this population, you decide to do a little research to learn what individuals might have used some centuries ago for the purposes of contraception. What was common in medieval times?

What was common in medieval times was the use of limes as a contraceptive. Recently, a historian tried this form of contraception and actually reported on it. Curious about medieval forms of contraception, the historian cut the top off of a lime and inserted it into her vagina, just like a modern diaphragm. She noted that it did not sting and neatly fitted over the cervix. Indeed it stayed there without any need for fixation devices. She could move about without feeling it and without suffering discomfort.[1]

According to oral tradition that has been handed down from medieval times, lime juice kills sperm and *Candida* and creates a hostile environment for most forms of venereal disease. Women who choose to go the lime approach, however, had better forewarn their gynecologist before a routine examination, otherwise someone is going to be surprised and puzzled by what they encounter.

J. A. Stockman III, MD

Reference

1. A lime as a contraceptive (editorial). *BMJ* 332:312, 2006.

Birth Spacing and Risk of Adverse Perinatal Outcomes: A Meta-analysis
Conde-Agudelo A, Rosas-Bermúdez A, Kafury-Goeta AC (Fundación Santa Fe de Bogotá, Columbia; Universidad Autonoma de Occidente, Cali, Columbia; Clínica Materno-Infantil Los Farallones, Cali, Columbia)
JAMA 295:1809-1823, 2006   14-18

Context.—Both short and long interpregnancy intervals have been associated with an increased risk of adverse perinatal outcomes. However, whether this possible association is confounded by maternal characteristics or socioeconomic status is uncertain.

Objective.—To examine the association between birth spacing and relative risk of adverse perinatal outcomes.

Data Sources.—Studies published in any language were retrieved by searching MEDLINE (1966 through January 2006), EMBASE, ECLA, POPLINE, CINAHL, and LILACS, proceedings of meetings on birth spacing, and bibliographies of retrieved articles, and by contact with relevant researchers in the field.

Study Selection.—Included studies were cohort, cross-sectional, and case-control studies with results adjusted for at least maternal age and socioeconomic status, reporting risk estimates and 95% confidence intervals (or data to calculate them) of birth spacing and perinatal outcomes. Of 130 articles identified in the search, 67 (52%) were included.

Data Extraction.—Information on study design, participant characteristics, measure of birth spacing used, measures of outcome, control for potential confounding factors, and risk estimates was abstracted independently by 2 investigators using a standardized protocol.

Data Synthesis.—A random-effects model and meta-regression analyses were used to pool data from individual studies. Compared with interpregnancy intervals of 18 to 23 months, interpregnancy intervals shorter than 6 months were associated with increased risks of preterm birth, low birth weight, and small for gestational age (pooled adjusted odds ratios [95% confidence intervals]: 1.40 [1.24-1.58], 1.61 [1.39-1.86], and 1.26 [1.18-1.33], respectively). Intervals of 6 to 17 months and longer than 59 months were also associated with a significantly greater risk for the 3 adverse perinatal outcomes.

Conclusions.—Interpregnancy intervals shorter than 18 months and longer than 59 months are significantly associated with increased risk of adverse perinatal outcomes. These data suggest that spacing pregnancies appropriately could help prevent such adverse perinatal outcomes.

▶ This is a very important report, which shows us the results of a systematic review and meta-analysis of studies that have attempted to investigate the association between interpregnancy interval and untoward perinatal health events. What we learn is that if the interval between pregnancies is less than 18 months or longer than 59 months, there will be an increased risk of adverse perinatal outcomes.

In some respects, it is easy to hypothesize why short intervals between pregnancies could have negative outcomes on the pregnancy. Several causal mechanisms have emerged to explain this risk, including postpartum hormone imbalances, maternal stress, and most plausibly, maternal nutritional depletion. For example, maternal stores of folate may not return to normal if a pregnancy occurs shortly on the heels of another. In support of this is the fact that neural tube defects are twice as common among children conceived within 6 months after a previous live birth compared with those conceived after 12 to 24 months. Some have even suggested that folate should be routinely administered in the postpartum period to minimize this problem. Unfortunately, short intervals are for the most part probably unintended, as are half of all pregnancies. Preventions that increase birth spacing seem to make sense, in particular, exclusive breast-feeding for as long as is reasonable.

The risk associated with long interpregnancy intervals is more difficult to explain. The risk of preeclampsia has been observed to increase significantly with longer interpregnancy intervals, with estimated odds ratios of 1.16 per additional year after pregnancy. Preeclampsia is a primary and significant cause of preterm delivery. Long intervals most likely are not chosen, but may result from the end of a partnership, infertility, reproductive losses in the interval, health problems in the mother or infant, or economic issues, all of which are tough to deal with in most cases. While longer intervals are likely to be beyond personal control, pregnancies occurring after an interval of 5 years may require more careful monitoring to avoid untoward outcomes.

J. A. Stockman III, MD

Cumulative Effective Doses Delivered by Radiographs to Preterm Infants in a Neonatal Intensive Care Unit
Donadieu J, Zeghnoun A, Roudier C, et al (Institut de Veille Sanitaire, St Maurice, France; Centre d'Assurance de Qualité ds Applications Technologiques dans le Domaine de la Santé (CAATS), Bourg la Reine, France; Universitée Paris-Descartes; et al)
Pediatrics 117:882-888, 2006   14–19

Objective.—We sought to determine the number and distribution of radiographs and the cumulative effective radiograph doses (cED) received by a population of preterm infants (PIs) hospitalized in an NICU.

Study Design.—We reviewed the files of all preterm infants (gestational age: <34 weeks) who were admitted to an NICU during an 18-month period and were discharged alive. A generalized additive model was used to study the relationship between cED and patient characteristics.

Results.—Four hundred fifty files were analyzed. The median gestational age was 30.1 weeks (range: 24.1-33.9 weeks), and the median birth weight was 1250 g (range: 520-2760 g). The median number of radiographs per infant was 10.6 (range: 0-95), and the median cED was 138 µSv (range: 0-1450 µSv). The cumulative dose exceeded 500 µSv in 7.6% of the cases.

Factors that influenced the cumulative effective dose were gestational age, birth weight, care procedures, and clinical adverse events.

Conclusions.—Given the potentially life-threatening complications of PIs, cumulative radiograph doses received in the ICU seem low with regard to environmental exposure and international recommendations. Additional studies are needed to evaluate the possible lifetime consequences of exposure to ionizing radiation at this age.

▶ This report emanates from France, but chances are had the study been done in the United States, similar results would have been found. There is growing concern about the amount of radiation small people receive from diagnostic studies, but fewer than a handful of reports have provided information on preterm infants, thus the importance of the study from France.

We see in this study that despite the large number of radiographs performed in NICUs, the actual radiation doses that any one infant receives are probably within acceptable ranges, except for the small percentage of infants who receive a fair amount of radiation because they require so many radiographs. It is noteworthy, however, that a single CT scan of the head (obviously not performed in the NICU) delivers more than 10 times the median radiation dose resulting from all standard radiographs that a given infant would receive in the NICU, whereas a combined CT of the head and abdomen delivers 30 times this dose. The authors of this report really do not give us any guidelines about how much radiation is acceptable and how much might do harm. There are virtually no data to provide such guidelines. They do caution us that given the uncertainties surrounding the precise radiosensitivity of extremely premature newborns, it does seem logical to try to minimize x-ray exposure, by limiting the radiograph field or by using shielding techniques. There is no need to include the thorax and abdomen together if all you are interested in is the chest. Clearly, CT scanning should be used sparingly, only as absolutely needed.

So, is MRI scanning any safer, overall, than CT scanning? If you are answering this question with all honesty, you would have to say that you really cannot be totally sure about the safety of MRI. Safety is a major concern as MR scanners have become much more ubiquitously used. Here in the US, there are more than 10,000 scanners currently up and operating with a push-through of about 10 million patients annually. At first glance, these scanners appear to have a fairly low rate of dangerous events with just 389 reports of MR safety incidents captured by the US Food and Drug Administration's manufacturer and user facility device experience (MAUDE) database over the most recent 10-year period. Of these incidents, 9 resulted in deaths. Most of these deaths were caused by failure of implantable devices such as pacemakers and insulin pumps. One death occurred when a patient was struck by a projectile drawn into the machine by its powerful magnetic field. Another occurred when an engineer was asphyxiated. Of all MR injuries, approximately 70% are burns, 10% are implant-related, and 10% result from flying projectiles.

The reason one cannot be totally certain about the real safety of MR scanners is the fact that it is not clear what type of MR-related complications are being reported, and current incident numbers probably are serious underestimates. Safety issues related to MR units largely result from failure to follow protocol. In a recent 16-month period, the Pennsylvania Patient Safety Reporting System recorded 88 MR incidents—fortunately, all "near misses" with no patient injuries. There were 33 screening errors, 28 contraindications for MR discovered during screening, 12 contraindications discovered during or after MR imaging, 12 pieces of incompatible equipment (potential projectiles) in MR rooms, and 3 potential burns and skin redness. If you are not familiar with the latter problem, this is caused by patients creating conductive loops by touching the sides of the scanner, perhaps with an ankle or wrist.

If you want to learn more about MR facility and safety issues, see the excellent review of this topic by Mitka.[1]

J. A. Stockman III, MD

Reference

1. Mitka M: Safety improvements urge for MRI facilities. *JAMA* 294:2145-2146, 2005.

15 Nutrition and Metabolism

Widespread Use of Soy-Based Formula Without Clinical Indications
Berger-Achituv S, Shohat T, Romano-Zelekha O, et al (Tel Aviv Univ, Israel; Ministry of Health and the Department of Public Health, Tel-Aviv, Israel)
J Pediatr Gastroenterol Nutr 41:660-666, 2005   15–1

Objectives.—In view of reports of the growing popularity of soy-based formula for infants, we examined soy consumption and its possible overuse during early infancy in central Israel.

Methods.—Mothers of 1803 infants aged 2, 4, 6 and 12 months attending well-baby clinics participated in a telephone survey covering background data, rate, duration, and pattern of soy-based formula use and the reasons for its initiation. The reasons were grouped into those based on the recommendations of the medical personnel and those based on mothers' initiative, and evaluated according to infants' age at soy-based formula initiation (0 to 1, 2 to 4 and 5 to 12 months). The symptoms that prompted soy-based formula use were assessed quantitatively.

Results.—The rate of soy-based formula use was 10.4% at 2 months and 31.5% at 12 months ($P < 0.001$); 70.6% ± 2.7% of the infants were given soy for >6 months. Regardless of infants' age, the role of the mothers in the decision to use soy-based formula was greater than that of the medical personnel, and increased significantly with age (χ^2 for trend = 0.018). A suspicion of cow's milk allergy was responsible for only 10.9% (7/64) of all soy initiations in infants aged 5 to 12 months. In all ages, occasional symptoms, mainly diarrhea (33.3%) and colic (19.8%), were the leading cause for recommending soy-based formula by medical personnel, whereas the personal preference without clinical justification was the leading cause among mothers.

Conclusions.—The use of soy-based formula in central Israel is extensive and continues for long periods, with rates far beyond clinical indications. Mothers play a greater role than medical personnel in the decision to initiate soy-based formula.

▶ Most residents in training (and probably most of the rest of us) have not been taught much about the history of soy formulas, nor is much written about their precise application. Soy-based formulas were first introduced back in 1929 as a nutritional substitute for infants with cow's milk allergy. Since that time, the list of possible uses for soy-based formulas has expanded quite remarkably. As recently as just a few years ago, Pollack et al[1] reported that 1 in every 3 infants in the United States experienced at least 1 formula change to a soy-based formula. Soy-based formulas largely consist of purified soy proteins and a mixture of vegetable oils and lactose-free carbohydrates. These formulas can be used for infants with primary lactase deficiency or galactosemia. Soy-based formula has also been used for the treatment of infants with acute diarrhea complicated by transient secondary lactase deficiency and infantile colic as well as for infants whose parents prefer a vegetarian diet. Most data indicate that healthy term infants fed soy-based formula will have similar growth and development compared with infants fed formula based on cow's milk or breast milk. Preterm infants, however, are a different story. When fed soy-based formula, many will show less weight gain and lower serum albumin levels. Soy formulas can also cause a variety of allergic reactions. It is not a bulletproof way to manage cow's milk allergy because somewhere between 10% and 40% of infants managed with soy formula will have some type of adverse reaction to soy. Over the years, concerns have emerged about high levels of aluminum and phytoestrogens found in soy-based formulas. The consequences of the latter, however, are poorly understood and may be of no significance.

What we learn from this article from Israel is probably not new: soy formula is commonly given to babies, and often, it is not because of an allergy related to cow's milk. Although these data are from Israel, they probably also reflect circumstances in the United States. One can only conclude that physicians, parents, or both reach for the soy for virtually any problem arising with infant feeding. In fact, few evidence-based studies exist to tell us what the proper indications might be for soy-based formula. Nonetheless, it appears to be the alternative formula of choice when there is a problem with feeding. Breast remains best, except in rare circumstances. Given that the full consequences of soy-based formula feeding are still largely unknown, we ought to be a bit more rigorous about what we recommend to our patients.

J. A. Stockman III, MD

Reference

1. Pollack FP, Khan N, Maisels MJ: Changing partners: The dance of the infant formula changes. *Clin Pediatr* 38:703-708, 1999.

May the Best Friend Be an Enemy if Not Recognized Early: Hypernatremic Dehydration Due to Breastfeeding
Yildizdaş HY, Satar M, Tutak E, et al (Çukurova Univ, Adana, Turkey)
Pediatr Emerg Care 21:445-448, 2005   15–2

Background.—Hypernatremic dehydration (HND) is an uncommon but serious condition in newborns. It is associated with a potential for seizures and permanent neurologic and vascular damage if not recognized and treated early. HND was thought to be unusual in breast-fed infants, but recent reports have identified breast-feeding malnutrition as a key factor in the pathophysiology of HND. Five cases of HND in breast-feeding neonates were presented, and the causes and treatment of HND were discussed.

Case 1.—Boy, 11 days, was admitted to the hospital for a thyroid screen test. He was born by cesarean section after an uneventful pregnancy to a mother with hyperthyroidism. He was dehydrated on physical examination, with a sunken anterior fontanelle and dry mucous membranes. He was hypoactive and not sucking. From a birth weight of 2700 g, he had a weight on admission of 1960 g. There was no history of fever, vomiting, or diarrhea, and he was exclusively breast-fed. Laboratory findings were indicative of HND. He was one-half orogastrically fed and hydrated with 3.3% dextrose containing 0.3% sodium chloride. He recovered and was discharged on the fourth day and has grown well.

Case 2.—Girl, 12 days, was seen in the emergency department with severe dehydration. She was born to a para 4, gravida 3 mother via normal spontaneous vaginal delivery at 38 weeks' gestation. Severe weight loss was recognized on admission day by a visitor who saw her at birth and advised the mother to take the infant to the hospital. Her physical examination was significant for lethargy, a sunken anterior fontanelle, dry mucous membranes, skin tenting, and capillary refill greater than 3 seconds. She was infused rapidly with 20 mL/kg of normal saline. She had lost approximately 38% of her birth weight. Laboratory findings were indicative of HND. The parents indicated that she was exclusively breast-feeding and had no previous health problems. Despite the infusion of maintenance fluid, the patient died on the ninth day of admission.

Case 3.—Boy, 4 days, was admitted to the hospital for fever and irritability. From a birth weight of 4300 g, his weight on admission was 3650 g. He had a sunken fontanelle, skin tenting, dry mucous membranes, and hypoactive reflexes. Laboratory findings were indicative of HND. He was hydrated with a 160-mL/kg dose of $D_{5-\frac{1}{4}}$ NS and was orally feeding by the second day. He was discharged on the third day of admission.

Case 4.—Boy, 5 days, was admitted to the outpatient clinic for hyperbilirubinemia. He was dehydrated on physical examination. His birth weight was 3950 g, but at admission his weight was 3220 g. Laboratory findings were indicative of HND. He was hospitalized for severe weight loss. He was breast-feeding, but the breast milk volume after pumping was insufficient for the daily needs of the baby. Biochemistry tests were within normal limits on the third day, and he was discharged. The patient was exclusively breast-fed until he was 4 months of age.

Case 5.—Girl, 6 days, was admitted to the hospital for poor feeding, irritability, and fever. She had lost 1000 g of birth weight (from 3500 g at birth to 2500 g on admission). Physical examination showed significant irritability, a sunken anterior fontanelle, very dry mucous membranes, skin tenting, and capillary refill of 6 seconds. Laboratory findings were indicative of HND. Rapid infusion of 20-mL/kg normal saline was initiated. Sodium bicarbonate and calcium gluconate were also administered for metabolic acidosis and hypocalcemia. She was discharged on the second day of admission and is breast-feeding and growing well.

Conclusions.—The most common problems related to breast-feeding are underfeeding and breast milk jaundice, but HND may also result from breast-feeding. The high sodium content of breast milk was at first thought to be the main cause of HND in these patients, but it was mainly the result of insufficient lactation caused by decreased milk removal.

▶ No one will argue that breast milk is the best source of nutrition for neonates, but no one should deny that no method of feeding is without potential problems. This report describes HND due to breast-feeding. HND is usually due to diarrhea, but it can result from excessive sodium intake such as with the use of improperly prepared infant formula. Although HND is unusual in breast-fed babies, it can occur. This is evidenced in the 5 cases reported here from Turkey. Each of these babies was only a few days to 2 weeks old. A significant part of the problem was the inability of parents to recognize or identify their infant as being dehydrated. As is true here, in Turkey there is a problem with routine postpartum follow-up of newborns after short postpartum nursery stays. Not everyone is able to successfully breast-feed without some help, and this seems to be the major cause of the problem reported.

While on the topic of breast-feeding, is there any relationship between exclusive breast-feeding and blood pressure later in life? Babies who are exclusively breast-fed are protected from hypertension later in life to an extent that is similar to that afforded by salt restriction and physical activity in adult life. An analysis of the European Heart Study, which included more than 2000 school children, not only showed that children who were breast-fed had lower blood pressures, but also found a dose relationship and independence of confounding factors—prompting the authors to suggest a true causal association between breast-feeding and the prevention of adult onset hypertension.[1]

J. A. Stockman III, MD

Reference

1. Lawlor DA, Riddoch CJ, Page AS, et al: Infant feeding and components of the metabolic syndrome: Findings from the European Youth Heart Study. *Arch Dis Childhood* 90:582-588, 2005.

Ghrelin, Leptin and IGF-I Levels in Breast-fed and Formula-fed Infants in the First Years of Life

Savino F, Fissore MF, Grassino EC, et al (Università di Torino, Italy)
Acta Paediatr 94:531-537, 2005   15–3

Aim.—To establish ghrelin, leptin and IGF-I serum levels in breastfed (BF) and formula-fed (FF) infants during the first period of life.

Methods.—A cross-sectional study was conducted on fasting blood venous samples obtained from exclusively BF (n = 106) and FF (n = 100) infants to measure total ghrelin (RIA test), leptin (RIA test) and IGF-I (chemiluminescence). Anthropometrical measurements of weight, length and cranial circumference were performed.

Results.—During the first 4 mo of life, FF infants compared to BF ones showed higher ghrelin levels (2654.86 vs 2132.96 pg/ml; $p<0.032$), higher IGF-I levels (3.73 vs 3.15 ng/ml; $p=0.00$) and lower leptin levels (0.68 vs 1.16 ng/ml; $p<0.04$). Leptin values were higher in females than in males (0.80 vs 0.47 ng/ml; $p<0.03$), while no gender-related difference was found for ghrelin and IGF-I. No differences were found in anthropometrical measurements comparing the two groups of infants. A multiple regression analysis showed an inverse correlation between ghrelin and leptin values ($p<0.04$) and between IGF-I and leptin levels ($p=0.00$).

Conclusion.—Our finding suggests that breastfeeding influences hormones such as ghrelin, leptin and IGF-I in infancy, mainly during the first 4 mo of life. Further evidence is needed to confirm and clarify the role of a protective link from mother to infants as seen in our observations.

▶ A number of articles have suggested a protective role of breast-feeding on the development of future obesity later in childhood and adolescence. The long-term persistence of the effect through adulthood has not been carefully evaluated but may well be there. Interestingly, the growth curves of breast-fed and formula-fed healthy, term infants differ in the first few months and are characterized by a higher rate of growth among those who are breast-fed until around 6 to 8 weeks of age, when the growth trend switches toward formula-fed infants. This trend ultimately translates to a major positive difference in the weight/length ratio at 12 months for those who are formula-fed.[1]

So why do breast-fed babies seem to do better than their bottle-fed peers when it comes to a more ideal weight velocity throughout most of infancy? Some have attributed the benefits to the differing composition of fats and proteins in breast milk, but the evidence for this explanation is thin at best. Perhaps more importantly, it has been shown that breast-fed babies have the unique ability to self-regulate both their breast milk and energy intake from solid foods. Some who have fed their infants breast milk in early infancy and who breast-feed for longer periods have reported less restrictive behavior regarding childhood feeding at a year of age.[2]

This article teaches us more than we ever knew before about the mediators of satiety in babies. Among these mediators are leptin, ghrelin, insulin-like growth factors, and many others that are currently under active investigation (eg, adiponectin, various peptides, and cytokine-like compounds). Savino et al report observations on higher levels of leptin and lower levels of ghrelin and IGF-I in breast-fed babies compared with formula-fed ones. Whether the balance of these various hormones, which would favor moderation of weight gain, relates to some substance in breast milk that is different from bottle milk remains to be seen. It is also possible that the behavior of breast-feeding itself might favor a balance of these mediators and lead to a more ideal weight. Ghrelin is the most recent modulator of appetite that has been described in some detail. This is an acylated 28-amino-acid peptide first discovered some 7 years ago. This peptide exerts a wide range of metabolic effects. It stimulates growth hormone secretion and other pituitary hormones such as adrenocorticotropic hormone and prolactin, probably by acting on hypothalamic and pituitary levels. Some have suggested that this mediator might actually help to regulate weight gain in utero. Administration of ghrelin will increase appetite and promote food intake in human beings. Blood levels rise during fasting and fall after eating, which suggests that this peptide is a short-term regulator of energy balance. Contrarily, leptin decreases immediately after fasting but generally acts as a long-term peptide to suppress appetite. Leptin is a protein secreted by fat cells themselves.

Whatever is going on in the first year of life with regard to appetite regulators, breast-feeding seems to favor ideal weight gain. You can bet, as time passes, that we will learn much more about the intricacies and complexities of how our appetites are controlled. Some day, hopefully in the not too distant future, there will be a leptin-like drug that those who have difficulty controlling their weight can take to help ease the difficulties associated with dieting.

An article from Australia by Burke et al (see Abstract 15–4) confirms that babies who are breast-fed for more than 12 months are, in fact, leaner than their peers at a year of age. Breast-feeding is best for virtually all babies, if the option exists.

One additional insight into breast milk: You are a firm believer in vitamin C as an agent that can prevent the ravages of the common cold. A patient asks you a question, however, that stumps you. She wishes to know whether she, a lactating mother, can increase the vitamin C content of her breast milk by drinking fresh orange juice. She hopes to protect her baby against the common cold. Ignoring the debate about the pros and cons of vitamin C in the prophylaxis of respiratory infection, can you provide advice to this breast-feeding mother about whether drinking fresh orange juice would increase the amount of ascorbic acid in her breast milk? A study in the American Journal of Clinical Nutrition provides the answer and has shown that the production of ascorbic acid in human milk increases in women who have a low level to start with, as is true of many African-American women.[3] Over a period of 6 weeks, such women will increase production of ascorbic acid in their breast milk from an average of 16 mg/kg to 32 mg/kg by taking 3 servings of orange juice a week and from 21 mg/kg to 46 mg/kg by taking 5 servings. The effect of drinking orange juice on women who are already vitamin C sufficient is negligible.

J. A. Stockman III, MD

References

1. Dewey KG, for the World Health Organization Working Group on Infant Growth: Growth of breast-fed infants deviates from current reference data: A pooled analysis of US, Canadian and European data sets. *Pediatrics* 96:495-505, 1995.
2. Taveras EM, Scanlon KS, Birch L, et al: Association of breast feeding with maternal control of infant feeding at age one year. *Pediatrics* 114:e577-e583, 2004.
3. Ascorbic acid supplementation and regular consumption of fresh orange juice increase the ascorbic acid content of human milk: Studies in European and African lactating women. *Am J Clin Nutr* 81:1088-1093, 2005.

Breastfeeding and Overweight: Longitudinal Analysis in an Australian Birth Cohort

Burke V, Beilin LJ, Simmer K, et al (Univ of Western Australia, Perth; Women's and Infants' Research Found, Perth, Australia)
J Pediatr 147:56-61, 2005   15–4

Objective.—To examine adiposity in relation to breastfeeding using longitudinal analysis in an Australian birth cohort.

Study Design.—Repeated surveys from 16 weeks gestation to 8 years in a cohort (N = 2087) recruited through antenatal clinics. Overweight was defined by National Center for Health Statistics 95th percentiles for weight-for-length at 1 year and body mass index (BMI) at 3, 6, and 8 years. Overweight was examined using Generalized Estimating Equations with results summarized as OR. BMI Z scores were analyzed in mixed models.

Results.—At 1 year, infants breastfed >12 months were the leanest group (mean Z score -0.16, 95% CL -0.28, -0.04; not breastfed 0.16, 95% CL 0.02, 0.29; breastfed $\leq$4 months 0.31, 95% CL 0.22, 0.40; 5-8 months 0.17, 95% CL 0.06, 0.27; 9-12 months 0.11, 95% CL 0.01, 0.22). From 1 to 8 years, children breastfed $\leq$4 months had the greatest risk of overweight (OR 1.29, 95% CL 0.89, 1.97) and the highest prevalence of maternal obesity, smoking, and lower education.

Conclusions.—Infants breastfed >12 months were leaner at 1 year but not at 8 years. Breastfeeding $\leq$4 months was associated with greatest risk of overweight and adverse maternal lifestyle. Familial factors may modify associations between breastfeeding and adiposity beyond infancy.

▶ No one will argue that breast feeding is not good for a baby. New information now suggests it is also very healthy for a mother. Breast feeding may turn out to protect women from type 2 diabetes for up to 15 years. Data from 2 long-running cohorts, including 150,000 women nurses, suggest that among women who have borne a child, each extra year they spend breastfeeding reduces their risk of type 2 diabetes by about 15%.

In the study of breastfeeding nurses, the benefits of breastfeeding were confined to women who had their last baby fewer than 15 years before. These benefits seem to be independent of other risk factors for diabetes, including body mass index, family history of diabetes, and lifestyle indicators such as diet, exercise, and smoking. Breastfeeding did not protect women with gestational diabetes, perhaps because their underlying risk of diabetes is simply too high to respond to lifestyle changes. For other women, the benefits started to accrue after the first 6 months of breastfeeding.

It is hardly clear that the findings among American nurses can be extrapolated to the US population as a whole. Female nurses are not particularly representative of other US women. As a whole, they are better educated and more likely to breastfeed. But in these women, at least, sustained breastfeeding seems to provide some significant protection against the risk of diabetes.[1]

J. A. Stockman III, MD

Reference

1. Stuebe AM, Rich-Edwards JW, Willett WC, et al: Duration of lactation and incidence of type 2 diabetes. *JAMA* 294:2601-2610, 2005.

Prevalence of Overweight and Obesity in the United States, 1999-2004
Ogden CL, Carroll MD, Curtin LR, et al (Ctrs for Disease Control and Prevention, Hyattsville, Md; Ctrs for Disease Control and Prevention, Atlanta, Ga)
JAMA 295:1549-1555, 2006   15–5

Context.—The prevalence of overweight in children and adolescents and obesity in adults in the United States has increased over several decades.

Objective.—To provide current estimates of the prevalence and trends of overweight in children and adolescents and obesity in adults.

Design, Setting, and Participants.—Analysis of height and weight measurements from 3958 children and adolescents aged 2 to 19 years and 4431 adults aged 20 years or older obtained in 2003-2004 as part of the National Health and Nutrition Examination Survey (NHANES), a nationally representative sample of the US population. Data from the NHANES obtained in 1999-2000 and in 2001-2002 were compared with data from 2003-2004.

Main Outcome Measures.—Estimates of the prevalence of overweight in children and adolescents and obesity in adults. Overweight among children and adolescents was defined as at or above the 95th percentile of the sex-specific body mass index (BMI) for age growth charts. Obesity among adults was defined as a BMI of 30 or higher; extreme obesity was defined as a BMI of 40 or higher.

Results.—In 2003-2004, 17.1% of US children and adolescents were overweight and 32.2% of adults were obese. Tests for trend were significant for male and female children and adolescents, indicating an increase in the prevalence of overweight in female children and adolescents from 13.8% in 1999-2000 to 16.0% in 2003-2004 and an increase in the prevalence of overweight in male children and adolescents from 14.0% to 18.2%. Among men, the prevalence of obesity increased significantly between 1999-2000 (27.5%) and 2003-2004 (31.1%). Among women, no significant increase in obesity was observed between 1999-2000 (33.4%) and 2003-2004

(33.2%). The prevalence of extreme obesity (body mass index ≥40) in 2003-2004 was 2.8% in men and 6.9% in women. In 2003-2004, significant differences in obesity prevalence remained by race/ethnicity and by age. Approximately 30% of non-Hispanic white adults were obese as were 45.0% of non-Hispanic black adults and 36.8% of Mexican Americans. Among adults aged 20 to 39 years, 28.5% were obese while 36.8% of adults aged 40 to 59 years and 31.0% of those aged 60 years or older were obese in 2003-2004.

Conclusions.—The prevalence of overweight among children and adolescents and obesity among men increased significantly during the 6-year period from 1999 to 2004; among women, no overall increases in the prevalence of obesity were observed. These estimates were based on a 6-year period and suggest that the increases in body weight are continuing in men and in children and adolescents while they may be leveling off in women.

▶ These data speak for themselves. The results of the 2003-2004 NHANES indicate that an estimated two thirds of US adults are overweight or obese, and some 17% of US children are overweight. In the authors' analysis of NHANES data from 1999-2004, they found an increasing prevalence of overweight in children aged 2 to 19 years and an increasing prevalence of obesity in men, but not women; however, women had nearly double the rate of severe obesity compared with men.

These new obesity data tell us that the United States is outstripping the rest of the world in terms of the rate of increase in obesity at all ages. This US problem puts the entire world at jeopardy, as the earth will eventually tilt on its axis and spin out of control, flinging itself elsewhere into our universe, all as a result of the ponderosity of our population.

Last, do you know the origin of the word obesity? It comes from the Latin *obesus*, meaning one who has become plump through eating. The term "obesity" first appears in a medical context in Thomas Venner's *Via Recta* in 1620. Venner described obesity as an occupational hazard of the genteel classes. The therapy for afflicted individuals to restore their physique was to pay attention to the Hippocratic concept of regimen: balancing diet, sleep, and other factors to create and maintain health. In the 18th and 19th centuries, writers preferred the term "corpulence" over obesity. The first real diet book was by William Banting (actually a pamphlet): *A Letter on Corpulence Addressed to the Public*. This was in 1863 and the book was a bestseller. Before the term "dieting" became popular, to go on a diet was called "banting."

It wasn't actually until the 1950s that obesity was truly recognized as a disease that required therapeutic intervention. In 1959, the Metropolitan Life Insurance Company made the very first attempt to define an ideal weight, and hence to create medical criteria for intervention in obesity. A decade later, body-mass index was proposed as a more "scientific" measure of obesity with the magical number 30 defining the problem.

For the aficionados of Latin, *obesus* has one other meaning: "coarse" or "vulgar." The intent was to imply a lack of self-control and self-respect on the part of those who were overweight. Like it or not, the same social stigmata has filtered down through three millennia.[1]

J. A. Stockman III, MD

Reference

1. Barnett R: Obesity. *Lancet* 365:1843, 2005.

Can Waist Circumference Identify Children With the Metabolic Syndrome?

Hirschler V, Aranda C, de Luján Calcagno M, et al (Durand Hosp of Buenos Aires, Argentina; Univ of Buenos Aires, Argentina)
Arch Pediatr Adolesc Med 159:740-744, 2005   15–6

Objective.—To determine in children the association between waist circumference (WC) and insulin resistance determined by homeostasis modeling (HOMA-IR) and proinsulinemia and components of the metabolic syndrome, including lipid profile and blood pressure (BP).

Methods.—Eighty-four students (40 boys) aged 6 to 13 years and matched for sex and age underwent anthropometric measurements; 40 were obese; 28, overweight; and 16, nonobese. Body mass index (BMI), WC, BP, and Tanner stage were determined. An oral glucose tolerance test, lipid profile, and insulin and proinsulin assays were performed. Children were classified as nonobese (BMI < 85th percentile), overweight (BMI, 85th-94th percentile), and obese (BMI $\geq$ 95th percentile).

Results.—There was univariate association ($P < .01$) between WC and height ($r = 0.73$), BMI ($r = 0.96$), Tanner stage ($r = 0.67$), age ($r = 0.56$), systolic BP ($r = 0.64$), diastolic BP ($r = 0.61$), high-density lipoprotein cholesterol level ($r = 0.45$), triglyceride level ($r = 0.28$), proinsulin level ($r = 0.59$), and HOMA-IR ($r = 0.59$). Multiple linear regression analysis using HOMA-IR as the dependent variable showed that WC (β coefficient = 0.050 [95% confidence interval, 0.028 to 0.073]; $P = .001$) and systolic BP (β coefficient = 0.033 [95% confidence interval, 0.004 to 0.062]; $P = .004$) were significant independent predictors for insulin resistance adjusted for diastolic BP, height, BMI, acanthosis nigricans, and high-density lipoprotein cholesterol level.

Conclusion.—Waist circumference is a predictor of insulin resistance syndrome in children and adolescents and could be included in clinical practice as a simple tool to help identify children at risk.

▶ Data have been emerging from the adult literature to suggest that waist circumference can be used to predict insulin resistance. For example, in a recent article by Wahrenberg et al[1] in adults, a waist circumference of less than 100 cm excludes individuals of both sexes from being at risk of insulin resistance. In fact, in adults, the data are so good that a simple measurement of waist circumference replaces body mass index, waist:hip ratio, and other measures of total body fat as a predictor of insulin resistance and explains more than 50% of the variation in insulin sensitivity alone.

The story, of course, in children is different in the sense that one must use an age-appropriate waist circumference in association with height to determine whether a waist circumference is out of line for a youngster. One can also complement this with the physical examination. The presence of acanthosis nigricans, if present on a physical examination, is a strong positive predictor of hyperinsulinemia. This skin finding alone is an extremely positive marker for an increased risk of type 2 diabetes mellitus. It is also an independent risk factor for this condition. The use of acanthosis nigricans, however, as a sole indicator of hyperinsulinemia will cause one to miss about half of all children with significant hyperinsulinemia; thus, one can see the value of a simple determination of waist circumference in addition to a good look at the skin.

We still do not know why truncal obesity correlates with the onset of type 2 diabetes mellitus and the metabolic syndrome. The coupling of insulin resistance with abdominal obesity strongly suggest a biological link at the fat cell level. Hyperinsulinemia activates 11-beta-hydroxysteroid dehydrogenase in omental adipose tissue, thus generating active cortisol and promoting a cushingoid fat distribution. This is probably why waist circumference becomes such an excellent, and simple, tool for excluding insulin resistance and for identifying those at greater risk (and, therefore, identifying those who would benefit most from lifestyle adjustments).

One concluding insight into a practical issue related to obesity in the form of a query: when giving an intramuscular injection, how critical is it to note whether the patient is significantly obese? We actually do not know this answer in pediatrics, since no one has performed a study to determine any correlation between weight and the depth of subcutaneous tissue (between the skin and the muscle). A study has been done in adults, however, which provides significant information in this regard. In Great Britain, an investigation was performed that examined CT scan findings from 100 consecutive adults (39 men, 61 women, average age 47.8 years) who had computed tomography scans of the pelvis. The depth of adipose tissue was measured and ranged from 2.5mm to 62.6mm (mean 19.0mm). In 12 patients, the depth was more than 35mm, the extent of a standard intramuscular needle. Unfortunately, in this report, the depth of adipose tissue was not correlated with body mass index.

It is clear that those who are overweight may not have a successful intramuscular injection if standard needles are used for this purpose. It would be terrific if someone were to do a similar study to the one carried out in Great Britain using data from children who had CT scans of the pelvis performed. It would be even better if such a study did attempt correlations with body mass index in order to allow a care provider to judge which child might, or might not, need a longer needle by which to give an intramuscular injection without having to do anything more than measuring a child's weight and height to determine a predictive BMI.[2]

J. A. Stockman III, MD

References

1. Wahrenberg H, Hertel K, Leijonhufvud B-M, et al: Use of waist circumference to predict insulin resistance: Retrospective study. *BMJ* 330:1363-1364, 2005.
2. Nisbet AC: Intramuscular intragluteal injections in the increasingly obese population: Retrospective study. *BMJ* 332:637-638, 2006.

Nontraditional Cardiovascular Risk Factors in Pediatric Metabolic Syndrome

Retnakaran R, Zinman B, Connelly PW, et al (Univ of Toronto; Mount Sinai Hosp, Toronto; Univ of Western Ontario, London, Canada)
J Pediatr 148:176-182, 2006   15–7

Objective.—To study the relationships between nontraditional cardiovascular (CV) risk factors and components of the metabolic syndrome in Native Canadian children, a population at risk of future CV disease.

Study Design.—CV risk factors were evaluated in a population-based study of a Canadian Oji-Cree community, involving 236 children aged 10 to 19 years.

Results.—Using an age- and sex-specific case definition, 18.6% of the children met criteria for pediatric metabolic syndrome. As the number of metabolic syndrome component criteria increased, C-reactive protein, leptin, and ratio of apolipoprotein B to apolipoprotein A1 levels rose (all $P <$ .0001) and adiponectin concentration decreased ($P = .0006$). Principal factor analysis using both traditional and nontraditional CV risk factors revealed 5 underlying core traits, defined as follows: adiposity, lipids/adiponectin, inflammation, blood pressure, and glucose.

Conclusions.—Nontraditional CV risk factors accompany the accrual of traditional risk factors early in the progression to pediatric metabolic syndrome. Furthermore, inclusion of these factors in factor analysis suggests that 5 core traits underlie the early development of an enhanced CV risk factor profile in Native children.

▶ This report provides an assessment of the metabolic syndrome in native Canadian adolescents taking part in the Sandy Blake Health and Diabetes Project. It is the first report of the metabolic syndrome in a native Indian population, a group that has been experiencing alarming increases in obesity as well as type 2 diabetes and CV disease. The Canadian situation virtually mimics the situation here in the United States. Using a fairly well accepted definition of metabolic syndrome, these investigators reported a prevalence of the metabolic syndrome in 18.6% in the native adolescent population.

It would be important for readers of the YEAR BOOK OF PEDIATRICS to read the editorial that accompanied this report. The editorial reminds us that despite the explosion of literature on the metabolic syndrome, its definition continues to evolve, and some people do not believe it exists at all. Three health organizations have created clinical criteria in an attempt to define this syndrome in adults. These include the World Health Organization, the National Cholesterol

Education Program Expert Panel on Detection, Evaluation, and Treatment of High Blood Cholesterol in Adults (Adult Treatment Panel III [ATP III]), and the American Association of Clinical Endocrinologists. The definitions differ significantly. The American Association of Clinical Endocrinologists lists 12 clinical criteria for the diagnosis of what they specifically refer to as insulin resistance syndrome. No required number of these criteria is specified for diagnosis. This is left to clinical judgment. Once diabetes intervenes, the diagnosis of insulin resistance syndrome becomes inapplicable. In contrast, the World Health Organization and the ATP III specify a minimum number of risk factors required for the diagnosis of metabolic syndrome and do not exclude those with type 2 diabetes mellitus. In fact, the World Health Organization explicitly requires the presence of insulin resistance. In contrast, the ATP III does not include insulin resistance in its definition, focusing instead on 5 metabolic risk factors as a way to identify obese persons at greatest risk for medical complications. Both the World Health Organization and ATP III definitions require the presence of at least 3 risk factors for a diagnosis of metabolic syndrome. Although there are shared risk factors between the World Health Organization and ATP III definitions, the defining cutoff points differ. Almost all the pediatric metabolic syndrome studies use a definition based on age- and sex-specific percentiles for various cutoff points of the 5 ATP III risk factors. Unfortunately, various studies use different cutoff points for these risk factors. For example, the pediatric definitions often use the 90th percentile cutoff for waist circumference, but for 18-year-olds, the adult cutoff is somewhere between the 75th and 90th percentile for boys and slightly above the 75th percentile for girls. An 18-year-old could be classified as having central obesity based on adult definitions of metabolic syndrome, but would not be considered to have central obesity by a pediatrician. Go figure.

Despite the rancorous debate about the definition of the metabolic syndrome, it does in fact exist, no matter what the naysayers (now a vanishing minority) say. Obesity is the core of the problem, and its treatment may be at the core of the solution.

J. A. Stockman III, MD

Decreased Serum Adiponectin: An Early Event in Pediatric Nonalcoholic Fatty Liver Disease
Louthan MV, Barve S, McClain CJ, et al (Univ of Louisville, Ky; Univ of Louisville Med Ctr, Ky; Louisville VA Med Ctr, Ky)
J Pediatr 147:835-838, 2005   15–8

Objective.—To evaluate the relative concentrations of cytokines in pediatric nonalcoholic fatty liver disease (NAFLD).

Study Design.—Thirty children were evaluated at a fasting morning visit to a pediatric research unit.

Results.—Compared with normal-weight children (n = 12) and children who were overweight (n = 11), children who had presumed NAFLD (elevated Alanine aminotransferase [ALT] with negative work-up) (n = 7) had significantly lower mean serum adiponectin levels ($P = .004$). Adiponectin negatively correlated with body mass index ($r = -0.60$, $P = .001$), insulin ($r = -0.74$, $P < .001$), glucose ($r = -0.52$, $P = .004$), and ALT ($r = -0.53$, $P = .003$). There was no difference between normal-weight, obese, and presumed NAFLD subjects in mean serum tumor necrosis factor α and interleukin-6 and -8 concentrations nor in tumor necrosis factor α and interleukin-8 and -10 levels in an ex vivo lipopolysaccharide-stimulated system.

Conclusions.—Serum adiponectin is reduced in children with elevated ALT, similar to adults. However, children with presumed NAFLD do not have elevated pro-inflammatory cytokine levels. This suggests that depressed adiponectin plays a more proximal role than elevated levels of circulating pro-inflammatory cytokines in the development of NAFLD in children.

▶ A brief survey of friends suggests that many, if not most, pediatricians are not all that familiar with obesity-associated chronic liver disease. This was first recognized in adults in the 1980s. We now know that anywhere from 6% to 25% of significantly overweight children will have obesity-associated chronic liver disease, making it potentially the most common of all pediatric liver diseases. The term NAFLD is commonly used to define the illness, and in its mildest form, there is simple fatty infiltration of the liver (steatosis), similar to what one sees in individuals taking steroids. This can progress to nonalcoholic steatohepatitis, which involves inflammation and, eventually, fibrosis and cirrhosis.

The article by Louthan et al from Louisville provides us with information regarding who is at risk of NAFLD. Serum levels of adiponectin, an anti-inflammatory adipocytokine, are negatively associated with increasing fatness in children. In adults, adiponectin levels have been shown to be predictive of future development of insulin resistance and type 2 diabetes. Low adiponectin levels are associated with increased hepatic fat, and adiponectin levels are decreased in adults with nonalcoholic steatohepatitis. As this article shows, obese children with elevated liver enzymes do, in fact, have low adiponectin levels.

If you are not familiar with adiponectin, it is an important fat cell–secreted cytokine that has anti-inflammatory properties. The inverse association between the serum adiponectin level and body mass index suggests that obesity, for whatever reason, causes a reduced level of adiponectin, which, in turn, allows inflammatory mediators to damage the liver. It may very well be that adiponectin is the most important factor related to elevated liver enzymes. Adiponectin may be useful as a screening test for those youngsters who are overweight who are at greatest risk of the long-term complications of obesity. Who would have ever thought that obesity might replace alcohol as the primary cause of cirrhosis in the United States?

Having just briefly mentioned alcohol, who eats a more healthy variety of foods, wine drinkers or beer drinkers? How would you perform a study to determine the answer to this question? A study undertaken in Denmark to determine what the food buying habits are of people who buy wine or beer provides the answers. The study design was quite fascinating. Data were taken from approximately 3.5 million transactions chosen at random from 98 outlets of 2 large Danish supermarket chains (Bilka and Føtex) over the period September 2002 to February 2003. Data from these supermarkets are collected routinely into a large databank that allows inventory control. The data were "mined" to see exactly what types of foods were purchased by wine buyers and by beer buyers (both wine and beer are available in supermarkets in Denmark). The Danish study found some quite interesting results. Customers who bought wine, but not beer, comprised 5.8% of the total number of customers whose data were recorded and those who bought beer, but not wine, constituted 6.6% of the total number. It was obvious that wine buyers bought more olives, fruits, vegetables, poultry, cooking oil, and lowfat products than people who bought beer. Beer buyers bought more ready cooked dishes, sugar, cold cuts, chips, pork, butter, sausages, lamb, and soft drinks. Wine buyers were more likely to buy "Mediterranean" food items, whereas beer buyers tended to buy "traditional" food items.

The results of the study from Denmark support findings from the United States and France showing that wine drinkers tend to eat fruits, vegetables, and fish and use cooking oil more often and saturated fat less often than those who prefer other alcoholic drinks.[1] These findings are significant since it has been presumed that drinking wine is heart healthy, when in fact it may be that it isn't the wine itself, but the other healthy foods that one buys, if one is a wine drinker, that make all the difference. In many parts of the world, wine drinkers have a higher level of education, higher income, better psychological functioning, and better subjective health than people who do not drink wine.[2] Similar results have been found in a California population: people who prefer wine tend to be better educated, healthy, lean, young, or middle-aged women with just a moderate alcohol intake, whereas those who prefer beer tend to be less educated, healthy young men with a higher alcohol intake.[3]

J. A. Stockman III, MD

References

1. Johansen D, Friis K, Skovenborg E, et al: Food buying habits of people who buy wine or beer: Cross-sectional study. *BMJ* 332:519-521, 2006.
2. Mortensen F, Jensen H, Sanders S, et al: Better psychological functioning and higher social status may largely explain the apparent health benefits of wine. *Arch Intern Med* 161:1844-1848, 2001.
3. Klatsky AL, Armstrong MA, Kipp H: Correlates of alcohol beverage preference: Traits of persons who choose wine, liquor, or beer. *Br J Addict* 85:1279-1289, 1990.

Underdiagnosis of Pediatric Obesity and Underscreening for Fatty Liver Disease and Metabolic Syndrome by Pediatricians and Pediatric Subspecialists

Riley MR, Bass NM, Rosenthal P, et al (Stanford Univ, Palo Alto, Calif; Univ of California, San Francisco)
J Pediatr 147:839-842, 2005   15–9

Objectives.—To evaluate how often general pediatricians, pediatric endocrinologists, and gastroenterologists diagnose children as overweight and how often interventions are provided, including nutritional counseling and screening for nonalcoholic fatty liver disease (NAFLD) and metabolic syndrome.

Study Design.—The study was a retrospective chart review of outpatient visits at 2 academic hospitals.

Results.—A total of 2256 patient visits were analyzed, including 715 visits by overweight children. Of those 715 visits, 31% resulted in a diagnosis of overweight. Diagnosis of overweight and nutritional counseling were least likely to occur during gastroenterology visits (22% and 13%, respectively, $P < .01$). Screening for metabolic syndrome was most likely to occur during endocrinology visits (34%; $P < .01$). Screening for NAFLD was most likely to occur during gastroenterology visits (23%; $P < .01$). Children age < 5 years and those with a body mass index percentile (BMI%) of 85% to 94% were least likely to receive diagnosis and intervention for overweight.

Conclusions.—The majority of overweight children were not diagnosed and did not receive relevant and recommended evaluations and interventions. Specific attention should be focused on providing diagnosis and interventions for overweight children, especially those age < 5 years and with a BMI% of 85% to 94%.

▶ In the commentary to Abstract 15–8, I noted that most pediatricians are not all that familiar with the relationship between obesity and fatty liver disease, the latter being a component of the evolving spectrum of the metabolic syndrome. This study from Stanford tells us not only that we are not familiar with fatty liver problems but also that we are severely underdiagnosing and managing obesity in our patient populations. Even when the problem is recognized, few overweight children are screened for obesity-related conditions such as NAFLD and the metabolic syndrome. Because both of these conditions are asymptomatic and because of their long-term associated morbidity, early diagnosis and intervention are critical. Currently, no published guidelines exist for the screening of NAFLD and the metabolic syndrome in obese children.

It is time for someone within our pediatric community, be it within the American Academy of Pediatrics or the North American Society for Pediatric Gastroenterology, Hepatology, and Nutrition, to set forth clear guidelines about what we should be looking for, and when, in our population of overweight children.

J. A. Stockman III, MD

Metabolic Hormonal, Oxidative, and Inflammatory Factors in Pediatric Obesity-Related Liver Disease

Mandato C, Lucariello S, Licenziati MR, et al (Univ of Naples "Federico II," Italy; Pediatria AORN Cardarelli Hosp, Naples, Italy; Second Univ of Naples, Italy)
J Pediatr 147:62-66, 2005   15–10

Objective.—To examine the role of metabolic, hormonal, oxidative, and inflammatory factors in pediatric obesity-related liver disease.

Study Design.—In 50 obese children (age 7 to 14 years) with (n = 20, group 1) or without (n = 30, group 2) hypertransaminasemia and ultrasonographic liver brightness, we studied insulin resistance (fasting glucose/insulin ratio [FGIR]) and serum levels of leptin, iron, transferrin, ferritin, C-reactive protein (CRP), white blood cell (WBC) count, tumor necrosis factor (TNF)-α, interleukin (IL)-6, C282Y and H63D mutations, and erythrocytic glutathione peroxidase (GPX) activity.

Results.—FGIR (6.7 ± 4.1 vs 9.2 ± 5.2; P = .02), serum ferritin (88.8 ± 36.0 vs 39.9 ± 24.0 ng/mL; P = .0001), serum CRP (5.4 ± 6.0 vs 1.1 ± 1.6 mg/dL; P = 0.004), and GPX (8.4 ± 0.9 vs 5.0 ± 0.5 U/g Hb; P = .05) were significantly higher and more frequently deranged in group 1 than in group 2. FGIR, ferritin, and CRP values were simultaneously deranged in 41% of the group 1 patients and in none of the group 2 patients (P = .098). Serum leptin, iron, and transferrin, WBC, TNF-α, IL-6, and C282Y and H63D mutations were similar in the 2 groups.

Conclusions.—Insulin resistance, oxidative stress, and low-grade systemic inflammatory status are implicated in pediatric obesity-related liver disease. These findings may be useful in planning pathophysiologically based therapeutic trials for hepatopathic obese children who are unable to follow hypocaloric diets.

▶ Being overweight during childhood has a variety of associated adverse consequences. If one looks at the Bogalusa Study,[1] more than 60% of overweight children 5 to 10 years of age have at least 1 risk factor for cardiovascular disease. This would include elevated blood pressure or serum insulin levels or dyslipidemia. One in 4 of these youngsters will have 2 or more risk factors. Type 2 diabetes among pediatric patients accounts for as much as 45% of all newly diagnosed diabetes in the United States and is significantly more common in ethnic and racial groups with higher rates of obesity. These include Native Americans, blacks, and Mexican Americans. In addition to being associated with a higher risk of cardiovascular disease later in life and type 2 diabetes in childhood, obesity is known to cause sleep apnea and gallbladder disease, both of which have tripled in incidence in the last 25 years.

What has not been fully appreciated in the past is the relationship between obesity and liver disease in children. The problem we are talking about is nonalcoholic fatty liver disease. This is a disorder with a spectrum of presentations ranging from simple hepatic steatosis, which is likely a common and benign problem, to progressive necrosis and inflammation of the liver resulting in fibrosis. Nonalcoholic fatty liver disease is being recognized more and more frequently in children. Various studies have shown that elevated liver enzymes vary in frequency between 10% and 25% in obese children, and liver brightness on ultrasonography is even more common (22.5% to 77%).[2]

Exactly why obese children develop liver problems has remained unclear. Elevated levels of inflammatory mediators and high WBC counts are markers of low-grade systemic inflammatory reactions common in both obese adults and children. This article confirms that obese children have a moderately increased inflammatory status as shown by elevated CRP values in comparison with healthy individuals. These values are significantly more pronounced in children with liver involvement. It is also possible that the insulin resistance and oxidative stresses induced by obesity may play a role in obesity-related liver disease in children.

Given the fact that the epidemic of obesity in the United States is a relatively recent phenomenon in children, it may be several decades before we learn exactly how harmful the hepatic abnormalities seen in such youngsters will be when they are 50, 60, or 70 years of age—if they live that long. Time will tell.

J. A. Stockman III, MD

References

1. Deshmukh-Taskar P, Nicklas TA, Morales M: Tracking of overweight status from childhood to young adulthood: The Bogalusa Heart Study. *Eur J Clin Nutr* 60:48-57, 2006.
2. American Diabetes Association: Standards of medical care for patients with diabetes mellitus. *Diabetes Care* 26:33-50, 2003.

Effect of Orlistat on Weight and Body Composition in Obese Adolescents: A Randomized Controlled Trial

Chanoine J-P, Hampl S, Jensen C, et al (British Columbia Children's Hosp, Vancouver, Canada; Children's Mercy Hosps and Clinics, Kansas City, Mo; Baylor College of Medicine, Houston; et al)
JAMA 293:2873-2883, 2005

15–11

Context.—The prevalence of overweight and obesity in children and adolescents is increasing rapidly. In this population, behavioral therapy alone has had limited success in providing meaningful, sustained weight reduction, and pharmacological treatment has not been extensively studied.

Objective.—To determine the efficacy and safety of orlistat in weight management of adolescents.

Design, Setting, and Patients.—Multicenter, 54-week (August 2000-October 2002), randomized, double-blind study of 539 obese adolescents (aged 12-16 years; body mass index [BMI] ≥2 units above the 95th percentile) at 32 centers in the United States and Canada.

Interventions.—A 120-mg dose of orlistat (n = 357) or placebo (n = 182) 3 times daily for 1 year, plus a mildly hypocaloric diet (30% fat calories), exercise, and behavioral therapy.

Main Outcome Measures.—Change in BMI; secondary measures included changes in waist and hip circumference, weight loss, lipid measurements, and glucose and insulin responses to oral glucose challenge.

Results.—There was a decrease in BMI in both treatment groups up to week 12, thereafter stabilizing with orlistat but increasing beyond baseline with placebo. At the end of the study, BMI had decreased by 0.55 with orlistat but increased by 0.31 with placebo (P = .001). Compared with 15.7% of the placebo group, 26.5% of participants taking orlistat had a 5% or higher decrease in BMI (P = .005); 4.5% and 13.3%, respectively, had a 10% or higher decrease in BMI (P = .002). At study end, weight had increased 0.53 kg with orlistat and 3.14 kg with placebo (P<.001). Dual-energy x-ray absorptiometry showed that this difference was explained by changes in fat mass. Waist circumference decreased in the orlistat group but increased in the placebo group (-1.33 cm vs $+0.12$ cm; P<.05). Generally mild to moderate gastrointestinal tract adverse events occurred in 9% to 50% of the orlistat group and in 1% to 13% of the placebo group.

Conclusions.—In combination with diet, exercise, and behavioral modification, orlistat statistically significantly improved weight management in obese adolescents compared with placebo. The use of orlistat for 1 year in this adolescent population did not raise major safety issues although gastrointestinal adverse events were more common in the orlistat group.

▶ Every article dealing with obesity and the pediatric age population begins by drawing us the picture of how common this issue is. All of us know the problem. What we do not know is what the solution to the problem is. This article provides us with a partial solution: a pharmacologic approach to the problem. We learn that after a year of treatment, adolescents taking 120 mg of the gastrointestinal lipase inhibitor, orlistat, 3 times a day, decreased their BMI by 0.55. In this study, diet, exercise, and behavioral modification were compared with diet, exercise, behavioral modification, and orlistat therapy. Although the adolescents in the comparative arm did lose weight during the first 12 weeks of the trial, diet, behavioral changes, and exercise alone were insufficient to sustain the weight loss over time.

So what do we learn from this article when it comes to the management of obesity in adolescents? We surely know there is no perfect "cure." On average, teens in the orlistat-treated group began to regain their weight after this study was completed. Although orlistat use in adults for more than 1 year appears to be safe, no data exist about its safety for prolonged periods in adolescents. If the changes in body fat and BMI are sustainable only with the ongoing use of medication, then weight management for these adolescents might conceivably require the use of orlistat, or similar medications, for many years. Orlistat is not cheap. It has been estimated that the average wholesale cost of the drug runs about $175 a month. The drug has been approved by the United States Food and Drug Administration for use by adolescents as part of the management of obesity and, therefore, is likely to be covered as a therapeutic. This is more than one can say about nutritional and behavioral counseling.

Without question, much more data are needed on the long-term benefits and risks of intestinal lipase inhibitors. They should never be given without attempts at nutritional control and exercise. No one has found any magic, stand-alone pill for obesity. It is certainly not orlistat all by itself.

J. A. Stockman III, MD

Evidence Based Physical Activity for School-Age Youth
Strong WB, Malina RM, Blimkie CJR, et al (Med College of Georgia, Augusta; Tarleton State Univ, Stephenville, Tex; McMaster Univ, Hamilton, Ontario, Canada; et al)
J Pediatr 146:732-737, 2005   15–12

Objectives.—To review the effects of physical activity on health and behavior outcomes and develop evidence-based recommendations for physical activity in youth.

Study Design.—A systematic literature review identified 850 articles; additional papers were identified by the expert panelists. Articles in the identified outcome areas were reviewed, evaluated and summarized by an expert panelist. The strength of the evidence, conclusions, key issues, and gaps in the evidence were abstracted in a standardized format and presented and discussed by panelists and organizational representatives.

Results.—Most intervention studies used supervised programs of moderate to vigorous physical activity of 30 to 45 minutes duration 3 to 5 days per week. The panel believed that a greater amount of physical activity would be necessary to achieve similar beneficial effects on health and behavioral outcomes in ordinary daily circumstances (typically intermittent and unsupervised activity).

Conclusion.—School-age youth should participate daily in 60 minutes or more of moderate to vigorous physical activity that is developmentally appropriate, enjoyable, and involves a variety of activities.

▶ Strong et al make very clear recommendations for the amount of physical activity in youth necessary to improve health and other outcomes. The recommendations that are made reflect information digested from more than 300 studies performed in recent years. The conclusion is that, for the average American school-aged child, participation daily in 60 minutes or more of moderate to vigorous physical activities would, in fact, be ideal. The article notes that, while swimming is great, weight-bearing activities are more likely to prevent osteoporosis, particularly of the lower extremities and spine.

It takes a wishful believer to think that the significant majority of all youngsters here in the United States would exercise at a moderate or vigorous level for 60 minutes every day. The great challenge is how to achieve such a goal. The trend that has occurred in recent years in the curricula of our schools certainly does not favor success. One of the most important barriers to increased physical activity of youth is the reduction in physical education programs in our schools. Hopefully, educators and those who ultimately pay the price tag for our schools will read this article by Strong et al and become believers in the need to get kids moving. To learn more about where we go with physical activity recommendations, see the excellent editorial by Dietz.[1]

We tend to think diet and exercise are the most significant ingredients in maintaining a healthy weight. Sleep is also important. Since the mid 1960s, the rate of obesity here in the US has tripled to 1 in 3 adults and is similarly an epidemic in children. Over the same period, US citizens have deducted, on average, about 2 hours from their nightly slumber. Recently, investigators have looked to see if there was a connection. Studies at the University of Chicago have shown that blood concentrations of hunger and satiety hormones, as well as food preferences, do in fact depend on how well rested individuals are. Leptin is a well-described satiety hormone. Leptin levels are roughly 20% lower in men who sleep only 4 hours a night in comparison to those who sleep 9 hours nightly. Conversely, hunger hormones such as ghrelin climb more than 25% in those who are sleep deprived. If one looks at appetite, in a study of those who were sleep deprived versus those who had adequate amounts of sleep, those who were sleep deprived had appetites that increased by some 24%. It has also been found that sleep loss increases the activity the vagus nerve, the trunk line for signals between the gut and the brain. During stress, the brain signals the gut to alter its release of appetite-controlling hormones, which might be the mechanism by which sleep loss changes eating behavior.

In case you did not know, humans are the only animals to voluntarily ignore their sleep needs. We often stay up, play, work, socialize, or watch television well beyond the signals that tell us to hit the sack. Could it be that the epidemic of obesity here in the United States in fact is related to sleep deprivation, at least in part? Perhaps.[2] Common sense might tell you that lying around a lot in bed decreases your metabolic rate. On the other hand, even more common sense would say that if you are awake longer during the day, and night, chances are you are eating more, or at least you certainly have the time to.

J. A. Stockman III, MD

References

1. Dietz WH: Physical activity recommendations: Where do we go from here? *J Pediatr* 146:719-720, 2005.
2. Raloff J: Still hungry? Fattening revelations—and new mysteries—about the hunger hormone. *Science News* 167:216-220, 2005.

Relation Between the Changes in Physical Activity and Body-Mass Index During Adolescence: A Multicentre Longitudinal Study
Kimm SYS, Glynn NW, Obarzanek E, et al (Univ of New Mexico, Albuquerque; Univ of Pittsburgh, Pa; Natl Heart, Lung, and Blood Inst, Bethesda, Md; et al)
Lancet 366:301-307, 2005   15–13

Background.—The role of physical activity in preventing obesity during adolescence remains unknown. We examined changes in activity in relation to changes in body-mass index (BMI) and adiposity in a cohort of 1152 black and 1135 white girls from the USA, who were followed up prospectively from ages 9 or 10 to 18 or 19 years.

Methods.—BMI and sum of skinfold thickness were assessed annually, whereas habitual activity was assessed at years 1 (baseline), 3, 5, and 7-10. Each girl's overall activity status was categorised as active, moderately active, or inactive. Longitudinal regression models examined associations between changes in activity and in overall activity status with changes in BMI and in sum of skinfold thickness.

Findings.—Each decline in activity of 10 metabolic equivalent [MET]-times per week was associated with an increase in BMI of 0.14 kg/m² (SE 0.03) and in sum of skinfold thickness of 0.62 mm (0.17) for black girls, and of 0.09 kg/m² (0.02) and 0.63 mm (0.13) for white girls. At ages 18 or 19 years, BMI differences between active and inactive girls were 2.98 kg/m² (p<0.0001) for black girls and 2.10 kg/m² (p<0.0001) for white girls. Similar results were apparent for sum of skinfold thickness. For moderately active girls, changes in BMI and sum of skinfold thickness were about midway between those for active and inactive girls.

Interpretation.—Changes in activity levels of US girls during adolescence significantly affected changes in BMI and adiposity. Thus, preventing the steep decline in activity during adolescence is an important method to reduce obesity.

▶ It comes as no surprise that investigators now report that changes in physical activity in late childhood and adolescence are related to changes in measures of body fatness in US girls who are followed for up to a decade. The differences between the most and least active girls in this article in terms of body weight gain over a decade are 4 kg in whites and 6 to 9 kg in blacks. The reasons for this are straightforward. In contrast with many previous studies, this study was large and well-designed. The association between physical activity and weight gain was detectable because of the age of the participants. Currently, the lifestyle of the average teen is obesogenic, and every study in recent years has shown that physical activity on the part of freshman high school students is much greater than on the part of seniors. As little as 50 kcal a day equivalent decline in physical activity will, over time, gradually lead to obesity. Studies have shown that, for the adult population, just an extra 100 kcal a day in terms of physical activity would prevent obesity in virtually all adults. In this sense, even a little is a lot when it comes to getting off the sofa and moving about.

The article by Strong et al (see Abstract 15–12) is from the Department of Pediatrics, Medical College of Georgia, a department that has pioneered in studies of risk factors related to obesity. It tells us exactly how much physical activity is necessary to maintain cardiovascular fitness and to minimize risk factors for long-term disease related to being overweight.

We close this commentary on obesity with a clinical scenario. See how you would address this situation. You have an extraordinarily large teenager in your patient population. His obesity is truly morbid. One day he presents with severe abdominal pain and you wish to obtain a CT scan of the abdomen. You are concerned, however, that the CT unit in your hospital is too small for your patient to fit into. What are your alternatives? The answer is clear. If you have a large zoo or a veterinary school in your area, that may be your solution. Take, for example, a snippet from a British Primary Care Trust's newsletter that had the following wording: "MRI scanners (for large patients): This is to inform all GPs that the veterinary department of the Zoological Society of London does not have CT or MRI scanners for scanning oversized patients; GPs are advised to contact the Equine/Large Animal Units at either Cambridge University Veterinary School or the Animal Health Trust in Newmarket".[1]

This editor was once on faculty at a children's hospital near a local zoo where a baby chimp was dropped by his mother, becoming unconscious. Since we were only a couple of blocks away and the problem was urgent, a hospital scanner was freed up to make a diagnosis of an epidural hematoma, which was promptly drained in the surgical suite of the hospital's research laboratories.

J. A. Stockman III, MD

Reference

1. MR scanning (editorial). *BMJ* 331:464, 2005.

Survival of Infants With Neural Tube Defects in the Presence of Folic Acid Fortification

Bol KA, for the National Birth Defects Prevention Network (Colorado Dept of Public Health and Environment, Denver; et al)
Pediatrics 117:803-812, 2006   15–14

Objective.—Neural tube defects (NTDs) are preventable through preconceptional and periconceptional folic acid intake. Although decreases in the prevalence of NTDs have been reported since folic acid fortification of United States grain products began, it is not known whether folic acid plays a role in reducing the severity of occurring NTDs. Our aim was to determine whether survival among infants born with spina bifida and encephalocele has improved since folic acid fortification and to measure the effects of selected maternal, pregnancy, and birth characteristics on first-year (infant) survival rates.

Methods.—A retrospective cohort study was conducted and included 2841 infants with spina bifida and 638 infants with encephalocele who were born between 1995 and 2001 and were registered in any of 16 participating birth defects monitoring programs in the United States. First-year survival rates for both spina bifida and encephalocele cohorts were measured with Kaplan-Meïer estimation; factors associated with improved chances of first-year survival, including birth before or during folic acid fortification, were measured with Cox proportional-hazards regression analysis.

Results.—Infants with spina bifida experienced a significantly improved first-year survival rate of 92.1% (adjusted hazard ratio: 0.68; 95% confidence interval: 0.50-0.91) during the period of mandatory folic acid fortification, compared with a 90.3% survival rate for those born before fortification. Infants with encephalocele had a statistically nonsignificant increase in survival rates, ie, 79.1% (adjusted hazard ratio: 0.76; 95% confidence interval: 0.51-1.13) with folic acid fortification, compared with 75.7% for earlier births.

Conclusions.—Folic acid may play a role in reducing the severity of NTDs in addition to preventing the occurrence of NTDs. This phenomenon contributes to our understanding of the efficacy of folic acid. Additionally, as survival of NTD-affected infants improves, health care, education, and family support must expand to meet their needs.

▶ We have known for some time that the enrichment of grains here in the United States and the supplementation with folic acid of pregnant women have had a major effect in reducing the number of children born with NTDs. Now we see that folic acid fortification may actually play a role in reducing the severity of NTDs as well.

For those interested in reading more about food enrichment with folic acid, its strengths and deficiencies, see the superb commentary by Brent and Oakley.[1] We are reminded that the article by Bol et al is a stern wake-up call that too many children continue to develop spina bifida because our enriched grains do not have enough folic acid. In the United States, folic acid fortification of grain is at the level of 140 µg of folic acid per 100 g of grain. In the United Kingdom, Australia, and New Zealand, twice as much folic acid is used to fortify grain. There are no known side effects to such fortification, and the cost difference to achieve higher fortification levels is essentially trivial. The Brent and Oakley commentary encourages us to persuade all women of reproductive age to consume 400 µg of folic acid daily, which is readily available in multivitamin supplements and in many breakfast cereals. The prevention of spina bifida and anencephaly that has occurred because of folic acid fortification has saved the country approximately a quarter of a billion dollars annually in medical care costs. A few bucks more invested in such fortification would yield an even better return on investment.

J. A. Stockman III, MD

Reference

1. Brent RL, Oakley GP: Triumph and/or tragedy: The present Food and Drug Administration program of enriching grains with folic acid. *Pediatrics* 117:930-931, 2006.

Autoantibodies to Folate Receptors in the Cerebral Folate Deficiency Syndrome

Ramaekers VT, Rothenberg SP, Sequeira JM, et al (Univ Hosp Aachen, Germany; State Univ of New York, Brooklyn; Univ Children's Hosp, Zurich, Switzerland; et al)
N Engl J Med 352:1985-1991, 2005   15–15

Abstract.—In infantile-onset cerebral folate deficiency, 5-methyl-tetrahydrofolate (5MTHF) levels in the cerebrospinal fluid are low, but folate levels in the serum and erythrocytes are normal. We examined serum specimens from 28 children with cerebral folate deficiency, 5 of their mothers, 28 age-matched control subjects, and 41 patients with an unrelated neurologic disorder. Serum from 25 of the 28 patients and 0 of 28 control subjects contained high-affinity blocking autoantibodies against membrane-bound folate receptors that are present on the choroid plexus. Oral folinic acid normalized 5MTHF levels in the cerebrospinal fluid and led to clinical improvement. Cerebral folate deficiency is a disorder in which autoantibodies can prevent the transfer of folate from the plasma to the cerebrospinal fluid.

▶ Chances are moderately good that you have never heard of the cerebral folate deficiency syndrome. As this article points out, the syndrome is defined as any neuropsychiatric condition associated with low levels of 5MTHF, the active folate metabolite in CSF, in association with normal folate metabolism outside the CNS, as reflected by normal hematologic values, normal serum homocysteine levels, and normal levels of folate in serum and red blood cells. The infantile-onset cerebral folate deficiency syndrome is a neurologic disorder that develops 4 to 6 months after birth and results in marked irritability, slow head growth, psychomotor retardation, cerebellar ataxia, pyramidal tract signs in the legs, and dyskinesias (in the form of choreoathetosis and ballismus). Some patients will have seizures. A little bit later in life, visual disturbances are seen and may result in optic atrophy and blindness. The only identifiable biochemical abnormality consistently observed in these children is a low level of 5MTHF in the CSF.

What we see in this study of 28 children with cerebral folate deficiency is the finding of an unusual neurodegenerative disorder in association with autoantibodies against folate receptors that block the transport of folate through the choroid plexus into the CNS. The choroid plexus is rich in folate receptors, and the blockade by the autoantibodies deprives the baby's developing brain of this essential vitamin. This results in low CSF folate levels but normal blood values. All the clinical signs of the disorder directly relate to the CNS deprivation of folate.

Given that babies with this disorder develop normally at least until 6 months of age and that mothers of these babies show no autoantibodies, one can speculate that the production of autoantibodies against the folate receptor occurs postpartum in the baby. The authors of this article go out on a limb to suggest that the autoantibodies are induced by soluble folate-binding proteins in human or bovine milk and result from sensitization by unknown antigens. Please think about this rare disorder any time you see a baby who seems to be having a progressive neurologic disorder. The disorder is important to detect early because folinic acid at pharmacologic dosages can bypass autoantibody-blocked folate receptors and enter the CSF by way of the reduced folate carrier. Such administration restores folate levels within the CNS and can ameliorate the neurologic disorder to a significant degree.

J. A. Stockman III, MD

Congenital Glutamine Deficiency With Glutamine Synthetase Mutations

Häberle J, Görg B, Rutsch F, et al (Universitätsklinikum Münster, Germany; Heinrich-Heine-Univ Düsseldorf, Germany; Centre Hospitalier Universitaire Bretonneau, Tours, France; et al)
N Engl J Med 353:1926-1933, 2005 15–16

Background.—Glutamine synthetase catalyzes the conversion of glutamate and ammonia to glutamine and is important in ammonia detoxification, inter-organ nitrogen flux, and acid–base regulation. High glutamine synthetase activity is found in the human liver, brain, and muscle. Diminished glutamine synthetase expression or a secondary deficiency of glutamine synthetase has been described but is rare. Two unrelated patients with congenital systemic glutamine synthetase deficiency as a result of a mutation in the glutamine synthetase gene are described.

Case 1.—Male infant, the second child of consanguineous Turkish parents, was resuscitated at birth. He was found to be neurologically compromised, with marked flaccidity, and also to have cardiac insufficiency. He died after 2 days of life. Cerebral MRI showed a markedly immature brain with hypersensitivity of the white matter, enlarged lateral ventricles, and almost complete agyria. On postmortem examination, the brain weighed only 202 g, but evidence of visceral malformations was not present.

Case 2.—Female infant, the third child of consanguineous Turkish parents, experienced convulsions and respiratory failure requiring intubation and ventilation on the first day of life. In the first weeks of life she had voluminous yellowish stools and progressive weight loss, despite enteral feeding. After 2 weeks, a generalized, blistering erythematous rash developed that, on histologic examination, supported a diagnosis of epidermal necrolysis. Brain MRI showed markedly attenuated gyri. The patient died during the fourth week of life from multiorgan failure.

Conclusions.—Glutamine was largely absent in the serum of both patients, although the glutamate levels were normal. The levels of both glutamine and glutamate were normal in the parents, for whom urine and serum samples were investigated. The most striking features in these 2 patients with congenital systemic glutamine deficiency were marked brain malformations with abnormal gyration and marked white matter lesions. This disorder should be considered in neonates with similar brain malformations. Obtaining serum glutamine levels in such neonates would aid in screening for congenital systemic glutamine deficiency.

▶ The topic of congenital glutamine deficiency may seem like a terribly obscure one to include in the YEAR BOOK OF PEDIATRICS. Potentially wider implications exist, however, for what is probably a quite rare metabolic disorder. Häberle et al report on 2 unrelated infants who had dramatically reduced levels of glutamine because of a deficiency of glutamine synthetase, the enzyme that catalyzes the conversion of glutamate to glutamine. Both infants had a profound cerebral disease that included malformations of the brain, and both died during the neonatal period. Molecular studies showed that each of the infants was homozygous for a different mutation in the glutamine synthetase gene. This article is of significance in that it adds a genetic disorder to the list of those that should be considered in any neonate or, perhaps, even in older infants with undiagnosed neurologic disease. In addition, these cases stimulate our thinking about the role of glutamine synthetase and glutamine itself with respect to brain functioning and development.

Glutamine is by far the most abundant free amino acid in the body. It is involved in cell viability, cellular energy metabolism, and the availability of glutamate neurotransmitters in neurons. It is made available largely by glutamine synthetase-catalyzed amidation of glutamate. Thus, glutamine deficiency resulting from defective glutamine synthetase is highly likely to be detrimental in many different ways. Glutamine deficiency obviously can produce problems long before birth. This is evidenced by the sad situation of the 2 infants reported above. Such prenatal damage is unusual because a fetus with a metabolic disorder is usually protected in utero by the metabolically normal mother through placental exchange of metabolites, so the fetus becomes affected only after birth. In the cases described, the glutamine supplied by the mother may not have adequately compensated for severe fetal glutamine deprivation. To read more about medical metabolic disorders related to glutamine, see the excellent review by Levey.[1]

Until I had read an article from Turkey[2] in which glutamine supplementation was found to reduce the duration of common diarrheal syndromes, I was not all that familiar with the relationship between glutamine and the health of the gastrointestinal (GI) tract. It turns out that glutamine has been the focus of intensive research for almost 2 decades. It is the most abundant circulating amino acid and is the major substrate for inter-organ nitrogen and carbon transfer. It is the principal metabolic fuel for the small intestine. L-glutamine is approved by the Food and Drug Administration as a protein supplement and is available in health food stores. It is mainly used by body builders for anabolic purposes. As importantly, it has significant effects in the GI tract. It stimulates intestinal salt and water absorption as well as crypt cell proliferation.

At one time, within the GI community, glutamine seemed to be the cure-all for many intestinal diseases. However, the field of "glutaminology" is peppered with negative clinical studies and numerous pessimistic editorials questioning its clinical usefulness. Virtually all studies show that it does not do anything to affect disease activity, for example, in patients with Crohn's disease. Nonetheless, studies such as the one by Yalçin et al[2] may lead to the acceptance of glutamine as a component of therapy for diarrheal disease. If you want to read more about glutamine and the GI tract, see the excellent editorial by Rhoads.[3] He draws an analogy between the influence of glutamine on the intestinal cell by thinking of the small intestinal enterocyte as an automobile. He suggests that glutamine keeps the car fueled so that it can absorb sodium and maintain its tight junctions. Glutamine will not convert a Ford Escort into a Ferrari; however, if, in the presence of glutamine, salt and water absorption increase, crypt cells undergo mitosis, the enterocyte becomes more resistant to injury via heat shock protein induction, and the intestinal barrier becomes more resistant to endotoxin. To further this analogy, Rhoads suggests that a low serum glutamine concentration or a low tissue level is equivalent to taking one's foot off the accelerator. Under these conditions, the car stalls and loses all function, which, in the intestinal cell, translates into apoptosis (programmed cell death).

J. A. Stockman III, MD

References

1. Levey HL: Metabolic disorders in the center of genetic medicine. *N Engl J Med* 353:1968-1970, 2005.
2. Yalçin SS, Yurdakök K, Tezcan I, et al: Effect of glutamine supplementation on diarrhea, interleukin-8 and secretory immunoglobulin A in children with acute diarrhea. *J Pediatr Gastroenterol Nutr* 38:494-501, 2004.
3. Rhoads M: Glutamine is the gas pedal but not the Ferrari. *J Pediatr Gastroenterol Nutr* 38:474-476, 2004.

Transplantation of Umbilical-Cord Blood in Babies With Infantile Krabbe's Disease
Escolar ML, Poe MD, Provenzale JM, et al (Univ of North Carolina, Chapel Hill; Duke Univ, Durham, NC; Jefferson Med College, Philadelphia, Pa; et al)
N Engl J Med 352:2069-2081, 2005   15–17

Background.—Infantile Krabbe's disease produces progressive neurologic deterioration and death in early childhood. We hypothesized that transplantation of umbilical-cord blood from unrelated donors before the development of symptoms would favorably alter the natural history of the disease among newborns in whom the disease was diagnosed because of a family history. We compared the outcomes among these newborns with the outcomes among infants who underwent transplantation after the development of symptoms and with the outcomes in an untreated cohort of affected children.

Methods.—Eleven asymptomatic newborns (age range, 12 to 44 days) and 14 symptomatic infants (age range, 142 to 352 days) with infantile Krabbe's disease underwent transplantation of umbilical-cord blood from unrelated donors after myeloablative chemotherapy. Engraftment, survival, and neurodevelopmental function were evaluated longitudinally for four months to six years.

Results.—The rates of donor-cell engraftment and survival were 100 percent and 100 percent, respectively, among the asymptomatic newborns (median follow-up, 3.0 years) and 100 percent and 43 percent, respectively, among the symptomatic infants (median follow-up, 3.4 years). Surviving patients showed durable engraftment of donor-derived hematopoietic cells with restoration of normal blood galactocerebrosidase levels. Infants who underwent transplantation before the development of symptoms showed progressive central myelination and continued gains in developmental skills, and most had age-appropriate cognitive function and receptive language skills, but a few had mild-to-moderate delays in expressive language and mild-to-severe delays in gross motor function. Children who underwent transplantation after the onset of symptoms had minimal neurologic improvement.

Conclusions.—Transplantation of umbilical-cord blood from unrelated donors in newborns with infantile Krabbe's disease favorably altered the natural history of the disease. Transplantation in babies after symptoms had developed did not result in substantive neurologic improvement.

▶ Please add infantile Krabbe's disease to the increasingly long list of diseases treatable with umbilical-cord blood transplantation. This autosomal recessive disease is due to a deficiency of the lysosomal enzyme galactocerebrosidase. Lack of the enzyme results in a failure of myelination in the central and peripheral nervous systems. Death is the result. More than 60 different mutations have resulted in the enzyme deficiency. The rationale for stem cell transplantation to treat infantile Krabbe's disease is straightforward. The procedure has been of benefit in the early stages of juvenile Krabbe's disease. Children so treated have had improved neurologic outcomes and improved overall survival rates. Older patients with Krabbe's so treated have been managed with bone marrow transplants, but many children lack a matched donor. Banked umbilical-cord blood from unrelated donors solves this problem. In the article abstracted, patients with Krabbe's disease diagnosed prenatally or at birth because of a family history were able to undergo transplantation as newborns. In addition, more than a dozen children without a family history of the disease underwent cord blood transplantation later in infancy after the onset of their clinical symptoms. When transplantation occurred in the immediate newborn period, the natural history of the disease was markedly improved. When cord blood transplantation occurred later, no reversal of existing neurologic disease was seen.

The Institute of Medicine (IOM) has called for a national network of cord blood stem cell banks that could ultimately provide transplantable hematopoietic progenitor cells for most patients who might benefit from such transplants. On April 14, 2005, the IOM recommended that the Department of Health and Human Services establish a National Cord Blood Policy Board to create rules for donation, collection, and use of cord blood, which is now routinely discarded. Cord blood is now considered to be superior to bone marrow as a source of transplantable stem cells for allogeneic transplants because its progenitor cells have a lower rejection rate than do those derived from bone marrow.

As of late 2005, some 50,000 units of cord blood are currently being stored in approximately 40 blood banks across the United States. To have a fully replete cord blood banking system, we would need about 150,000 units of cord blood to be available. A national network of cord blood of this size would care for at least 90% of the some 11,700 patients who could benefit from a transplant currently.

Emerging evidence suggests that umbilical cord blood may be the solution for how to generate embryonic stem cells without having to utilize fertilized embryos for this purpose. The money necessary to set up a national network of cord blood banks to achieve the desired inventory goals is not massive (probably on the order of less than $50 million), and the return on the investment would be extremely favorable. To read more on the cord blood stem cell network report of the IOM, see http://www.nap.edu/catalog/11269.html.

J. A. Stockman III, MD

Population-Based Study of Incidence and Risk Factors for Cerebral Edema in Pediatric Diabetic Ketoacidosis

Lawrence SE, Cummings EA, Gaboury I, et al (Children's Hosp of Eastern Ontario, Ottawa, Canada; Dalhousie Univ, Halifax, Nova Scotia, Canada; Chalmers Research Group, Ottawa, Ontario, Canada; et al)
J Pediatr 146:688-692, 2005   15–18

Objectives.—To determine incidence, outcomes, and risk factors for pediatric cerebral edema with diabetic ketoacidosis (CEDKA) in Canada.

Study Design.—This was a case-control study nested within a population-based active surveillance study of CEDKA in Canada from July 1999 to June 2001. Cases are patients with DKA <16 years of age with cerebral edema. Two unmatched control subjects per case are patients with DKA without cerebral edema.

Results.—Thirteen cases of CEDKA were identified over the surveillance period for an incidence rate of 0.51%; 23% died and 15% survived with neurologic sequelae. CEDKA was present at initial presentation of DKA in 19% of cases. CEDKA was associated with lower initial bicarbonate ($P = .001$), higher initial urea ($P = .001$), and higher glucose at presentation ($P = .014$). Although there was a trend to association with higher fluid rates and treatment with bicarbonate, these were not independent predictors.

Conclusions.—CEDKA remains a significant problem with a high mortality rate. No association was found between the occurrence of CEDKA and treatment factors. The presence of cerebral edema before treatment of DKA and the association with severity of illness suggest that prevention of DKA is the key to avoiding this devastating complication.

▶ The development of cerebral edema in patients being managed for DKA remains one of the truly dread complications of therapy in pediatrics. Estimates of the incidence of cerebral edema in such circumstances range from 0.4 to 3.1 per 100 treated cases. Recent reports from Great Britain and the United States have shown a mortality rate between 21% and 24% for this condition and significant neurologic sequelae in 21% to 35%.[1] In this article from Canada, we learn exactly what happens in a group of youngsters studied prospectively who develop cerebral edema. In Canada, the incidence of this problem appears to run at 0.51%; 23% of patients die, and 15% survive with neurologic sequelae. About 1 patient in 5 actually presents with cerebral edema as the initial sign of DKA. The latter finding shows how important it is to prevent DKA, which is the only strategy in the absolute prevention of cerebral edema as a complication of the disorder.

This is the last entry in the Nutrition and Metabolism chapter. We will close with a very practical question about nutrition. Just how bad is it for you to skip breakfast and lunch? If you think about it, it has been only until relatively recently in human evolution that we have eaten 3 meals (plus, perhaps, snacks) daily. Our ancestors consumed food much less frequently and often had to subsist on 1 large meal per day or go for several days at a time without food at all. In the evolutionary schema, humans evolved current practices preceded by many millennia of intermittent feeding rather than what we do now, which is more like continuous grazing. Data suggest that although eating 3 or more meals a day may promote rapid growth and sexual maturation in children, it just may not be the healthiest pattern for adults. Three "squares" a day, in fact, tends to lead to obesity.

Just what is the science, however, behind meal frequency and health? Studies that have attempted to determine the effects of meal frequency on health have resulted in mixed conclusions. For example, an early survey study suggested an association between reduced meal frequency and risk for diabetes and cardiovascular disease (obesity, hypercholesterolemia, and glucose intolerance).[2] In another study, healthy men ate either 3 standard meals or 17 small snacks every day. After 2 weeks on this diet, participants on the snacking diet had reduced fasting total cholesterol, LDL cholesterol, and insulin concentrations, whereas blood glucose and insulin responses to a glucose challenge did not differ.[3]

There is one natural experiment that gives some insight into the medical implications of meal patterning. Different populations of people practice intermittent fasting worldwide, usually as part of their religion. As an example, during the period of Ramadan, which lasts 1 month, Muslims do not eat during the day and typically consume most of their food in the evening. Analyses of blood from people before, during, and after Ramadan have revealed several effects of this meal-skipping diet on health indicators and disease risks, including increased HDL cholesterol and decreased LDL cholesterol concentrations and lowered platelet aggregation, suggesting a reduced risk of cardiovascular disease during Ramadan.[4,5]

The preceding is about all the data available for humans, but if we believe what happens to rats and mice, we ought to eat more like they do. For example, it has been shown that rats and mice frequently eat but 1 meal a day, if that. A study of rats has shown that rats maintained on a meal-skipping diet (alternate day feeding) with unlimited access to food when they feed, consume 30% to 40% less food over time than do those who are allowed to continuously graze.[6] As importantly, a study of mice and rats maintained on an intermittent fasting regimen (repeated cycles of 24 hours with no food followed by 24 hours with free access to food) lived up to 30% longer than those fed ad libitum.[7]

So which is it? Packing it in once a day or grazing in the refrigerator all day? We need more information on this topic. Anyone want to volunteer?

J. A. Stockman III, MD

References

1. Glaser N, Barnett P, McCaslin I, et al: Risk factors for cerebral edema in children with diabetic ketoacidosis. *N Engl J Med* 344:264-269, 2001.
2. Fabry P, Hejl Z, Fodor J, et al: The frequency of meals and its relation to overweight, hypercholesterolemia and decreased glucose tolerance. *Lancet* 284:614-615, 1964.
3. Jenkins JD, Wolever TM, Vuksan V, et al: Nibbling versus gorging: Metabolic advantages of increased meal frequency. *N Engl J Med* 321:929-934, 1989.
4. Aybak M, Turkoglu A, Sermeta et al: The effect of Ramadan fasting on platelet aggregation in healthy male subjects. *Eur J Appl Physiol Occup Physiol* 73:552-556, 1996.
5. Adlouni A, Ghalim N, Benslimane A, et al: Fasting during Ramadan induces a marked increase in high-density-lipoprotein cholesterol and decrease in low-density lipoprotein cholesterol. *Ann Nutr Metab* 41:242-249, 1997.
6. Wan R, Camandola S, Mattson MP: Intermittent fasting improves cardiovascular and neuroendocrine responses to stress. *J Nutr* 133:1921-1929, 2003.
7. Goodrick CL, Ingram DK, Reynolds MA, et al: Differential effects of intermittent feeding and voluntary exercise on body weight and life span in adult rats. *J Gerontol* 38:36-45, 1983.

16 Oncology

Day Care in Infancy and Risk of Childhood Acute Lymphoblastic Leukaemia: Findings From UK Case-Control Study
Gilham C, for the UKCCS Investigators (Inst of Cancer Research, Sutton, England; et al)
BMJ 330:1294-1297, 2005   16-1

Objective.—To test the hypothesis that reduced exposure to common infections in the first year of life increases the risk of developing acute lymphoblastic leukaemia.

Design and Setting.—The United Kingdom childhood cancer study (UKCCS) is a large population based case-control study of childhood cancer across 10 regions of the UK.

Participants.—6305 children (aged 2-14 years) without cancer; 3140 children with cancer (diagnosed 1991-6), of whom 1286 had acute lymphoblastic leukaemia (ALL).

Main Outcome Measure.—Day care and social activity during the first year of life were used as proxies for potential exposure to infection in infancy.

Results.—Increasing levels of social activity were associated with consistent reductions in risk of ALL; a dose-response trend was seen. When children whose mothers reported no regular activity outside the family were used as the reference group, odds ratios for increasing levels of activity were 0.73 (95% confidence interval 0.62 to 0.87) for any social activity, 0.62 (0.51 to 0.75) for regular day care outside the home, and 0.48 (0.37 to 0.62) for formal day care (attendance at facility with at least four children at least twice a week) (P value for trend < 0.001). Although not as striking, results for non-ALL malignancies showed a similar pattern (P value for trend < 0.001). When children with non-ALL malignancies were taken as the reference group, a significant protective effect for ALL was seen only for formal day care (odds ratio = 0.69, 0.51 to 0.93; P = 0.02). Similar results were obtained for B cell precursor common ALL and other subgroups, as well as for cases diagnosed above and below age 5 years.

Conclusion.—These results support the hypothesis that reduced exposure to infection in the first few months of life increases the risk of developing acute lymphoblastic leukaemia.

► This is an intriguing study suggesting a relationship between the risk of childhood ALL and early childhood infection rates. Currently, leukemia will develop in about 1 in 2000 children before the age of 17 and most of these cases will be ALL. We do know some of the precedent risk factors for this disorder. For example, children with Down's syndrome and certain other genetic syndromes are more susceptible to leukemia, but such conditions are involved with a distinct minority of leukemia cases. Being big at birth and being a boy will slightly increase the risk for leukemia. A number of external factors may also be associated with an increased risk of leukemia. For example, in the 1950s, a large case-control study of childhood cancer in the United Kingdom found that radiographs of a mother's abdomen during pregnancy increased the risk of a baby subsequently developing ALL by almost 50%. Practically no pregnant woman intentionally has abdominal radiographic studies these days as a result of this report.

During the past decade or so, a number of studies have suggested the possibility that an unusual pattern of exposure to infection increases the risk of ALL. One study showed that rapid population growth, especially into previously isolated rural areas, could promote epidemics of common infections, most likely viral, associated with an increased incidence of childhood leukemia.[1] In this report, in settings with extreme population mixing (new towns, commuter belts, major construction sites, and areas used for wartime evacuation or for military camps), an increased incidence of leukemia was found. Other investigators have confirmed these findings, suggesting that it is entirely possible that ALL may be caused by at least 2 events: 1 before birth, which is then followed by a challenge from infection. Recent molecular evidence has corroborated this theory. About a quarter of children with ALL have fusion of *TEL* and *AML1* genes and these chromosomal translocations have usually developed before birth. Many more babies, however, have these preleukemic cells in their cord blood than actually develop leukemia, so postnatal events may be necessary to trigger the disease. Epidemiologic studies indirectly support the theory that early protection from infection actually increases a child's risk of leukemia by allowing a later greater risk of infection at a more vulnerable time conducive to leukemia. Studies have had to use surrogates, such as daycare, for early exposure to infections. Many have found that babies who go to daycare at a young age have a lower risk of developing ALL. This report by Gilham et al strengthens this evidence. It found a dose relation: babies had a greater protection from leukemia when they had more contact with other infants.

Studies have shown that exposure to multiple potential allergens very early in life frequently diminishes the ultimate lifetime risk of allergic reactions to these allergens (such as to dog and cat dander). It may well be that getting "down and dirty" early in life, being exposed to multiple infections as soon as possible, is also protective to some degree against the development of childhood leukemia.

See the following study by Draper et al (Abstract 16–2) that discusses magnetic fields and the risk of ALL.

J. A. Stockman III, MD

Reference

1. Kinlen LJ: Infection, childhood leukemia and the Seascale cluster. *Radiol Prot Bull* 226:9-18, 2000.

Childhood Cancer in Relation to Distance From High Voltage Power Lines in England and Wales: A Case-Control Study
Draper G, Vincent T, Kroll ME, et al (Univ of Oxford, England; Natl Grid Transco plc, London)
BMJ 330:1290-1293, 2005   16–2

Objective.—To determine whether there is an association between distance of home address at birth from high voltage power lines and the incidence of leukaemia and other cancers in children in England and Wales.

Design.—Case-control study.

Setting.—Cancer registry and National Grid records.

Subjects.—Records of 29 081 children with cancer, including 9700 with leukaemia. Children were aged 0-14 years and born in England and Wales, 1962-95. Controls were individually matched for sex, approximate date of birth, and birth registration district. No active participation was required.

Main Outcome Measures.—Distance from home address at birth to the nearest high voltage overhead power line in existence at the time.

Results.—Compared with those who lived > 600 m from a line at birth, children who lived within 200 m had a relative risk of leukaemia of 1.69 (95% confidence interval 1.13 to 2.53); those born between 200 and 600 m had a relative risk of 1.23 (1.02 to 1.49). There was a significant ($P < 0.01$) trend in risk in relation to the reciprocal of distance from the line. No excess risk in relation to proximity to lines was found for other childhood cancers.

Conclusions.—There is an association between childhood leukaemia and proximity of home address at birth to high voltage power lines, and the apparent risk extends to a greater distance than would have been expected from previous studies. About 4% of children in England and Wales live within 600 m of high voltage lines at birth. If the association is causal, about 1% of childhood leukaemia in England and Wales would be attributable to these lines, though this estimate has considerable statistical uncertainty. There is no accepted biological mechanism to explain the epidemiological results; indeed, the relation may be due to chance or confounding.

▶ For more than 20 years, extremely low-frequency magnetic fields, which are produced by alternating electric currents, such as those found in high-voltage power lines, electric appliances, and wiring, have been suspected of increasing the risk of childhood leukemia. In 2000, a meta-analysis of 9 studies did not find any increase in a child's risk of leukemia in magnetic fields averaging under 0.4 fT, but above this level the risk doubled.[1] One should note that a magnetic field of 0.4 fT is very weak, amounting to only about 1% of the earth's magnetic field, which affects all of us all of the time. Studies of animals and of cells in culture have found no evidence of a plausible biological mechanism whereby very weak magnetic fields could influence the development of leukemia.

Draper et al performed a very large case-controlled study that found that a child's risk of leukemia increased steadily in relation to the proximity to high-voltage power lines of the home in which they lived at birth.

Unfortunately, this study did not include estimates or measures of the magnetic field from either the power lines or other sources. It provides little evidence that the increased risk closer to power lines is due to magnetic fields. It is entirely possible, since the risk of childhood leukemia is known to vary geographically, that the increased risk closer to power lines simply reflects some other factor that varies geographically. If, indeed, magnetic fields are capable of causing leukemia in children, they would account for only a tiny percentage of all cases.

Obviously we still do not know the cause of childhood leukemia but are reasonably sure that it involves damage to DNA before birth—probably in response to infection, chemical exposure, ionizing radiation, or other environmental exposures. These preleukemic cells are converted into overt disease after birth if children are susceptible because of their genetic makeup and early protection from infection, and they experience 1 or more other events—perhaps, a delayed challenge from infection, as suggested in the comment to Abstract 16–1. Needless to say, we need a much better understanding of these links between our environment and our genes.

For more on this topic, see the excellent editorial by Dickenson.[2]

J. A. Stockman III, MD

References

1. Ahlbom A, Day N, Feychting M, et al: A pooled analysis of magnetic fields and childhood leukemia. *Br J Cancer* 83:692-698, 2000.
2. Dickenson HO: The causes of childhood leukemia. Delayed exposure to infection may trigger leukemia after prenatal damage to DNA (editorial). *BMJ* 330:1279-1280, 2005.

Risk of Cancer After Low Doses of Ionising Radiation—Retrospective Cohort Study in 15 Countries

Cardis E, and the International Study Group (Internatl Agency for Research on Cancer, Lyon, France; Univ of Mainz, Germany; Natl Cancer Inst, Bethesda, Md; et al)
BMJ 331:77-80, 2005   16–3

Objectives.—To provide direct estimates of risk of cancer after protracted low doses of ionising radiation and to strengthen the scientific basis of radiation protection standards for environmental, occupational, and medical diagnostic exposures.

Design.—Multinational retrospective cohort study of cancer mortality.

Setting.—Cohorts of workers in the nuclear industry in 15 countries.

Participants.—407,391 workers individually monitored for external radiation with a total follow-up of 5.2 million person years.

Main Outcome Measurements.—Estimates of excess relative risks per sievert (Sv) of radiation dose for mortality from cancers other than leukaemia and from leukaemia excluding chronic lymphocytic leukaemia, the main causes of death considered by radiation protection authorities.

Results.—The excess relative risk for cancers other than leukaemia was 0.97 per Sv, 95% confidence interval 0.14 to 1.97. Analyses of causes of death related or unrelated to smoking indicate that, although confounding by smoking may be present, it is unlikely to explain all of this increased risk. The excess relative risk for leukaemia excluding chronic lymphocytic leukaemia was 1.93 per Sv (<0 to 8.47). On the basis of these estimates, 1-2% of deaths from cancer among workers in this cohort may be attributable to radiation.

Conclusions.—These estimates, from the largest study of nuclear workers ever conducted, are higher than, but statistically compatible with, the risk estimates used for current radiation protection standards. The results suggest that there is a small excess risk of cancer, even at the low doses and dose rates typically received by nuclear workers in this study.

▶ This review was carried out in workers in the nuclear industry across 15 countries. It is included in the YEAR BOOK OF PEDIATRICS largely because it is important for us, as pediatricians, to recognize the consequences of low doses of ionizing radiation in at-risk groups. Should there ever be another nuclear plant radiation accident or a terrorist attack that exposes children to radiation, data from studies such as this will become extremely relevant. A recent National Research Council (NRC) report[1] finds that, although the risks of low-dose radiation are small, no safe level of radiation exposure exists. Radiation exposure doses at or below 0.1 Sv, which is about twice the yearly limit for nuclear workers and 40 times the natural background that adults and children are exposed to, carry significant risks. Right now, for typical folks here in the United States, 82% of radiation exposure stems from natural sources such as radon gas seeping from the earth. The rest is human made, coming mostly from medical procedures such as x-ray examinations. The NRC is now telling us that it does not take a great deal more than our average current exposure to begin to increase the risk of developing radiation-associated malignancies. The NRC believes that a single 0.1-Sv dose will cause cancer in 1 of 100 people over one's lifetime. Such risks must be taken into account when one considers full-body CT scanning on a routine basis, which is a recent fad that delivers a radiation dose of 0.012 Sv. A few CT scans and there you are with a truly real risk of the development of a malignancy, albeit in the 1% range.

The article by Sigurdson et al (Abstract 16–9) dealing with the risk of radiation-associated thyroid cancer shows that this risk remains elevated for up to 30 years when children are exposed to therapeutic radiation doses for the treatment of a childhood malignancy. When it comes to environmental exposure to radiation, the pediatric thyroid gland appears to be particularly vulnerable to the oncogenic effects of radiation. The dramatic increase (30-fold) of thyroid cancer in girls younger than 14 years in Belarus who were exposed to marginal levels of radioactive fallout after the Chernobyl nuclear reactor explosion is well documented.[2] Others have also observed that children younger than 5 years at the time of such exposure are the most vulnerable to the risks of ionizing radiation, and girls are at greater risk than boys.[3]

Please note that issues have arisen recently about radiation environmental exposures to children. Take the following scenario, fictitious but drawn from real life: You are a physician who is a captain in the army. You have been assigned to Iraq as an advisor assisting in the identification of conflict-related injuries in children. You receive a call from your commander relating the fact that several children have been identified who have been playing in a burnt-out Iraqi tank that had been "taken out" by tank-piercing bullets made from depleted uranium. The question posed to you is whether such exposure to radioactive materials will be of long-term harm to these children.

Depleted uranium is an incredibly dense metal and is now being used by the military as a projectile that is capable of piercing armor. Depleted uranium is a weakly radioactive manufacturing byproduct of nuclear fuel and warheads. Critics have charged that breathing airborne debris, created when these bullets strike armor, can cause leukemia, other cancers, and birth defects. A recent study, however, suggests that such concerns have little substance. It would appear that the risks for development of leukemia or the induction of birth defects appears to be very small, even among troops who have breathed heavy amounts of uranium-tainted dust. Data in follow-up of Gulf War exposure seem to verify this. Specifically, studies now show that the average US smoking adult faces a 7% lifetime risk of death from lung cancer, a risk that might climb to 8.5% if an individual breathed a heavy dose of uranium dust for a period of time. Calculations seem to imply that a child could play inside a vehicle destroyed by a depleted-uranium munition for some 300 hours and outside it for another 700 hours and face an added risk of 1 death in 1000 exposed individuals.

Whether studies such as mentioned will convince the critics of the military's use of depleted uranium remains to be seen. No one should believe, however, that any radioactive material is actually good for you.[4]

J. A. Stockman III, MD

References

1. Committee to Assess Health Risks From Exposure to Low Levels of Ionizing Radiation, National Research Council: *Health Risks From Exposure to Low Levels of Ionizing Radiation: BEIR VII—Phase 2.* Washington, DC, National Academies Press, prepublication copy, Nap.edu/catalog/11340.html.
2. Mahoney MC, Lawvere S, Falkner KL, et al: Thyroid cancer incidents, trends in Belarus: Examining the impact of Chernobyl. *Int J Epidemiol* 33:1025-1033, 2004.
3. Inskip PD: Thyroid cancer after radiotherapy for childhood cancer. *Med Pediatr Oncol* 36:568-573, 2001.
4. Raloff J: Low biofield hazard in depleted uranium. *Science News* 168:110, 2005.

Childhood Cancer Following Neonatal Oxygen Supplementation

Spector LG, Klebanoff MA, Feusner JH, et al (Univ of Minnesota, Minneapolis; Natl Inst of Child Health and Human Development, Rockville, Md; Children's Hosp and Research Ctr of Oakland, Calif)

J Pediatr 147:27-31, 2005   16–4

Objective.—To evaluate the relationship between neonatal oxygen supplementation (O_2) and childhood cancer in the Collaborative Perinatal Project (CPP).

Study Design.—The CPP consisted of 54,795 children born between 1959 and 1966 and followed to age 8 years. We used Cox proportional hazards modeling to examine the association between history of neonatal O_2 and cancer (n = 48).

Results.—The hazard ratio (HR) for any O_2 was 1.77 (95% confidence interval [CI] = 0.94 to 3.35). The HR for continuous duration of O_2 was near 1 and not significant. However, the HRs were 0.69 (95% CI = 0.17 to 2.88) and 2.87 (95% CI = 1.46 to 5.66) when comparing 0 to 2 and 3 or more minutes of O_2, respectively, to no O_2. The latter association was weaker (HR = 2.00; 95% CI = 0.88 to 4.54) and not significant ($P = 10$) when analysis was restricted to cancers diagnosed after age 1 year (n = 41).

Conclusions.—These findings are consistent with an association between O_2 for 3 minutes or longer and cancer in childhood, and should serve as a basis for further study.

▶ This editor was ready to consign this report to an entry suitable for inclusion in *Ripley's Believe It Or Not*, at least until he read an editorial that accompanied the report which made him at least think about the possibility of an association between neonatal oxygen administration and the subsequent risk of malignancy.[1]

It took an analysis of the huge database of the NCPP to show what the report by Spector et al shows, that is, a somewhat higher risk of cancer in children exposed to greater than 3 minutes of oxygen in the delivery room compared with children who receive no such exposure. It is true that the excess risk is small, but the data do suggest that if one were to look at a population of 10,000 unexposed children and compared them with 10,000 exposed children, the former will have 6 cancers by the age of 5, whereas the latter will have perhaps 17 or 18 cases. Needless to say, the overwhelming majority of all exposed children will not have cancer, just as lung cancer will never develop in 90% to 95% of smokers.

If there is a link between exposure to oxygen in the immediate newborn period and the development of cancer, what might cause this relationship? The authors speculate on 2 possibilities. The first is the known fact that exposure to oxygen at a particularly vulnerable point in one's life does produce a burst of oxidative stress. All pediatric hematologists recognize the relationship of oxidative stress to neonatal hemolysis, for example. A second speculation relates to the multiplicity of ways in which reactive oxygen species can damage DNA and possibly contribute to carcinogenesis. This is a bit more of a speculation because studies have shown that antioxidant compounds, such as vitamin E, cannot prevent cancer.[2]

Please add to your thinking the possibility that there may be a relationship between the use of oxygen in the delivery room and a subsequent risk of developing pediatric malignancies, and add this to the mounting data suggesting that room air, overall, is less risky in the delivery room in comparison to the use of oxygen for resuscitation purposes. With respect to the latter statement, data are evolving to indicate that levels of oxygen in premature infants not previously considered to be hyperoxic, in fact, may be dangerous to eyes, lungs, or brain. Two recent studies have indicated that if one looks at all of the literature comparing room air with 100% oxygen for resuscitation, room air is superior on several measures, including mortality.[3,4]

One final comment: If you are still not a believer about the evidence mounting against the use of oxygen in newborn resuscitation, recognize that the data from Spector et al's study are totally consistent with a recent large Swedish case-control study that looked at greater than 500 leukemia cases and found a significant odds ratio of 2.6 for resuscitation with 100% oxygen with face mask and bag after birth, which further increased to 3.5 when manual ventilation lasted for 3 minutes or more![5] How much more data do we need to convince ourselves that there are better ways to resuscitate neonates than by bathing them in pure oxygen?

J. A. Stockman III, MD

References

1. Paneth N. Evidence mounts against use of pure oxygen in newborn resuscitation. *J Pediatr* 147:4-6, 2005.
2. Bjelakovic G, Nikolova D, Simonetti RG, et al: Antioxidant supplements for prevention of gastrointestinal cancers: A systematic review and meta-analysis. *Lancet* 364:1219-1228, 2004.
3. Davis PG, Tan A, O'Donnell CP, et al: Resuscitation of newborn infants with 100% oxygen or air: A systematic review and meta-analysis. *Lancet* 364:1329-1333, 2004.
4. Saugstad OD, Ramji S, Vento M: Resuscitation of depressed newborn infants with ambient air or pure oxygen: A meta-analysis. *Biol Neonate* 87:27-34, 2005.
5. Naumburg E, Bellocco R, Cnattingious S, et al: Supplementary oxygen and risk of childhood lymphatic leukemia. *Acta Paediatr* 91:1328-1333, 2002.

West Nile Virus Infection in a Teenage Boy With Acute Lymphocytic Leukemia in Remission
Hindo H, Buescher ES, Frank LM, et al (Children's Hosp of The King's Daughters, Norfolk, Va; Commonwealth of Virginia, Richmond; Children's Hosps, Minneapolis)
J Pediatr Hematol Oncol 27:659-662, 2005   16–5

Background.—West Nile virus (WNV) was first isolated from the blood of a Ugandan woman in 1937. Since then outbreaks of WNV infection have occurred in Israel in the 1950s, in France in the early 1960s, in South Africa in the 1970s, in India in the early 1980s, and in Romania and Russia in the 1990s. The first case of WNV infection in the Western Hemisphere was reported in New York City in 1999. Since then WNV activity and infection have been reported in nearly all of the United States. The most common mode of transmission of the virus is a mosquito bite. WNV is an important cause of encephalitis. Although there have been many reports of WNV encephalitis in susceptible adults, mainly elderly, immunocompromised persons, there have been few case reports involving susceptible pediatric hosts. The purpose of this report was to describe an adolescent with acute lymphocytic leukemia and WNV encephalitis.

Case Report.—A 14-year-old male North Carolina resident was admitted to hospital in Virginia with ataxia and altered mental status in August 2003. He had been diagnosed with acute lymphocytic leukemia 15 months earlier. His leukemia was in remission when his most recent course of chemotherapy was completed a week before the case hospitalization. His last blood transfusion was in April 2003. He had no history of prior neurologic illness, and had no known tick exposure. He had not consumed any raw or unpasteurized foods. The patient reported that he had received multiple mosquito bites 2 weeks before presentation.

About 1 week before admission he presented to a local emergency room with fever, rhinorrhea, and nasal congestion. Intramuscular ceftriaxone was administered, and the patient felt better overall, although the fever persisted. On the day of admission he had difficulty walking and had slurred and incoherent speech. At admission he was uncooperative and disoriented, and his speech was incoherent. His right eye was deviated medially, and he had horizontal nystagmus and complained of diplopia. He had an erythematous malar rash. Within a few hours, he developed seizures and respiratory decompensation that required antiepileptic agents and intubation and mechanical ventilation. The most likely differential diagnosis was thought to include a viral encephalitis and meningoencephalitis. An MRI of the brain showed a slight increase in the size of the right thalamic region without contrast enhancement. This area was further enlarged on CT 31 hours later. Nerve conduction studies showed slowing of motor and sensory nerves. By 48 hours after admission the patient was comatose, unresponsive to pain, and without response to cold caloric testing. Confirmation of WNV infection was obtained using RT-PCR on nucleic acid extracts from specimens collected 6 days after the onset of illness. Repeated courses of IVIG produced in Israel had no effect. The patient died in January 2004 with no sign of neurologic recovery.

Conclusions.—The epidemiology of West Nile virus in North America has evolved dramatically over the past 5 years, and it is likely that the virus will persist in the United States for the foreseeable future. It is important that physicians are cognizant of the level of WNV activity in their communities and maintain a high level of suspicion when presented with a patient with acute mental status changes and fever.

▶ This report documents that even those with leukemia can contract the same diseases from which everyone else in a community may be getting ill. It was back in 1999 that the first cases of West Nile Virus (WNV) infection were detected in New York State. Since its recognition in New York, WNV infection has spread across North America and has become a major public health concern here in the US. The case of this youngster with leukemia shows how problematic WNV can be, particularly in someone who is immunosuppressed.

The most common mode of transmission of WNV to humans is through the bite of an infected mosquito. Reports of WNV transmission through organ transplantation and blood transfusions have also been documented. It is also possible that the virus can be transmitted via breast milk. Four years ago, blood collection agencies began to screen for WNV in blood donations using mini-pool nucleic acid amplification tests. These tests are fairly good but can miss low levels of viremia. The leukemia patient described had received a blood transfusion 4 months prior to his illness. It should be noted, however, that all patients reported who have had transfusion-associated transmission receive blood products within 28 days of the onset of their illness. The incubation period of WNV is typically 2 to 14 days, but theoretically can be longer in immunosuppressed patients. Approximately 1 in 5 infected patients will develop afebrile illness. The fever known as West Nile fever is characterized by chills, malaise, headache, backache, arthralgia, myalgia, swollen lymph nodes, and retro-orbital pain. Hepatomegaly, conjunctivitis, splenomegaly, myocarditis, pancreatitis, and hepatitis have also been described. Many patients, of course, develop encephalitis. A polio-like flaccid paralysis syndrome has also been recognized as a unique manifestation of WNV disease. Lumbar puncture shows a lymphocytic pleocytosis. Protein concentrations are elevated but glucose concentrations are normal. CT of the brain is usually normal but MRI will show nonspecific enhancement of the meninges or periventricular areas.

There is no known treatment for WNV infection although some advocate the use of IVIG. Since there seems to be no end to the future of this infection here in the United States, be aware of it at the times of the year when mosquitoes are biting.

J. A. Stockman III, MD

Metabolic Syndrome in Children and Adolescents With Acute Lymphoblastic Leukemia After the Completion of Chemotherapy
Kourti M, Tragiannidis A, Makedou A, et al (Aristotle Univ of Thessaloniki, Greece)
J Pediatr Hematol Oncol 27:499-501, 2005   16–6

Summary.—The metabolic syndrome is a cluster of potent risk factors for cardiovascular diseases. To provide information on the late complications of chemotherapy for acute lymphoblastic leukemia (ALL), the authors prospectively studied the frequency of overweight, obesity, and metabolic syndrome in survivors of ALL in the initial years after the completion of therapy. Children and adolescents were classified as having the metabolic syndrome if they met three or more of the following criteria: hypertriglyceridemia, low levels of high-density lipoprotein (HDL), high fasting glucose, obesity, and hypertension. Obesity was defined on the basis of Body Mass Index (BMI) (kg/m²) standard deviation scores or z-scores. Cutoff points for triglycerides and HDL were taken from equivalent pediatric percentiles with the cutoff points proposed by the Adult Treatment Panel III (ATPIII). Hyperglycemia was defined using the ATPIII cutoff points. Elevated systolic or diastolic blood pressure was defined as a value greater than the 95th percentile for age, gender, and height. Fifty-two subjects (29 male and 23 female) with a median age of 15.2 years (range 6.1–22.6 years) were evaluated. Median interval since completion of therapy was 37 months (range 13–121 months). All of them had been treated according to the ALL-BFM 90 chemotherapy protocol and none had received cranial radiotherapy. Of the 52 subjects, 25 (48%) were overweight (BMI z-score >1.5) and 3 (5.76%) were obese (BMI z-score >2); among them, 1 was severely obese (BMI z-score >2.5). Three criteria for the metabolic syndrome (high triglyceride levels, glucose intolerance, and obesity) were fulfilled by three subjects (5.76%). Twenty-nine subjects (55.7%) had at least one risk factor for metabolic syndrome. Hyperglycemia and hypertension were infrequent. Prompt recognition of the risk factors for metabolic syndrome and intervention seem mandatory to ensure early prevention of cardiovascular disease in survivors of ALL.

▶ When this editor was a fellow in pediatric hematology/oncology more than 30 years ago, it was very common to see survivors of childhood leukemia who a few years after cessation of treatment were plump little youngsters. Little did we know then that these children, in fact, were setups for what subsequently we now know to be the "metabolic syndrome." Had we known then what we know now, these youngsters would have been carefully followed up to prevent the onset of the manifestations of the metabolic syndrome, including diabetes and cardiovascular disease. Although the association of certain risk factors (such as visceral obesity, dyslipidemia, hyperglycemia, and hypertension) has been known for more than 80 years, the clustering of these signs and symptoms received scant attention until 1988 when Reaven[1] described syndrome X: insulin resistance, high blood sugar, hypertension, low HDL cholesterol, and raised very low-density lipoprotein (VLDL) triglycerides. The ultimate importance of metabolic syndrome is that it helps to identify individuals at high risk for both type 2 diabetes and cardiovascular disease. As we see from the report abstracted, this now includes survivors of childhood leukemia.

Currently, the controversy continues about what actually constitutes the definition of the metabolic syndrome. This definition is hardly settled in either the pediatric population or in the adult population, although the International Diabetes Foundation has provided the following criteria: central obesity (ethnicity specific) plus any 2 of the following: raised triglycerides, reduced HDL cholesterol, raised blood pressure, and raised fasting glucose.[2] It should be stressed that these new International Diabetes Foundation criteria defining metabolic syndrome are not the final word, but hopefully will assist in identifying people at increased risk, and through further research will lead to more accurate predictive indices.

J. A. Stockman III, MD

References

1. Reaven G: Role of insulin resistance in human disease. *Diabetes* 37:1595-1607, 1988.
2. Alberti KGMM, Zimmet P, Shaw J: Metabolic syndrome: A new worldwide definition. *Lancet* 366:1059-1061, 2005.

Myelopathy Due to Intrathecal Chemotherapy: Report of Six Cases
Bay A, Oner AF, Etlik O, et al (Yuzuncu Yil Univ, Van, Turkey)
J Pediatr Hematol Oncol 27:270-272, 2005   16–7

Summary.—Intrathecal chemotherapy and systemic chemotherapy are used for both prophylaxis and treatment of central nervous system disease in hematologic malignancies. However, intrathecal treatment has some adverse effects, such as arachnoiditis, progressive myelopathy, and leukoencephalopathy. The authors describe six children in whom myelopathy and adhesive arachnoiditis developed after administration of intrathecal chemotherapy including methotrexate, cytosine arabinoside, and prednisolone. Urinary retention and incontinence, the main presenting complaints in all patients, developed within 12 hours after intrathecal therapy and spontaneously resolved within 7 days. Two patients were unable to walk. In these two, weakness in the lower extremities gradually recovered by 1 month but urinary incontinence did not improve. None of the children had sensory loss. On follow-up periodic recurrent urinary tract infection was noted in four patients. MRI findings corresponded to arachnoiditis. No response was recorded on tibial nerve somatosensory evoked potentials in all patients. Intrathecal chemotherapy, especially methotrexate, can cause spinal cord dysfunction in children with acute lymphoblastic leukemia and non-Hodgkin's lymphoma. Arachnoiditis should be kept in mind as a causative factor in recurrent urinary tract infection in patients receiving intrathecal chemotherapy.

▶ This is the first of 2 reports (Abstracts 16–7 and 16–8) telling us that as important as it is to adequately treat the CNS in children with acute lymphatic leukemia, such treatment is hardly risk free. We see, in this report, the CNS complications of intrathecal chemotherapy when used as part of the management of children with acute lymphoblastic leukemia, acute myeloblastic leukemia, and non-Hodgkin's lymphoma. Six children out of 150 developed evidence of a myelopathy. Urinary retention and incontinence and encopresis were the main presenting complaints in each patient. Symptoms generally began within half a day with urinary retention being the first complaint. This gradually subsided within a week to be replaced by urinary incontinence. Two of the 6 children were unable to walk. While the latter finding disappeared, the urinary tract findings did not.

Exactly why some children get into trouble after the intrathecal administration of chemotherapy is not known. A variety of neurotoxic effects of intrathecal methotrexate have been reported.[1] Arachnoiditis is a well-recognized adverse effect, but usually transient. Arachnoiditis leads to the development of headaches, back pain, meningismus, and fever in some patients. A progressive myelopathy is distinctly more rare and has been reported in patients receiving intrathecal methotrexate with or without Ara-C.

Exactly why intrathecal methotrexate causes a problem in some remains speculative. It has been suggested that the problem is related to the preservative used in the diluent or results from a local depletion of folate secondary to the drug itself. Arachnoiditis, however, has been seen when methotrexate has been administered with preservative-free diluents.

The most ominous consequence after intrathecal therapy is the onset of a progressive myelopathy. This may occur from minutes to as long as 6 months after a lumbar puncture in which chemotherapy is administered. A rapid progression to complete quadriplegia, brain stem dysfunction, and death has been reported. Lesser symptoms in the form of leg weakness, urinary retention or incontinence, and paresthesias may also occur along with sensory loss.

The diagnosis of intrathecal drug-induced myelopathy is made with MRI, the most sensitive radiologic technique to demonstrate the symmetric, patchy, nonenhancing white matter changes, which may actually occur even absent clinical symptoms. Once established, treatment options for myelopathy and arachnoiditis are fairly limited. It has been suggested that IV steroids or dextromethorphan could be helpful.[2]

The report that follows (Abstract 16–8) gives more information about the clinical and laboratory consequences of intrathecal chemotherapy on children with childhood leukemia.

J. A. Stockman III, MD

References

1. Koh S, Nelson MD, Kovanlika YAA, et al: Anterior lumbosacral radiculopathy after intrathecal methotrexate treatment. *Pediatr Neurol* 21:576-578, 1999.
2. Drachtman RA, Cole PD, Golden CB, et al: Dextromethorphan is effective in the treatment of subacute methotrexate neurotoxicity. *Pediatr Hematol Oncol* 19:319-327, 2002.

Prospective Evaluation of Clinical and Laboratory Effects of Intrathecal Chemotherapy on Children With Acute Leukemia

Keidan I, Bielorei B, Berkenstadt H, et al (Tel Aviv Univ, Israel)
J Pediatr Hematol Oncol 27:307-310, 2005   16–8

Summary.—The objective of this prospective 18-month study was to evaluate the clinical and laboratory effects of repeated intrathecal injections of chemotherapy in children with acute leukemia. All procedures were performed under general anesthesia, and complications were prospectively recorded. Laboratory measurements included lumbar puncture opening pressure, cerebrospinal fluid (CSF) chemistry, and cell count and morphology. Central venous pressure and ophthalmologic examinations were also performed. Forty-seven children underwent 247 intrathecal injections of chemotherapy. Adverse effects (13.7% of the procedures) included nausea and vomiting, back pain, and headache. One child each had transient cauda equina syndrome, transient communicating hydrocephalus, and persistent sacral plexus injury. The mean lumbar puncture opening pressure was significantly higher after intrathecal therapy than before (22 ± 8 vs. 15 ± 9 cm H_2O, $P = 0.02$) and higher than reported in age-matched children without leukemia. All CSF chemistries, cell count, and morphology were normal. The overall incidence of complications was 13.7%. Most were mild and resolved quickly, but significant neurologic complications did occur. Lumbar puncture opening pressure was significantly higher in children with acute leukemia after intrathecal chemotherapy.

▶ Without question, intrathecal chemotherapy is associated with acute, subacute, and delayed toxicities, and in some cases, major neurologic complications. Intrathecal methotrexate may be associated with an acute arachnoiditis characterized by headache, nausea, and vomiting, meningismus, and other signs of increased intracranial pressure, usually occurring 12 to 24 hours after intrathecal injection. More commonly, postlumbar puncture headache occurs, which is more common the larger the lumbar puncture needle used for the procedure. Data suggest that with a 22-gauge needle, the incidence runs between 12% and 15% compared with just 5% when a 25- or 27-gauge needle is used. Older children are more likely to have a headache after a lumbar puncture.

What we learn from this report from Israel is that approximately 14% of lumbar punctures in which intrathecal chemotherapy is provided will result in 1 or more adverse effects. Fortunately, most of the complications are mild and resolve fairly quickly, but not all. There are few findings on subsequent lumbar puncture to give a clue as to exactly what is occurring, suggesting the need for MRI to sort things out when serious physical findings are present.

No one is going to delete intrathecal chemotherapy as part of the management of childhood leukemia, despite the untoward consequences of this therapy. However we must attempt to minimize risks by using small-bore needles and preservative-free diluents and by carefully checking and rechecking the amount of chemotherapy that is being instilled. Our patients deserve at least this much care and caution.

J. A. Stockman III, MD

Primary Thyroid Cancer After a First Tumour in Childhood (the Childhood Cancer Survivor Study): A Nested Case-Control Study
Sigurdson AJ, Ronckers CM, Mertens AC, et al (Natl Cancer Inst, Bethesda, Md; Univ of Minnesota, Minneapolis; Univ of Texas, Houston; et al)
Lancet 365:2014-2023, 2005   16–9

Background.—Survivors of malignant disease in childhood who have had radiotherapy to the head, neck, or upper thorax have an increased risk of subsequent primary thyroid cancer, but the magnitude of risk over the therapeutic dose range has not been well established. We aimed to quantify the long-term risk of thyroid cancer after radiotherapy and chemotherapy.

Methods.—In a nested case-control study, 69 cases with pathologically confirmed thyroid cancer and 265 matched controls without thyroid cancer were identified from 14,054 5-year survivors of cancer during childhood from the Childhood Cancer Survivor Study cohort. Childhood cancers were diagnosed between 1970 and 1986 with cohort follow-up to 2000.

Findings.—Risk of thyroid cancer increased with radiation doses up to 20-29 Gy (odds ratio 9.8 [95% CI 3.2-34.8]). At doses greater than 30 Gy, a fall in the dose-response relation was seen. Both the increased and decreased risks were more pronounced in those diagnosed with a first primary malignant disease before age 10 years than in those older than 10 years. Furthermore, the fall in risk remained when those diagnosed with Hodgkin's lymphoma were excluded. Chemotherapy for the first cancer was not associated with thyroid-cancer risk, and it did not modify the effect of radiotherapy. 29 (42%) cases had a first diagnosis of Hodgkin's lymphoma compared with 49 (19%) controls. 11 (42%) of those who had Hodgkin's lymphoma had subsequent thyroid cancers smaller than 1 cm compared with six (17%) of those who had other types of childhood cancer (p=0.07).

Interpretation.—The reduction in radiation dose-response for risk of thyroid cancer after childhood exposure to thyroid doses higher than 30 Gy is consistent with a cell-killing effect. Standard long-term follow-up of patients who have had Hodgkin's lymphoma for detection of thyroid cancer should also be undertaken for survivors of any cancer during childhood who received radiotherapy to the thorax or head and neck region.

▶ With all the amazing advances that have been made in the treatment of childhood malignancies, we are seeing survival to the point at which long-term secondary consequences of therapy are becoming as important to survivorship as adequate treatment of the original disease. One of the long-term complications of cancer therapy in children is an increased risk of a secondary thyroid malignancy. This risk of subsequent primary thyroid cancer exists for some decades after receiving radiotherapy, in particular, as part of treatment for certain disorders including Hodgkin's lymphoma, acute leukemia, brain tumors, neuroblastomas, and non-Hodgkin's lymphoma. Most of these secondary thyroid cancers are curable, but the very fact that they develop is an extraordinarily problematic setback to a survivor of a childhood primary malignancy.

This article gives us truly solid information about what the risk is in terms of the development of a secondary thyroid cancer in long-term survivors of a variety of childhood malignancies. What we learn is that chemotherapy, in and of itself, does not affect the subsequent risk of thyroid cancer. Rather, any increased risk is almost solely the result of radiation exposure. The risk of subsequent thyroid cancer rises with an increasing radiation dose (greatest risk, 20-29 Gy) but, curiously, decreases at doses of more than 30 Gy. Presumably, at these high doses, the thyroid is actually sufficiently destroyed that it does not have the opportunity to develop a malignancy. These are the patients who ultimately require thyroid replacement. This drop in thyroid cancer risk at high doses appears to be quite real. The finding of an increasing thyroid cancer risk with a rising therapeutic radiation dose at low levels (ie, <15 Gy) and a declining risk at higher doses is consistent with the cell-killing hypothesis proposed by Lewis Gray back in 1964.[1] This "Gray" effect has been noted in both children and adults. For example, when a solid tumor malignancy is treated with radiotherapy, surrounding tissues that are being exposed to radiation actually have a resistance to the development of a malignancy if they are exposed to high spillover doses of radiation. The greatest risk of a secondary malignancy appears to be in the "Gray" zone, or the edges of the high-treatment exposure, where tissues do not experience the killing effect but do experience radiation-induced mutagenic effects.

This article also highlights the one malignancy during childhood that requires the most careful surveillance for the development of radiation-induced malignancies. This is Hodgkin's lymphoma. These patients should be watched like a hawk, particularly with respect to the development of secondary thyroid cancer. Yearly examination of the neck and the thyroid gland in all survivors previously given irradiation to the chest or head and neck region is imperative. An unresolved question is whether palpation alone as part of a physical examination is sufficient to detect a secondary malignancy. Some believe that ultrasound will detect more secondary thyroid malignancies and should be part of the routine follow-up of patients at risk; however, we need more data on this point.

See the article by Cardis et al (Abstract 16–3) to find out about the risk of cancer after low-dose exposure to environmental ionizing radiation. Also recognize that it would be wise to be wary of hair coloring products. It does appear that there is an increased risk of cancer associated with the frequent application of permanent hair dye (>200 lifetime applications).[2] Of particular note is a study that has reported significantly elevated risks of non-Hodgkin lymphoma (NHL) associated with increasing duration of use, the application of dark colors, and use before 1980.[3] Importantly, this risk of the development of NHL strongly depends on the color you are coloring your hair with (odds ratios of 2.0, 4.1, and 3.0 among users of brown/brunette, black, and red dyes respectively). Those who dye their hair blonde show no elevated risk of non-Hodgkin lymphoma!

Thus it is that if you must dye your hair, blonde it is.

J. A. Stockman III, MD

References

1. Gray LH: Radiation biology in cancer, in *Cellular Radiation Biology: A Collection of Works Presented at the 18th Annual Symposium on Experimental Cancer Research 1964*. Baltimore, Maryland, Williams and Wilkins, 1965, pp 7-25.
2. Takkouche B, Etminan M, Montes-Martinez A: Personal use of hair dyes and risk of cancer: A meta-analysis. *JAMA* 293:2516-2525, 2005.
3. Zhang Y, Holford TR, Leaderer B, et al: Hair-coloring product use and risk of non-Hodgkin's lymphoma: A population-based case-control study in Connecticut. *Am J Epidemiol* 159:148-154, 2004.

Prognostic Significance of Autoimmunity During Treatment of Melanoma With Interferon

Gogas H, Ioannovich J, Dafni U, et al (Natl and Kapodistrian Univ of Athens, Greece; Gen Hosp of Athens, Greece; Sotiria Gen Hosp, Athens, Greece; et al)

N Engl J Med 354:709-718, 2006   16–10

Background.—Immunotherapy for advanced melanoma induces serologic and clinical manifestations of autoimmunity. We assessed the prognostic significance of autoimmunity in patients with stage IIB, IIC, or III melanoma who were treated with high-dose adjuvant interferon alfa-2b.

Methods.—We enrolled 200 patients in a substudy of a larger, ongoing randomized trial. Blood was obtained before the initiation of intravenous interferon therapy, after 1 month of therapy, and at 3, 6, 9, and 12 months. Serum was tested for antithyroid, antinuclear, anti-DNA, and anticardiolipin autoantibodies, and patients were examined for vitiligo.

Results.—The median duration of follow-up was 45.6 months. Relapse occurred in 115 patients, and 82 patients died. The median relapse-free survival was 28.0 months, and the median overall survival was 58.7 months. Autoantibodies and clinical manifestations of autoimmunity were detected in 52 patients (26 percent). The median relapse-free survival was 16.0 months among patients without autoimmunity (108 of 148 had a relapse) and was not reached among patients with autoimmunity (7 of 52 had a relapse). The median survival was 37.6 months among patients without autoimmunity (80 of 148 died) and was not reached among patients with autoimmunity (2 of 52 died). In univariate and multivariate regression analyses, autoimmunity was an independent prognostic marker for improved relapse-free survival and overall survival ($P<0.001$).

Conclusions.—The appearance of autoantibodies or clinical manifestations of autoimmunity during treatment with interferon alfa-2b is associated with statistically significant improvements in relapse-free survival and overall survival in patients with melanoma.

▶ If you are not familiar with the increasing body of evidence suggesting that immunotherapy is appropriate for patients with moderate- to high-risk melanoma, read this report in detail. It applies equally to children and adults. Deep primary lesions or lesions associated with melanoma cells in regional lymph nodes represent a high risk for relapse or death. Patients with American Joint Committee on Cancer stage IIB, IIC, or III melanoma have a risk of relapse and death exceeding 40% at 5 years and are candidates for immunotherapy with interferon alfa-2b. Many large cooperative group trials looking at adjuvant therapy with high-dose interferon alfa-2b in patients with high-risk melanoma have consistently demonstrated statistically significant prolongation of relapse-free survival with adjuvant therapy compared with observation. Therapy with interferon alfa-2b is extremely rigorous and fraught with numerous side effects including fatigue, fever, arthralgias, anorexia, and toxic hepatic effects. It is usually given over many months, and patients receiving it are absolutely miserable in most cases.

The report by Gogas et al shows us some fascinating insights into how interferon alfa-2b might work. It would seem that all immunotherapies that can improve survival in patients with advanced melanoma induce the collateral appearance of autoimmunity. Hypothyroidism, hyperthyroidism, the antiphospholipid antibody syndrome, and vitiligo have been cited as being positive marker side effects of interferon alfa-2b effectiveness. These were actually favorable prognostic factors in patients with melanoma even before the advent of immunotherapy. Gogas et al now tell us that the development of autoimmunity in the form of these autoimmune side effects is associated with an approximate reduction by a factor of 50 in the risk of recurrence of melanoma.

Thus, if interferon alfa-2b is used in patients with high-risk melanoma, pray for side effects in terms of secondary autoimmune disease. Such a phenomenon seems to be a marker for a good prognosis. Interestingly, an association between the development of autoimmunity and the responsiveness to immunotherapy has been largely restricted to just 2 cancers: melanoma and renal cancer. Why these 2 tumors seem to be unusually sensitive to autoimmune regulation remains a mystery.

The immunotherapy of melanoma represents an exciting approach to the management of a malignancy. The work of these investigators and others suggests that there exists a population of patients with diminished immune regulation in whom autoimmunity will develop during effective immunotherapy, such as with interferon alfa-2b. If such patients have immune-sensitive tumors, they would be able to mount a protective antitumor immune response. The prospective identification of such patients not only will help clinicians select patients for immunotherapy, but also will spare other patients from exposure to side effects and ineffective treatment.

To read more about immunotherapy for cancer and autoimmunity, see the superb editorial on this topic by Coon and Atkins.[1]

J. A. Stockman III, MD

Reference

1. Coon H, Atkins M: Autoimmunity and immunotherapy for cancer (editorial). *N Engl J Med* 354:758-760, 2006.

Distinct Sets of Genetic Alterations in Melanoma

Curtin JA, Fridlyand J, Kageshita T, et al (Univ of California, San Francisco; Kumamoto Univ, Japan; Mem Sloan-Kettering Cancer Ctr, New York; et al)
N Engl J Med 353:2135-2147, 2005   16–11

Background.—Exposure to ultraviolet light is a major causative factor in melanoma, although the relationship between risk and exposure is complex. We hypothesized that the clinical heterogeneity is explained by genetically distinct types of melanoma with different susceptibility to ultraviolet light.

Methods.—We compared genome-wide alterations in the number of copies of DNA and mutational status of *BRAF* and *N-RAS* in 126 melanomas from four groups in which the degree of exposure to ultraviolet light differs: 30 melanomas from skin with chronic sun-induced damage and 40 melanomas from skin without such damage; 36 melanomas from palms, soles, and subungual (acral) sites; and 20 mucosal melanomas.

Results.—We found significant differences in the frequencies of regional changes in the number of copies of DNA and mutation frequencies in *BRAF* among the four groups of melanomas. Samples could be correctly classified into the four groups with 70 percent accuracy on the basis of the changes in the number of copies of genomic DNA. In two-way comparisons, melanomas arising on skin with signs of chronic sun-induced damage and skin without such signs could be correctly classified with 84 percent accuracy. Acral melanoma could be distinguished from mucosal melanoma with 89 percent accuracy. Eighty-one percent of melanomas on skin without chronic sun-induced damage had mutations in *BRAF* or *N-RAS*; the majority of melanomas in the other groups had mutations in neither gene. Melanomas with wild-type *BRAF* or *N-RAS* frequently had increases in the number of copies of the genes for cyclin-dependent kinase 4 (*CDK4*) and cyclin D1 (*CCND1*), downstream components of the RAS-BRAF pathway.

Conclusions.—The genetic alterations identified in melanomas at different sites and with different levels of sun exposure indicate that there are distinct genetic pathways in the development of melanoma and implicate *CDK4* and *CCND1* as independent oncogenes in melanomas without mutations in *BRAF* or *N-RAS*.

▶ The more we learn about melanomas, the more complex the information. The study of Curtin et al describes distinct patterns of genetic alterations in what they tell us are 4 groups of primary melanomas as they define them: acral, mucosal melanomas on skin with chronic sun-induced damage, and melanomas on skin without chronic sun-induced damage. The first 2 of these areas (palm/soles and mucosal surfaces) are parts of the body that are not exposed to sun. Differences shown in both chromosomal aberrations and the frequency of chromosomal mutations of specific genes suggest that melanomas develop by different mechanisms in response to different selective influences, such as the sun. For example, melanomas occurring on the palms and soles and on mucosal surfaces are uniquely characterized by a much higher frequency of focal amplifications of certain genes in comparison with melanomas that arise on skin with chronic sun-induced damage or on skin without chronic sun-induced damage, indicating that melanomas occurring on palms/soles and mucosal surfaces are mechanistically similar to each other and different from other types of melanomas. Melanomas presenting on sites with chronic exposure to the sun typically occur late in life and are associated with other UV-related neoplasms such as solar keratoses, suggesting that high cumulative rates of UV light are required for these types of skin lesions. In contrast, melanomas presenting on skin that is intermittently exposed to sun are typically found in persons who have a large number of moles but fewer solar keratoses, and tend to occur at a younger age. Moreover, these melanomas share an important genetic characteristic. The melanomas on skin that is intermittently exposed to sun have much more frequent mutations of the *BRAF* gene than do other types of melanoma.

The authors of this report are proposing that melanocytes of persons in whom melanomas develop on skin that is intermittently exposed to sun have an increased susceptibility to UV exposure that involves a high probability of acquiring *BRAF* mutations or of proliferating if such mutations occur. It may very well be that this subset of people has a window of vulnerability to exposure to UV light early in life. In contrast, patients without susceptible melanocytes will require a sufficiently high cumulative UV dose to induce melanoma, so that sun-damaged skin would be present, and the development would involve mechanisms that do not include *BRAF* mutations. These would be individuals whose tumors predominantly occur on sites that are chronically exposed to the sun, such as the face and upper arms.

So what does all this mean? If you have seen one melanoma, you have seen one melanoma, at least until we know more about the cancer biology of these tumors. Melanomas occurring on different parts of the body may have a different molecular biology associated with them. Therapies are now being directed against mutated genes such as *BRAF*. If the data from this report hold true, only a subset of patients with melanoma would be responsive to such therapies.

J. A. Stockman III, MD

Chromosome 1p and 11q Deletions and Outcome in Neuroblastoma
Maris JM, for the Children's Oncology Group (Univ of Pennsylvania, Philadelphia; et al)
N Engl J Med 353:2243-2253, 2005   16–12

Background.—Neuroblastoma is a childhood cancer with considerable morbidity and mortality. Tumor-derived biomarkers may improve risk stratification.

Methods.—We screened 915 samples of neuroblastoma for loss of heterozygosity (LOH) at chromosome bands 1p36 and 11q23. Additional analyses identified a subgroup of cases of 11q23 LOH with unbalanced 11q LOH (unb11q LOH; defined as loss of 11q with retention of 11p). The associations of LOH with relapse and survival were determined.

Results.—LOH at 1p36 was identified in 209 of 898 tumors (23 percent) and LOH at 11q23 in 307 of 913 (34 percent). Unb11q LOH was found in 151 of 307 tumors with 11q23 LOH (17 percent of the total cohort). There was a strong association of 1p36 LOH, 11q23 LOH, and unb11q LOH with most high-risk disease features (P<0.001). LOH at 1p36 was associated with amplification of the *MYCN* oncogene (P<0.001), but 11q23 LOH and unb11q LOH were not (P<0.001 and P=0.002, respectively). Cases with unb11q LOH were associated with three-year event-free and overall survival rates (±SE) of 50±5 percent and 66±5 percent, respectively, as compared with 74±2 percent and 83±2 percent among cases without unb11q LOH (P<0.001 for both comparisons). In a multivariate model, unb11q LOH was independently associated with decreased event-free survival (P=0.009) in the entire cohort, and both 1p36 LOH and unb11q LOH were independently associated with decreased progression-free survival in the subgroup of patients with features of low-risk and intermediate-risk disease (P=0.002 and P=0.02, respectively).

Conclusions.—Unb11q LOH and 1p36 LOH are independently associated with a worse outcome in patients with neuroblastoma.

▶ Neuroblastoma is one of the more curious of the childhood malignancies. In some children with extensive disease, the prognosis is excellent, yet in others, the prognosis is terrible. Much of the difference has to do with one's genes. The Children's Oncology Group stratifies children with neuroblastoma into 3 subtypes with expected low, intermediate, and high risk of death from the malignancy. This stratification system involves the use of the clinical factors of age at diagnosis, tumor stage, and the results of the Shimada method of histopathologic classification, as well as the biological factors of amplification status of the *MYCN* oncogene and DNA index. Amplification of *MYCN*, which plays a critical part in the neurodevelopment, occurs in 20% of cases of neuroblastoma. In fact, amplification of *MYCN* was one of the first tumor-derived genetic markers that was shown to be of clinical value, and it continues to provide important prognostic information. Whereas patients in the low-risk subgroup have an overall survival rate of more than 95%, patients in the high-risk subgroup have a rate of long-term survival of less than 40% despite dose-intensive, multimodal therapy. These differences reflect, in part, the genetic heterogeneity of neuroblastoma. For example, many high-risk tumors have *MYCN* amplification, but more than 60% do not, suggesting that there are other genetic pathways in the development of high-risk neuroblastoma.

It would appear that chromosomal aberrations account for much of the prognosis children have with neuroblastoma. We learn from this report from the Children's Hospital of Philadelphia that LOH at chromosome bands 1p36 and 11q23 is independently associated with a worse outcome in patients with neuroblastoma. Such loss of 1p36 seems to occur in about one fourth of cases of primary neuroblastoma and is highly associated with a poor outcome. Some 17% of primary neuroblastomas have loss of unb11q. This too is independently associated with a decreased length of survivorship.

We close this commentary with a question. When it comes to malignancies in the pediatric age group, is there any one malignancy in particular that has as an adverse risk factor being taller than your peers? For some time now it has been suggested that osteosarcoma may be associated with a taller stature. Some have considered this relationship controversial. It no longer is based on a large study conducted recently in Italy.[1] These findings indeed make sense. High-grade central osteosarcoma, the most common primary bone cancer, which frequently occurs in children and adolescents, tends to present at sites of rapid bone growth. For those under the age of 21, osteosarcoma accounts for approximately 60% of all bone tumors. Numerous chemicals are known to induce osteosarcoma. Radiation exposure is also related to the development of this malignancy. Approximately 1% of those with Paget's disease develop osteosarcoma, and there is an association with a number of inherited syndromes, including hereditary bilateral retinoblastoma, Li-Fraumeni syndrome, Bloom syndrome, and Rothmund-Thompson syndrome. Add to these predilections for osteosarcoma height, in excess. The relationship between body size and the risk of osteosarcoma actually makes some sense. The phenomenon is true not just in humans, but also in canines. Bet you were not aware that osteosarcoma is much more common in dogs than in man, and the dogs that are most affected are large or giant breeds. The risk of developing osteosarcoma in dogs weighing more than 35 kg is as much as 185 times that in dogs weighing less than 10 kg. The relationship in humans between body size and the risk of developing osteosarcoma may be related to the observed fact that certain neoplasms depend on growth factors and growth receptors, acting through autocrine or paracrine mechanisms for tumor growth. Take for example, insulin-like growth factor I. It is a potent mitogen for human osteosarcoma cells in the laboratory.

Height does have its advantages. You can see a lot more. Height also has its disadvantages, including a higher risk of certain types of malignancy and also a greater probability of being elected as president of the United States, the latter a well-known fact in the literature.

To read more about the translation of genetic profiles to clinical challenges in children with neuroblastoma, see the excellent review by Kushner and Cheung.[2]

J. A. Stockman III, MD

References

1. Longhi A, Pasini A, Cicognani A, et al: Height as a risk factor for osteosarcoma. *J Pediatr Hematol Oncol* 27:314-318, 2005.
2. Kushner BH, Cheung N-K: Neuroblastoma: From genetic profiles to clinical challenge. *N Engl J Med* 353:2215-2217, 2005.

Lexofloxacin to Prevent Bacterial Infection in Patients With Cancer and Neutropenia
Del Favero A, for the Gruppo Italiano Malattie Ematologiche dell'Adulto (GIMEMA) Infection Program (Policlinico Monteluce, Perugia, Italy; et al)
N Engl J Med 353:977-987, 2005   16–13

Background.—The prophylactic use of fluoroquinolones in patients with cancer and neutropenia is controversial and is not a recommended intervention.

Methods.—We randomly assigned 760 consecutive adult patients with cancer in whom chemotherapy-induced neutropenia (<1000 neutrophils per cubic millimeter) was expected to occur for more than seven days to receive either oral levofloxacin (500 mg daily) or placebo from the start of chemotherapy until the resolution of neutropenia. Patients were stratified according to their underlying disease (acute leukemia vs. solid tumor or lymphoma).

Results.—An intention-to-treat analysis showed that fever was present for the duration of neutropenia in 65 percent of patients who received levofloxacin prophylaxis, as compared with 85 percent of those receiving placebo (243 of 375 vs. 308 of 363; relative risk, 0.76; absolute difference in risk, −20 percent; 95 percent confidence interval, −26 to −14 percent; P=0.001). The levofloxacin group had a lower rate of microbiologically documented infections (absolute difference in risk, −17 percent; 95 percent confidence interval, −24 to −10 percent; P<0.001), bacteremias (difference in risk, −16 percent; 95 percent confidence interval, −22 to −9 percent; P<0.001), and single-agent gram-negative bacteremias (difference in risk, −7 percent; 95 percent confidence interval, −10 to −2 percent; P<0.01) than did the placebo group. Mortality and tolerability were similar in the two groups. The effects of prophylaxis were also similar between patients with acute leukemia and those with solid tumors or lymphoma.

Conclusions.—Prophylactic treatment with levofloxacin is an effective and well-tolerated way of preventing febrile episodes and other relevant infection-related outcomes in patients with cancer and profound and protracted neutropenia. The long-term effect of this intervention on microbial resistance in the community is not known.

▶ This report by Del Favero et al and the one that follows by Cullen et al (Abstract 16–14) involve adults who are receiving cancer chemotherapy. It is likely that the data derived from these studies will ultimately be incorporated into pediatric protocols; thus the inclusion of the findings of these 2 reports in the YEAR BOOK OF PEDIATRICS.

A number of randomized clinical trials have suggested that prophylaxis with fluoroquinolones may be better than placebo or trimethoprim-sulfamethoxazole in reducing bacteremic infections caused by gram-negative bacilli, with ciprofloxacin being the compound most widely used. Most, however, have accepted the evidence from these studies as not particularly convincing. In fact, only 3 studies have been placebo-controlled, double-blind, randomized clinical trials, and none were sufficiently large to provide conclusive evidence of the real efficacy of prophylaxis. Also, none of the studies addressed the important question of whether prophylaxis should be considered for all patients with cancer and neutropenia, since the risk of infection may differ among such patients. It was pretty clear from these studies, however, that prophylaxis with fluoroquinolones did not reduce the risk of infections caused by gram-positive microorganisms.

The reports by Del Favero et al and Cullen et al are the best to date in looking at the issue of infection in patients with neutropenia as the result of cancer therapy. Del Favero et al studied patients at high risk, including inpatients undergoing therapy for leukemia or an autologous hematopoietic stem-cell transplantation. Cullen et al studied outpatients who were receiving multiple cycles of chemotherapy, but not cytokine growth factors or an autologous hematopoietic stem-cell transplant. The prophylactic intervention was thus deployed differently in these 2 studies, given the differences in perceived risk. Del Favero et al administered levofloxacin from about the time of the initiation of chemotherapy until engraftment, and Cullen et al used levofloxacin therapy for the 7 days estimated to coincide with the nadir of the white blood cell count during each cycle of chemotherapy (maximum, 6 cycles). Both groups used a similar primary endpoint: the occurrence of fever. As expected, infection was definitively documented in a minority of episodes of febrile neutropenia, since there are many causes of fever in this patient population.

So what were the data? Cullen et al report multiple, substantial benefits of their prophylactic strategy, including a significant decrease in the relative risk of a first febrile episode by 56%, of any febrile episode by 29%, of probable infection during the first cycle of chemotherapy by 28%, and of hospitalization during any cycle by 36%. These data are impressive. However, the absolute reductions in the risk of these events were 4.4%, 4.4%, 5.4%, and 3.6%, respectively. The use of levofloxacin prophylaxis protected 35 patients against the primary endpoint of fever. To achieve this benefit, approximately 20,000 doses of levofloxacin had to be administered. If one examines these data somewhat differently, according to the cycles of chemotherapy, the absolute risk of a febrile episode is 4.3% per cycle in the placebo group and 2.9% per cycle in the levofloxacin group. The number of patients treated per cycle to avoid 1 febrile episode is approximately 70. Prophylactic levofloxacin seemed to have no protective effect against the risk of severe infection or death, and was associated with an absolute increase in the incidence of side effects (occurring in 78 patients, compared with 40 patients in the placebo group).

So how about the study of Del Favero et al? These investigators also reported a reduction in the rate of febrile episodes, positive cultures, bacteremias, and infections with gram-negative rods with the use of levofloxacin prophylaxis, but no survival benefit. The rate of febrile episodes was unusually high: 85% in the placebo group and 65% in the levofloxacin group. The number of patients who needed to be treated to avoid a single episode of febrile neutropenia was estimated to be 5. The levofloxacin group had a lower rate of *Escherichia coli* bacteremia than did the placebo group (1.2% vs 3.0%), but this was associated with an increased rate of levofloxacin resistance (77% vs 17%). Thus, the use of levofloxacin prophylaxis led to a decrease in the overall rate of documented bacterial infection but a substantial increase in the rate of documented infections with significantly resistant organisms. You win one; you lose one.

So what do we really learn from these reports? The most important lesson is the need to weigh the potential for the emergence, amplification, and dissemination of antibiotic-resistant organisms. The prophylactic use of fluoroquinolones has already been associated with the emergence of resistant gram-negative rods in patients undergoing cancer chemotherapy, thus implying that the resistance threshold is not at all high. Once a resistant clone of organisms has been established, it is difficult to control. This suggests that if one is to use prophylactic antibiotics, perhaps their use should be restricted to those who are at greatest risk for complications of febrile neutropenia.

To learn more about prophylactic antibiotic use in cancer patients, see the editorial by Baden.[1] It is strongly recommended that if prophylactic antibiotic therapy is to be adopted at a cancer center, it should be accompanied by vigorous infection-control practices and careful monitoring for the emergence of resistant organisms. The studies by Del Favero et al and Cullen et al do provide evidence of the potential significant benefit of levofloxacin prophylaxis, a benefit that comes at a high price, however. Stay tuned to see how all this plays out in the pediatric population.

J. A. Stockman III, MD

Reference

1. Baden LR: Prophylactic antimicrobial agents and the importance of fitness (editorial). *N Engl J Med* 353:1052-1054, 2005.

Antibacterial Prophylaxis After Chemotherapy for Solid Tumors and Lymphomas
Cullen M, for the Simple Investigation in Neutropenic Individuals of the Frequency of Infection After Chemotherapy +/- Antibiotic in a Number of Tumours (SIGNIFICANT) Trial Group (Univ Hosp Birmingham Cancer Centre, England; et al)
N Engl J Med 353:988-998, 2005   16–14

Background.—The role of prophylactic antibacterial agents after chemotherapy remains controversial.

Methods.—We conducted a randomized, double-blind, placebo-controlled trial in patients who were receiving cyclic chemotherapy for solid tumors or lymphoma and who were at risk for temporary, severe neutropenia (fewer than 500 neutrophils per cubic millimeter). Patients were randomly assigned to receive either 500 mg of levofloxacin once daily or matching placebo for seven days during the expected neutropenic period. The primary outcome was the incidence of clinically documented febrile episodes (temperature of more than 38°C) attributed to infection. Secondary outcomes included the incidence of all probable infections, severe infections, and hospitalization but did not include a systematic evaluation of antibacterial resistance.

Results.—A total of 1565 patients underwent randomization (784 to placebo and 781 to levofloxacin). The tumors included breast cancer (35.4 percent), lung cancer (22.5 percent), testicular cancer (14.4 percent), and lymphoma (12.8 percent). During the first cycle of chemotherapy, 3.5 percent of patients in the levofloxacin group had at least one febrile episode, as compared with 7.9 percent in the placebo group (P<0.001). During the entire chemotherapy course, 10.8 percent of patients in the levofloxacin group had at least one febrile episode, as compared with 15.2 percent of patients in the placebo group (P=0.01); the respective rates of probable infection were 34.2 percent and 41.5 percent (P=0.004). Hospitalization was required for the treatment of infection in 15.7 percent of patients in the levofloxacin group and 21.6 percent of patients in the placebo group (P=0.004). The respective rate of severe infection was 1.0 percent and 2.0 percent (P=0.15), with four infection-related deaths in each group. An organism was isolated in 9.2 percent of probable infections.

Conclusions.—Among patients receiving chemotherapy for solid tumors or lymphoma, the prophylactic use of levofloxacin reduces the incidence of fever, probable infection, and hospitalization. no comment

---

Parental Suicide After the Expected Death of a Child at Home
Davies DE (Univ of Alberta, Edmonton, Canada)
BMJ 332:647-648, 2006   16–15

Background.—Opioids and other controlled drugs are often prescribed by physicians to make patients in a variety of states more comfortable. However, once in the community, these drugs are not monitored or audited, and patients and their families are responsible for handling these drugs safely. End-of-life care has received greater attention in the international literature in recent years, and the field of palliative care has emerged as an important aspect of end-of-life care. This increased scrutiny has in many cases changed the setting in which palliative care services are provided, and often this care is now provided in the home. A potential hazard in this system is presented in this report.

> *Case 1.*—A boy with congenital rhabdoid tumor of the face received palliative care at home for progressive disease. The boy developed sudden signs of airway obstruction 2 days before his death. Lorazepam had been prescribed, and was titrated until it helped. He died the day before his first birthday. The mother refused to have his body removed from the house on the night of his death and refused to release the body to a funeral home. Attempts to encourage the parents to return the baby's drugs were unsuccessful. The parents repeatedly denied any plans for suicide. The mother was found the next day and was pronounced dead on arrival at the hospital. Toxicology tests at

autopsy showed high concentrations of opioids and benzodiaz-epines; however, a review of the drugs found in her home after her death did not identify any discrepancy in the amounts predicted to be remaining after the baby's treatment. The last visual review of the boy's drugs was 2 days before he died.

Case 2.—An 8-year-old girl received palliative care at home for ad-vanced metastatic Wilms' disease. Escalating doses of morphine eventually had minimal effect, and the patient was subsequently changed to enteral methadone. As her condition deteriorated, she be-came unwilling to take oral medications. Methadone was prepared for parenteral use, controlled by a central venous catheter with con-tinuous background infusion and patient-controlled boluses. The patient remained alert until she died. In the days after the girl's death, her mother was found unconscious at home. She had taken the child's enteral methadone. The family had been advised to return all drugs to the pharmacy on the day that their child died by the home care nurse who visited them. The mother was admitted to a hospital's ICU and survived.

Conclusions.—The widespread development of palliative care has al-lowed more and more dying patients to stay at home, with a concurrent in-crease in the medical use of 4 common opioids from 73% to 402% in 6 years. At this time there is little guidance from the law or from public policy as to the handling of remaining opioid drugs in patients' home after they die, ex-cept for reminders to families to return them for safe disposal. In rare cases families may use these residual drugs for self harm, despite denial of suicidal intentions.

▶ There is no question that the death of a child brings profound distress and intense grief to an entire family. That such grief can lead to suicide is known, but the 2 cases reported show a particular hazard after a child has died at home. In both cases the mothers either committed or tried to commit suicide with drugs prescribed for the palliative care of their children.

Data suggest that parental vulnerability and an increased risk of suicide fol-lowing the death of a child is highest in the first month after the child's demise. Studies have also shown that anxiety and depression can last for as long as 4 to 9 years after the loss of a child from cancer. The situation is different when a child has died from a chronic disease as opposed to death as the result of sui-cide, homicide, violence, or an accident. The challenges that arise when a child's death is prolonged are somewhat unique. Caring for a child with a chronic fatal disease such as cancer may involve intense and prolonged treat-ment, the sustaining of hope, and the denial of the potential for death as the parent fights for the child's survival in a protracted battle with the disease. An-ticipatory grieving as the probability of death becomes more real may lead par-ents to feel guilt about giving in to such a possibility—as though they are some-how abandoning the child. Recognizing that there will be an end to this suffering is ambivalent; it again means admitting the reality of death. The parent, usually the mother, may invest her own life so intensely that she hopes to keep the child alive, by force of will, if all else fails. There are also the questions. Why did this child become ill in this way? The "if only something" had been done differently. This intense involvement may lead to an almost symbiotic relationship between the mother and the dying child in such circumstances, reflecting the wish to bring the child back from the brink, and, in some circumstances, the mother's inner belief that she cannot live if her child dies.

A care provider must recognize that all these issues need to be considered in assessing a parent's, family's, and child's needs through the period of preparation for the realities of the youngster's death and its aftermath. Caring just for the child is not enough. Looking after the caregiver before, during, and in the aftermath of the death is an integral part of comprehensive care. All too often, pediatric oncology services are no long accessible to a grieving parent following the death of their child. Primary care providers need to fill this gap. Support from others who have survived such an experience can be tremendously helpful to parents and such support should be provided whenever possible.

J. A. Stockman III, MD

Limitations on Physical Performance and Daily Activities Among Long-term Survivors of Childhood Cancer
Ness KK, Mertens AC, Hudson MM, et al (Univ of Minnesota, Minneapolis; Univ of Tennessee, Memphis; Fred Hutchinson Cancer Research Ctr, Seattle; et al)
Ann Intern Med 143:639-647, 2005   16–16

Background.—Survivors of childhood cancer may experience important disease- and treatment-related late effects, including functional limitations.

Objective.—This study evaluated performance limitations and restricted abilities to participate in personal care, to engage in routine activities like shopping or housework, and to attend work or school (participation restrictions) in a cohort of survivors of childhood cancer.

Setting.—Epidemiologic survey and 26 institutions that treat childhood cancer.

Patients.—Participants included 11 481 persons who were treated for primary brain cancer, leukemia, Hodgkin disease, non-Hodgkin lymphoma, kidney tumor, neuroblastoma, soft-tissue sarcoma, or malignant bone tumor before the age of 21 years and who survived at least 5 years after diagnosis. The comparison group included 3839 siblings of survivors of childhood cancer.

Measurement.—Medical data were abstracted, and participants or parents (if the participants were <18 years of age at survey completion) completed a 24-page questionnaire.

Results.—Compared with siblings, survivors were more likely to report performance limitations (risk ratio, 1.8 [95% CI, 1.7 to 2.0]) and to report restricted participation in personal care skills (risk ratio, 4.7 [CI, 3.0 to 7.2]), routine activities (risk ratio, 4.7 [CI, 3.6 to 6.2]), and the ability to attend work or school (risk ratio, 5.9 [CI, 4.5 to 7.6]). Survivors of brain (26.6%) and bone (36.9%) cancer were most likely to report performance limitations, restricted ability to do routine activities (20.9% and 8.5%, respectively), and restricted ability to attend work or school (20.0% and 11.2%, respectively). Survivors of brain cancer were also most likely to report restricted abilities to perform personal care (10.5%).

Limitations.—There was the potential for participants to be healthier or more physically capable than nonparticipants or for persons to be more motivated to participate in this study if they had functional deficits. In addition, the nature of the questionnaire did not allow specific physical limitations to be measured.

Conclusion.—Long-term survivors of childhood cancer are at increased risk for functional limitations in physical performance and in participation in activities needed for daily living.

▶ Over time, we have learned about many of the long-standing impairments related to survivorship of childhood cancer. These include impairments in intellectual, emotional, and physical domains that diminish functioning over time and are capable of restricting a survivor's ability to participate fully in daily activities necessary for self-care, home management, or work. The Childhood Cancer Survivor Study is a long-standing study that has examined the sequelae of treatment for childhood cancer. The study is funded by grant CA 55727 from the National Cancer Institute, which provides support for data collection.

The Childhood Cancer Survivor Study now tells us that the greatest risks for performance limitations in survivors of childhood cancer may be found among those who have survived brain tumors, bone cancer, neuroblastoma, soft tissue sarcoma, and Hodgkin lymphoma. Survivors of brain and bone cancer seem to have the highest prevalence of significant long-term impairments. More than one third of the survivors of bone cancer report physical limitations, and some 11% report that poor health has restricted their ability to attend work or school. Performance limitations are also a significant problem in survivors of neuroblastoma, primarily because such patients can have a multitude of late effects affecting the musculoskeletal and neurologic system. As many as 6% of neuroblastoma survivors report difficulty with routine activities such as shopping or housework.

Hodgkin lymphoma survivors are nearly twice as likely as siblings to report performance limitations, but are not as likely as survivors of brain cancer, bone cancer, or neuroblastoma to report difficulty with activities of daily living, routine activities, or interference with work or school attendance. Late effects in survivors of Hodgkin lymphoma are more likely to include impairments of the cardiac or pulmonary systems.

Although not all late effects can be avoided or eliminated, their impact in survivors of childhood cancer on physical performance and participation in routine activities can be influenced by rehabilitation measures designed specifically to restore function or remediate loss in physical performance. Survivors are at risk for many years after cessation of their therapy. All too often these kids grow up to be adults whose long-term problems are not recognized for what they are, and no therapies (prophylactic or otherwise) are provided. We have to do more for these patients.

J. A. Stockman III, MD

Performance Limitations and Participation Restrictions Among Childhood Cancer Survivors Treated With Hematopoietic Stem Cell Transplantation: The Bone Marrow Transplant Survivor Study

Ness KK, Bhatia S, Baker KS, et al (Univ of Minnesota, Minneapolis; City of Hope Natl Med Ctr, Duarte, Calif)
Arch Pediatr Adolesc Med 159:706-713, 2005   16–17

Background.—Hematopoietic stem cell transplantation (HCT) may result in important disease- and treatment-related late effects. This study estimated physical, emotional, and educational limitations (performance limitations) and restrictions in the ability to perform personal care or routine daily activities (physical participation restrictions) and restrictions in the ability to participate in social roles (social participation restrictions) in a cohort of cancer survivors treated with HCT during childhood.

Methods.—Study participants included 235 persons who had a malignancy or hematologic disorder, were treated with HCT before the age of 21 years, and survived at least 2 years after transplantation. A comparison group was recruited and frequency matched for age, sex, and ethnicity. Medical data were abstracted, and patients or parents (if <18 years at survey completion) completed a mailed 24-page questionnaire.

Results.—Adult survivors of childhood cancer were more likely than the comparison group to report limitations in physical (prevalence odds ratio [OR], 2.2; 95% confidence interval [CI], 1.3-3.7) and emotional domains (OR, 2.9; 95% CI, 1.4-5.8) and to report physical participation restrictions (OR, 3.9; 95% CI, 1.9-8.2). Adult survivors were also less likely than the comparison group to be married (OR, 0.4; 95% CI, 0.2-0.6). Child survivors were more likely than similarly aged children to have participated in special education (OR, 3.0; 95% CI, 1.5-6.0), to report physical participation restrictions (OR, 10.8; 95% CI, 2.2-53.9), and to have behaviors that indicated impaired social competence (OR, 2.0; 95% CI, 0.9-4.2).

Conclusion.—This study demonstrated that persons treated with HCT as children were at increased risk for performance limitations that restricted participation in routine daily activities and interpersonal relationships.

▶ This report reminds us that not all is rosy in the survivorship after HCT. Thousands of these procedures are being performed yearly and currently well more than 100,000 individuals are long-term (5 years or more) survivors of HCT here in the United States. What we learn from this study, which has examined the long-term consequences in more than 200 persons who were treated with HCT before the age of 21 years, is that adult survivors are twice as likely to have physical limitations and 3 times as likely to have emotional problems compared with control subjects. Those survivors who are still in childhood are 3 times more likely to need special education and 11 times more likely to have significant degrees of physical limitation.

None of the findings in this report should imply that we should not push forward with using HCT to save lives. We need to learn how to use this technique better. We need to determine ways of detecting long-term side effects early, so that we can intervene to improve the lives of these children as they grow older. While there is a substantial subset of individuals after HCT that will experience significant functional limitations, the majority of survivors do go on to lead independent and productive lives, free of long-term complications.

J. A. Stockman III, MD

17 Ophthalmology

Clinical and Bacterial Characteristics of Acute Bacterial Conjunctivitis in Children in the Antibiotic Resistance Era
Buznach N, Dagan R, Greenberg D (Soroka Univ Med Ctr, Beer-Sheva, Israel; Ben-Gurion Univ of the Negev, Beer-Sheva, Israel)
Pediatr Infect Dis J 24:823-828, 2005   17–1

Background.—Acute conjunctivitis is the most common eye disorder in young children. Bacteria are responsible for 54–73% of all cases. The goals of the study were to identify the rates of *Haemophilus influenzae*, *Streptococcus pneumoniae* and *Moraxella catarrhalis* in cases of bacterial conjunctivitis in children and to define antibiotic resistance rates.

Methods.—During a 2-year study period, conjunctival swabs of children 2–36 months old were collected prospectively. Nontypable *H. influenzae*, *S. pneumoniae* and *M. catarrhalis* were defined as the study pathogens. Analyzed variables included demography, clinical presentation, bacteriologic results and susceptibility patterns.

Results.—There were 428 patients enrolled. Of all cultures, 55% (237 of 428) yielded at least 1 of the study pathogens. *H influenzae* and *S. pneumoniae* were isolated from 29 and 20% of cultures, respectively. β-Lactamase production was found in 29% of *H. influenzae* isolates, and penicillin nonsusceptibility was observed in 60% of *S. pneumoniae* isolates. The most common *S. pneumoniae* serotypes were: 19F (14%); 6A and 14 (11% each). Nontypable *S. pneumoniae* was found in 12%. The 7-valent pneumococcal conjugate vaccine (PCV-7) could potentially cover 44% of all isolates. Conjunctivitis-otitis syndrome was found in 32% of patients, of whom 82% of cultures yielded *H. influenzae*.

Conclusions.—Antibiotic resistance rates are alarmingly high. Conjunctivitis-otitis syndrome, predominantly caused by *H. influenzae*, is quite common. The potential coverage of the PCV-7 in conjunctivitis is relatively lower than that reported in other pneumococcal infections. Our findings should alert physicians on the choice of appropriate antibiotic treatment, on the frequent copresence of acute otitis media and on the potential role of conjunctivitis in the spread of antibiotic-resistant pathogens.

▶ This report is an extremely important one, but has to be viewed in the context of the observation that many, if perhaps not most, cases of conjunctivitis in children are viral in origin. The issue for the practitioner is whether he or she is willing to culture every case of conjunctivitis to pick up those that are bacterial in origin and that might, just possibly might, benefit from the administration of antibiotics. As far as the bacterial causes of conjunctivitis are concerned, nontypeable *H influenzae* remains the most frequently isolated pathogen in children, accounting for as many as 44% to 68% of all cases of bacterial conjunctivitis. *S pneumoniae* and *M catarrhalis* cause 7% to 44% and 1% to 6% of cases, respectively. There is, of course, an association between bacterial conjunctivitis and acute otitis media, an association known as the conjunctivitis-otitis syndrome. In such cases, *H influenzae* is the predominant pathogen causing the problem. Acute otitis media is seen in some 20% to 70% of cases of bacterial conjunctivitis.

This report is important because it tells us a bit about antibiotic resistance to the common pathogens that cause conjunctivitis in this day and age. We learn from this report that about half of children presenting with conjunctivitis have a bacterial pathogen detectable on culture, with *H influenzae* and *S pneumoniae* accounting for 29% and 20% of positive cultures, respectively. β-Lactamase production was found in almost 30% of *H influenzae* isolates, and penicillin nonsusceptibility was observed in the majority of *S pneumoniae* isolates.

In the report abstracted, 96% of the *H influenzae* isolates and 97% of the *S pneumoniae* isolates were susceptible to chloramphenicol. This finding reinforces the traditional choice of topical chloramphenicol in Israel (the site of the report) as an appropriate and effective empiric treatment of bacterial conjunctivitis in children. The authors note that when systemic antibiotic treatment is needed, such as in the conjunctivitis-otitis syndrome, the prevalence of penicillin-nonsusceptible *S pneumoniae* and β-lactamase–producing *H influenzae* should be considered in choosing the most suitable empiric treatment. Here in the United States, topical polymyxin B with gentamicin, polymyxin B with bacitracin, sodium sulfacetamide, and gentamicin are the predominant antibiotics used for conjunctivitis. This is based on our reluctance, in the United States, to use topical chloramphenicol given the risks of this agent even when used nonsystemically.

Readers of the YEAR BOOK should be aware of a report that recently appeared in the *Lancet*.[1] This report from Great Britain compared the efficacy of chloramphenicol eye drops with placebo eye drops for the treatment of all comers with acute infective conjunctivitis in children. This study showed that most children presenting with acute infective conjunctivitis in a primary care setting get better by themselves and do not need treatment with an antibiotic. This is in a country where chloramphenicol is the treatment of choice for acute conjunctivitis in children. It should be noted that the United Kingdom's Medicines and Healthcare Products Regulatory Agency (MHRA) has recently announced that chloramphenicol eye drops can be sold through pharmacies without a prescriptions.[2] With the worldwide continuously emerging problem of antibiotic resistance, it is unfathomable why the MHRA would ever recommend that antibiotic eye drops be available without prescription in the United Kingdom.

This commentary closes with a bit of eye trivia. Do you know what percentage of eye injuries presenting to emergency rooms are the result of a strike from a champagne cork? Believe it or not, somebody has actually done a study to address this question.[3] There is a registry of eye injuries here in the United States as well as one in Hungary and comparisons were made between causes of eye injury here in the US and Hungary. It turns out that 1.4% of eye injuries in Hungary are ascribed to champagne corks, compared with just 0.07% here in the United States. The consequences, by the way, of such injury can be very serious. It is calculated that a cork from an exploding bottle can strike the eye of an opener at a speed of 50 km/h and at a pressure of 100 atmospheres.[4]

J. A. Stockman III, MD

References

1. Rose PW, Harnden A, Brueggemann AB, et al: Chloramphenicol treatment for acute infective conjunctivitis in children in primary care: A randomized, double-blind placebo-controlled trial. *Lancet* 366:37-43, 2005.
2. Medicines and Healthcare Products Regulatory Agency: Antibiotic eye drops available over the counter, http://www.mhra.gov.uk/home/groups/comms-po/documents/news/con002092.pdf, accessed January 16, 2006.
3. Kuhn F, Mester V, Berta A, et al: Epidemiology of severe eye injuries: United States Eye Injury Registry (USEIR) and Hungarian Eye Injury Registry (HEIR). *Ophthalmologe* 95:332-334, 1998.
4. Archer D, Galloway N: Champagne cork injury to the eye. *Lancet* 2:47-49, 1967.

Clinical Decision Support and Appropriateness of Antimicrobial Prescribing: A Randomized Trial
Samore MH, Bateman K, Alder SC, et al (VA Salt Lake City Health Care System, Utah; Univ of Utah, Salt Lake City; HealthInsight, Salt Lake City, Utah; et al)
JAMA 294:2305-2314, 2005   17–2

Context.—The impact of clinical decision support systems (CDSS) on antimicrobial prescribing in ambulatory settings has not previously been evaluated.

Objective.—To measure the added value of CDSS when coupled with a community intervention to reduce inappropriate prescribing of antimicrobial drugs for acute respiratory tract infections.

Design, Participants and Setting.—Cluster randomized trial that included 407,460 inhabitants and 334 primary care clinicians in 12 rural communities in Utah and Idaho (6 with 1 shared characteristic and 6 with another), and a third group of 6 communities that served as nonstudy controls. The preintervention period was January to December 2001 and the postintervention period was January 2002 to September 2003. Acute respiratory tract infection diagnoses were classified into groups based on indication for antimicrobial use. Multilevel regression methods were applied to account for the clustered design.

Intervention.—Six communities received a community intervention alone and 6 communities received community intervention plus CDSS that were targeted toward primary care clinicians. The CDSS comprised decision support tools on paper and a handheld computer to guide diagnosis and management of acute respiratory tract infection.

Main Outcome Measure.—Community-wide antimicrobial usage was assessed using retail pharmacy data. Diagnosis-specific antimicrobial use was compared by chart review.

Results.—Within CDSS communities, 71% of primary care clinicians participated in the use of CDSS. The prescribing rate decreased from 84.1 to 75.3 per 100 person-years in the CDSS arm vs 84.3 to 85.2 in community intervention alone, and remained stable in the other communities ($P = .03$). A total of 13,081 acute respiratory tract infection visits were abstracted. The relative decrease in antimicrobial prescribing for visits in the antibiotics "never-indicated" category during the post-intervention period was 32% in CDSS communities and 5% in community intervention-alone communities ($P = .03$). Use of macrolides decreased significantly in CDSS communities but not in community intervention–alone communities.

Conclusion.—CDSS implemented in rural primary care settings reduced overall antimicrobial use and improved appropriateness of antimicrobial selection for acute respiratory tract infections.

▶ The authors of this report describe a randomized trial to test the effectiveness of a CDSS to reduce inappropriate prescribing of antibiotics for acute respiratory infections in rural settings, assessing prescribing through retail pharmacy data and chart review. They have designed a cluster randomized trial involving communities divided into 2 groups. One group received a community intervention that included meetings, news releases, distribution of educational materials, a mailing to parents of young children, and news articles about antibiotic use. The other group received the same community-level intervention as well as a clinical decision support tool given to primary care clinicians, either on paper or in an electronic version accessible through a personal digital assistant, whichever they preferred. These tools were accompanied by lectures, meetings, one-on-one interactions with physicians from the study team, and a voluntary continuing medical education session. Over a period of 2 years, the prescribing of antibiotic drugs declined by 10% in these communities in contrast with a 1% decline elsewhere. Nonetheless, antibiotics were still prescribed for more than 24% of diagnoses that one would not have expected an antibiotic to be prescribed for.

All interventions for improving rates of appropriate use of antibiotics must be introduced in the context of efforts to raise awareness among the public and to further educate prescribers. Such interventions, as well as algorithms and guidelines to improve antibiotic use, must be transparently evidence based. Increased use of an electronic health record may serve as a framework for some of these practice changes. The electronic health record also may help answer the need for better, more universal, readily available data for designing and evaluating interventions that include patient-linked microbiological testing and results, diagnoses, and prescriptions. Needless to say, pay-for-performance initiatives, hopefully based on evidence-based decision making, will play some role as well.

To read more on the topic of the appropriate use of antibiotics, see the excellent editorial by Weber.[1]

J. A. Stockman III, MD

Reference

1. Weber JT: Appropriate use of antimicrobial drugs. A better prescription is needed (editorial). *JAMA* 294:2354-2356, 2005.

Epidemiology and Diagnosis of Hospital-Acquired Conjunctivitis Among Neonatal Intensive Care Unit Patients

Haas J, Larson E, Ross B, et al (Columbia Univ, New York; New York-Presbyterian Hosp Weill Cornell Med Ctr)
Pediatr Infect Dis J 24:586-589, 2005   17–3

Background.—Few recent reports describe the epidemiology and risk factors for health care-associated conjunctivitis among neonatal intensive care unit (NICU) patients in developed countries. Reporting may be inaccurate in this population given that the National Nosocomial Infection Surveillance System (NNIS) definition is largely dependent on a positive culture, whereas clinical practice often consists of empiric treatment.

Objectives.—We describe the epidemiology of conjunctivitis among neonates in 2 level III-IV NICUs and compare the NNIS definition with our study definition: eye drainage and empiric treatment with or without a culture.

Methods.—Patient demographics, clinical, device usage and conjunctivitis data collected prospectively from March 2001 through January 2003 were analyzed.

Results.—Conjunctivitis occurred in 5% (n = 154/2935) of infants, of whom 51% (n = 79) were in NICU 1 and 49% (n = 75) in NICU 2. Predominant pathogens included coagulase-negative staphylococci (25%), *Staphylococcus aureus* (19%) and *Klebsiella spp.* (10%). Significant predictors of conjunctivitis included low birth weight, use of ventilator or nasal cannula continuous positive airway pressure and study year. Ophthalmologic examination was an additional predictor of infection in NICU 1. Eye examination data were unavailable for NICU 2. Only 62% of cases that met the study definition for conjunctivitis met the NNIS definition, because many infants received empiric treatment.

Conclusions.—Clinical conjunctivitis was associated with low birth weight and patient care factors that could lead to contamination of the eye with respiratory tract secretions. The NNIS definition failed to detect 38% of clinical infections. Consideration should be given to revising the definition of conjunctivitis for the NICU population.

▶ Most of us have become accustomed to the fact that conjunctivitis is one of the most frequently occurring acquired infections in the NICU. Health care–acquired conjunctivitis in such a setting is defined as a conjunctivitis that occurs 48 hours or more after birth or after hospitalization in a neonate. It is caused by bacterial or viral pathogens unrelated to maternal infection. In most instances, such conjunctivitis is readily treated with topical antimicrobial agents without any further consequence, and for this reason, more often than not, cultures are not obtained as part of the evaluation of such babies. For this reason, there is precious little information about the epidemiology and diagnosis of hospital-acquired conjunctivitis among neonates in ICUs. That is why this article is so important.

We learn from this article, one of the largest studies ever conducted to examine endemic conjunctivitis in NICUs, that some 5% of babies will experience this problem. Low birth weight appears to be a consistent and significant independent risk factor for the development of conjunctivitis, most likely because tiny immature babies spend considerable time with their eyes either closed or covered, which is a circumstance that allows bacteria to proliferate. Also, small babies have immature lacrimal systems producing scanty amounts of tears. That and the fact that there is infrequent opening and closing of the eyes, which acts as a pump to facilitate tear distribution across the surface of the eye and to wash material away through lacrimal ducts, explain a good bit of why NICU inhabitants have such a high prevalence of conjunctivitis.

The organisms most commonly causing conjunctivitis in the series reported are coagulase-negative staphylococci, *S aureus, Klebsiella, Pseudomonas aeruginosa,* and *Enterococcus.* Fortunately, most of these organisms can be treated topically, although the authors of this article do suggest that it would be good to perform a culture if babies have red eyes or eye discharge.

If one wants to minimize the prevalence of conjunctivitis in NICUs, several approaches can accomplish this. One cannot change birth weight, but strict adherence to infection control techniques when examining babies would go a long way in decreasing the prevalence of this disease. Protecting the eyes of intubated babies during respiratory care is important because hands-on approaches to respiratory care often contaminate babies' eyes and/or the environment around a baby. Interestingly, an eye examination for retinopathy of prematurity turns out to be a risk factor for conjunctivitis. We have to ask our ophthalmology friends to be very careful during their eye examinations. All instruments used for such purposes need to be sterile.

There is one form of eye infection that newborns will not get. See if you can answer the following question: Why is the combination of diving in fresh water and the wearing of contact lenses incompatible? A recent case report of a diving instructor who wore soft contact lenses while diving in the waters of a unused quarry answers this question.[1] The young lady developed serious inflammation with a corneal infiltrate. Corneal biopsy confirmed the presence of acanthamoeba. Treatment with appropriate agents improved her keratitis, although she could have easily lost vision.

Acanthamoeba is a cystic protozoan that is ubiquitous in fresh water and highly resilient. The most common ocular problem it causes is corneal infection (keratitis). Although diving in salt water while wearing contact lenses does not pose a risk of infection with this organism, fresh water diving carries a high risk.

J. A. Stockman III, MD

Reference

1. Lockwood A: Keratitis resulting from diving in fresh water. *BMJ* 331:1152, 2005.

The Incidence and Course of Retinopathy of Prematurity: Findings From the Early Treatment for Retinopathy of Prematurity Study

Good WV, for the Early Treatment for Retinopathy of Prematurity Cooperative Group (Smith-Kettlewell Eye Research Inst, San Francisco)
Pediatrics 116:15-23, 2005   17–4

Objectives.—To estimate the incidence of retinopathy of prematurity (ROP) in the Early Treatment for Retinopathy of Prematurity (ETROP) Study and compare these results with those reported in the Cryotherapy for Retinopathy of Prematurity (CRYO-ROP) Study.

Methods.—The ETROP Study, as part of its protocol, screened 6998 infants at 26 centers throughout the United States. Serial eye examinations were conducted for infants born weighing <1251 g, making it possible to estimate the frequency of ROP in different birth weight and gestational age categories. ROP was categorized according to the International Classification for ROP.

Results.—The incidence of any ROP was 68% among infants of <1251 g. The findings were compared with those for infants born in 1986 and 1987 in the CRYO-ROP Study. The overall incidences of ROP were similar in the 2 studies, but there was more zone I ROP in the ETROP Study. Among infants with ROP, more-severe ROP (prethreshold) occurred for 36.9% of infants in the ETROP Study and 27.1% of infants in the CRYO-ROP Study. The gestational age of onset of ROP of different severities has changed very little since the CRYO-ROP Study was conducted.

Conclusions.—ROP remains a common important problem among infants with birth weights of <1251 g. The incidence of ROP, time of onset, rate of progression, and time of onset of prethreshold disease have changed little since the CRYO-ROP natural-history study.

▶ We learn from this report that things have not changed much in the last decade or two with respect to the prevalence of ROP. The recent development of peripheral retinal ablative therapy using laser photocoagulation has resulted in the possibility of markedly decreasing the incidence of poor visual outcome, but the sequential evolutionary nature of ROP creates a requirement that at-risk preterm infants be examined at specific proper times to detect the changes of ROP before they become permanently destructive. Recently, the American Academy of Pediatrics published its policy statement on the screening examination of premature infants for ROP.[1]

You should read the policy statement on screening for ROP in order to understand the rationales and principles upon which the screening programs are based. The goal of an effective screening program must be to identify the relatively few preterm infants who require treatment for ROP from among the much larger number of at-risk infants, minimizing the number of stressful examinations required for these sick infants. Please also recognize that infants at risk for ROP may be at significant risk for other seemingly unrelated visual disorders such as strabismus, amblyopia, and cataract. Ophthalmologic follow-up for these potential problems after discharge from the neonatal ICU is clearly indicated.

While on the subject of physical examination techniques, pediatricians use the red reflex to assess a variety of eye problems in children. When was the red reflex first described? What is the actual source within the eye of the red reflex? The use of the red reflex as a screening tool was originally described by a Swiss ophthalmologist, Brückner, in 1962.[2] Brückner described a test he called the "translumination test" comparing the red reflex in both eyes simultaneously. He noted the ease with which one could perform the test in the pediatric population; the test can be performed without having to touch an anxious child. Brückner described the test's use in uncovering atrophy of the optic nerve, anisometropia, cataract, intraocular hemorrhage, retinal detachment, intraocular tumor, and strabismus. The performance of a red reflex as a test has a high sensitivity in detecting amblyopia and the several conditions that cause amblyopia.

Although all pediatricians should be familiar with the best manner to perform a red reflex, the American Academy of Pediatrics tells us how this is best done. To perform the red reflex test, the examiner should stand approximately 80 cm to 1 m (2-3 feet) away from the patient and look through the aperture of the direct ophthalmoscope. The largest white-light circle of the ophthalmoscope should be aimed directly along the patient's face and pupils. By focusing the dial, the patient's face should be brought into focus. The patient should be looking directly at the examiner. Both pupils should be illuminated simultaneously so that the red reflex from each eye is viewed at the same time to allow for comparison. The red reflex is not the result of light bouncing off the retina, but rather off the choroid with its pigments and vasculature. The choroid lies between the retina and the sclera as a middle layer. The retina itself is transparent. While Brückner originally described the normal reflex as red, the average "red" reflex tends to be slightly yellow/orange/red or a combination of these colors. To read more about the red reflex, see the superb review by McLaughlin and Levin.[3]

J. A. Stockman III, MD

References

1. American Academy of Pediatrics: Screening examination of premature infants for retinopathy of prematurity. *Pediatrics* 117:572-576, 2006.
2. Roe LD, Guyton DL: The light that leaks: Brückner and the red reflex. *Surv Ophthalmol* 28:665-670, 1984.
3. McLaughlin C, Levin AV: The red reflex. *Pediatr Emerg Care* 22:137-140, 2006.

18 Respiratory Tract

Epidemiology of Cystic Fibrosis-Related Diabetes
Marshall BC, for the Advisors, Investigators, and Coordinators of the Epidemiologic Study of Cystic Fibrosis (Univ of Utah, Salt Lake City; Genentech, Inc, South San Francisco; Univ of Minnesota, Minneapolis; et al)
J Pediatr 146:681-687, 2005   18–1

Objectives.—Cystic fibrosis-related diabetes (CFRD) has emerged as an important complication of CF. To better understand who is at risk of developing CFRD, to gain insight into the impact of CFRD on pulmonary and nutritional status, and to assess the association of CFRD with various practice patterns and comorbid conditions, we characterized the Epidemiologic Study of Cystic Fibrosis (ESCF) patient population.

Study Design.—Analyses were performed on the 8247 adolescents and adults who were evaluated at one of 204 participating sites during 1998. CFRD was defined as the use of insulin or an oral hypoglycemic agent at any time during the year.

Results.—Previously reported risk factors for CFRD including age, gender (female), and pancreatic insufficiency were confirmed in this study. Patients with CFRD had more severe pulmonary disease, more frequent pulmonary exacerbations, and poorer nutritional status as compared with those without diabetes. CFRD also was associated with liver disease.

Conclusions.—CFRD is a common complication in adolescents and adults that is associated with more severe disease.

▶ Endocrine pancreatic insufficiency occurs with increasing frequency after the age of 10 years in youngsters with CF. CFRD is a distinct form of diabetes that shares features of both type 1 and type 2 diabetes. The cause of this problem is a relative insulin deficiency related to the destruction of the pancreas. Some insulin resistance has also been reported in the CF population, but this probably plays a relatively minor role in the cause of most cases of diabetes related to CF. Given the markedly improved survivorship of patients with CF these days, one can expect to see a very high prevalence of the disorder in the CF population.

This article shows us exactly what the risk factors are for the development of diabetes in patients with CF. Girls seem to be at greater risk. Those who have greater pulmonary disease and who have poorer nutrition are also at greatest risk.

If you are interested in reading more about the diagnosis and management of CF, see the excellent review of this topic by Smyth.[1] Dr Smyth reviews all the best evidence for diagnosing as well as managing CF.

One unrelated comment having to do with wheezing (a common symptom in patients with cystic fibrosis): How would you solve this interesting diagnostic puzzle? Little Suzie, a 7-year-old, has reactive airway disease. She comes to the office with her father with a strange tale. The father states that whenever Suzie uses her nebulizer in the kitchen while her mother is cooking on a gas stovetop, the flame of the gas heaters turns from light blue to bright yellow-orange. The father has called the gas company and maintenance engineers have come over and have found no fault with the stovetop. The father asks you what is going on here and demands an answer since he has already bought 2 new stovetops and the problem continues. He blames it on your prescription writing. How would you respond?

The first thing you would do is probably look up an article in Thorax.[2] There you would read about 3 patients who became alarmed when the flame of gas burners changed colors when they used their nebulizers for bronchodilator treatments. Two called out gas maintenance engineers and the third bought a new gas cook top. It turns out that there was a fairly simple explanation. The sodium in the fine saline mist will turn a open gas flame bright orange-yellow, even if the flame is more than 6 feet away. The color change remains for as long as 10 minutes after nebulization is discontinued. One can see it now. Medication product inserts will have to warn people about this side effect of nebulizers. Then again, perhaps one can use one's nebulizer to entertain cocktail party guests around the fireplace.

J. A. Stockman III, MD

References

1. Smyth RL: Diagnosis and management of cystic fibrosis. *Arch Dis Child Educ Pract Ed* 90:ep1-ep6, 2005.
2. Effect of nebulizers on open flames (editorial). *Thorax* 60:1068, 2005.

Genetic Modifiers of Lung Disease in Cystic Fibrosis
Knowles MR, for the Gene Modifier Study Group (Univ of North Carolina, Chapel Hill; et al)
N Engl J Med 353:1443-1453, 2005   18–2

Background.—Polymorphisms in genes other than the cystic fibrosis transmembrane conductance regulator (*CFTR*) gene may modify the severity of pulmonary disease in patients with cystic fibrosis.

Methods.—We performed two studies with different patient samples. We first tested 808 patients who were homozygous for the $\Delta F508$ mutation and were classified as having either severe or mild lung disease, as defined by the lowest or highest quartile of forced expiratory volume in one second (FEV_1), respectively, for age. We genotyped 16 polymorphisms in 10 genes reported by others as modifiers of disease severity in cystic fibrosis and tested for an association in patients with severe disease (263 patients) or mild disease (545). In the replication (second) study, we tested 498 patients, with various *CFTR* genotypes and a range of FEV$_1$ values, for an association of the *TGFβ1* codon 10 CC genotype with low FEV$_1$.

Results.—In the initial study, significant allelic and genotypic associations with phenotype were seen only for *TGFβ1* (the gene encoding transforming growth factor β1), particularly the −509 and codon 10 polymorphisms (with P values obtained with the use of Fisher's exact test and logistic regression ranging from 0.006 to 0.0002). The odds ratio was about 2.2 for the highest-risk *TGFβ1* genotype (codon 10 CC) in association with the phenotype for severe lung disease. The replication study confirmed the association of the *TGFβ1* codon 10 CC genotype with more severe lung disease in comparisons with the use of dichotomized FEV$_1$ for severity status (P=0.0002) and FEV$_1$ values directly (P=0.02).

Conclusions.—Genetic variation in the 5' end of *TGFβ1* or a nearby upstream region modifies disease severity in cystic fibrosis.

▶ We all recognize the variability that exists among patients with cystic fibrosis, even those showing the same molecular genotype. Such variation probably relates, as the report abstracted shows, to variation in susceptibility and modifier genes. Susceptibility genes (genes with functional variants that affect the causes of disease) are routinely being identified for simple Mendelian diseases, and more recently, for common genetic disorders. Modifier genes are distinct from susceptibility genes, in that they are genetic variants that affect the clinical manifestation of disease (as opposed to the risk of disease). The identification of modifier genes has proven quite elusive.

It was back in 1989 that the genetic mutations causing cystic fibrosis were identified. These mutations are in the *CFTR* gene. Since then, enormous interest has developed in studies that attempt to correlate the clinical presentation of patients with cystic fibrosis who have the *CFTR* mutation with environmental factors, specific mutations within *CFTR*, and variants in modifier genes. In the report abstracted, the Gene Modifier Study Group reports data designed to identify variants in genes other than *CFTR* that may influence the severity of pulmonary disease in patients with cystic fibrosis. They included only patients who are homozygous for the most common genotypic abnormality in cystic fibrosis, ΔF508. Although this is only 1 of more than 1300 known mutations in *CFTR*, it is far and away the most common, and restricting their study to this group of patients essentially eliminates variables other than modifier genes in the expression of the severity of pulmonary disease in the patients with cystic fibrosis who were studied.

Pulmonary manifestations vary greatly among patients who are homozygous for the ΔF508 mutation. The report of the Gene Modifier Study Group describes a 2-stage study. In the first stage, 10 genes that were previously reported as potential modifiers in earlier studies were further evaluated for the relationship between the presence of variance in these genes and the progression of pulmonary disease. Of these genes, the investigators found that 2 variants in the *TGFβ1* gene occurred in homozygous states more often in patients with cystic fibrosis who had more severe impairment of lung function than in those with mild impairment. The research group then performed a second study for replication of these findings in a large number of patients with cystic fibrosis, including both patients who are homozygous for the ΔF508 variant and those with other *CFTR* genotypes. Again, the modifier gene related to TGF was associated with more severe lung disease. This modifier gene is now called the "codon 10 CC genotype." This genotype is more than twice as common in patients with severe lung disease than in those with mild disease.

The identification of gene modifiers and their interactions in cystic fibrosis and other diseases has only just begun. What has been reported by the Gene Modifier Study Group is a modifier gene that is responsible for only a small portion of the variability in lung disease, and this modifier gene may actually only operate in the presence of other genetic or environmental factors. Efforts started by the Gene Modifier Study Group and other consortia are essential for the establishment of large, well-defined samples for screening and validation of new genes that modulate the clinical manifestation of human diseases. Hopefully, such studies will yield new insights regarding therapeutic interventions.

Monk Mendel would likely be a little astonished at how his theory of inheritance of genetic disorders has mutated to become infinitely more complex than he could have possibly imagined. For more on the topic of genetic modifiers of cystic fibrosis, see the superb review by Haston and Hudson.[1] See also the report that follows (Abstract 18–3), which describes the decline in birth rates (in Canada) since the onset of genetic testing for cystic fibrosis. It is likely that we soon will be seeing a similar trend here in the United States.

J. A. Stockman III, MD

Reference

1. Haston CK, Hudson TJ: Finding genetic modifiers of cystic fibrosis. *N Engl J Med* 353:1509-1511, 2005.

Cystic Fibrosis Birth Rates in Canada: A Decreasing Trend Since the Onset of Genetic Testing

Dupuis A, Hamilton D, Cole DEC, et al (Univ of Toronto; Dalhousie Univ, Halifax, Nova Scotia, Canada)
J Pediatr 147:312-315, 2005   18–3

Objective.—To estimate cystic fibrosis (CF) birth rates in Canada from 1971 to 2000 and to assess the population impact of genetic testing in families with a history of CF, after identification of the CF transmembrane conductance regulator gene in 1989.

Study Design.—Age-at-diagnosis data were obtained from the Canadian Cystic Fibrosis Foundation Patient Data Registry and Canadian births for the corresponding years from Canadian Vital Statistics. Estimates of the CF birth rate in each year were based on a nonparametric model that allows the birth rate to vary across the years and adjusts for censoring of currently undiagnosed patients.

Results.—The overall CF birth rate from 1971-1987 was 1/2714 with no increasing or decreasing trend. Beginning in 1988, 1 year before identification of the CF transmembrane conductance regulator gene, estimated CF birth rates followed a linear decline to an estimated rate of 1/3608 in 2000. CF birth rates may have stabilized in the last few years, but further decline may occur with implementation of carrier screening in the general population.

Conclusions.—These results demonstrate the temporal association of genetic testing and declining CF birth rates in Canada. They may assist in decisions relating to the allocation of resources for prenatal and neonatal CF screening programs.

▶ The ΔF508 mutation now accounts for slightly over 70% of all the mutations causing CF. This mutation, as noted previously in this chapter, is just one of more than 1300 mutations capable of causing the clinical entity we call CF. From the onset of genetic screening and detection of CF, some have suspected that there has been a decline in the number of new cases. Accurate estimates of CF birth rates are important in evaluating epidemiologic trends and predicting the future burden of disease. Such estimates are difficult to obtain because delayed diagnosis or late onset of symptoms results in a later age at diagnosis in a substantial proportion of patients. The Canadian Cystic Fibrosis Foundation's Patient Data Registry Report for 2000 notes that 40% of patients alive in 2000 were diagnosed after the first year of age, 9.6% after their 10th birthday, and 2% were diagnosed after age 30, consistent with reports for the CF population here in the United States. The difference between the existing population of patients with CF and future populations has to do with prenatal testing and genetic testing. Both are now in place in most wealthy countries. With the localization of the *CFTR* gene to chromosome 7, a reliable approach based on closely linked restriction fragment length polymorphisms was developed and used to genotype fetal DNA from chorionic villus biopsy specimens. Although population screening for CF mutations has not taken place on any wide basis, carrier screening of large at-risk populations is now being advocated. Some have recommended that screening be offered to all women as an integral part of prenatal care. This is the case in Canada and as we see, the result has been a decreasing birth rate of individuals who are homozygous for CF.

The data from Canada are not dissimilar to what has been seen in other parts of the world. A steady decline in CF birth rates was noted in Great Britain between the early 1980s and early 1990s, corresponding to a period when neonatal screening along with genetic counseling and later prenatal diagnosis was established.[1] Similarly, in northwest France, the decline in CF birth prevalence rates from 1/2364 in the 1980s to 1/3055 in the 1990s coincided with the institution of screening programs.[2]

If one looks across other genetic disorders, such as hemophilia, in which screening and prenatal detection techniques were developed, one has also observed similar declines in the prevalence of these disorders. Clearly, the information yielded by such techniques is being utilized by families in their decision making to have a child.

Another important aspect of neonatal screening is that it allows the identification of cases of CF in its preclinical phases and also allows the detection of milder forms of CF that otherwise would not be diagnosed. See the report which follows (Abstract 18–4) that provides additional insights about pregnancies affected by CF and what babies look like in the neonatal period who are ultimately diagnosed with CF.

J. A. Stockman III, MD

References

1. Green MR, Weaver TL, Heeley AF, et al: Cystic fibrosis identified by neonatal screening: Incidence, genotype and early natural history. *Arch Dis Child* 68:464-467, 1993.
2. Scotet V, Gillet D, Dugueperoux I, et al: Spacial and temporal distribution of cystic fibrosis and of its mutations in Brittany, France: A retrospective study from 1960. *Hum Genet* 111:247-254, 2002.

Gestational and Neonatal Characteristics of Children With Cystic Fibrosis: A Cohort Study

Festini F, Taccetti G, Repetto T, et al (Univ of Florence, Italy)
J Pediatr 147:316-320, 2005

18–4

Objective.—To examine whether the birth weight (BW) and the risks of being pre-term, low birth weight (LBW), and small for gestational age (SGA) of children with cystic fibrosis (CF) are different from nonaffected children.

Study Design.—Retrospective cohort study. We examined all the children with CF born in Tuscany, Italy, from 1991 to 2002 (n = 70) comparing them to the entire population of non-CF-affected children born in the same period (n = 290,059).

Results.—The mean BW of newborns with CF was 246.2 g lower than the mean BW of the non-CF neonatal population (P = .0003). Children with CF had a higher risk of being born pre-term (RR 2.62, P = .001), LBW (RR 2.66, P = .0009), and SGA (RR = 1.74, P = .04) than the non-CF-affected children. The mean BW of term newborns with CF was 205.7 g lower than that of term non-CF-affected babies (P = .0002).

Conclusions.—Our data show an association between CF and reduced BW and show a greater risk of being pre-term for babies with CF.

► This is not the first report that has looked at the neonatal characteristics of youngsters affected with CF, but it is one that has examined this topic in great detail. The data show, for the first time, that there is a subset of children with CF who are at significantly greater risk of being born preterm, weighing less than 2500 g at birth, and who are at greater risk for being born SGA. It has been hypothesized that in children with CF, fetal growth may be impaired owing to an inadequate functioning of the exocrine pancreas, which results in reduced intrauterine nutrition and lower birth weight. In case you are not aware, amniotic fluid supplies anywhere from 10% to 14% of the nutritional needs of a fetus. Not everything comes directly from the placental circulation in terms of nutrition.

Another theory for the LBW of newborns with CF relates to maternal factors. Expression of the CF transmembrane regulator (CFTR) protein on the maternal part of the placenta has been demonstrated and may affect placental ionic exchange, with the possible result of reducing fetal nutrition.

Thus, we need to be on top of the nutrition of patients with CF early on, early meaning in utero. The report that follows (Abstract 18–5) tells us about how we can modify behavior and nutrition to improve growth in toddlers and preschoolers with CF.

One concluding comment about early detection of infections of the airways that may assist patients at risk for such problems: A simple analysis of exhaled air may be all that is needed in some cases. Scientists in New Zealand have devised a breath test for detecting a fungal lung infection. Using gas chromatography and mass spectroscopy, it is possible to detect a substance called 2-pentylfuran in the breath of people infected with *Aspergillus fumigatus*. Thus, exhaled air can be a biomarker of pulmonary pathogens.

Aspergillus fumigatus is capable of causing severe and life-threatening infections in people with compromised immune systems. Obviously, a breath-test–based study is far less invasive than lung biopsy to make the diagnosis of a fungal infection. It should not be long before biomarkers in exhaled air will be used for rapid diagnosis of other serious lung disorders.[1]

J. A. Stockman III, MD

Reference

1. Seppa N: Breath test could detect bad microbe. *Science News* 168:302, 2005.

Randomized Clinical Trial of Behavioral and Nutrition Treatment to Improve Energy Intake and Growth in Toddlers and Preschoolers With Cystic Fibrosis

Powers SW, Jones JS, Ferguson KS, et al (Cincinnati Children's Hosp Med Ctr, Ohio; Univ of Cincinnati, Ohio; Greenville Hosp System Children's Hosp, SC)
Pediatrics 116:1442-1450, 2005   18–5

Objective.—To conduct a randomized clinical trial comparing a behavioral and nutrition intervention (BEH) with a usual care control condition (CTL) for children (ages 18 months to 4 years) with cystic fibrosis (CF) and pancreatic insufficiency. This trial was designed to (1) evaluate a randomized comparison of BEH with CTL over 8 weeks, (2) provide a replication of the impact of BEH by inviting the CTL group to receive BEH after 8 weeks, and (3) examine the maintenance of BEH at 3- and 12-month follow-up.

Methods.—Of 14 eligible children, 10 were randomly assigned and initiated treatment (71% recruitment rate). Four participants were randomly assigned to BEH, and 6 were assigned to CTL (5 of whom chose to crossover to BEH). BEH included nutrition counseling to increase energy intake (via types of foods and addables/spreadables) and child behavioral management training to teach parents differential attention and contingency management skills. CTL was consistent with the 2002 CF Foundation Consensus Conference Guidelines for nutritional care.

Results.—BEH led to greater increases in energy intake pre- to posttreatment than CTL as measured by calories per day (842 kcal/day vs −131 kcal/day change). On receiving BEH, the change in energy intake was replicated with the CTL group (892 kcal/day change). At 3- and 12-month follow-up, energy intake was maintained (672 kcal/day increase from baseline and 750 kcal/day increase from baseline, respectively). Children in this study met or exceeded normal weight and height velocities from pretreatment to the 3-month follow-up (mean weight: 1.4 kg/6 months; mean height: 5.1 cm/6 months) and from posttreatment to the 12-month follow-up (mean weight: 2.5 kg/12 months; mean height: 8.3 cm/12 months).

Conclusions.—Toddlers and preschoolers who have CF and received BEH were able to meet the energy intake recommendations for this disease and maintain these gains up to 12 months after treatment. In addition, these children demonstrated weight and height velocities from pretreatment to 12-month follow-up, consistent with the goal of normal growth. BEH is a promising, evidence-based, early nutritional intervention for children with CF. An upcoming multisite clinical trial will test BEH versus an attention control condition using a larger sample ($N = 100$), providing additional evidence about the efficacy of this treatment for energy intake and growth in young children with CF.

▶ Several management techniques markedly increase the life span of patients with CF. One of these is early diagnosis and institution of proper nutritional management. The sooner one gets on top of this, the more likely it is that the other complications of CF are minimized. Nutrition is the foundation upon which all other therapies for CF pivot. Currently, the median predicted survival age of patients with CF is 33.5 years, and about 40% of patients with CF are currently older than 18. There is, however, considerable variability in the age at death among the CF population. Much of this variation can be explained by individual patient differences in genetic constitution and environmental or sociodemographic exposures, but there is growing appreciation of the degree to which average patient outcomes differ among accredited CF care centers. There are, in fact, some centers that achieve uniformly superior results across all performance measures, all other things being equated. These centers are not necessarily the largest or best known. They differ in size and geographic location, and they do not share a specific unique treatment method. What they have in common is a highly developed system of care that is well adapted to local conditions and allows the consistent and methodologic application of therapies based on the best evidence available. One of the best relates to the need to maintain adequate nutritional status.

If you are not familiar with the system of care for children with CF here in the United States, most of this care occurs within centers accredited by the CF Foundation. The CF Foundation was created in 1955 by a consortium of parents and physicians with the primary goal of encouraging CF-related research.

The work of the CF Foundation quickly broadened to support clinical care and to foster teaching about the disease. The CF Foundation is highly respected. It guides the research agenda in the area of CF by interacting with the NIH, and more recently, industry, to solicit funding for a significant proportion of all CF research. It works to ensure the general availability of high-quality medical care for patients with CF through its accreditation system.

Currently, there are nearly 120 CF Foundation–accredited CF care centers in the United States. The accreditation process requires an onsite evaluation to ensure the presence of a multidisciplinary provider team, social workers, respiratory therapists, and physical therapists, as well as the adequacy of microbiologic techniques, sweat chloride testing, and other care services. With the increasing survivorship of patients with CF, care centers have expanded to include adult CF care centers as well. There are more than 90 of the latter in the United States.

One reason why CF care has resulted in improved outcomes is that every patient diagnosed in the United States who is cared for in an accredited CF center has his or her clinical data entered into a national patient registry. This registry has allowed analyses of outcomes as improvements in therapies have evolved. Back in the 1940s, the median age at death of patients with CF was 0.5 years. This had increased to just 1 year by 1950. By the 1980s, the median age of death was 18. That average age of death in just a quarter of a century had improved to over 33 years by the turn of the millennium.

The system that has been evolving for the care of children with CF offers an inkling of how subspecialists can organize and share data that lead to significant improvements in outcomes. A recent review of what has been accomplished in CF was published by Schechter and Margolis.[1] The many accomplishments observed in the care of patients with CF serve as an example applicable to other pediatric subspecialties that wish to take better advantage of existing knowledge to improve health outcomes for children for whom they provide care.

J. A. Stockman III, MD

Reference

1. Schechter MS, Margolis P: Improving subspecialty healthcare: Lessons from cystic fibrosis. *J Pediatr* 147:295-301, 2005.

Combination Antibiotic Susceptibility Testing to Treat Exacerbations of Cystic Fibrosis Associated With Multiresistant Bacteria: A Randomised, Double-blind, Controlled Clinical Trial

Aaron SD, Vandemheen KL, Ferris W, et al (Univ of Ottawa, Ontario, Canada; Children's Hosp of Eastern Ontario, Ottawa, Canada; St Michael's Hosp, Toronto; et al)
Lancet 366:463-471, 2005   18–6

Background.—We did a randomised, double-blind, controlled clinical trial to prospectively assess whether use of combination antibiotic susceptibility testing improved clinical outcomes in patients with acute pulmonary exacerbations of cystic fibrosis who were infected with multiresistant bacteria.

Methods.—251 patients with cystic fibrosis who were chronically infected with multiresistant gram negative bacteria gave sputum at 3-month intervals for conventional culture and sensitivity tests and for combination antibiotic susceptibility tests using multiple combination bactericidal antibiotic testing (MCBT). Patients who developed an exacerbation of pulmonary disease were randomised to receive a 14-day course of any two blinded intravenous antibiotics chosen on the basis of either results from conventional sputum culture and sensitivity testing or the result of MCBT. The primary outcome was time from randomisation until the patient's next pulmonary exacerbation. Analysis was by intention-to-treat. This study is registered as an International Standard Randomised Controlled Trial, number ISRCTN60187870.

Findings.—132 patients had a pulmonary exacerbation and were randomised during the 4.5-year study period. The time to next pulmonary exacerbation was not prolonged in the MCBT-treated group (hazard ratio 0.86 in favour of the conventionally-treated group, 95% CI 0.60-1.23, p=0.40). There was no difference between the groups in treatment failure rate. After 14 days of intravenous antibiotic therapy, changes in lung function, dyspnoea, and sputum bacterial density were similar in both groups.

Interpretation.—Antibiotic therapy directed by combination antibiotic susceptibility testing did not result in better clinical and bacteriological outcomes compared with therapy directed by standard culture and sensitivity techniques. The non-bactericidal effects of antibiotic therapy might play an important part in determining improvement in patients with cystic fibrosis pulmonary exacerbations.

▶ Most studies now suggest that some 20% to 25% of individuals with cystic fibrosis, particularly as they grow into adulthood, are chronically infected with multiresistant bacteria in their airways. The conundrum in managing such patients has been what combination of antibiotics to select if the bacterial organisms are multiresistant or panresistant to antibiotics on routine sensitivity testing. This question is of particular concern for patients with severe cystic fibrosis, in whom further loss of any lung function could lead to disastrous consequences, including a markedly shortened survivorship. This article from Canada tells us that antibiotic therapy as directed by combination antibiotic susceptibility testing does not appear to produce particularly better clinical outcomes when compared with standard culture insensitivity testing techniques. Why this is so is not entirely clear but may have to do with factors other than the straightforward relationship between antibiotic sensitivity and successful treatment. For example, recent evidence suggests that *Pseudomonas aeruginosa* may grow as a biofilm in the airways of patients with cystic fibrosis. Bacterial biofilms are dense communities of bacteria, encased in an exopolysaccharide, that adhere to biological or prosthetic surfaces. Conventional clinical microbiological testing only involves the culture of growing bacteria that are free floating, not those in biofilms. Bacteria growing in biofilms have been shown to be significantly more resistant to antimicrobials than are those that are free growing. Ultimately, cultures of bacteria grown as biofilms might provide more accurate antibiotic susceptibility results on which to base clinical practice. Clinical trials of this approach are badly needed.

While on the topic of antibiotic resistance, be aware of something that recently occurred in France. In the latest step to wean its citizens from their antibiotic habit, France has banned 12 popular sore throat remedies that contain topical antibiotics. The drugs—lozenges, mouthwashes, and sprays—have not been shown to do anything good, and the French Health Products Safety Agency has banned such products. Since 2001, the French government has campaigned to drive down the country's use of antibiotics, particularly because the French population is the highest user of antibiotics in Europe. There has been an explosion in that country of treatment resistance in pneumonia cases and hospital-acquired infections. The government first prohibited the use of several medically important antibiotics and sore throat remedies in 2003. The latest ban affects 4 others whose overuse posed a much smaller risk to public health. Although some may find it hard to believe, France is actually getting tough when it comes to sore throats, but it still leads the list of over-prescribers.[1] When it comes to total antibiotic use among outpatients in western European countries that are members of the European Union, a 3-fold difference in antibiotic use has been found. France, for example, has physicians that write an average of 33 daily prescriptions per 1000 population, in comparison to The Netherlands (the lowest prescription writing country), where fewer than 10 daily prescriptions are written per 1000 inhabitants. In rank order, from highest prescription writing to lowest prescription writing are the following countries:

1. France
2. Greece
3. Luxembourg
4. Portugal
5. Italy
6. Belgium
7. Slovakia
8. Croatia
9. Poland
10. Iceland
11. Ireland
12. Spain
13. Finland
14. Bulgaria
15. Czech Republic
16. Slovenia
17. Sweden
18. Hungary
19. Norway
20. United Kingdom
21. Denmark

22. Germany
23. Latvia
24. Austria
25. Estonia
26. Netherlands

As one might suspect, there was a direct correlation between antibiotic resistance and antibiotic prescription writing in European countries.[2]

J. A. Stockman III, MD

References

1. Adieu antibiotics (editorial). *Science* 309:872, 2005.
2. Mayor S: Antibiotic resistance is highest in south and east Europe. *BMJ* 330:383, 2005.

Smoking in the Movies Increases Adolescent Smoking: A Review
Charlesworth A, Glantz SA (Univ of California, San Francisco)
Pediatrics 116:1516-1528, 2005   18–7

Objective.—Despite voluntary restrictions prohibiting direct and indirect cigarette marketing to youth and paid product placement, tobacco use remains prevalent in movies. This article presents a systematic review of the evidence on the nature and effect of smoking in the movies on adolescents (and others).

Methodology.—We performed a comprehensive literature review.

Results.—We identified 40 studies. Smoking in the movies decreased from 1950 to ~1990 and then increased rapidly. In 2002, smoking in movies was as common as it was in 1950. Movies rarely depict the negative health outcomes associated with smoking and contribute to increased perceptions of smoking prevalence and the benefits of smoking. Movie smoking is presented as adult behavior. Exposure to movie smoking makes viewers' attitudes and beliefs about smoking and smokers more favorable and has a dose-response relationship with adolescent smoking behavior. Parental restrictions on R-rated movies significantly reduces youth exposure to movie smoking and subsequent smoking uptake. Beginning in 2002, the total amount of smoking in movies was greater in youth-rated (G/PG/PG-13) films than adult-rated (R) films, significantly increasing adolescent exposure to movie smoking. Viewing antismoking advertisements before viewing movie smoking seems to blunt the stimulating effects of movie smoking on adolescent smoking.

Conclusions.—Strong empirical evidence indicates that smoking in movies increases adolescent smoking initiation. Amending the movie-rating system to rate movies containing smoking as "R" should reduce adolescent exposure to smoking and subsequent smoking.

▶ Figure 1 tells the entire story. Film producers and film directors, although initially getting the message a decade or more ago that smoking is not something to be viewed in movies that teens see, have now gone off the wagon. A random sample of top-grossing films from 1950 through 2002 indicates that the amount of smoking decreased from an average of 10.7 events per hour in 1950 to a low of 4.9 events per hour in 1980-1982, then began to increase rapidly to 10.9 events per hour by 2002. Some 87% of the most popular films between 1988 and 1997 showed tobacco occurrences, with two thirds of the movies showing tobacco use by at least 1 major character. Leading actors smoked in 60% of the popular films from 2002 to 2003. As one might suspect, tobacco use in almost all films is unrelated to movie genre; it is rarely relevant to a scene and is even less likely to be a major focus of a scene. We also learn from this report that at least until the mid 1990s, the number of smoking occurrences in films increased with the rating of the film, with an R-rated film featuring significantly more smoking than films rated G (general audiences, all ages admitted), PG (parental guidance suggested, some material may not be suitable for children), and PG-13 (parents strongly cautioned, some material may be inappropriate for children under 13). Unfortunately, beginning in the mid 1990s, there was a "down rating" of movies resulting in PG-13 ratings for many films that would have been previously rated R. There was a consequent increase in the prevalence of smoking in such films as well.

There is no need to see actors smoke. Only when things blow up from time to time do we see any improvements in filmmaking and then only for short periods. It was only after the US Congress held hearings on smoking in the movies in 1989 in response to the revelation that Philip-Morris paid to place Marlboros in the film *Superman II* did the tobacco industry amend its voluntary advertising code to prohibit paid brand placement. The Master Settlement Agreement also prohibited paid product placement in movies. Despite these agreements by the tobacco industry, the amount of smoking in the movies increased rapidly during the late 1990s, reversing the earlier downward trend.

If you do not believe there is a link between the amount of smoking seen in films these days and early initiation of smoking by adolescents, see the report that follows (Abstract 18–8).

Last, recognize that smoking may be a cause of birth defects. It is well known that women thinking of starting a family have likely heard that smoking may increase their risks of infertility, ectopic pregnancy, and spontaneous abortion. Now they have another reason to stay clear of cigarettes. In the largest study of its kind, plastic surgeons found that smoking during pregnancy increases the risk of having a child with excess, webbed, or missing fingers and toes. It appears that smoking half of a pack of cigarettes a day, or less, significantly increases the risk of having a child born with such digit defects.[1] By analyzing the US Natality database from 2001 and 2002, and examining the records of more than 6.8 million live births (more than 84% of all US births), Chang et al identified 5,171 children born with congenital digital abnormalities. It was found that the more cigarettes a pregnant woman smoked, the greater the risk of having a child with a toe or finger deformity. Smoking 1 to 10 cigarettes per day during pregnancy was associated with a 29% increased risk, 11-20 cigarettes per day was associated with a 38% increased risk, and 21 or more cigarettes per day was associated with a 78% increased risk. These statistics did not change even when adjusted for potential confounding factors such as maternal anemia, maternal cardiac disease, lung disease, diabetes, and hypertension.

One of the problems of the potential relationship between prenatal smoking and neonatal digit defects is the fact that limb formation begins at around 4 weeks' gestation. This means that if a mother starts into a pregnancy smoking, her baby will already have the problem before she realizes she is pregnant, even if she stops smoking at that point. For that very reason, any woman of childbearing age who thinks she may want to have children should really think about stopping smoking well in advance of becoming pregnant.

J. A. Stockman III, MD

Reference

1. Man LX, Chang B: Smoking and the risk of distal extremity deformities. *Plastic Reconstr Surg* 117:301-308, 2006.

Exposure to Movie Smoking: Its Relation to Smoking Initiation Among US Adolescents

Sargent JD, Beach ML, Adachi-Mejia AM, et al (Dartmouth Med School, Lebanon, NH; Dartmouth College, Hanover, NH; Westat, Rockville, Md)
Pediatrics 116:1183-1191, 2005   18–8

Objective.—Regional studies have linked exposure to movie smoking with adolescent smoking. We examined this association in a representative US sample.

Design/Methods.—We conducted a random-digit-dial survey of 6522 US adolescents aged 10 to 14 years. Using previously validated methods, we estimated exposure to movie smoking, in 532 recent box-office hits, and examined its relation with adolescents having ever tried smoking a cigarette.

Results.—The distributions of demographics and census region in the unweighted sample were almost identical to 2000 US Census estimates, confirming representativeness. Overall, 10% of the population had tried smoking. Quartile (Q) of movie smoking exposure was significantly associated with the prevalence of smoking initiation: 0.02 of adolescents in Q1 had tried smoking; 0.06 in Q2; 0.11 in Q3; and 0.22 in Q4. This association did not differ significantly by race/ethnicity or census region. After controlling for sociodemographics, friend/sibling/parent smoking, school performance, personality characteristics, and parenting style, the adjusted odds ratio for having tried smoking were 1.7 (95% confidence interval [CI]: 1.1, 2.7) for Q2, 1.8 (95% CI: 1.2, 2.9) for Q3, and 2.6 (95% CI: 1.7, 4.1) for Q4 compared with adolescents in Q1. The covariate-adjusted attributable fraction was 0.38 (95% CI: 0.20, 0.56), suggesting that exposure to movie smoking is the primary independent risk factor for smoking initiation in US adolescents in this age group (Fig 2).

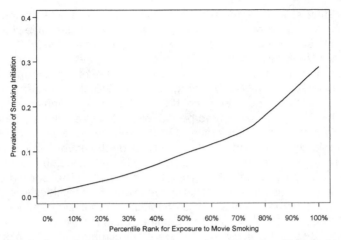

FIGURE 2.—Crude association between exposure to movie smoking and smoking initiation. (Courtesy of Sargent JD, Beach ML, Adachi-Mejia AM, et al: Exposure to movie smoking: Its relation to smoking initiation among US adolescents. *Pediatrics* 116:1183-1191, 2005. Reproduced by permission of *Pediatrics*.)

Conclusions.—Smoking in movies is a risk factor for smoking initiation among US adolescents. Limiting exposure of young adolescents to movie smoking could have important public health implications.

▶ This report is one of the most powerful, if not the most powerful, study of a nationally representative sample of young adolescents demonstrating the strong association between exposure to films in which there are characters who smoke and the early initiation of smoking. The authors even go out on a limb and say that exposure to movie smoking is a primary risk factor accounting for as much as one third of adolescents who begin to smoke at 10 to 14 years of age.

If you believe the data linking smoking in films to early onset of initiation of smoking, perhaps the producers of films depicting characters who smoke should bear the health-related costs of smoking in our society. If you are not familiar with some of the estimates of what a pack of cigarettes should really cost if all the health care costs were built into the price, it appears that $40 per pack is the real cost that a 24-year-old smoker should consider as the true purchase price each time he or she lights up a new pack of cigarettes. In one's lifetime, this amounts to $220,000 for men and $106,000 for women. That smoking costs a substantial amount in terms of health care services, lives lost, etc, should not surprise those who follow the ongoing saga of tobacco as public health enemy number one. This is not to say that all the news is bad in terms of dollars and cents. Smoking actually saves Medicare money by killing smokers at earlier ages even after the smoker's payroll tax contributions to the program are included. Smoking is also found to save the Social Security program about $1519 per female smoker and $6549 per male smoker for exactly the same reason.

If you want to read more about the real price of smoking, see the excellent book by Sloan et al.[1]

Fortunately, sales of cigarettes in the United States have fallen and, in fact, are at their lowest point for more than half a century.[2] Sales have slumped by around 21% since 1998, the year of the introduction of the Master Settlement Agreement. 2005 saw a 4.2% decline in sales of cigarettes over the previous year, according to data from the Tobacco Committee of the National Association of Attorney Generals (www.naag.org). The 378 billion cigarettes sold in 2005 was the lowest number since 1951, although the population has more than doubled over the same time period. Most of the decline in the last half century appears to be directly related to the 1998 Master Settlement Agreement on tobacco, which imposed restrictions on the advertising, promoting, and marketing of cigarettes by tobacco companies, including prohibiting the targeting of cigarette advertising at young people. The agreement also stopped the advertising of cigarettes in public transport facilities as well as the use of cigarette brand names on merchandising. While cigarette sales in the United States appear to be on the decline, the World Health Organization databank shows that worldwide sales were still climbing at the turn of the millennium and had reached record numbers at 5,500 billion cigarettes a year, from 1,000 billion in 1940 and 10 billion in 1880 (www.who.int/tobacco/en/atlas8.pdf). It should come as no surprise that China is now the major consumer of cigarettes. More than one third of all cigarettes smoked worldwide are consumed in China.

J. A. Stockman III, MD

References

1. Sloan FA, Ostermann J, Picone G, et al: *The Price of Smoking.* Cambridge, Mass, MIT Press, 2004.
2. Dobson R: US cigarette consumption falls to its lowest point since 1951. *BMJ* 332:687, 2006.

Televised State-Sponsored Antitobacco Advertising and Youth Smoking Beliefs and Behavior in the United States, 1999-2000
Emery S, Wakefield MA, Terry-McElrath Y, et al (Univ of Illinois at Chicago; Cancer Council Victoria, Melbourne, Australia; Univ of Michigan, Ann Arbor; et al)
Arch Pediatr Adolesc Med 159:639-645, 2005   18–9

Background.—Recent state budget crises have dramatically reduced funding for state-sponsored antitobacco media campaigns. If campaigns are associated with reduced smoking, such cuts could result in long-term increases in state health care costs.

Methods.—Commercial ratings data on mean audience exposure to antitobacco advertising that appeared on network and cable television across the largest 75 media markets in the United States for 1999 through 2000 were combined with nationally representative survey data from school-based samples of youth in the contiguous 48 states. Multivariate regression models were used to analyze associations between mean exposure to state antitobacco advertising and youth smoking-related beliefs and behaviors, controlling for individual and environmental factors usually associated with youth smoking and other televised tobacco-related advertising.

Results.—Mean exposure to at least 1 state-sponsored antitobacco advertisement in the past 4 months was associated with lower perceived rates of friends' smoking (odds ratio [OR], 0.72; 95% confidence interval [CI], 0.58-0.88), greater perceived harm of smoking (OR, 1.25; 95% CI, 1.11-1.42), stronger intentions not to smoke in the future (OR, 1.43; 95% CI, 1.17-1.74), and lower odds of being a smoker (OR, 0.74; 95% CI, 0.63-0.88).

Conclusions.—To our knowledge, this study is the first to explore the potential impact of state-sponsored antitobacco media campaigns while controlling for other tobacco-related advertising and other tobacco control policies. State-sponsored antitobacco advertising is associated with desired outcomes of greater antitobacco sentiment and reduced smoking among youth. Recent cuts in these campaigns may have future negative health and budgetary consequences.

▶ Despite promises from state leaders to spend a significant portion of the 1998 Tobacco Master Settlement Agreement funds on antitobacco efforts, only an estimated 3% of state Master Settlement Agreement funds are now used for such purposes. Only a few states earmark tobacco excise tax revenue to support state tobacco control programs. Most funds from the Master Settlement Agreement are used by states to fill short-term budget deficits. Some examples of spending from the fund are far removed from tobacco control or health purposes, such as financing support for tobacco farmers, debt service on flood control projects, and industrial bonds. In fact, 5 states and the District of Columbia use zero dollars from their settlement money for tobacco control. This diversion of funds from the Master Settlement Agreement distribution and other settlement money has been called "moral treason" by Michael Moore, not the filmographer, but rather the Mississippi Attorney General who filed the first state tobacco lawsuit in 1994.

The diversion of dollars from the Master Settlement Agreement is unfortunate, since as the report abstracted shows, when such dollars are targeted to support antitobacco advertising, the advertising works to reduce teen smoking. In fact, there has been a substantial and unprecedented national decline in adolescent smoking since the late 1990s. The Monitoring the Future Project has been continuously tracking cigarette smoking using nationally representative samples of high school seniors in the United States. The 2003 estimate of teen smoking of 24.4% represents a decline of almost 33% over a 6-year period, largely a result of early tobacco cessation efforts.

The report of Emery et al adds to a large body of literature on the critical role that antiadvertising plays in tobacco prevention. It supports the finding of many other reports, including the United States Community Preventative Services Task Force, that mass media counteradvertising campaigns are effective in preventing tobacco use initiation. Advertising and antiadvertising do work.

This is the last entry in the Respiratory Tract chapter, so we will close with a query to test your knowledge of cigarette smoke. Which is more toxic, directly inhaled cigarette smoke or the smoke inhaled that is emanating from the tip of a lit cigarette?

Unpublished research by the tobacco industry shows that inhaled "sidestream" cigarette smoke—the smoke that rises from the tip of the burning cigarette between puffs—is more toxic than the "mainstream" smoke inhaled directly by the smoker. Inhaled, fresh sidestream smoke, which makes up about 85% of secondhand smoke, turns out to be four times more toxic per gram of total particulate matter than inhaled mainstream smoke. Data on sidestream cigarette smoke appeared in 2005 in a report in *Tobacco Control*,[1] which described the research conducted by Philip Morris Tobacco in the 1980s. While publically denying that sidestream cigarette smoke was a danger, Philip Morris privately performed extensive in vivo toxicologic testing of sidestream smoke at its secret Institut Für Biologische Forschung in Germany. When this research was reanalyzed (there were 40 million pages of tobacco industry documents related to this), it showed that sidestream smoke caused 2 to 6 times more tumors in laboratory animals and was found to inhibit normal weight gain in developing mice. In addition, mice showed damage to their respiratory epithelium.

It is clear that sidestream smoke, particularly when compared to filtered "light" cigarette inhaled smoke, is quite a bit more toxic. Most data now confirm that secondhand smoke causes about 53,000 deaths a year here in the United States, largely as the result of lung cancer. It is a shame that the tobacco industry failed to initially publish their findings and that it took an investigative reporter to ferret out the information 20 years after the cancer experiments were undertaken.[2]

Scientists who study the effects of smoke on mice should be considered candidates for the Ig Nobel Award. If you are not familiar with the Ig Nobel Awards (short term "Igs"), they are awarded for science that "makes you laugh, then makes you think" and "cannot and should not be reproduced." This past year's winners were awarded their Ig Nobel prizes by true Nobel laureates at the 15th Ig Nobel ceremony in Boston. Among the prizewinners was someone who described a cure for narcolepsy; this winner, from the Massachusetts Institute of Technology, invented Clocky, an alarm clock with wheels that runs away and hides after it goes off, insuring that people have to get out of bed to turn it off. It appears to be of particular help to individuals with narcolepsy. An investigator from Massey University in New Zealand was awarded the agricultural historical award for describing the health hazards of sodium chlorate, which in 1931, caused an outbreak of exploding trousers among farmers in rural New Zealand.[3] It seems that a certain Mr Buckley, who wasn't actually wearing his trousers when they exploded, witnessed a string of detonations in his pants after he had hung them to dry in front of a fire. Similar occurrences, however, were unfortunately occurring when trousers were actually being occupied at the time of immolation. The mystery of the exploding britches was solved when it was learned that the farmers used sodium chlorate—which becomes violently explosive when combined with organic fibers, such as cotton or wool—a herbicide to kill ragwort weed.

The winner of the Ig Nobel Medicine Award was given to an inventor from Missouri, who had designed "neuticles"—that is, prosthetic dog testicles, available in 3 sizes and 3 degrees of firmness, intended to help dogs that might feel disgraced after being neutered. Lastly, professors of physics from the University of Queensland, Australia, won the physics award for an experiment started in 1927 that proves that tar is not a solid at room temperature, even though it appears solid and can be smashed to bits with a hammer. The experiment, in which a congealed glob of tar was placed in a glass funnel, showed that tar actually can slowly drip at the rate of one drop every 9 to 12 years.

If you wish to learn more about the 2005 Ig Nobel Awards, see the review by Lenzer.[4]

J. A. Stockman III, MD

References

1. Shick S, Glantz S: Philip Morris toxicological experiments with fresh sidestream smoke: More toxic than mainstream smoke. *Tobacco Control* 14:396-404, 2005.
2. Dobson R: Smoke from cigarette tip is more toxic than main inhaled smoke. *BMJ* 331:1425, 2005.
3. Watson J: The significance of Mr. Richard Buckley's exploding trousers: Reflections on an aspect of technological change in New Zealand dairy-farming between the World Wars. *Agricultural History* 78(3): Summer, 46-60, 2004.
4. Lenzer J: Mr Buckley's exploding trousers and other scientific observations. *BMJ* 331:865, 2005.

19 Therapeutics and Toxicology

An Evaluation of *Echinacea angustifolia* in Experimental Rhinovirus Infections

Turner RB, Bauer R, Woelkart K, et al (Univ of Virginia, Charlottesville; Karl-Franzens-Universitaet, Graz, Austria; Med Univ of South Carolina, Charleston; et al)

N Engl J Med 353:341-348, 2005   19–1

Background.—Echinacea has been widely used as an herbal remedy for the common cold, but efficacy studies have produced conflicting results, and there are a variety of echinacea products on the market with different phytochemical compositions. We evaluated the effect of chemically defined extracts from *Echinacea angustifolia* roots on rhinovirus infection.

Methods.—Three preparations of echinacea, with distinct phytochemical profiles, were produced by extraction from *E. angustifolia* roots with supercritical carbon dioxide, 60 percent ethanol, or 20 percent ethanol. A total of 437 volunteers were randomly assigned to receive either prophylaxis (beginning seven days before the virus challenge) or treatment (beginning at the time of the challenge) either with one of these preparations or with placebo. The results for 399 volunteers who were challenged with rhinovirus type 39 and observed in a sequestered setting for five days were included in the data analysis.

Results.—There were no statistically significant effects of the three echinacea extracts on rates of infection or severity of symptoms. Similarly, there were no significant effects of treatment on the volume of nasal secretions, on polymorphonuclear leukocyte or interleukin-8 concentrations in nasal-lavage specimens, or on quantitative-virus titer.

Conclusions.—The results of this study indicate that extracts of *E. angustifolia* root, either alone or in combination, do not have clinically significant effects on infection with a rhinovirus or on the clinical illness that results from it.

▶ *E angustifolia* is about as ubiquitous as tobacco products here in the United States. Echinacea made from the roots, the whole plant, or the aerial parts of *E angustifolia* is formulated as a powdered plant material, alcoholic tinctures, tea preparations, or as pressed juice (of the aerial parts). Consistent extraction procedures are not specifically required, so what one buys as echinacea could vary as a product containing a little or a lot. In this article, the amount of echinacea used was consistent with the amount used by Native Americans of the American Midwest—a quantity recently endorsed by the World Health Organization for the treatment of the common cold.[1] As we see from this article, the World Health Organization got it wrong. Echinacea seems to have no beneficial effect, at least in experimental rhinovirus infection.

So why has echinacea gotten to be so popular? Herbal texts list the use of echinacea by at least 13 tribes of Native Americans for the treatment of such widely diverse conditions as sore throats and gums, coughing, dyspepsia, toothaches, bowel complaints, hydrophobia, and snake bites. The potential for the distortion of knowledge about this herb arose between the late 1600s and the mid 1800s when native people shared information about the uses of herbs with explorers, traders, and healers. Descriptions, accurate or inaccurate, were translated into French, Spanish, and English, and from each of those languages into many others. Eventually, 19th century physicians adopted herbs into their eclectic medicine therapies, along with water cures, homeopathy, and manipulation. Emerging as a panacea in 20th century Europe, echinacea somehow became popular for the treatment of respiratory illness in Germany. In the early 1900s here in the United States, echinacea was used as an "oral anti-infective" and was applied locally for wound healing. When antibiotics came along, it quickly fell into disfavor; then, in the 1960s, the herbal supplement boom brought echinacea back into the limelight as a cold remedy.

Between 1950 and 1990, more than 200 clinical reports studied the effectiveness of echinacea, but most of these were small and inadequate for reaching conclusions. Positive findings on nonspecific stimulation of immune-cell division and cytokine release were observed, but these findings had no clinical correlations associated with them.

In the last 7 years, the National Institutes of Health (NIH) has spent close to $2 billion in grants for research into alternative therapies. It is legitimate to ask why we are doing randomized clinical trials of folkway uses of herbs when people are dying of malaria simply because hospitals do not stock existing, effective drugs. As noted in a commentary by Sampson,[2] we might as well have the NIH spend the money on investigations into the psychology of personal beliefs in irrational proposals, in the study of erroneous thinking, and in the study of the mechanisms behind errant sociomedical trends, including the alternative medicine movement.

If you have never seen the echinacea plant, it is a beautiful light purple flowering plant. While worthwhile to look at with your eyes, it is not as worthwhile to put in your mouth.

J. A. Stockman III, MD

References

1. World Health Organization: Radix echinacea, in WHO *Monographs on Selected Medicinal Plants*, vol 1. Geneva, World Health Organization, 1999, pp 125-135.
2. Sampson W: Studying herbal remedies. *N Engl J Med* 353:337-339, 2005.

Unit-Dose Packaging of Iron Supplements and Reduction of Iron Poisoning in Young Children

Tenenbein M (Univ of Manitoba, Winnipeg, Canada)
Arch Pediatr Adolesc Med 159:557-560, 2005   19–2

Background.—Iron poisoning is a major cause of unintentional poisoning death in young children. The US Food and Drug Administration proclaimed a regulation for unit-dose packaging of iron supplements in 1997.

Objective.—To determine whether the requirement for unit-dose packaging of iron supplements decreases the incidence of iron ingestion and the incidence of deaths due to iron poisoning in children younger than 6 years.

Methods.—This is a preintervention-postintervention study of the US federally mandated requirement for unit-dose packaging of iron supplements. The 10 years prior to the intervention were compared with the 5 years after its promulgation. The incidences of iron ingestion and of iron poisoning deaths for children younger than 6 years were obtained from the annual reports of the American Association of Poison Control Centers (Washington, DC).

Results.—The average number of iron ingestion calls per 1000 of all calls to poison control centers regarding children younger than 6 years decreased from 2.99 per 1000 to 1.91 per 1000 (odds ratio, 1.29 [95% confidence interval, 1.27-1.32]; $P<.001$). The number of deaths decreased from 29 to 1 (odds ratio, 13.56 [95% confidence interval, 1.85-99.52]; $P = .03$).

Conclusions.—These are the first data that show a decrease in the incidence of nonintentional ingestion of a specific drug by young children and a decrease in mortality from poisoning by this drug after the introduction of unit-dose packaging. There was a decrease in the incidence of iron ingestion and a dramatic decrease in the number of deaths due to iron poisoning. This validates unit-dose packaging as an effective strategy for the prevention of iron poisoning and iron poisoning deaths in young children. This highly effective intervention should be considered for other medications with a high hazard for morbidity and mortality when taken as an overdose.

▶ It is about time that we are sure, or at least have reasonable assurance, that attempts to decrease the frequency of iron poisoning in young children have borne fruit. Far back in 1972, the Poison Prevention Packaging Act was enacted. Despite this, iron tablets seem to have slipped through the regulatory system, at least until sometime in the 1990s. Even though iron was included as a medicine for which child-resistant packaging compliance was mandated, young children in the 1980s and early 1990s were obtaining enough iron from open bottles, incompletely secured child-resistant closures, transferred products, or child-resistant closure exempt container sizes to do themselves harm. Adult-formulation iron was one of the leading causes of serious childhood pharmaceutical poisonings. Fortunately, this situation has changed. This report shows a decrease in the frequency of US poison centers taking calls related to adult formulations of iron injested by children. Not only this occurred, but the number of deaths in children related to iron poisoning declined from 29 during the period from 1988 to 1997 to just 1 in the period from 1998 to 2002. There seems to be a direct correlation with the 1997 regulations promulgated by the Food and Drug Administration requiring the use of unit-dose packaging for adult-formulation iron. The way iron is now packaged, in effect, represents a physical barrier to inquisitive toddlers, slowing them down enough by having to unwrap each pill, either frustrating their efforts or alerting a parent or parents to discover the source of their curiosity before any serious harm has taken place.

I hope progress will continue in minimizing the risk of a child being exposed inadvertently to adult medications. It is true that there has been a significant decline in childhood iron poisonings. It is only logical to believe that tamper-proof packaging is the likely source of the benefit, but this remains unproven. In October 2003, the United States Appellate Court declared the Food and Drug Administration's 1999 regulations requiring the use of unit-dose packaging for adult-formulation iron to be illegal. Should US manufacturers choose to change their packaging back to recloseable containers, and if child-resistant unit-dose packaging is truly effective, one might expect to see an unfortunate increase in both serious pediatric iron poisonings and fatalities. As of this writing, the pharmaceutical industry has foregone the opportunity to reverse their packaging policies and has adhered to prior child-resistant unit-dose packaging as the standard for iron medications.

When this editor was a resident in training in Philadelphia some 30 years ago, physicians saw lots of iron poisoning, including some deaths. At that time, there were a few excellent poison centers around the United States (we always called New York City for their advice). Fortunately, there are many poison centers now, and a new national toll-free telephone number for poison centers has been established and promoted by the American Association of Poison Control Centers in Washington. The number is 1-800-222-1222. The national toll-free telephone number allows easier access to immediate help anywhere in the United States and can be used by anyone. It is so good, most of us would use it even if it were a 900 number.

One final insight having to do with iron, this in the form of a question. Anyone who has ridden a subway realizes that there seems to be a fair amount of dust underground. What does this dust consist of? A study of the London underground gives us the answer and shows exactly what the composition of dust is in the subterranean atmosphere of the tube.[1] It has now been shown that the concentrations of dust on station platforms are 270-480 $\mu g/m^3$ and 14,000-29,000 particles/cm^3. Approximately 70% of the dust is comprised, by mass, of iron oxide. There are also small amounts of quartz and traces of other metals. This study was reported prior to the terrorist attacks in London in the summer of 2005.

You can guess where the iron oxide comes from. It is probably from the metal on metal of the subway rail and the steel wheels of the carriages. The amount of dust found is not thought to represent any environmental hazard to humans.

J. A. Stockman III, MD

Reference

1. Seaton A, Cherrie J, Dennekamp M, et al: The London Underground: Dust and hazards to health. *Occup Environ Med* 62:355-362, 2005.

Febuxostat Compared with Allopurinol in Patients With Hyperuricemia and Gout

Becker MA, Schumacher HR Jr, Wortmann RL, et al (Univ of Chicago; Univ of Pennsylvania, Philadelphia; Univ of Oklahoma, Tulsa; et al)

N Engl J Med 353:2450-2461, 2005   19–3

Background.—Febuxostat, a novel nonpurine selective inhibitor of xanthine oxidase, is a potential alternative to allopurinol for patients with hyperuricemia and gout.

Methods.—We randomly assigned 762 patients with gout and with serum urate concentrations of at least 8.0 mg per deciliter (480 μmol per liter) to receive either febuxostat (80 mg or 120 mg) or allopurinol (300 mg) once daily for 52 weeks; 760 received the study drug. Prophylaxis against gout flares with naproxen or colchicine was provided during weeks 1 through 8. The primary end point was a serum urate concentration of less than 6.0 mg per deciliter (360 μmol per liter) at the last three monthly measurements. The secondary end points included reduction in the incidence of gout flares and in tophus area.

Results.—The primary end point was reached in 53 percent of patients receiving 80 mg of febuxostat, 62 percent of those receiving 120 mg of febuxostat, and 21 percent of those receiving allopurinol (P<0.001 for the comparison of each febuxostat group with the allopurinol group). Although the incidence of gout flares diminished with continued treatment, the overall incidence during weeks 9 through 52 was similar in all groups: 64 percent of patients receiving 80 mg of febuxostat, 70 percent of those receiving 120 mg of febuxostat, and 64 percent of those receiving allopurinol (P=0.99 for 80 mg of febuxostat vs. allopurinol; P=0.23 for 120 mg of febuxostat vs. allopurinol). The median reduction in tophus area was 83 percent in patients receiving 80 mg of febuxostat and 66 percent in those receiving 120 mg of febuxostat, as compared with 50 percent in those receiving allopurinol (P=0.08 for 80 mg of febuxostat vs. allopurinol; P=0.16 for 120 mg of febuxostat vs. allopurinol). More patients in the high-dose febuxostat group than in the allopurinol group (P=0.003) or the low-dose febuxostat group discontinued the study. Four of the 507 patients in the two febuxostat groups (0.8 percent) and none of the 253 patients in the allopurinol group died; all deaths were from causes that the investigators (while still blinded to treatment) judged to be unrelated to the study drugs (P=0.31 for the comparison between the combined febuxostat groups and the allopurinol group).

Conclusions.—Febuxostat, at a daily dose of 80 mg or 120 mg, was more effective than allopurinol at the commonly used fixed daily dose of 300 mg in lowering serum urate. Similar reductions in gout flares and tophus area occurred in all treatment groups.

▶ Certainly, kids do not commonly get gout, but from time to time, they are seen with disorders that may raise the uric acid level in blood, either on a short- or long-term basis. A new drug, febuxostat, can be used to manage hyperuricemia. The emergence of any new medication to lower serum urate levels is welcome because no other drug has been approved for this use in the United States since the introduction of allopurinol and because the drugs currently available have limitations related to their toxicity or modest ineffectiveness.

Hyperuricemia has a number of causes. It usually results from inadequate renal excretion of uric acid relative to its production. The imbalance is often due to a defect in the complex excretory mechanisms of the kidney. In youngsters, overproduction is also a problem because of hereditary disorders of purine metabolism or other clinical disorders, as well as exogenous factors including diet and certain medications that will overwhelm excretory mechanisms. Agents such as probenecid lower uric acid levels by increasing the renal clearance of uric acid, whereas agents such as allopurinol and its metabolite, oxypurinol, inhibit the oxidation of xanthine to uric acid, decreasing its production. Unfortunately, a good fifth of patients treated with allopurinol will have some side effect, including gastrointestinal intolerance, skin rashes, and a diminished white blood cell count. More serious side effects, including toxic epidermal necrolysis, bone marrow suppression, hepatitis, and vasculitis, can also occur. Thus, febuxostat comes none too soon.

Febuxostat is an orally administered nonpurine analogue inhibitor of xanthine oxidase. This drug is metabolized mainly in the liver, unlike allopurinol, which is excreted in the kidney. The capability of febuxostat to lower serum urate levels is not altered in the presence of renal insufficiency.

Febuxostat is not a perfect drug. In the current article, we see a high dropout rate in those receiving the drug for reasons that are not entirely defined. We need to know more, for example, about why it causes an elevation in liver enzyme profiles and whether this is really a serious problem.

Precious little information exists on febuxostat use in children. Chances are that indications for its administration will probably be the same as those for allopurinol. It is anticipated that the benefit–risk ratio of these drugs may favor febuxostat. However, the relative cost of allopurinol versus febuxostat may influence the decision to use one or the other. Allopurinol is basically "dirt cheap" in comparison with its newer sister drug. Stay tuned for more information on drugs to lower uric acid levels.

This YEAR BOOK OF PEDIATRICS contains little on poisonings, so we will add a bit more on the topic by closing this commentary with a question, this regarding arsenic. Just how likely is it that someone can survive a massive ingestion of arsenic?

Not likely, but it has been reported. For example, recently, the case of a 43-year-old man who attempted suicide by drinking 54g of arsenic trioxide appeared in the literature.[1] The patient, a chemist by profession, prepared this amount of arsenic trioxide in his factory laboratory using a commercial solution of arsenic trichloride as a base. He was admitted to the hospital 5 hours after the ingestion and was pale and sweaty, but his vital signs were normal. He was initially treated with gastric lavage and charcoal, but soon began to vomit, had diarrhea, thirst, pharyngeal constriction, and paresthesias of the legs. A blood-arsenic level performed during the first day of hospitalization was 132 µg/L (normal <5 µg/L). The arsenic level in urine was 67,500 µg/L (normal <50 µg/L). These are lethal levels. The patient was given supportive therapy in terms of IV fluids, and dimercaprol, a chelating agent, was administered intramuscularly. A plain film of the abdomen showed large radio-opaque masses in the gastric antrum and a speckled pattern throughout the intestine. Figuring the patient would not last long without something dramatic being done; surgeons did a laparotomy, clamped the pylorus, and manually removed the arsenic from the stomach wall.

The patient stabilized after the surgical procedure and did well for 2 additional days, but then became severely agitated and disoriented. The level of arsenic in his blood rose to 160 µg/L and a plain film of the abdomen now showed radio-opaque arsenic remaining in the ascending colon near the ileocecal valve. This was extracted with a colonoscope. Symptoms waxed and waned for the next month until day 29 when he was able to be successfully extubated. His only residual problem was a distal polyneuropathy of the legs.

Arsenic trioxide is one of the most toxic forms of arsenic. Death is believed to be inevitable if the ingested amount is over 2 mg/kg (200-300 mg in an adult). This fellow took more than 150 times that dose. Treatment is largely supportive and includes the use of chelators. The need for surgery and endoscopy is a rare phenomenon because patients usually die before one can think about such management. The patient described is probably the first (and may be the last) individual to ever survive ingesting more than 50g of arsenic trioxide.

J. A. Stockman III, MD

Reference

1. Duenas-Laita A, Pere-Miranda M, Gonzalez-Lopez MA, et al: Acute arsenic poisoning. *Lancet* 365:1982, 2005.

Association Between Parental Satisfaction and Antibiotic Prescription for Children With Cough and Cold Symptoms
Christakis DA, Wright JA, Taylor JA, et al (Univ of Washington, Seattle; Dept of Health Services, Seattle)
Pediatr Infect Dis J 24:774-777, 2005   19–4

Background.—Providers' interest in satisfying parents may provide an impetus for unnecessary antibiotic use in children.

Objectives.—To determine (1) whether receipt of antibiotics at a visit for cough and cold symptoms was associated with increased satisfaction and (2) whether nonreceipt of antibiotics at an initial visit but subsequent receipt of antibiotics in the course of the same illness episode was associated with decreased satisfaction.

Methods.—Prospective cohort study of patients 2–10 years of age presenting to a university-affiliated pediatric clinic with cough and cold symptoms. Parents were enrolled at the index visit and then followed up by phone at least 7 days later (mean time to follow-up, 14.9 days). Satisfaction with the index visit on a 10 point scale was the primary outcome. The primary predictors were whether antibiotics were prescribed at the index visit and, if not, whether they were prescribed since that visit. Linear and median regression were used to adjust for income, child age, parental race and individual provider.

Results.—A total of 539 parents were enrolled in the study, and 378 (70%) completed follow-up interviews. The mean age of participating children was 4.67 years (SD 2.16). Overall 47% of patients received antibiotics at the index visit, and 8% of those that did not reported receiving them between the index visit and the follow-up assessment. In the regression model, receiving antibiotics at the index visit trended toward being associated with higher satisfaction scores (0.28; $P = 0.08$). Among those who did not receive antibiotics initially, receiving them subsequently was associated with significantly lower median satisfaction scores for the index visit (-3.0; $P < 0.01$).

Conclusions.—Receiving antibiotics after an initial visit for cough and cold symptoms at which antibiotics were not prescribed is associated with decreased satisfaction. Use of contingency prescriptions may be an important intervention.

▶ Few studies to date have prospectively and carefully measured patient satisfaction based on whether or not antibiotics are prescribed, and none have assessed parent satisfaction if antibiotics were not initially, but subsequently, prescribed. What we learn from this report is that almost half of all patients between the ages of 2 and 10 years seen in a large pediatric center were prescribed antibiotics, often for something as simple as a common cold. As importantly, it was observed that not receiving antibiotics at the time of initial visit and subsequently getting a prescription for them during the same illness episode was associated with significantly lower satisfaction on the part of families. Thus, it would appear that family satisfaction with a visit is a driver of provider antibiotic use, particularly if providers are concerned that parents may have to make a return visit if antibiotics are not prescribed initially. Some have advocated for the use of contingency prescriptions whereby a parent is given a prescription at an initial visit and told to fill it only if their child is not better in a couple of days. Such an approach is discussed elsewhere in the YEAR BOOK OF PEDIATRICS and has been found to be associated with improved patient satisfaction and reduced antibiotic usage, at least in adults. Such an approach does also seem to increase parent satisfaction among parents expecting antibiotics for their children.[1]

Without question, writing a prescription and telling a parent not to have it filled for at least a couple of days is far better than indiscriminately writing prescriptions when you truly think a patient may have a viral disorder. The National Health Service in Great Britain recommends, for otitis media, that the best way to manage the problem is to ask the patient to come back in 2 or 3 days if not better, when a prescription is then automatically dispensed without an examination unless the child is sufficiently ill to require one. That would be a hard sell here in the United States.

J. A. Stockman III, MD

Reference

1. Mangione-Smith R, McGlynne A, Elliott MN, et al: Parent expectations for antibiotics, physician-parent communication and satisfaction. *Arch Pediatr Adolesc Med* 155:800-806, 2001.

Antibiotic Treatment of Children With Sore Throat
Linder JA, Bates DW, Lee GM, et al (Harvard Med School, Boston; Children's Hosp, Boston)
JAMA 294:2315-2322, 2005   19–5

Context.—Of children with sore throat, 15% to 36% have pharyngitis caused by group A β-hemolytic streptococci (GABHS). Performance of a GABHS test prior to antibiotic prescribing is recommended for children with sore throat. Penicillin, amoxicillin, erythromycin, and first-generation cephalosporins are the recommended antibiotics for treatment of sore throat due to GABHS.

Objectives.—To measure rates of antibiotic prescribing and GABHS testing and to evaluate the association between testing and antibiotic treatment for children with sore throat.

Design, Setting, and Participants.—Analysis of visits by children aged 3 to 17 years with sore throat to office-based physicians, hospital outpatient departments, and emergency departments in the National Ambulatory Medical Care Survey and National Hospital Ambulatory Medical Care Survey, 1995 to 2003 (N = 4158) and of a subset of visits with GABHS testing data (n = 2797).

Main Outcome Measures.—National rates of antibiotic prescribing, prescribing of antibiotics recommended and not recommended for GABHS, and GABHS testing.

Results.—Physicians prescribed antibiotics in 53% (95% confidence interval [CI], 49%-56%) of an estimated 7.3 million annual visits for sore throat and nonrecommended antibiotics to 27% (95% CI, 24%-31%) of children who received an antibiotic. Antibiotic prescribing decreased from 66% of visits in 1995 to 54% of visits in 2003 ($P = .01$ for trend). This decrease was attributable to a decrease in the prescribing of recommended antibiotics (49% to 38%; $P = .002$). Physicians performed a GABHS test in 53% (95% CI, 48%-57%) of visits and in 51% (95% CI, 45%-57%) of visits at which an antibiotic was prescribed. GABHS testing was not associated with a lower antibiotic prescribing rate overall (48% tested vs 51% not tested; $P = .40$), but testing was associated with a lower antibiotic prescribing rate for children with diagnosis codes for pharyngitis, tonsillitis, and streptococcal sore throat (57% tested vs 73% not tested; $P<.001$).

Conclusions.—Physicians prescribed antibiotics to 53% of children with sore throat, in excess of the maximum expected prevalence of GABHS. Although there was a decrease in the proportion of children receiving antibiotics between 1995 and 2003, this was due to decreased prescribing of agents recommended for GABHS. Although GABHS testing was associated with a lower rate of antibiotic prescribing for children with diagnosis codes of pharyngitis, tonsillitis, and streptococcal sore throat, GABHS testing was underused.

▶ The results of this report are both impressive and disturbing. All of us know that if we are even remotely thinking about using an antibiotic to treat pharyngitis in a child, we should be doing a screen for strep. Nonetheless, about 50% more antibiotics are being prescribed than would be expected to be prescribed based on the prevalence of GABHS in children presenting with a sore throat/pharyngitis diagnosis. Roughly half of such patients are given antibiotics despite the fact that only about one quarter will be GABHS positive. This not only means that we are overprescribing antibiotics, but also that we are underusing rapid GABHS tests or cultures.

The evaluation and treatment of most children with sore throat are reasonably straightforward. The treatment is largely symptomatic. Current guidelines suggest that we can restrict GABHS testing to those children who are likely to have GABHS pharyngitis: those older than 3 years with acute onset of sore throat, fever, headache, pain on swallowing, abdominal pain, nausea, vomiting, or tender anterior cervical lymphadenopathy.[1] Children with symptoms suggestive of viral infections, such as coryza, conjunctivitis, hoarseness, cough, stomatitis, or diarrhea, are unlikely to have GABHS and generally do not need to be tested. If a child is initially treated with antibiotics pending test results, antibiotics should be stopped if the GABHS test result is negative. The antibiotic of choice for pharyngitis caused by GABHS remains penicillin, which is narrow-spectrum, inexpensive, and to which GABHS is still universally susceptible.

The bottom line is clear. We overprescribe antibiotics for sore throat in children. We use broad-spectrum antibiotics when they are not appropriate. We should be limiting antibiotic prescribing to children with sore throat who have positive GABHS screening tests or cultures. This is a feasible goal for all of us in primary care.

One final comment about antibiotic use here in the United States. You would think everyone would be happier with a reduced rate of prescribing given the expenses associated with the filing of prescriptions these days. While it would be impractical to order antibiotics from Canada, there are a number of other drugs that we prescribe which can be purchased much more inexpensively in Canada, although it is not currently legal to do so. A recent article compared the prices of brand-name drugs purchased online from Canadian-based Internet pharmacies with prices charged here in the United States by major US drug chain pharmacies.[2] The savings can be substantial if one buys online from Canada. The following table gives an example of 5 drugs and the yearly savings in US dollars for these drugs:

Drug	Savings Per Year ($ US)
Lipitor (20mg)	$416.40
Nexium (20mg)	772.47
Prilosec (20mg)	720.71
Singulair (10mg)	376.56
Zyrtec (10mg)	444.89

For the average individual, there are enough savings by purchasing drugs in Canada to afford a nice weekend for two in the beautiful town of Quebec City.

J. A. Stockman III, MD

References

1. American Academy of Pediatrics: Group A streptococcal infections, in Pickering LK (ed): *Redbook: 2003 Report of the Committee of Infectious Diseases*, ed 26. Elk Grove Village, Ill, American Academy of Pediatrics, 2003, pp 573-584.
2. Quon BS, Firsz TR, Eisenberg MJ: A comparison of brand-name drug prices between Canadian-based Internet pharmacies and major US drug chain pharmacies. *Ann Intern Med* 143:347-403, 2005.

Antibiotic Prescribing for Children With Nasopharyngitis (Common Colds), Upper Respiratory Infections, and Bronchitits Who Have Health-Professional Parents

Huang N, Morlock L, Lee C-H, et al (Natl Yang Ming Univ, Taipei, Taiwan; Johns Hopkins Bloomberg School of Public Health, Baltimore, Md; Bureau of Natl Health Insurance, Taipei, Taiwan)
Pediatrics 116:826-832, 2005   19–6

Objective.—Antibiotic resistance might be reduced if patients could be better informed regarding the lack of benefits of antibiotics for children with viral infections and avoid antibiotic prescriptions in these circumstances. This study investigated whether children having health professionals as parents, a group whose parents are expected to have more medical knowledge and expertise, are less likely than other children to receive antibiotics for nasopharyngitis (common colds), upper respiratory tract infections (URIs), and acute bronchitis.

Methods.—Retrospective analyses were conducted by using National Health Insurance data for children of physicians, nurses, pharmacists, and non–health personnel, who had visited hospital outpatient departments or physician clinics for common colds, URIs, and acute bronchitis in Taiwan in 2000. A total of 53,733 episodes of care for common colds, URIs, and acute bronchitis in a nationally representative sample of children (aged ≤18 years) living in nonremote areas were analyzed.

Results.—The study found that, after adjusting for characteristics of the children (demographic, socioeconomic, and health status) and the treating physicians (demographic, practice style, and setting), children with a physician (odds ratio [OR]: 0.50; 95% confidence interval [CI]: 0.36-0.68) or a pharmacist (OR: 0.69; 95% CI: 0.52-0.91) as a parent were significantly less likely than other children to receive antibiotic prescriptions. The likelihood of receiving an antibiotic for the children of nurses (OR: 0.91; 95% CI: 0.77-1.09) was similar to that for children in the comparison group.

Conclusions.—This finding supports our hypothesis that better parental education does help to reduce the frequency of injudicious antibiotic prescribing. Medical knowledge alone, however, may not fully reduce the overuse of antibiotics. Physician-parents, the expected medically savvy parents, can serve as a benchmark for the improvement potentially achievable in Taiwan through a combination of educational, regulatory, communication, and policy efforts targeted at more appropriate antibiotic prescribing in ambulatory settings.

▶ Antimicrobial resistance is a serious public threat that is exacerbated by the gradual withdrawal of the pharmaceutical industry from new antimicrobial agent development. Overuse of antimicrobial agents fosters the spread of antimicrobial-resistant organisms. Despite recent trends that demonstrate reduced outpatient use of antimicrobial agents, prescribing continues to significantly exceed prudent levels. Approximately 50% of courses of ambulatory antimicrobial drugs are prescribed for patients with viral respiratory infections and, therefore, are not clinically indicated. Behavioral facilitators of antimicrobial overuse and barriers to prudent use operate on both clinicians and patients. Patient demand, perceived or actual, creates challenges that distinguish this problem from other quality-of-care concerns.

Whether and to what extent educational efforts targeting patients can effectively and safely reduce unnecessary antibiotic use and ambulatory care remain unclear. The report from Taiwan suggests that among all children, those with physician parents are least likely to receive potentially inappropriate antibiotic prescriptions, and their chance of being prescribed antibiotics with questionable value is significantly lower than children in general. Basically, what this means is that children whose parents possess medical expertise are less likely to receive potentially inappropriate prescriptions and are therefore more likely to receive better quality of care, with the punch line being that care providers know what to do when they have the "total family" under their influence. Nonetheless, in this study, children of physicians still received antibiotics all too frequently for viral illnesses, suggesting that parent education alone is not likely to eliminate all prescribing of antibiotics with questionable value in the ambulatory care settings.

As long as we in the United States have a "free market" approach to medicine, wherein there are virtually no consequences to either care providers or to those families receiving care should an antibiotic be prescribed inappropriately, we will continue to see overprescribing. In Great Britain, the National Health Service has very strict guidelines on antibiotic prescription writing, and with universal electronic medical record accessibility, disincentives to using antibiotics inappropriately are readily applied. Such a circumstance will happen no time soon here in the United States, and thus we need to find alternatives that are effective in minimizing the inappropriate use of antibiotics.

J. A. Stockman III, MD

Effect of Handwashing on Child Health: A Randomised Controlled Trial
Luby SP, Agboatwalla M, Feikin DR, et al (Ctrs for Disease Control and Prevention, Atlanta, Ga; Health Oriented Preventive Education, Karachi, Pakistan; Aga Khan Univ, Karachi, Pakistan; et al)
Lancet 366:225-233, 2005   19–7

Background.—More than 3.5 million children aged less than 5 years die from diarrhoea and acute lower respiratory-tract infection every year. We undertook a randomised controlled trial to assess the effect of handwashing promotion with soap on the incidence of acute respiratory infection, impetigo, and diarrhoea.

Methods.—In adjoining squatter settlements in Karachi, Pakistan, we randomly assigned 25 neighbourhoods to handwashing promotion; 11 neighbourhoods (306 households) were randomised as controls. In neighbourhoods with handwashing promotion, 300 households each were assigned to antibacterial soap containing 1.2% triclocarban and to plain soap. Fieldworkers visited households weekly for 1 year to encourage handwashing by residents in soap households and to record symptoms in all households. Primary study outcomes were diarrhoea, impetigo, and acute respiratory-tract infections (ie, the number of new episodes of illness per person-weeks at risk). Pneumonia was defined according to the WHO clinical case definition. Analysis was by intention to treat.

Findings.—Children younger than 5 years in households that received plain soap and handwashing promotion had a 50% lower incidence of pneumonia than controls (95% CI −65% to −34%). Also compared with controls, children younger than 15 years in households with plain soap had a 53% lower incidence of diarrhoea (−65% to −41%) and a 34% lower incidence of impetigo (−52% to −16%). Incidence of disease did not differ significantly between households given plain soap compared with those given antibacterial soap.

Interpretation.—Handwashing with soap prevents the two clinical syndromes that cause the largest number of childhood deaths globally—namely, diarrhoea and acute lower respiratory infections. Handwashing with daily bathing also prevents impetigo.

▶ If you have not been a strong advocate for your patients to wash their hands (mothers and fathers included), this report should be more than enough to convince you. The data are there. Controlled trials of handwashing promotion in child care centers have reported an almost 15% reduction in upper-respiratory tract infections, at least in Canada.[1] Specifically, in day care centers, there is a 12% reduction in upper-respiratory tract infection in children 24 months or younger in Australia and a 32% reduction in colds in 1 child care center here in the United States.[2,3] In school age children, 5 to 12 years, here in the United States, a handwashing promotion program in selected classrooms was associated with a 21% decrease in absences from respiratory illness.[4] Another program at a US Navy training center that included directives to wash hands 5 times a day resulted in a 45% reduction in total outpatient visits for respiratory illness.[5] Thus the data are there.

If all these data are not convincing of the need for advocacy in handwashing, see the report abstracted from the collaborative effort between the Centers for Disease Control and Prevention (CDC) and the health-oriented preventive education program in Pakistan. The fieldworkers in Pakistan visited at least weekly to distribute free soap and educate households, particularly mothers, encouraging handwashing. Soap and education decreased the occurrences of impetigo by 34%, diarrhea by 53%, and pneumonia by 50%. Clinic visits by children for diarrhea decreased by 56%, and there was a 26% reduction in hospitalization for diarrhea. The only problem with the recommendation to frequently wash the hands with soap and water is the cost associated with this in Pakistan. Although the cost of soap there is relatively low (US $0.17-$0.25 a bar, or about $1.00 a week), the average income is less than $15.00 a week, leading one to suspect that the buying of soap would be of relatively low priority. The situation here in the United States, obviously, is very different

An excellent commentary accompanied this report.[6] The author of that commentary closed the comment with the following suggestion: "The time has come to shout from the rooftops that hand-hygiene promotion should be a worldwide priority for health and healthcare, and I call on policy makers, medical and nursing schools, chief medical and executive officers, and all healthcare workers and community members with potential to be a role model, to help highlight, support, prioritize, and fund research and intervention to improve hand hygiene behavior." Well said!

This last commentary in the Therapeutics and Toxicology chapter of the YEAR BOOK concludes with a question about the pharmaceutical industry. What prior occupation on your resume will put you at the top of the most desirable candidate list to be a pharmaceutical sales representative promoting drugs to physicians? It turns out that drug companies here in the United States prefer hiring ex-cheerleaders as sales representatives to promote drugs to doctors, as reported in the *New York Times*, November 28, 2005, page 1. This story claimed that drug companies were turning to cheerleaders as sales people because not only are they good looking, but they have enthusiastic, outgoing personalities. A review has shown that several hundred former cheerleaders had become drug sale representatives when the *Times* investigated this situation.

Needless to say, the major pharmaceutical industry trade association organization responded quickly to the *New York Times* piece with the Senior Vice President of the Pharmaceutical Research and Manufacturers of America complaining that the article re-enforced a sexist stereotype. In a letter to the editor, he said that former cheerleaders formed only a small percentage of the drug sales force. Companies train their sales representatives to have doctors educate themselves by reading journals and reviewing the clinical data, he said . . . yeah, right! So why are the reps doing summersaults?

J. A. Stockman III, MD

References

1. Carabin H, Gyokos TW, Soto JC, et al: Effectiveness of a training program in reducing infections in toddlers attending daycare centers. *Epidemiology* 10:219-227, 1999.
2. Roberts L, Smith W, Jorm L, et al: Effect of infection control measures on the frequency of respiratory infection in child care: A randomized control trial. *Pediatrics* 105:738-742, 2000.
3. Nieffenegger JP: Proper handwashing promotes wellness in childcare. *J Pediatr Health Care* 11:26-31, 1997.
4. Master D, Hess SH, Dickson H: Scheduled handwashing in an elementary school population. *Fam Med* 29:336-339, 1997.
5. Ryan MA, Christian RS, Rohlrabe J: Handwashing and respiratory illness among adults in military training. *Am J Prev Med* 21:79-83, 2001.
6. Pittet D: Clean hands reduce the burden of disease. *Lancet* 366:185-187, 2005.

Subject Index

C

Author Index